W0090529

Oxford Clinical Practice Series

COMPLICATIONS AFTER GASTROINTESTINAL SURGERY

Oxford Clinical Practice Series

COMPLICATIONS AFTER GASTROINTESTINAL SURGERY

Edited by

Samiran Nundy
and
Dirk J. Gouma

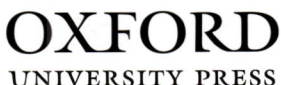

OXFORD
UNIVERSITY PRESS

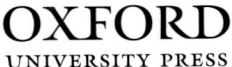

OXFORD
UNIVERSITY PRESS

Oxford University Press is a department of the University of Oxford.
It furthers the University's objective of excellence in research, scholarship,
and education by publishing worldwide. Oxford is a registered trademark of
Oxford University Press in the UK and in certain other countries.

Published in India by
Oxford University Press
YMCA Library Building, 1 Jai Singh Road, New Delhi 110 001, India

© Oxford University Press 2017

The moral rights of the authors have been asserted.

First Edition published in 2017

All rights reserved. No part of this publication may be reproduced, stored in
a retrieval system, or transmitted, in any form or by any means, without the
prior permission in writing of Oxford University Press, or as expressly permitted
by law, by licence, or under terms agreed with the appropriate reprographics
rights organization. Enquiries concerning reproduction outside the scope of the
above should be sent to the Rights Department, Oxford University Press, at the
address above.

You must not circulate this work in any other form
and you must impose this same condition on any acquirer

ISBN-13: 978-0-19-947518-6
ISBN-10: 0-19-947518-0

Typeset in Adobe Garamond Pro 10.5/13
by Tranistics Data Technologies, Kolkata 700 091
Printed in India by Replika Press Pvt. Ltd

Oxford University Press makes no representation, express or implied, that the
drug dosages in this book are correct. Readers must therefore always check the
product information and clinical procedures with the most up-to-date published
product information and data sheets provided by the manufacturers and the
most recent codes of conduct and safety regulations. The authors and the
publishers do not accept responsibility or legal liability for any errors in the text
or for the misuse or misapplication of material in this work. Except where
otherwise stated, drug dosages and recommendations are for the non-pregnant
adult who is not breast-feeding.

Links to third party websites are provided by Oxford in good faith and for
information only. Oxford disclaims any responsibility for the materials
contained in any third party website referenced in this work.

Contents

PART III   ORGAN-SPECIFIC PROBLEMS

Oesophagus and Stomach

Intestines

Liver, Gallbladder and Bile Ducts

Pancreas

Foreword

This is a very important book that concentrates on the complications of gastrointestinal surgery. There are many textbooks that describe the clinical and surgical features of gastrointestinal surgery, but with the increasing narrow specialisation of surgeons and new very expensive endoscopic and robotic instruments, individual patients worldwide may be worse off than they would have been before the introduction of these specialist advances. A fearful patient in pain may be admitted to a hospital as an emergency where an appropriate trained specialist surgeon may not be available, but the pathology may be or may become serious, thus needing urgent attention. Delayed treatment or poor surgery is likely to lead to lethal complications. The patient's life may depend on early identification of what has gone wrong and instructions on how to deal with it in varying conditions of availability of expertise and specialised equipment.

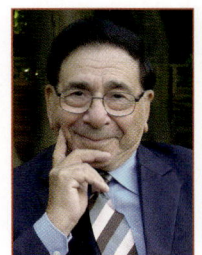

Samiran Nundy and Dirk J. Gouma have compiled a comprehensive text with the help of many renowned specialists. It covers almost all complications that may be encountered in gastrointestinal surgery, with an explanation of not only advanced diagnostic equipment but also the easily forgotten basic clinical skills, using which an experienced surgeon may anticipate complications before expensive diagnostic techniques can be employed.

I am delighted to recommend this book and congratulate my old registrar Professor Nundy and his colleague Dr. Gouma for their achievement.

Sir Roy Yorke Calne, FRCP, FRCS, FRS
Emeritus Professor of Surgery, Cambridge University,
Cambridge, United Kingdom

Editors and Contributors

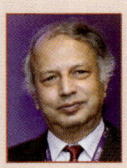 **Samiran Nundy**

Emeritus Consultant, Sir Ganga Ram Hospital, New Delhi; Dean, GRIPMER (The Ganga Ram Institute for Postgraduate Medical Education and Research), New Delhi, India

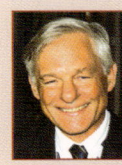 **Dirk J. Gouma**

Emeritus Chairman and Professor of Surgery, Academic Medical Center, University of Amsterdam, Amsterdam, the Netherlands

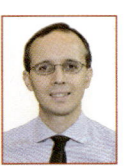 **Marco E. Allaix**

Assistant Professor, Department of Surgical Sciences, University of Torino, Italy

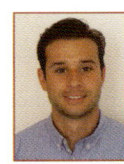 **Wernard A.A. Borstlap**

PhD Candidate; Coordinator FIT-Trial, Department of Surgery, Academic Medical Centre, Amsterdam, the Netherlands

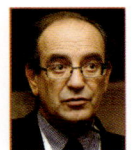 **Claudio Bassi**

Professor, Department of General and Pancreatic Surgery, Pancreas Institute, University of Verona Hospital Trust, Policlinico GB Rossi, Verona, Italy

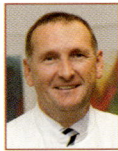 **Markus Büchler**

Professor of Surgery; Chairman, Department of Surgery and General, Visceral and Transplantation Surgery, Heidelberg University Hospital, Heidelberg, Germany

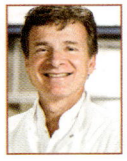 **Willem A. Bemelman**

Professor, Department of Surgery, Academic Medical Centre, Amsterdam, the Netherlands

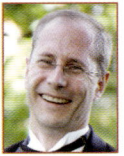 **Sean Burmeister**

Senior Consultant, Surgical Gastroenterology/Hepatobiliary Unit, University of Cape Town and Groote Schuur Hospital, Observatory, Cape Town, South African

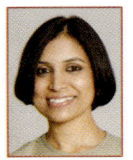 **Aparna Govil Bhasker**

Section Chief, Minimal Access Bariatric Surgery, Saifee Hospital; Consultant Surgeon, Centre for Obesity and Digestive Surgery, Mumbai, India

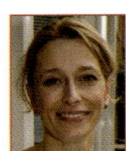 **Chrstianne J. Buskens**

Gastrointestinal Surgeon, Department of Surgery, Academic Medical Centre, Amsterdam, the Netherlands

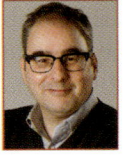 **Marc J.M. Bonten**

Professor of Molecular Epidemiology of Infectious Diseases, University Medical Center Utrecht, Division Laboratory and Pharmacy, Medical Microbiology, Utrecht, the Netherlands

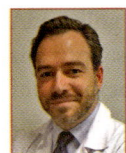 **Santiago Sánchez Cabús**

Head, Pancreatic Surgery, Department of Hepatopancreaticobiliary Surgery and Transplantation, Clínic Institute of Digestive and Metabolic Diseases (ICMDiM), Hospital Clínic de Barcelona; Associate Professor of Surgery, Universitat de Barcelona, Catalonia, Spain

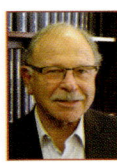 **Philippus C. Bornman**

Emeritus Professor of Surgery, University of Cape Town and Groote Schuur Hospital, Observatory, Cape Town, South Africa

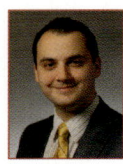

Eugene P. Ceppa

Assistant Professor of Surgery, Indiana University School of Medicine, Indianapolis, Indiana, United States of America

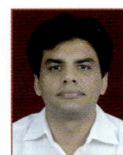

Neeraj Chaudhary

Associate Consultant, Department of Surgical Gastroenterology and Liver Transplantation, Jaypee Hospital, Noida, India

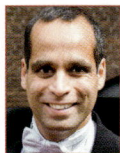

Thomas G.V. Cherpanath

Cardiologist-Intensivist, Department of Intensive Care, Academic Medical Center, Amsterdam, the Netherlands

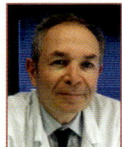

Daniel Cherqui

Professor of Surgery; Hepatopancreaticobiliary and Transplant Surgeon; Surgical Director Liver Transplantation, Hepatobiliary Center, Paul Brousse Hospital – Université Paris Sud, Villejuif, France

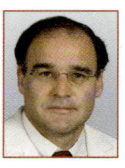

Pierre-Alain Clavien

Chairman, Department of Surgery and Transplantation, University Hospital Zurich, Switzerland

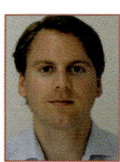

Robert J.S. Coelen

Surgical Resident, Postdoctoral Researcher, Department of Surgery, Academic Medical Center, Surgical Laboratory, Amsterdam, the Netherlands

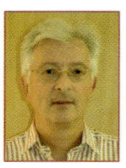

Andrew Davenport

Consultant Renal Physician/Honorary Reader, UCL Centre for Nephrology, Royal Free Hospital, London, United Kingdom

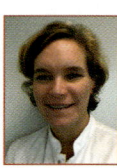

Els J.M. Nieveen van Dijkum

Associate Professor in Surgery, Department of Surgery, Academic Medical Center, Amsterdam, the Netherlands

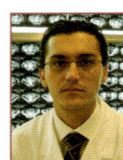

Mirko D'Onofrio

Associate Professor of Radiology, Department of Radiology, Pancreas Institute, University of Verona Hospital Trust, Policlinico GB Rossi, Verona, Italy

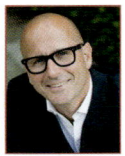

Eric Hans Eddes

Gastrointestinal Surgeon, Department of Surgery, Deventer Hospital; CEO, DICA, Leiden, the Netherlands

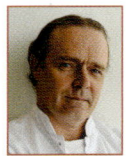

Casper H.J. van Eijck

Professor in General Surgery, Department of Surgery, Erasmus Medical Center, Rotterdam, the Netherlands

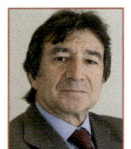

Laureano Fernández-Cruz

Emeritus Professor of Surgery, Department of Surgery, IMD Hospital Clinic y Provincial de Barcelona, University of Barcelona, Spain

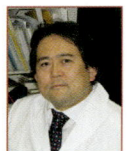

Takeo Fukagawa

Chief, Department of Gastric Surgery, National Cancer Center Hospital, Tokyo, Japan

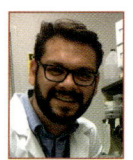

Georgios Gemenetzis

Postdoctoral Fellow, Department of Surgery, Johns Hopkins University School of Medicine, Baltimore, Maryland, United States of America

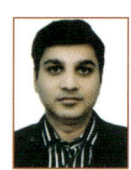

Neerav Goyal

Senior Consultant, Department of Liver Transplantation and Hepatopancreaticobiliary Surgery, Apollo Indraprastha Hospital, New Delhi, India

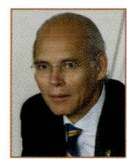

Jan Willem W.M. Greve

Medical Director, Dutch Obesity Clinics South, Department of Surgery, Zuyderland Medical Center, Heerlen, the Netherlands

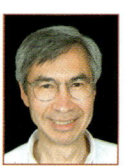

Thomas M. van Gulik

Hepatopancreaticobiliary Surgeon, Professor of Surgery, Department of Surgery, Surgical Laboratory, Amsterdam, the Netherlands

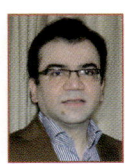

Subhash Gupta

Senior Consultant, Department of Liver Transplantation and Hepatopancreaticobiliary Surgery, Apollo Indraprastha Hospital, New Delhi, India

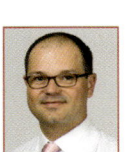

Georg Györi

Consultant for Transplant Surgery, Department of Surgery, Medical University of Vienna, Vienna, Austria

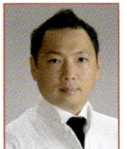

Tomoyuki Irino

Research Fellow, Upper Gastrointestinal Surgery, Gastrocentrum, Centre for Digestive Diseases, Karolinska University Hospital, Stockholm, Sweden

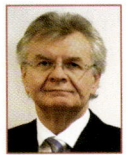

Jakob R. Izbicki

Chairman, Professor of Surgery, Department of General, Visceral and Thoracic Surgery, University Hospital Hamburg-Eppendorf Hamburg, Germany

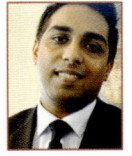

Ammar A. Javed

Clinical Research Fellow and Program Coordinator (Pancreatic Surgery), Department of Surgery, Center for Research Excellence and Surgical Trials (CREST), Johns Hopkins University School of Medicine, Baltimore, Maryland, United States of America

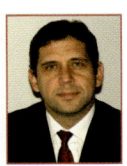

Eduard Jonas

Professor and Head of Surgical Gastroenterology, Division of General Surgery, University of Cape Town and Groote Schuur Hospital, Observatory, Cape Town, South Africa

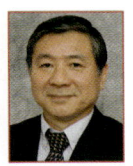

Hitoshi Katai

Director, Department of Gastric Surgery, National Cancer Center Hospital, Tokyo, Japan

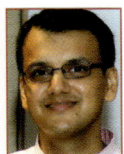

Monty U. Khajanchi

Assistant Professor, Department of General Surgery, Seth G.S. Medical College and King Edward Memorial Hospital, Mumbai, India

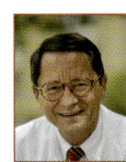

Ernst Klar

Chairman and Professor of Surgery, Department of General, Thoracic, Vascular and Transplantation Surgery, University of Rostock, Rostock, Germany

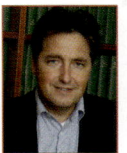

Jan A.J.W. Kluytmans

Professor of Microbiology and Infection Control, University Medical Centre Utrecht, Division Julius Center for Health Sciences and Primary Care, Utrecht, the Netherlands

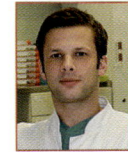

Florian Kuehn

Consultant Surgeon, Department of General, Thoracic, Vascular and Transplantation Surgery, University of Rostock, Rostock, Germany

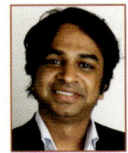

Goutham Kumar

Consultant, Department of Liver Transplantation and Hepatopancreaticobiliary Surgery, Apollo Indraprastha Hospital, New Delhi, India

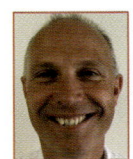

Wim K. Lagrand

Cardiologist-Intensivist, Department of Intensive Care Adults, Academic Medical Center, Amsterdam, the Netherlands

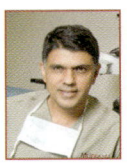

Muffazal Lakdawala

Chairman, Institute of Minimal Access Surgical Sciences, Saifee Hospital; Director, Centre for Obesity and Digestive Surgery, Mumbai, India

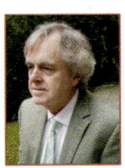

Johan F. Lange

Professor of Surgery; Coordinator R.E.P.A.I.R. Research Group; Coordinator Academic Colorectal Center, Erasmus University Medical Center-Havenziekenhuis, Rotterdam, the Netherlands

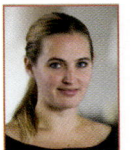

Nicoline J. van Leersum

Researcher, Department of Surgery, Leiden University Medical Center; Teamleader, Innovation at DICA, Leiden, the Netherlands

Editors and Contributors

xiv

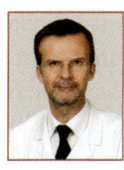
Mickael Lesurtel
Professor of Surgery, Department of Surgery and Liver Transplantation, Croix Rousse University Hospital, University of Lyon, Lyon, France

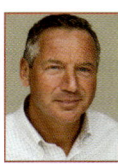
Marcel M. Levi
Professor, Department of Medicine, University College London Hospitals, London, United Kingdom

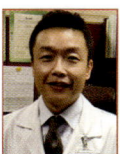
Chung-Wei Lin
Attending Physician, Department of Surgery and Surgical Oncology, Koo Foundation Sun Yat-Sen Cancer, Taipei, Taiwan

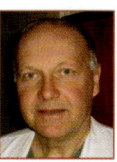
Lars Lundell
Professor, Consultant in Surgery, Gastrocentrum, Centre for Digestive Diseases, Karolinska University Hospital, Stockholm, Sweden

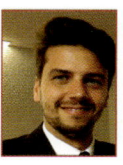
Giovanni Marchegiani
PhD Student, Department of General and Pancreatic Surgery, Pancreas Institute, University of Verona Hospital Trust, Policlinico GB Rossi, Verona, Italy

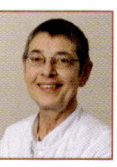
E.M.H. (Lisbeth) Mathus-Vliegen
Gastroenterologist, Professor in Clinical Nutrition, Department of Gastroenterology and Hepatology, Academic Medical Centre, University of Amsterdam, Amsterdam, the Netherlands

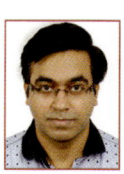
Abhishek Mitra
Lecturer, Department of Gastrointestinal and Hepatopancreaticobiliary Surgical Oncology, Tata Memorial Hospital, Mumbai, India

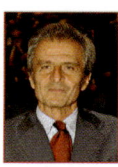
Mario Morino
Chair, Department of Surgical Sciences, University of Torino, Italy

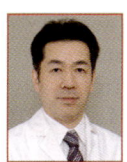
Shinji Morita
Chief, Department of Gastric Surgery, National Cancer Center Hospital, Tokyo, Japan

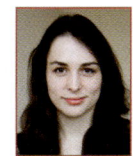
Tessa Mulder
PhD Candidate, University Medical Centre Utrecht, Division Julius Center for Health Sciences and Primary Care, Utrecht, the Netherlands

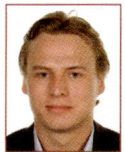
Gijsbert D. Musters
Surgical Resident, Department of Surgery, Academic Medical Centre, Amsterdam, the Netherlands

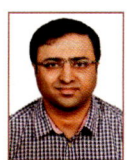
Raghavendra Nagaraja
Consultant, Surgical Gastroenterology, Vikram Jyoth Hospital, Mysore, India

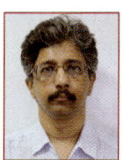
Sanjay S. Nagral
Coordinator and Senior Consultant, Deptartment of Surgical Gastroenterology, Jaslok Hospital & Research Centre; Head, Department of Surgery, KB Bhabha Municipal General Hospital, Mumbai, India

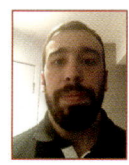
Ary Serpa Neto
Professor, Department of Critical Care Medicine, Hospital Israelita Albert Einstein, São Paulo, Brazil

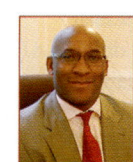
Abuchi Okaro
Associate Attending Surgeon, Department of Gastrointestinal Surgery, Hospital of St. John's and St. Elizabeth, London, United Kingdom

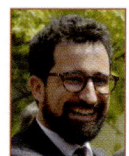
Salvatore Paiella
PhD Student, Department of General and Pancreatic Surgery, Pancreas Institute, University of Verona Hospital Trust, Policlinico GB Rossi, Verona, Italy

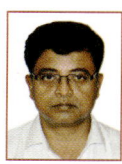

Sujoy Pal

Professor, Department of Gastrointestinal Surgery & Liver Transplantation, All India Institute of Medical Sciences, New Delhi, India

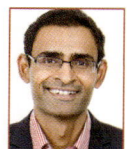

Sanjay Pandanaboyana

Consultant Hepatopancreaticobiliary and Transplant Surgeon, Hepatopancreaticobiliary/Upper Gastrointestinal Unit, Department of General Surgery, Auckland City Hospital; Department of Surgery, Faculty of Medical and Health Sciences, University of Auckland, Auckland, New Zealand

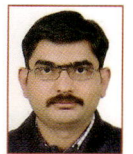

Rajesh Panwar

Assistant Professor, Department of Gastrointestinal Surgery & Liver Transplantation, All India Institute of Medical Sciences, New Delhi, India

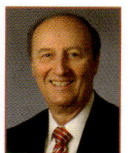

Henry A. Pitt

Chief Quality Officer, Temple University Health System; Associate Vice Dean for Clinical Affairs, Lewis Katz School of Medicine, Temple University, Philadelphia, Pennsylvania, United States of America

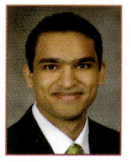

Nakul P. Raykar

Resident, Department of Surgery, Beth Israel Deaconess Medical Center; Fellow, Program in Global Surgery and Social Change, Harvard Medical School, Boston, Massachusetts, United States of America

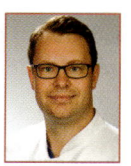

Matthias Reeh

Associate Professor of Surgery, Department of General, Visceral and Thoracic Surgery, University Hospital Hamburg-Eppendorf Hamburg, Germany

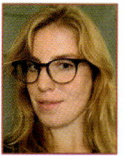

Eva Roos

PhD Candidate, Department of Surgery, Academic Medical Center, Surgical Laboratory, Amsterdam, the Netherlands

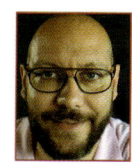

Ioannis Rouvelas

Senior Consultant in Surgery, Gastrocentrum, Centre for Digestive Diseases, Karolinska University Hospital Stockholm, Sweden

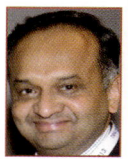

Nobhojit Roy

Professor and Head, Department of Surgery, BARC Hospital, HBNI University (Govt. of India); Public Health Specialist, School of Habitat, Tata Institute of Social Sciences, Mumbai, India

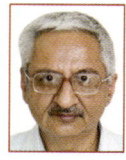

Peush Sahni

Professor and Head, Department of Gastrointestinal Surgery & Liver Transplantation, All India Institute of Medical Sciences, New Delhi, India

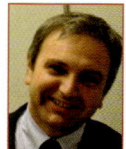

Roberto Salvia

Associate Professor of Surgery, Department of General and Pancreatic Surgery, Pancreas Institute, University of Verona Hospital Trust, Policlinico GB Rossi, Verona, Italy

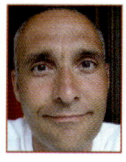

Marcus J. Schultz

Professor of Intensive Care Medicine, Laboratory of Experimental Intensive Care and Anesthesiology, Academic Medical Center, Amsterdam, the Netherlands

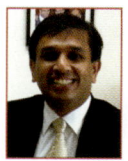

Shailesh V. Shrikhande

Chief of Gastrointestinal and Hepatopancreaticobiliary Surgical Oncology, Tata Memorial Hospital, Mumbai, India

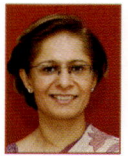

Bhawna Sirohi

Consultant Medical Oncologist, Department of Medical Oncology, Barts Cancer Institute, London, United Kingdom

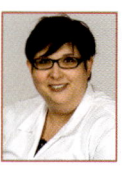

Ksenija Slankamenac

Attending Surgeon, Department of Surgery, University Hospital Zurich, Switzerland

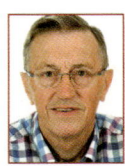

Peter B. Soeters

Emeritus Professor of Surgery, Maastricht University Medical Centre, Maastricht, the Netherlands

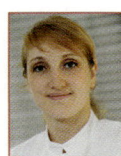

Anna-Katharina Stadler

Resident in Surgery, Department of General, Visceral and Transplantation Surgery, Heidelberg University Hospital, Heidelberg, Germany

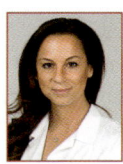

Roxane D. Staiger

Research Fellow, Department of Visceral and Transplant Surgery, University Hospital Zurich, Switzerland

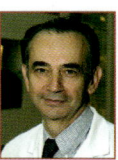

Steven M. Strasberg

Pruett Professor of Surgery, Section of Hepatopancreaticobiliary Surgery, Washington University, St. Louis, Missouri, United States of America

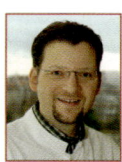

Oliver Strobel

Associate Professor of Surgery, Department of General, Visceral and Transplantation Surgery, Heidelberg University Hospital, Heidelberg, Germany

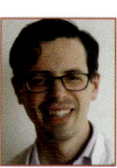

Pieter J. Tanis

Consultant, Gastrointestinal and Oncological Surgeon, Department of Surgery, Academic Medical Centre, Amsterdam, the Netherlands

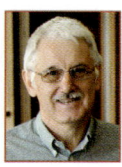

Sandie R. Thomson

Professor and Head of the Division, Division of Medical Gastroenterology, University of Cape Town and Groote Schuur Hospital, Observatory, Cape Town, South Africa

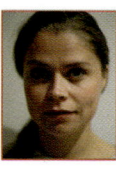

Johanna A.M.G. Tol

Surgical Resident, Department of Surgery Academic Medical Center, Amsterdam, the Netherlands

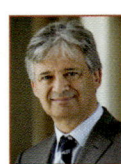

Rob A.E.M. Tollenaar

Professor of Surgery, Leiden University Medical Center, Department of Surgery; Chair, DICA, Leiden, the Netherlands

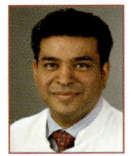

Yogesh K. Vashist

Associate Professor of Surgery, Department of Surgery, Kantonspital Aarau, Aarau, Switzerland

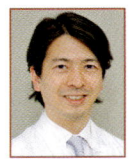

Takeyuki Wada

Attending Surgeon, Department of Gastric Surgery, National Cancer Center Hospital, Tokyo, Japan

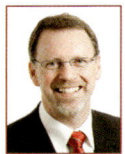

John A. Windsor

FRSNZ Professor of Surgery and Consultant Hepatopancreaticobiliary Surgeon, Hepatopancreaticobiliary/Upper Gastrointestinal Unit, Department of General Surgery, Auckland City Hospital; Department of Surgery, Faculty of Medical and Health Sciences, University of Auckland, Auckland, New Zealand

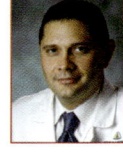

Christopher L. Wolfgang

Chief, Hepatobiliary and Pancreas Surgery; Professor of Surgery, Pathology and Oncology; Paul K. Neumann Professor of Pancreatic Cancer Research; Member, Miller-Coulson Academy of Clinical Excellence, Johns Hopkins University School of Medicine, Baltimore, Maryland, United States of America

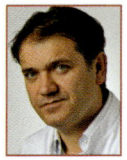

Michel W.J.M. Wouters

Surgeon, Department of Surgery, Antoni van Leeuwenhoek Hospital; Chair, Scientific Bureau, DICA, Leiden, the Netherlands

Abbreviations

ACE	Angiotensin-converting enzyme	JT	Jejunostomy tube
ACS–NSQIP	American College of Surgeons National Surgical Quality Improvement Program	LBM	Lean body mass
		LDLT	Living-donor liver transplantation
		LHV	Left hepatic vein
ARDS	Acute respiratory distress syndrome	LLG	Left lobe graft
ARISCAT	Assess Respiratory Risk in Surgical Patients in Catalonia	LLSG	Left lateral segment graft
		LOHS	Length of hospital stay
AS	Anastomotic stricture	LOS	Length of stay
ASA	American Society of Anesthesiologists	MHV	Middle hepatic vein
ASPEN	American Society of Parenteral and Enteral Nutrition	MNA	Mini Nutritional Assessment
		MUST	Malnutrition Universal Screening Tool
BIA	Bioimpedance analysis	NAS	Nonanastomotic stricture
BMI	Body mass index	NIV	Noninvasive ventilation
CCI	Comprehensive Complication Index	NJT	Nasojejunal feeding tube
CCPG	Canadian clinical practice guidelines	NMA	Network meta-analysis
CT	Computed tomography	NPWT	Negative-pressure wound therapy
DCD	Donation after cardiac death	NRI	Nutritional Risk Index
DDLT	Deceased-donor liver transplantation	NRS	Nutritional Risk Screening
DGE	Delayed gastric emptying	NRS-2002	Nutritional Risk Screening-2002
DHA	Docosahexaenoic acid	O/E	Observed/expected
DUS	Duplex ultrasonography	ONS	Oral nutrient supplement
ECG	Electrocardiogram	PBW	Predicted body weight
EN	Enteral nutrition	PEEP	Positive end-expiratory pressure
EPA	Eicosapentaenoic acid	PN	Parenteral nutrition
ERAS	Enhanced Recovery after Surgery	PNF	Primary nonfunction
ERCP	Endoscopic retrograde cholangiopancreatography	POPF	Postoperative pancreatic fistula
		PPC	Postoperative pulmonary complication
ESPEN	European Society of Parenteral and Enteral Nutrition	PPH	Postpancreatic haemorrhage
		PTCD	Percutaneous transhepatic cholangiodrainage
FFA	Free fatty acid		
FFM	Fat-free mass	PVT	Portal vein thrombosis
GCCI	Gentamicin-containing collagen implants	RCT	Randomised controlled trial
		RHV	Right hepatic vein
GI	Gastrointestinal	RLG	Right lobe graft
GJT	Gastrojejunostomy tube	RNA	Ribonucleic acid
GRWR	Graft-to-recipient weight ratio	RPSG	Right posterior segment graft
HAT	Hepatic artery thrombosis	SCCM	Society of Critical Care Medicine
HPB	Hepatopancreatobiliary	SCR	Surgical clinical reviewer
HVOO	Hepatic vein outflow obstruction	SFSS	Small-for-size syndrome
IBW	Ideal body weight	SGA	Subjective global assessment
ICU	Intensive care unit	SSI	Surgical site infection
IMF	Immunomodulating formula	VAC	Vacuum-assisted closure therapy
IRR	Interrater reliability	VHA	Veterans Health Administration

1

Introduction

S. Nundy and D.J. Gouma

Gastrointestinal (GI) surgery is now among the most sought after subspecialties for training worldwide, and the kind of patients we see, the spectrum of diseases and the stages at which they present to us vary widely in different countries around the world and also within the same country.

Gastrointestinal surgical operations are performed for a range of benign and malignant conditions, in both the elective and emergency settings. Therefore, it is important not only to become familiar with the normal postoperative course for these patients but also to detect complications early and manage them in a manner that is rational and based on published evidence, by using the local resources that are available. These operative procedures have recently become more and more complex and include living donor liver transplantation, pancreatic resections and operations for massive bleeding, and there have been advances in the ancillary procedures such as endoscopy, laparoscopy, imaging and interventional radiology.

During the past decades, there was an increasing realisation that outcome after GI surgery is dependent on not only the technical performance of the surgeons but also the availability of new instrumental technology and developments in other disciplines such as anaesthesiology, intensive care, gastroenterology and radiology. These developments have changed the process of patient care within hospitals, so that it is now undertaken by multidisciplinary teams and needs an efficient overall organisation of medical and surgical care.

We, therefore, thought that there was a need to publish, in a single volume, what might be the current postoperative management options for these patients. *Complications after Gastrointestinal Surgery* is a book that discusses the diagnosis and management of patients who have not followed a 'normal' course after GI procedures.

This book covers the entire spectrum of GI diseases and includes a wide range of subjects. It starts with chapters about the pathophysiology and development of several general complications, and the clinical aspects and the general management of these complications. In the second part of the book, more new developments are discussed, which are general institutional issues, such as management in limited-resource situations, the impact of centralisation, the definition and grading of complications, impact of checklists, nationwide audits and the role of the American College of Surgeons National Surgical Quality Improvement Program (ACS–NSQIP). The last part focuses on organ-specific problems that occur after operations of the oesophagus, stomach, small intestine, colon, liver, gallbladder, bile ducts and pancreas.

It was our aim to bring together, in a single volume, the opinions of experts from around the world, to highlight the current best clinical practice for the early detection and management of complications after GI surgery, in both the developing and developed worlds.

Our intended readers are not only GI and general surgeons but also gastroenterologists, critical care consultants and postgraduate students in both medicine and surgery, and we hope that they will find this 'international' approach informative and useful.

It would not have been possible to produce this book in such a short time without an extensive use of the internet. Both editors, one from India and the other from the Netherlands, the publisher and the opinion leaders from as far afield as New Zealand, Japan, Europe, South Africa, the United States and India were able to exchange ideas, problems and suggestions almost every day, and this has culminated into a book, of which everyone involved in its production is proud.

We hope that it will become a standard work of reference in the future.

Part I

General Aspects of Management of Surgical Complications

Cardiopulmonary Complications in Gastrointestinal Surgery Patients

T.G.V. Cherpanath, A.S. Neto,
W.K. Lagrand and M.J. Schultz

ABSTRACT

Postoperative cardiac and pulmonary complications negatively affect patient outcome and substantially increase healthcare costs. Reducing the incidence of these nonsurgical complications is thus of the utmost importance. This chapter provides an overview of how to predict, prevent and treat cardiopulmonary complications during the pre-, intra- and postoperative phases in patients with gastrointestinal surgery.

KEYWORDS

Postoperative, gastrointestinal surgery, cardiac complications, pulmonary complications

INTRODUCTION

Development of major postoperative nonsurgical complications has a strong impact on the resources used and outcomes in surgical patients.[1,2] Indeed, costs of care increase dramatically due to the postoperative complications themselves as well as the subsequent prolonged hospitalisation.[1] More importantly, patients who develop nonsurgical complication have an increased risk of dying.[2] Approximately 10% of patients undergoing major surgery, including gastrointestinal surgery, are at increased risk of postoperative nonsurgical complications, accounting for 80% of all postoperative deaths and long-term reduced functional independence in survivors.[1,2] With more than 60 million gastrointestinal surgery procedures undertaken worldwide each year,[1,3] it is obvious that even a small reduction in the incidence of major postoperative nonsurgical complications can have an enormous impact.

Major postoperative cardiac complications, including hypotension and disturbed cardiac performance, cardiac arrhythmias and myocardial ischaemia and infarction, account for at least one-third of all perioperative deaths and result in prolonged hospitalisation.[3–5] Large prospective cohort studies have shown that chronic cardiac conditions such as coronary artery disease provide a substrate for cardiac complications during and after surgery.[6] Likewise, development of major postoperative pulmonary complications, including bronchial secretions and productive cough, pulmonary infiltrates and pneumonia, aspiration, bronchospasm, pleural effusions, barotraumas and atelectasis, acute pulmonary oedema, acute respiratory failure and the more severe acute respiratory distress syndrome (ARDS), accounts for up to one-fifth of all postoperative deaths within 30 days after surgery and results in prolonged hospitalisation.[2,7,8] Recent knowledge is that the way in which intraoperative ventilation is applied can have a strong effect on the risk for postoperative pulmonary complications.[9,10]

This chapter provides an overview of not only the risk factors associated with postoperative cardiopulmonary complications but also how to prevent these complications during and after surgery, with focus on gastrointestinal surgery, where possible. Most attention is given to the prevention of cardiopulmonary complications, since management of most of the cardiopulmonary complications requires expertise from medical specialties beyond surgery, and a detailed description of highly specialised care for specific complications is beyond the scope of this book.

CARDIAC COMPLICATIONS

Definition

A formal definition of cardiac complications after gastrointestinal surgery is currently lacking. Although cardiac problems mainly consist of three components, that is, myocardial ischaemia and infarction, arrhythmia and heart failure, the first is by far the most important factor after major surgery, including gastrointestinal surgery.[11] Notably, arrhythmias and heart failure frequently result from myocardial ischaemia and infarction. Therefore, we focus mainly on the prevention and management of myocardial ischaemia and infarction in the context of gastrointestinal surgery.

Incidence and Impact of Cardiac Complications

Cardiac complications during gastrointestinal surgery are not uncommon. The reported incidence of cardiac complications is 5%,[12] which impacts healthcare costs and length of stay. Furthermore, noncardiac complications are more likely to occur in the presence of cardiac complications, both contributing to an increase in mortality.

Preoperative Recognition of Patients at Risk for Cardiac Complications

Prevention of postoperative cardiac complications includes preoperative screening. Patients at a certain risk for cardiac complications, depending on patient factors such as risk factors for coronary artery disease and factors associated with the surgical intervention, such as the expected duration of anaesthesia, should always undergo preoperative optimisation and perioperative treatment, if the surgical intervention can be delayed.

As the main cardiac complication during gastrointestinal surgery consists of myocardial ischaemia and infarction, it is of no surprise that risk factors for coronary artery disease such as diabetes, renal dysfunction and history of ischaemic disease and/or heart failure are all independent predictors. Therefore, it is important to screen patients before the surgical intervention, in order to evaluate perioperative cardiovascular risks, not only to optimise

perioperative care but also to plan for the longer term, if necessary. As mentioned above, type and urgency for surgery should be considered (i.e., the risk and benefit of performing the surgical procedure vs. the risk and benefit of not performing or postponing it). In case of an elective setting, the procedure may be performed after clinical risk stratification. A clear step-wise approach to preoperative cardiac assessment is delineated in the American College of Cardiology (ACC)/American Heart Association (AHH) guidelines.[13]

In the setting of an emergency surgery, a well-organised preoperative screening is usually not feasible, and a global determination of the relative merits of an immediate surgery versus the risk of waiting must be made, realising that the former setting entails a two to five times higher risk for cardiac complications as compared with the latter, that is, an elective, setting. The Revised Cardiac Risk Index uses a simple system to estimate the cardiac risk.[14] For a more complex risk assessment, the 'American College of Surgeons National Surgical Quality Improvement Program' (ACS–NSQIP) calculator (riskcalculator.facs. org) can be used. The ACS–NSQIP calculator includes 20 risk factors, including age and functional status. When patients are at low risk for cardiac complications, no further cardiovascular testing is deemed necessary before surgery. Nevertheless, a preoperative electrocardiogram (ECG) may be helpful in this patient group as well, serving as a baseline comparison tool.

All patients with moderate to high risk for cardiac complications should be assessed preoperatively. Special attention should be paid to ischaemic symptoms and functional status, as both necessitate further evaluation such as (pharmacological) stress testing, echocardiography and coronary imaging (angiography and computed tomography scanning). In general, additional preoperative testing and treatment are required only if indicated, as would be done in cases without pending gastrointestinal surgery, such as a significant stenosis of the left main coronary artery. Routine coronary angiography is not recommended.

When potential interventions are contemplated to reduce the cardiac complications during elective gastrointestinal surgery, some topics need to be addressed. Firstly, there has been much debate whether ß-blockade should be initiated before surgery. In addition, in case of ß-blocking agents, the optimal timing and the agent of choice need to be recognised.[15] We believe that there is insufficient evidence for the initiation of ß-blockade, especially when taking into account the emerging evidence of increased mortality.[16] However, in patients who were already on ß-blocking agents before surgery, continuation is recommended. The same holds true for aspirin and other antiplatelet drugs, as long as no severe coagulopathy is present and the type of gastrointestinal surgery does not encompass severe complications upon minor bleeding, as frequently is the case in neurosurgery. Continuation of angiotensin-converting-enzyme inhibitor (ACEi) therapy is reasonable;[13] if stopped before surgery, it should be restarted as soon as possible after the surgery. Statins should be continued or should be started when the 10-year cardiovascular risk threshold is exceeded.[17] It is even thought that statin initiation 2 to 3 days before surgery may encompass endothelial stabilisation, potentially contributing to a reduction in cardiac complications. Alpha-2 agonists are not recommended for the perioperative phase.

Patients with implantable cardioverter defibrillator (ICD) should be monitored continuously in case the ICD is reprogrammed or inactivated. In these cases, external defibrillation equipment should be available at the bedside and should be ready to use (pads on the patient). Active ICD treatment should be restarted as soon as possible after the surgery.

Finally, but certainly not unimportantly, antibiotics are to be given to reduce the risk of endocarditis in case of prior endocarditis and a mechanical prosthetic valve, according to a recent change in the guidelines.[18]

Intraoperative Care to Prevent Cardiac Complications

As myocardial ischaemia is the primary cause of cardiac complications during gastrointestinal surgery, perioperative ECG monitoring capable of analysing ST-segment deviations is recommended in patients at moderate to high cardiovascular risk. Haemodynamic monitoring may be indicated in patients undergoing gastrointestinal surgery.

Perioperative echocardiography is not recommended routinely but is reasonable in patients with unexplained haemodynamic instability. In addition, pulmonary artery catheters should not be used routinely but may be considered in case of unexplained or persisting haemodynamic instability.

Intravenous nitroglycerine was not found to be effective in diminishing myocardial ischaemia during surgery. Maintenance of a normal body temperature is considered reasonable, with the aim to reduce perioperative cardiac events.

The concept of intraoperative 'goal-directed fluid therapy' has been used in elective major gastrointestinal surgery. Intraoperative hypovolaemia, upon a decrease in blood volume of 15%, can already instigate a fall in splanchnic perfusion,[19] associated with severe complications such as anastomotic leakage and wound infection. A recent meta-analysis of randomised controlled trials shows that 'goal-directed fluid therapy' is associated with a significant reduction in the overall morbidity and length of stay in the intensive care unit and hospital.[20] However, there is a U-shaped relation between the amount of fluids infused and morbidity in surgical patients,[21] explaining the importance of a near-zero fluid balance in the perioperative setting.[22] It is vital to understand that fluid responsiveness—the increase in stroke volume or cardiac output upon fluid loading—does not mean that fluids need to be administered; this should be done on the basis of inadequate tissue perfusion due to haemodynamic compromise. A systematic review on cardiac-output-guided haemodynamic protocols using intravenous fluids and inotropic drugs during major gastrointestinal surgery did not show a reduction in mortality; however, decreased complication rates such as postoperative infection and shorter duration of hospital stay were noted.[23] Therefore, the National Institute for Health and Clinical Excellence of the United Kingdom recommends the use of perioperative 'goal-directed fluid therapy' in patients undergoing high-risk surgery, which includes major gastrointestinal surgery.[24] For this purpose, dynamic parameters such as stroke volume variation and pulse pressure variation can be used in contrast to a static parameter such as central venous pressure in gastrointestinal surgery.[25–28]

Volatile or intravenous anaesthesia may be used, and the decision for the anaesthetic modality is based on other than the prevention of myocardial ischaemia alone.[13,29] However, in a recent meta-analysis, an independent association has been found between the use of volatile anaesthetics (vs. intravenous anaesthetics) and the reduced incidence of pulmonary and extrapulmonary complications.[29] No irrefutable evidence has been presented showing the superiority of epidural versus general anaesthesia.

Postoperative Prevention of Cardiac Complications and Their Management

Adequate pain management is important to reduce the incidence of cardiac complications, in particular myocardial ischaemia (e.g., by neuraxial or epidural anaesthesia). As ibuprofen and naproxen can hinder the antiplatelet effect of aspirin and diclofenac may increase the risk of myocardial infarction in the absence of aspirin, these agents are usually not prescribed in patients at risk for cardiac ischaemia.

It is essential to be alert of cardiac complications after gastrointestinal surgery, as most complications occur in the early postoperative period, typically on Day 3. Electrocardiogram screening in selected patients may be considered, but it is recommended in high-risk patients with cardiac symptoms, such as dyspnoea, pain and arrhythmias. While haemoglobin levels as low as 6.4 g/dL can be accepted in the absence of vascular disease, higher triggers are used in patients with vascular disease (8.0 g/dL) and patients with peripheral, cerebral, and cardiac ischaemia (9.6 g/dL), according to one national guideline.[30]

When cardiac ischaemia is suspected, an ECG and cardiac biomarkers should be rapidly obtained. Routine postoperative screening by means of troponin is not recommended, but it should be reserved for those at high risk or those with signs of myocardial ischaemia. The elevation of cardiac biomarkers after gastrointestinal surgery may also be present without myocardial ischaemia due to an unstable plaque, so that pulmonary embolism and severe anaemia among others must also be contemplated.

Treatment of Postoperative Cardiac Complications

Postoperative cardiac complications frequenty require the expertise of a consulting cardiologist and should be addressed immediately. Postoperative cardiac arrhythmias mostly consist of atrial fibrillation, amongst other supraventricular arrhythmias, which could be treated in two ways: by aiming to restore sinus rhythm (i.e., 'rhythm control') or to accept atrial fibrillation with adequate ventricular frequency (i.e., 'rate control'). Besides the treatment of the arrhythmia with antiarrhythmic drugs, it is paramount to search for triggers, substrates and modulating factors that underlie the arrhythmia (e.g., myocardial ischaemia, hypoxia, hyper-/hypovolaemia, electrolyte disorders, medication, fever, anaemia, pain and anxiety).

Most of the times, postoperative heart failure originates from myocardial ischaemia. Severe heart failure, especially when resulting in forward failure, with the risk of development of shock and organ failure, usually requires admission to an intensive care unit for optimisation of fluid management and treatment with vasopressors and inotropes. Myocardial ischaemia should be diagnosed and treated accordingly, as described in the pre- and perioperative section.

PULMONARY COMPLICATIONS

Definition

A standard definition of the postoperative pulmonary complications is currently lacking. Most studies that report on postoperative pulmonary complications performed so far use composite endpoints,[7] including various postoperative pulmonary conditions such as excessive bronchial secretions, productive cough, pulmonary infiltrates, pneumonia, aspiration, bronchospasm, pleural effusions, barotrauma, atelectasis, acute pulmonary oedema, acute respiratory failure and ARDS. Frequently, unexpected need for supplementary oxygen is also included, even though this is usually considered a 'minor' complication.

Incidence

When using composite endpoints, the incidence of postoperative pulmonary complications ranges from 2 to 40%,[7] depending on whether not only minor complications such as unexpected need for supplementary oxygen are included in the composite but also the preoperative condition of patients, types of surgery and even types of anaesthesia are included. Recently, it was estimated that the incidence of postoperative pulmonary complications in general surgery patients and gastrointestinal surgery patients is 5 and 7%, respectively.[2]

Impact of Development of Postoperative Pulmonary Complications

The impact of postoperative pulmonary complications can be quite substantial. The impact of each individual postoperative pulmonary complication on the outcome of surgical patients is not fully elucidated, but it is clear that a more severe pulmonary complication such as ARDS has a larger impact than a simpler complication such as the need for supplementary oxygen. Nevertheless, one in five general surgery patients who develop a postoperative pulmonary complications dies in the first 30 days after the intervention.[2] The impact is even higher in gastrointestinal surgery patients, where one in three patients who develop a postoperative pulmonary complications dies.[2] In addition, the development of postoperative pulmonary complications in these patients is strongly related to the short- and long-term mortality and to hospital stay (Figure 2.1).[2,8]

Preoperative Recognition of Patients at Risk for Pulmonary Complications

Prevention of postoperative pulmonary complications includes preoperative screening: patients at a certain risk for pulmonary complications, depending on patient factors, such as age, obesity and preoperative oxygen levels,

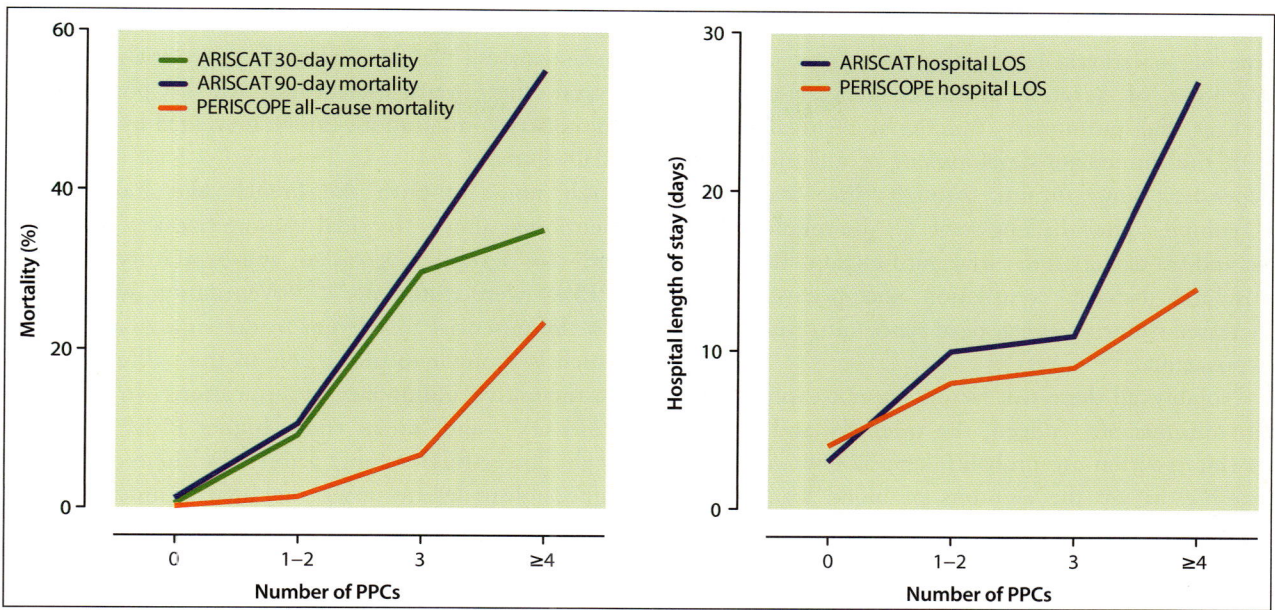

Figure 2.1 Relationship between number of postoperative pulmonary complications (PPC), hospital length of stay (LOS) (in days) and mortality (in %) in cohorts from 'Assess Respiratory Risk in Surgical Patients in Catalonia' (ARISCAT) and 'Prospective Evaluation of a Risk Score for Postoperative Pulmonary Complications in Europe' (PERISCOPE) studies.
Courtesy: Ary Serpa Neto.

and factors associated with the surgical intervention, such as the type of incision and the expected duration of the procedure, should undergo preoperative optimisation if the surgical intervention can be delayed.

Prediction of postoperative pulmonary complications is possible by using only a few perioperative variables, as researchers from Spain developed their so-called 'Assess Respiratory Risk in Surgical Patients in Catalonia' (ARISCAT) score.[2] The ARISCAT score is based on a small set of objective, easily assessable factors with excellent discriminative ability: age, preoperative pulse oximetry, preoperative anaemia and presence of respiratory infection. Patients with a score less than 26 have a low risk for the development of postoperative pulmonary complications. A score between 26 and 44 is associated with an intermediate risk and a score of more than 44 is associated with a high risk for the development of postoperative pulmonary complications. Robustness of the ARISCAT score was recently confirmed in settings outside Spain.[8]

The type of surgical insult also contributes to the risk for the development of postoperative pulmonary complications.[7] Abdominal and thoracic surgical interventions close to the diaphragm can result in at least three types of injury, all associated with postoperative pulmonary complications: (1) functional disruption of the respiratory muscles, caused by the incision,

(2) effect of postoperative pain by limiting the movement of the respiratory muscles, and (3) the inhibition reflex of the phrenic nerve and other nerves that innervate the respiratory muscles.[7]

Among the preventive measures to be adopted in order to decrease the chance of postoperative pulmonary complications are smoking cessation, use of bronchodilators in patients with chronic lung disease and a good nutritional state.

Intraoperative Factors Associated with Pulmonary Complications

Factors related to the 'intensity' of the surgical intervention, the length of the procedure, blood loss and other factors, all are associated with the development of postoperative pulmonary complications. Immune depression caused by surgical trauma is an important mediator that can lead to an increased risk of infectious complications after surgery.[7] According to the ARISCAT score[2] mentioned above, the surgical incision site (peripheral, upper abdominal or intrathoracic), procedures lasting more than 2 hours and the need for an emergency surgery are important factors related to the development of postoperative pulmonary complications.

There are several intraoperative anaesthesia-related factors that could play a role in the development of postoperative pulmonary complications. Firstly, the type of anaesthesia is an important factor in clinical outcomes of surgical patients. General anaesthesia reduces the pulmonary functional residual capacity, with the immediate development of atelectasis in the dependent lung regions through three mechanisms: (1) compression of the lung tissue, (2) absorption of alveolar air, and (3) reduction in surfactant function. The resulting mismatch between ventilation and perfusion causes increased shunting effect, dead space and, consequently, hypoxaemia.[31]

Notably, all these risk factors are not easily, if not at all, minimisable. Indeed, the intensity and length of the intervention are probably kept as low and short as possible, as are the amounts of blood transfused. In addition, major abdominal surgery usually requires general anaesthesia.

Protective Ventilation to Prevent Postoperative Pulmonary Complications

Mechanical ventilation is almost always mandatory during major surgery. There are several ways to reduce the risk of lung injury caused by mechanical ventilation. For a long time, use of high tidal volumes (i.e., 10–15 mL/Kg) during intraoperative ventilation was encouraged in order to prevent hypoxaemia and atelectasis.[32] Increased understanding of how high tidal volumes could cause so-called 'volutrauma' of the lungs in intensive care unit patients[33] triggered research in intraoperative ventilation strategies that could reduce the risk for pulmonary complications after surgery. Two recently published randomised controlled trials in patients undergoing gastrointestinal surgery confirmed the benefits of so-called 'lung-protective' intraoperative ventilation with low tidal volumes. In the multicentre 'Intraoperative PROtective VEntilation (IMPROVE) trial of 400 nonobese patients planned for major abdominal surgery in France,[34] lung-protective ventilation with tidal volumes of 6 to 8 mL/Kg was compared with conventional ventilation with tidal volume of 10 to 12 mL/Kg. The incidence of postoperative pulmonary complications dropped from 27.5 to 10.5% with the use of lung-protective ventilation. In a single-centre randomised controlled trial[35] of 56 patients scheduled for open abdominal surgery lasting more than 2 hours in Italy, lung-protective ventilation with tidal volumes of 7 mL/Kg was compared with conventional ventilation with tidal volumes of 9 mL/Kg. The modified 'Clinical Pulmonary Infection Score' was lower, pulmonary functional tests and arterial oxygenation levels were better and chest radiographs showed fewer abnormalities in patients receiving lung-protective ventilation. A series of meta-analyses,[9,10,36] including these two trials, as well as several other investigations confirmed that postoperative pulmonary complications can be prevented by using low tidal volumes.

Of note, in both the French and Italian trials mentioned above, the tidal volume size was compared and the levels of positive end-expiratory pressure (PEEP) were different.[34–36] Ventilation with PEEP has the potential to prevent intraoperative atelectasis, which is thought to play a role in the pathogenesis of postoperative pulmonary complications. In both the IMPROVE and Italian trials, higher PEEP was used in the lower-tidal-volume arm.[34,35] Therefore, it was impossible to determine whether benefit came only from the use of low tidal volumes. However, one recently published international multicentre randomised controlled trial (the 'PROtective Ventilation using HIgh vs. LOw PEEP' [PROVHILO] trial) showed no benefit from PEEP of 12 cm H_2O versus PEEP of 2 cm H_2O during intraoperative ventilation with low tidal volumes in 900 patients planned for open abdominal surgery.[37] A recently published meta-analysis suggests that the benefit of lung protection is mainly achieved with the use of low tidal volumes and not with the level of PEEP.[36]

Recent investigations suggest that a low amplitude of the airway pressure (or driving pressure—the difference between the upper airway pressure and PEEP) may be even more important than a low tidal volume.[38–40] The driving pressure is dependent not only on the tidal volume size but also on the effects of PEEP (not the level of PEEP), as PEEP could recruit lung tissue (leading to a low driving pressure) or cause lung overdistension (leading to high driving pressure). Actually, the driving pressure could be the key ventilatory variable related to the outcome of surgery patients,[41] but it is still uncertain how exactly to set the ventilator so that the lowest or best driving pressure could be achieved in an individual patient.

Postoperative Prevention of Pulmonary Complications

Adequate pain management through multimodal analgesic protocols and sufficient evacuation of pulmonary secretions by patient through prevention of rest-sedation and postoperative residual neuromuscular blockade and placement of the patient in the upright position are some general measures that can decrease the risk of pulmonary complications and shortened hospital stay.[42]

Postoperative noninvasive ventilation (NIV) has been suggested as a tool to prevent or treat postoperative hypoxaemia.[43] While two earlier randomised controlled trials in postoperative patients showed that NIV was not effective for the management of postextubation respiratory failure,[44,45] a very recent multicentre randomised controlled trial in 293 patients after abdominal surgery in France showed that NIV reduced the risk of reintubation within 7 days.[46] However, upper digestive stitching requires great prudence with the use of NIV. Indeed, there is a risk for intradigestive air insufflation when high insufflation pressures are applied.[47] High-flow nasal cannula oxygen therapy[48] may also benefit postoperative patients. In patients after cardiac surgery, high-flow nasal oxygen therapy reduced the need for the escalation of respiratory support.[49,50] Randomised controlled trial evidence for the benefit of high-flow nasal oxygen therapy in patients after abdominal surgery is presently lacking.

Finally, it has been suggested that incentive spirometry in patients undergoing abdominal surgery could reduce the incidence of postoperative pulmonary complications.[51] An algorithm for the management of patients undergoing abdominal surgery in the perioperative period is shown in Algorithm 2.1.

Treatment of Postoperative Pulmonary Complications

Postoperative pulmonary complications should always be promptly treated, and some of these require specific actions. Postoperative respiratory failure could be treated with a trial of NIV[46]; however, tracheal reintubation should not be delayed. If a patient cannot continue without ventilation, lung-protective ventilation with low tidal volume is a must,[52] as is the use of PEEP.[53] Prone ventilation and muscle relaxation should be considered early in patients with severe ARDS.[54,55] Notably, ARDS is not a postoperative complication 'on its own,' and usually, its cause in a surgical complication is known (e.g., leaking anastomose and abdominal abscess); undoubtedly, this should always be treated first, if possible.

Patients who develop atelectasis may need supplemental oxygen. Removal of any obstruction in the larger airways (e.g., pulmonary secretions and sputum), adequate pain control, early mobilisation and NIV may all help in solving this problem.[56] Any pulmonary infections should be adequately treated. If sepsis develops, the Surviving Sepsis Campaign guidelines should be followed.[57] Pneumothorax and large pleural effusions should be treated with thoracic drainage. Patients with small pleural effusions with no

		Preoperative phase	Intraoperative phase	Postoperative phase	Treatment
Postoperative complications	**Cardiac**	• Cardiac risk screening (e.g., the ACS–NSQIP calculator) • Cardiac stress test, echocardiography or coronary imaging (when ischaemic symptoms) • Cardiac optimisation • Continue β-blockade, ACE inhibitor, aspirin and statin	• Use goal-directed fluid strategies • Maybe: use of volatile anaesthetics during surgery	• ECG and troponin screening (high-risk patients) • Adequate analgesia • Restricted transfusion of packed red cells	• Treat arrhythmias • Treat myocardial ischaemia • Treat cardiac shock with optimisation of the fluid status, vasopressors and/or inotropes (usually requires ICU admission)
	Pulmonary	• PPC risk screening (e.g., the ARISCAT score) • Stop smoking • Continuation/start bronchodilators (in chronic pulmonary disease)	• Use of lung low tidal volumes (6–8 mL/Kg PBW) during intraoperative ventilation • Maybe: use low PEEP (0–2 cm H₂O) • Maybe: use low driving pressure (<13 cm H₂O)	• Prophylactic NIV (high-risk patients) • Incentive spirometry • Adequate analgesia • Maybe: high-flow nasal oxygen	• NIV, and invasive ventilation if NIV fails • ARDS treatment consisting of low tidal volumes (6–8 mL/Kg PBW), prone ventilation, and maybe muscle paralysis (requires ICU admission) • Always: consider a surgical complications and/or infection as a reason for respiratory failure

Algorithm 2.1 Algorithm for the management and treatment of patients undergoing abdominal surgery.

Abbreviations: ACS–NSQIP, American College of Surgeons National Surgical Quality Improvement Program; ACE, angiotensin-converting enzyme; PPC, postoperative pulmonary complications; ARISCAT, Assess Respiratory Risk in Surgical Patients in Catalonia; PBW, predicted body weight; PEEP, positive end-expiratory pressure; ECG, electrocardiogram; ICU intensive care unit; ARDS, acute respiratory distress syndrome; NIV, noninvasive ventilation.

Courtesy: Ary Serpa Neto.

clinical impact could be clinically followed. Finally, it is important to consider that severe complications usually require admission of patient to an intensive care unit, where care is provided by physicians experienced in treating patients who have a high chance of rapid deterioration.

CONCLUSIONS

This chapter provides an overview of postoperative cardiopulmonary complications after surgery. While most literature does not focus on gastrointestinal surgery per se, we consider all findings relevant for patients who are planned to undergo gastrointestinal surgery. Consequently, we follow all recommendations, as they exist for the general surgery patients. Key is early recognition of patients at risk for postoperative cardiopulmonary complications, that is, before surgery, as this allows optimisation of each patient if time allows so. Simple interventions could prevent, or at least minimise, the risk for certain complications. When a postoperative complication develops, whether it concerns a cardiac complication or a pulmonary complication, it requires the expertise of other specialties, usually cardiologists and intensive care physicians.

REFERENCES

1. Pearse RM, Moreno RP, Bauer P, et al. Mortality after surgery in Europe: a 7-day cohort study. *Lancet* 2012;380: 1059–65.
2. Canet J, Gallart L, Gomar C, et al. Prediction of postoperative pulmonary complications in a population-based surgical cohort. *Anesthesiology* 2010;113:1338–50.
3. Protective Ventilation Network. LAS VEGAS website. [Accessed 2016 March 18]. Available from: https://sites.google.com/site/lasvegasstudy/home.
4. Devereaux PJ, Sessler DI. Cardiac complications in patients undergoing major noncardiac surgery. *N Engl J Med* 2015;373:2258–69.
5. Botto F, Alonso-Coello P, Chan MT, et al. Myocardial injury after noncardiac surgery: a large, international, prospective cohort study establishing diagnostic criteria, characteristics, predictors, and 30-day outcomes. *Anesthesiology* 2014;120:564–78.
6. Gupta PK, Gupta H, Sundaram A, et al. Development and validation of a risk calculator for prediction of cardiac risk after surgery. *Circulation* 2011;124:381–7.
7. Canet J, Mazo V. Postoperative pulmonary complications. *Minerva Anestesiol* 2010;76:138–43.
8. Mazo V, Sabaté S, Canet J, et al. Prospective external validation of a predictive score for postoperative pulmonary complications. *Anesthesiology* 2014;121:219–31.
9. Güldner A, Kiss T, Serpa Neto A, et al. Intraoperative protective mechanical ventilation for prevention of postoperative pulmonary complications: a comprehensive review of the role of tidal volume, positive end-expiratory pressure, and lung recruitment maneuvers. *Anesthesiology*. 2015;123:692–713.
10. Serpa Neto A, Schultz MJ, Gama de Abreu M. Intraoperative ventilation strategies to prevent postoperative pulmonary complications: systematic review, meta-analysis, and trial sequential analysis. *Best Pract Res Clin Anaesthesiol* 2015;29:331–40.
11. van Diepen S, Bakal JA, McAlister FA, Ezekowitz JA. Mortality and readmission of patients with heart failure, atrial fibrillation, or coronary artery disease undergoing noncardiac surgery: an analysis of 38047 patients. *Circulation* 2011;124:289–96.
12. Devereaux PJ, Yang H, Yusuf S, et al. Effects of extended-release metoprolol succinate in patients undergoing non-cardiac surgery (POISE trial): a randomized controlled trial. *Lancet* 2008;371:1839–47.
13. Fleisher LA, Fleischmann KE, Auerbach AD, et al. 2014 ACC/AHA guideline on perioperative cardiovascular evaluation and management of patients undergoing noncardiac surgery: executive summary. A report of the American College of Cardiology/American Heart Association Task Force on Practice Guidelines. *Circulation* 2014;130:2215–45.
14. Lee TH, Marcantonio ER, Mangione CM, et al. Derivation and prospective validation of a simple index for prediction of cardiac risk of major noncardiac surgery. *Circulation* 1999;100:1043–9.
15. Wijeysundera DN, Duncan D, Nkonde-Price D, et al. Perioperative beta blockade in noncardiac surgery: a systematic review for the 2014 ACC/AHA guideline on perioperative cardiovascular evaluation and management of patients undergoing noncardiac surgery. *J Am Coll Cardiol* 2014;64:2406–25.
16. Brown DL. Perioperative β-blockade reduces nonfatal MI but increases mortality in noncardiac surgery. *Ann Intern Med* 2015;162:10.
17. Pandya A, Sy S, Cho S, Weinstein MC, Gaziano TA. Cost-effectiveness of 10-year risk thresholds for initiation of statin therapy for primary prevention of cardiovascular disease. *JAMA* 2015;314:142–50.
18. Habib G, Lancellotti P, Antunes MJ, et al. 2015 ESC Guidelines for the management of infective endocarditis. *Eur Heart J* 2015;36:3075–128.
19. Giglio MT, Marucci M, Testini M, Brienza M. Goal-directed haemodynamic therapy and gastrointestinal complications in major surgery: a meta-analysis of randomized controlled trials. *Br J Anaesth* 2009;103: 637–46.
20. Rollins KE, Lobo DN. Intraoperative goal-directed fluid therapy in elective major abdominal surgery. A meta-analysis of randomized controlled trials. *Ann Surg* 2015;263:465–76.
21. Bellamy MC. Wet, dry or something else? *Br J Anaesth* 2006;97:755–7.

22. Doherty M, Buggy DJ. Intraoperative fluids: how much is too much? *Br J Anaesth* 2012;109:69–79.

23. Pearse RM, Harrison DA, MacDonald N, et al. Effect of a perioperative, cardiac output-guided hemodynamic therapy algorithm on outcomes following major gastrointestinal surgery: a randomized clinical trial and systematic review. *JAMA* 2014;311:2181–90.

24. National Institute for Health and Clinical Excellence. CardioQ-ODM Oesophageal Doppler Monitor. London, UK; 2011 [Accessed 2016 February 26]. Available from: https://www.nice.org.uk/guidance/mtg3.

25. Biais M, Nouette-Gaulain K, Cottenceau V, Revel P, Sztark F. Uncalibrated pulse contour-derived stroke volume variation predicts fluid responsiveness in mechanically ventilated patients undergoing liver transplantation. *Br J Anaesth* 2008;101:761–8.

26. Zimmermann M, Feibicke T, Keyl C, et al. Accuracy of stroke volume variation compared with pleth variability index to predict fluid responsiveness in mechanically ventilated patients undergoing major surgery. *Eur J Anaesthesiol* 2010;27:555–61.

27. Solus-Biguenet H, Fleyfel M, Tavernier B, et al. Non-invasive prediction of fluid responsiveness during major hepatic surgery. *Br J Anaesth* 2006;97:808–16.

28. Derichard A, Robin E, Tavernier B, et al. Automated pulse pressure and stroke volume variations from radial artery: evaluation during major abdominal surgery. *Br J Anaesth* 2009;103:678–84.

29. Uhlig C, Bluth T, Schwarz K, et al. Effects of volatile anesthetics on mortality and postoperative pulmonary and extra-pulmonary complications in patients undergoing surgery: a systematic review and meta-analysis. *Anesthesiology* 2016;124:1230–45.

30. CBO. Richtlijn Bloedtransfusie. [Accessed 2016 March 18]. Available from: https://nvic.nl/sites/default/files/CBO%20Richtlijn%20Bloedtransfusie.pdf.

31. Kavanagh BP. Perioperative atelectasis. *Minerva Anestesiol* 2008;74:285–7.

32. Bendixen HH, Hedley-Whyte J, Laver MB. Impaired oxygenation in surgical patients during general anesthesia with controlled ventilation. A concept of atelectasis. *N Engl J Med* 1863;269:991–6.

33. Slutsky AS. Lung injury caused by mechanical ventilation. *Chest* 1999;116:9S–15S.

34. Futier E, Constantin JM, Paugam-Burtz C, et al. A trial of intraoperative low-tidal-volume ventilation in abdominal surgery. *N Engl J Med* 2013;369:428–37.

35. Severgnini P, Selmo G, Lanza C, et al. Protective mechanical ventilation during general anesthesia for open abdominal surgery improves postoperative pulmonary function. *Anesthesiology* 2013;118:1307–21.

36. Serpa Neto A, Hemmes SN, Barbas CS, et al. Protective versus conventional ventilation for surgery: a systematic review and individual patient data meta-analysis. *Anesthesiology* 2015;123:66–78.

37. PROVE Network Investigators for the Clinical Trial Network of the European Society of Anaesthesiology, Hemmes SN, Gama de Abreu M, et al. High versus low positive end-expiratory pressure during general anaesthesia for open abdominal surgery (PROVHILO trial): a multicentre randomised controlled trial. *Lancet* 2014;384:495–503.

38. Amato MBP, Meade MO, Slutsky AS, et al. Driving-pressure as a mediator of survival in patients with acute respiratory distress syndrome (ARDS). *N Engl J Med* 2015;372:747–55.

39. Estenssoro E, Dubin A, Laffaire E, et al. Incidence, clinical course, and outcomes in 217 patients with acute respiratory distress syndrome. *Crit Care Med* 2002;30:2450–56.

40. Boissier F, Katsahian S, Razazi K, et al. Prevalence and prognosis of cor pulmonale during protective ventilation for acute respiratory distress syndrome. *Intensive Care Med* 2013;39:1725–33.

41. Serpa Neto A, Hemmes SNT, Barbas CSV, et al; PROVE Network Investigators. Association between driving pressure and development of postoperative pulmonary complications in patients undergoing mechanical ventilation for general anaesthesia: a meta-analysis of individual patient data. *Lancet Respir Med* 2016;4:272–80.

42. Reilly JJ Jr. Preoperative and postoperative care of standard and high risk surgical patients. *Hematol Oncol Clin North Am* 1997;11:449–59.

43. Esteban A, Frutos-Vivar F, Ferguson N, et al. Noninvasive positive-pressure ventilation for respiratory failure after extubation. *N Engl J Med* 2004;350:2452–60.

44. Keenan S, Powers C, McCormack D, Block G. Noninvasive positive-pressure ventilation for postextubation respiratory distress: a randomized controlled trial. *JAMA* 2002;287:3238–44.

45. Nava S, Gregoretti C, Fanfulla F, et al. Noninvasive ventilation to prevent respiratory failure after extubation in high-risk patients. *Crit Care Med* 2005;33:2465–70.

46. Jaber S, Lescot T, Futier E, et al; NIVAS Study Group. Effect of Noninvasive ventilation on tracheal reintubation among patients with hypoxemic respiratory failure following abdominal surgery. A randomized controlled trial. *JAMA* 2016;315:1345–53.

47. International consensus conferences in intensive care medicine. Noninvasive positive pressure ventilation in acute respiratory failure. *Am J Respir Crit Care Med* 2001;163:283–91.

48. Ward JJ. High-flow oxygen administration by nasal cannula for adult and perinatal patients. *Respir Care* 2013;58:98–120.

49. Parke R, Mc Guinness S, Dixon R, Jull A. Open-label, phase II study of routine high-flow nasal oxygen therapy in cardiac surgical patients. *Brit J Anaesth* 2013;111:925–31.

50. Corley A, Bull T, Spooner AJ, Barnett AG, Fraster JF. Direct extubation onto high-flow nasal cannulae post-

cardiac surgery versus standard treatment in patients with a BMI ≥ 30: a randomised controlled trial. *Intensive Care Med* 2015;41:887–94.

51. do Nascimento Junior P, Módolo NS, Andrade S, Guimarães MM, Braz LG, El Dib R. Incentive spirometry for prevention of postoperative pulmonary complications in upper abdominal surgery. *Cochrane Database Syst Rev* 2014;2:CD006058.

52. Ventilation with lower tidal volumes as compared with traditional tidal volumes for acute lung injury and the acute respiratory distress syndrome. The Acute Respiratory Distress Syndrome Network. *N Engl J Med* 2000; 342:1301–8.

53. Briel M, Meade M, Mercat A, et al. Higher vs lower positive end-expiratory pressure in patients with acute lung injury and acute respiratory distress syndrome: systematic review and meta-analysis. *JAMA* 2010;303:865–73.

54. Guérin C, Reignier J, Richard JC, et al. Prone positioning in severe acute respiratory distress syndrome. *N Engl J Med* 2013;368:2159–68.

55. Papazian L, Forel JM, Gacouin A, et al. Neuromuscular blockers in early acute respiratory distress syndrome. *N Engl J Med* 2010;363:1107–363.

56. Hayden SP, Mayer ME, Stoller JK. Postoperative pulmonary complications: risk assessment, prevention, and treatment. *Cleve Clin J Med* 1995;62:401–7.

57. Dellinger RP, Levy MM, Rhodes A, et al. Surviving sepsis campaign: international guidelines for management of severe sepsis and septic shock: 2012. *Crit Care Med* 2013; 41:580–637.

3

Prevention and Management of Acute Kidney Injury

A. Davenport

ABSTRACT

The incidence of acute kidney injury (AKI) after major abdominal surgery is now recognised to be similar to that for cardiac surgery, of around 13.4%; however, there is major variation between centres and countries. The development of AKI is associated with increased postoperative complications, hospital stay and mortality. It is therefore important to identify risk factors for AKI preoperatively and, if possible, to appropriately resuscitate patients before surgery, withdraw medications that increase the risk for developing AKI and minimise exposure to known nephrotoxins.

KEYWORDS

Acute kidney injury, serum creatinine, nephrotoxins, biomarkers, comorbidity, dialysis

INTRODUCTION

The European Surgical Outcomes Study reported 4% mortality for patients undergoing major noncardiac surgery, with crude mortality rates varying widely between countries (from 1·2% [95% CI: 0·0–3·0] for Iceland to 21·5% [95% CI: 16·9–26·2] for Latvia).[1] Although preoperative comorbidity is a major risk factor for postoperative complications,[2] the development of postoperative acute renal failure, now termed acute kidney injury (AKI), is an independent risk factor associated with increased hospital stay, morbidity and mortality after major surgery.[3] In addition, postoperative AKI increases the risk of death not only in the short term but also after hospital discharge. It also increases the risk for chronic progressive kidney disease.[4]

The kidney plays a vital role in maintaining homeostasis, regulating water and sodium balance, acid–base balance and other electrolyte balances and excreting the waste products of metabolism. Acute kidney injury is characterised by a sudden rapid fall in the glomerular filtration rate (GFR), leading to a reduction in kidney function, which may manifest clinically as a failure to maintain fluid, electrolyte and acid–base homoeostasis.

The development of AKI is now recognised to increase the risk of mortality in a wide range of clinical settings.[5] The kidney plays an important role in clearing inflammatory mediators, and as such, AKI leads to an increase in circulating inflammatory cytokines and damage-associated molecular patterns.[6] This increase in the inflammatory milieu has effects on other distant organs, including the brain, lungs and heart.[7]

CLASSIFICATION OF ACUTE KIDNEY INJURY

Until relatively recently, there was no consensus classification of AKI. The definition varied from 25% increase in serum creatinine to a 50% or 100% increase within the time frame of anything as short as 24 hours, 48 hours, 72 hours or as long as a week or fall in urine output of <500 mL/day to <0.5 mL/Kg/h or requirement for renal replacement therapy (RRT). With such a variation in the definition of AKI, it was difficult to compare the results of studies to determine both the incidence and prevalence of AKI and also patient outcomes.

As such, a consensus definition and staging system was proposed not only to allow for both the earlier detection and management of AKI but also to unify reporting of AKI to establish the epidemiology of AKI. The introduction of new terminology was designed for all healthcare professionals, in order to allow ease of communication between different groups of clinicians. The first consensus classification was proposed by the Acute Dialysis Quality Initiative group, which introduced the concept of staging the severity of AKI by grading patients from 'at risk' (stage R), to 'injury' (stage I), to 'failure' (stage F), to 'loss of kidney function' (stage L) and finally to 'end-stage renal disease' (stage E).[8] This RIFLE staging system was based on both an increase in serum creatinine and a reduction in urine output (Table 3.1). This was modified a few years later by the Acute Kidney Injury Network (AKIN),[9] which introduced a more precise timing to the definition of AKI by defining changes in serum creatinine within a maximum of a 48-hour time period, whereas RIFLE used a longer time frame of 1 to 7 days and also dispensed with changes in GFR (Table 3.1). Although the AKIN's definition redefined the concept of AKI, it excluded patients who had a stepwise increase in serum creatinine, with each step meeting the criteria for a rise within any 48-hour time frame, and as such, the definition was reviewed by the Kidney Disease Improving Global

Outcomes (KDIGO's) consensus meeting and a further modification in definition of AKI was made, combining the elements of both the RIFLE and AKIN classifications[10] (Table 3.2 and Algorithm 3.1).

It is expected that the KDIGO's definition and staging system will be adopted into clinical practice. The advantage of an agreed, unified classification is to allow standardisation of data collection, thus permitting the definition of the epidemiology and outcomes for patients with AKI and allowing the comparison between studies and also the efficacy of treatments designed to reduce the incidence and severity of AKI.

Problems with Classification of Acute Kidney Injury

Most reports of AKI have concentrated on the definition of AKI that uses changes in serum creatinine rather than urine output, as laboratory measurements of serum creatinine are easier to analyse by retrospective observational studies. However, the definition of AKI then rests on a change in serum creatinine. Ideally, patients have a baseline serum creatinine, measured in the preceding 3 months, when kidney function was stable. However, many patients do

Table 3.1 Consensus definitions of acute kidney injury. Comparison of ADQI RIFLE grading and AKIN staging 1 to 3. For both RIFLE grading and AKIN staging, only one criterion (creatinine rise or fall in urine output) needs to be fulfilled. Class is based on the worst of serum creatinine change, fall in GFR or urine output criteria. Decrease in GFR is calculated from the increase in serum creatinine above baseline. For AKIN, the increase in creatinine must occur in a 48-hour window, whereas for RIFLE, AKI should be both abrupt (within 1–7 days) and sustained (>24 hours). When the baseline serum creatinine is increased above the normal reference range, an abrupt rise of at least 0.5 mg/dL to more than 4.0 mg/dL is sufficient for AKIN stage 3 or RIFLE class 'Failure'[2,3]

AKIN AKI staging	Common criteria	RIFLE grading
Stage 1	**Urine output**	**Grade R**
≥0.3 mg/dL increase in serum creatinine or >1.5 × 2.0 fold increase in serum creatinine	Less than 0.5 mL/Kg/h for more than 6 hours	Increase in serum creatinine by >1.5 fold or reduction in GFR by >25%
Stage 2		**Grade I**
>2.0–3.0 fold increase in serum creatinine within a 48-hour period	Less than 0.5 mL/Kg/h for >12 hours	Increase in serum creatinine by >2.0 fold or reduction in GFR by >50%
Stage 3		**Grade F**
>3.0 fold increase in serum creatinine or an absolute increase in serum creatinine to >4.0 mg/dL with an absolute increase of >0.5 mg/dL	Less than 0.3 mL/Kg/h for 24 hours or anuria for 12 hours	Increase in serum creatinine by >3.0 fold or an absolute increase in serum creatinine to >4.0 mg/dL with an increase of >0.5 mg/dL, or a reduction in GFR by >75%, or initiation of RRT

Abbreviations: ADQI: Acute Dialysis Quality Initiative; AKI: acute kidney injury; AKIN: Acute Kidney Injury Network; GFR: glomerular filteration rate; RIFLE: 'risk' (stage R), 'injury' (stage I), 'failure' (stage F), 'loss' (stage L) and 'end-stage renal disease' (stage E); RRT: renal replacement treatment.

Adapted from: Longo WE, Virgo KS, Johnson FE, et al. Risk factors for morbidity and mortality after colectomy for colon cancer. *Dis Colon Rectum* 2000;43:83–91.

Uchino S, Kellum JA, Bellomo R, et al; Beginning and Ending Supportive Therapy for the Kidney (BEST Kidney) Investigators. Acute renal failure in critically ill patients: a multinational, multicenter study *JAMA* 2005;294:813–8.

Table 3.2   Kidney disease improving global outcomes definition of acute kidney injury[3]

Stage	Serum creatinine criteria	Urine output criteria
1	1.5–1.9 times baseline *OR* ≥0.3 mg/dL (≥26.5 µmol/L) increase	<0.5 mL/Kg/h for 6–12 hours
2	2.0–2.09 times baseline	<0.5 mL/Kg/h for ≥12 hours
3	3.0 times baseline *OR* Increase in serum creatinine to ≥4.0 mg/dL (≥353.6 µmol/L) *OR* Initiation of renal replacement therapy *OR* In patients <18 years, decrease in eGFR to <35 mL/min per 1.73 m²	<0.3 mL/Kg/h for ≥24 hours *OR* Anuria for ≥12 hours

Abbreviation: eGFR: estimated glomerular filtration rate.

Reproduced with permission from: Summary of Recommendation Statements Kidney International Supplements 2012;2:8–12. doi: 10.1038/kisup.2012.7.

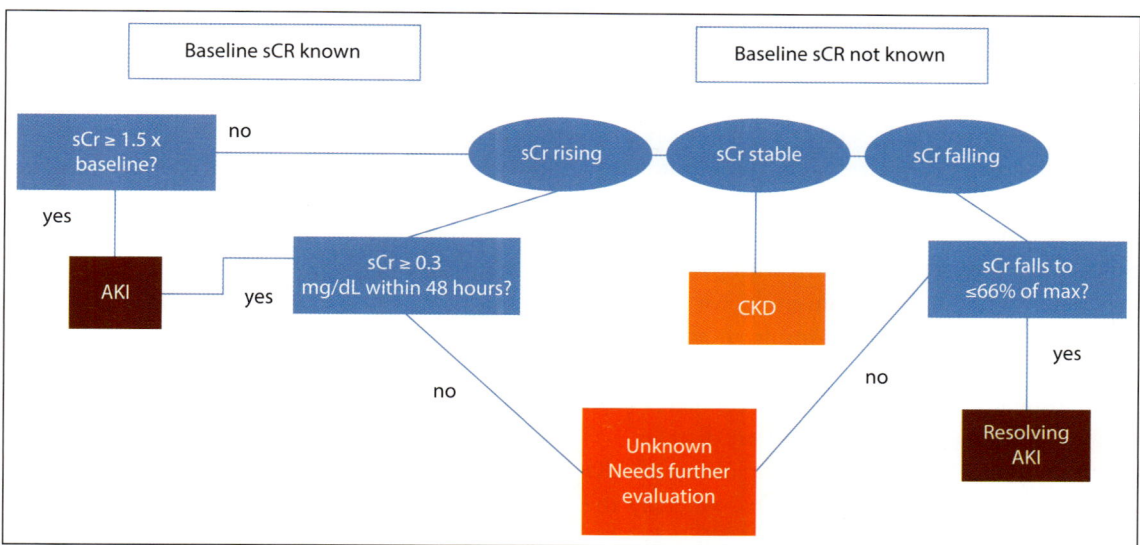

Algorithm 3.1   Simple algorithm based on changes in serum creatinine (sCR) and determining whether patient has acute kidney injury (AKI) or chronic kidney disease (CKD).

Courtesy: Andrew Davenport.

not have such a baseline measurement. To overcome this problem, serum creatinine should be measured at preadmission visits for elective procedures. However, for emergency admissions, some authorities suggest using a predicted creatinine value,[11] whereas others have advocated using the lowest serum creatinine result obtained during hospital admission. Although this may be acceptable for retrospective epidemiological studies, it means that the diagnosis of AKI and its staging become retrospective rather than in real time. As serum creatinine is measured as a concentration, serum creatinine will increase with dehydration and conversely fall with volume expansion. As such, when patients are acutely ill, they are usually volume-depleted—either dehydrated or have a relative reduction in circulating volume—due to redistribution of fluid from the plasma space secondary to increased endothelial permeability. Thus, serum creatinine concentration at the time of admission is typically increased and then falls with volume repletion. Hence, studies that have used the admission serum creatinine as the baseline have tended to underestimate the incidence of AKI, whereas those that have used the postresuscitation value have overestimated the incidence of AKI.[12,13]

As the definition of stage 1 AKI depends on a relatively small change in serum creatinine of 0.3 mg/dL (27 umol/L), the incidence of AKI will vary between centres because of different laboratory methods of measuring serum creatinine, as some laboratories overestimate their creatinine measurements and others make an underestimation.[14] Secondly, as most laboratories use a modified Jaffe picric acid assay, which is based on a colour change to measure creatinine, then substances that can alter the colour change can affect serum creatinine determinations. In clinical practice, the commonest interactions are found with bilirubin in the case of jaundiced patients and with hyperglycaemia in patients with poorly controlled diabetes. In both cases, these interactions lead to an underestimation of serum creatinine and therefore an overestimation of kidney function.[14]

Healthy people with normal kidney function have a reserve amount of kidney function and can have increased levels of GFR after exercise or after eating a high-protein meal, such that the GFR levels may increase from 100–120 mL/min up to 140–160 mL/min. On the contrary, patients who have chronic kidney disease will have lost this ability to increase their GFR in response to an appropriate stress.[15] Thus, for the same insult to the kidney, the rise in serum creatinine will be greater for patients who have lost their renal reserve, compared with patients with normal baseline function, and conversely, for the same increase in serum creatinine, the insult to the kidney will have been much more severe for patients starting with normal baseline kidney function, as compared with patients with some degree of chronic kidney disease.

The introduction of the consensus definition of AKI has led to the development of AKI alerts, whereby the clinical laboratory informs the requesting clinician that the level of serum creatinine has increased. The idea behind these electronic alerts is to speed up the recognition and awareness of AKI, so that clinicians can then take appropriate action, including withdrawing potentially nephrotoxic drugs, adjusting fluid management and avoiding unnecessary radiocontrast examinations. Despite these good intentions, AKI alerts have not as yet been demonstrated to reduce the incidence or improve the management of patients with AKI.[16] This may be because the alerts are set to trigger with stage 1 AKI and such small changes in serum creatinine may trigger numerous "false" alarms, so clinicians become overwhelmed with AKI alerts, and also after being alerted, clinicians fail to respond appropriately.[17] As such, further studies on AKI alerts are required to determine the most effective trigger point, coupled with advice on how then best to manage patients.

Although most studies reporting on AKI have used creatinine-based criteria for defining the incidence and prevalence of AKI, a minority of studies have used urine criteria, and these studies have shown that the incidence of AKI differs as to whether changes in serum creatinine or urine output have been used.[18] In addition, patient outcomes appear to be worse with increasing grading of AKI due to severity of oligoanuria, compared with corresponding grading of severity of AKI based on changes in serum creatinine.[19] Typically, changes in urine flow are more dynamic compared with changes in serum creatinine, in that a fall in urine flow precedes the increase in serum creatinine, and similarly, after an improvement in kidney function, an increase in urine flow typically occurs before a fall in serum creatinine.[20]

Although the consensus definition of AKI and staging system suggests that patients can be diagnosed with AKI, it must be recognised that AKI is simply a descriptive term and not a formal diagnosis. Thus, patients require further investigation to determine the cause of the AKI. In most cases of patients admitted acutely to hospital, this will be either volume-responsive or volume-unresponsive AKI, previously termed prerenal AKI and acute tubular necrosis, respectively. However, occasionally, AKI is due to another diagnosis that requires specific management.

NEWER BIOMARKERS FOR ACUTE KIDNEY INJURY

As serum creatinine may not increase for some 24 to 72 hours after an AKI insult, this has led to the search for other biomarkers to detect AKI at an earlier stage. For example, cystatin C tends to increase 24 hours or more before the rise in serum creatinine. Other urinary biomarkers investigated include neutrophil gelatinase-associated lipocalin (NGAL), interleukin (IL)-18, kidney injury molecule-1 and N-Acetyl-β-(D)-glucosaminidase. Some of these biomarkers can increase within 2 to 4 hours of AKI, and similarly, some biomarkers have been shown to predict the requirement for dialysis. However, these biomarkers are not as helpful in adult practice as in paediatric practice, as many adult patients have underlying chronic kidney disease.[21]

Some of these biomarkers are now commercially available, including urinary NGAL and the combination of insulin-like growth factor–binding protein 7 and tissue inhibitor of metalloproteinase-2. Although these biomarkers increase in the urine before changes in serum creatinine after a renal insult, the rate of rise and fall varies with different renal insults; however, they do not predict which patients will require dialysis.[22]

Table 3.3 Estimated glomerular filtration rate staging for chronic kidney disease. Patients may be additionally classified with a 'p' for proteinuria

Stage	eGFR (in mL/min per 1.73 m²)
Stage 1	>90
Stage 2	60–90
Stage 3a	45–60
Stage 3b	30–45
Stage 4	15–30
Stage 5	<15 or dialysis

Abbreviation: eGFR: estimated glomerular filtration rate.

Estimated Glomerular Filtration Rate

The majority of clinical chemistry laboratories now report not only serum creatinine but also estimated glomerular filtration rate (eGFR) values as a routine. The equations for estimating eGFR were developed from a cohort of patients with stable chronic kidney disease who had radiocontrast-measured GFR[23] (Table 3.3). Laboratories should standardise their serum creatinine assay against "gold" standards of creatinine measured by isotopic dilution methods.[14] As such, even though different laboratories will report different serum creatinine results from the same sample, the calculated eGFR reported should be the same.[23] The concept behind eGFR reporting is to make clinicians aware that patients may have chronic kidney disease, to prompt investigation, to review medications to avoid nephrotoxins and to consider cardiovascular risk profile and management.

Patients admitted to hospital will have eGFR results reported, but it should be borne in mind that the eGFR grading system was designed for stable outpatients and that dynamic changes in eGFR do not necessarily directly correlate with absolute changes in underlying renal function. As such, both the AKIN and KDIGO classification of AKI[12,13] removed changes in GFR from the earlier RIFLE classification.[11]

INCIDENCE OF ACUTE KIDNEY INJURY AND MORTALITY AFTER MAJOR ABDOMINAL SURGERY

A recent meta-analysis reported an overall incidence of AKI (all stages) after major surgery to be 13.4% (95% confidence limits: 10.9–16.4) based on RIFLE, AKIN or KDIGO classifications,[24] with the majority (i.e., 72%) of patients having AKI stage 1 or RIFLE-R, 17% having stage 2 or RIFLE-I and 11% having stage 3 or RIFLE-F. Although the incidence of AKI was 13.4%, only 0 to 3% of patients required RRT.[25–35] As such, the incidence of AKI after major abdominal surgery is similar to that after cardiac surgery and general vascular surgery.[10]

Developing AKI after major abdominal surgery increased the relative risk of death by 12.6 folds, but with wide 95% confidence limits of 6.8 to 23.4.[24] It is important to recognise that this increased risk of death is associated with all grades of AKI, and as the majority of patients were classified as AKIN/KDIGO stage 1 or RIFLE-R, even what may appear to be small or modest increases in serum creatinine are associated with a marked increased risk for mortality. In addition to the increased risk for mortality, developing AKI was also associated with increased other postoperative complications,[32,34] hospital stay[25,28,29,31,34] and healthcare costs.

GENERAL RISK FACTORS FOR DEVELOPING ACUTE KIDNEY INJURY POST MAJOR SURGERY

Retrospective analysis of cohorts of patients with AKI has shown that in hospital, AKI typically follows a sequence of insults, typically including volume depletion and sepsis in patients with pre-existing comorbidity, predominantly cardiac failure, diabetes and chronic kidney disease. This has led to risk factor prediction for hospital-acquired AKI, such as the renal 'angina' index[35] (Table 3.4).

Prediction models for developing AKI have been developed for cardiac surgery, and although there are models that assess the risk for developing AKI post general surgery, these have come from a previous era, before the newer classifications of AKI, when acute renal failure was defined as a much higher increase in serum creatinine (2 mg/dL or 176.8 umol/L) and, consequently, a much lower incidence of AKI of 1%.[36] More recently, models have been described for developing AKI post orthopaedic surgery,[37] which found that the independent

Table 3.4 Risk factors for developing acute kidney injury in adult patients, proposed by the Renal Angina Index[35]

Susceptibility	Exposure
Advanced age	Volume depletion
Congestive heart failure	Cardio-pulmonary bypass
Hypertension	Nephrotoxin exposure
Diabetes	Mechanical ventilation
Chronic kidney disease	Sepsis
	Vasopressors

Reprinted with permission from: Chawla LS, Goldstein SL, Kellum JA, Ronco C. Renal angina: concept and development of pretest probability assessment in acute kidney injury. *Crit Care* 2015;19:93.

factors associated with developing AKI included age at operation, male gender, diabetes, lower baseline eGFR, use of angiotensin-converting enzyme inhibitors or angiotensin receptor blockers, the number of prescribed drugs and the American Society of Anesthesiologists grade (Anaesthesiologists' grade that categorises patients into five categories: 1 = normal, healthy individual; 2 = mild systemic disease; 3 = severe systemic disease, not incapacitating; 4 = incapacitating systemic disease that is a threat to life and 5 = moribund person who is not expected to survive without the operation,[38] and whether the operation was elective, expedited or an emergency).[37]

Despite the increasing use of clinical practice guidelines and local protocol-based management algorithms for resuscitation of patients and treatment of sepsis, the incidence of AKI continues to increase in hospital practice. Clinical alerts have been developed and introduced into many hospitals; however, these clinical triggers based on hypo- or hypertension, bradycardia or tachycardia, pyrexia and increased respiratory rate are generally not triggered by those patients who develop AKI. This is because patients at risk of developing AKI are not typically sufficiently hypotensive to trigger these alerts but have a lower blood pressure than their normal baseline blood pressure, as these patients are usually hypertensive, with small vessel disease.[39] For example, a systolic blood pressure of 120 to 130 mmHg would not trigger any alert, yet it may be somewhat lower than the patient's normal systolic pressure of 160 mmHg, etc. Similarly, these alerts do not include measurements of urine output to detect oliguria at an early stage.

Prophylactic Antibiotics

Scottish hospitals changed their policy for surgical antibiotic prophylaxis from cephalosporins to 4 mg/Kg of gentamicin for surgical antibiotic prophylaxis. This change in policy resulted in an increase in the incidence of AKI, which was associated with a 94% increase in AKI for patients undergoing orthopaedic procedures, and 72.9% for gastrointestinal surgery, but the change in antibiotic policy was not associated with a significant increase in kidney injury for urological, vascular surgery or gynaecological surgery.[40] Regardless of antibiotic regimen, however, the rates of AKI were high (24%) after vascular surgery.

Contrast Nephropathy

The risk of developing contrast nephropathy depends on patient factors, the route of administration, type and dosage of contrast exposure[41,42] (Table 3.5). In theory, the

Table 3.5 Risk factors for developing acute contrast-induced kidney injury in adult patients, proposed by Mehran and colleagues. Congestive cardiac failure as New York Heart Classification Grade III/IV or a history of left ventricular failure: risk score ≤5 = low risk; 6–10 = medium risk; 11–15 = high risk and ≥16 = very high risk

Risk factor	Score
Congestive heart failure	5
Hypotension	5
Intra-aortic balloon pump	5
Age ≥75 years	4
Anaemia	3
Diabetes	3
Contrast volume	1/100 mL
eGFR	
40–60 mL/min/1.73 m^2	2
20–40 mL/min/1.73 m^2	4
<20 mL/min/1.73 m^2	6

Abbreviation: eGFR: estimated glomerular filtration rate.

Reproduced with permission from: Mehran R, Aymong ED, Nikolsky E, et al. A simple risk score for prediction of contrast-induced nephropathy after percutaneous coronary intervention Development and initial validation. *J Am Coll Cardiol* 2004;44:1393–9.

development of clinical practice guidelines, coupled with dissemination and risk assessment of patients, would lead to a change in clinical management, such as withdrawal of potentially nephrotoxic drugs and greater emphasis on the prevention of volume depletion,[43] which would then lead to a reduction in the incidence of AKI. Although there has been a reduction in the incidence of contrast-induced nephropathy over time and most patients at high risk of developing contrast nephropathy are correctly identified, there remains large variation in clinical practice in terms of ensuring adequate patient hydration.[44]

Intra-abdominal Pressure

Intra-abdominal pressure (IAP) varies with posture, and it is greatest when seated and lowest when supine. The normal IAP in adults lies between 5 mmHg and 7 mmHg.[45] However, in critically ill adults, an elevated IAP is defined as being greater than 8 mmHg and intra-abdominal hypertension as being more than 12 mmHg. It has been recognised for more than a century that increasing IAP can directly lead to renal compromise in the setting of abdominal compartment syndrome or other surgical conditions involving visceral oedema.[46]

Increased pressure within the abdominal compartment leads to a number of changes. Firstly, pressure on the inferior vena cava (IVC) may reduce venous return to the right side of the heart, resulting in a reduced cardiac output and increased systemic vasoconstriction. Changes in effective circulating volume, and also intra-abdominal inflammation and visceral organ oedema,[47,48] lead to increases in neurohumoral activation by a combination of changes in baroreceptor activation, thus causing increased sympathetic nervous system activity, catecholamine, renin-angiotensin and vasopressin release. These changes also lead to reduced section of cardiac natriuretic peptides, thus causing reduced glomerular filtration, renal tubular flow, urine output and renal sodium excretion. Increased IVC pressure is transmitted to the major renal veins, and renal vein pressure may also be increased by direct external pressure, which leads to increased intrarenal interstitial pressure, directly resulting in local intrarenal vasoconstriction, with reduction in both renal glomerular and tubular blood flow and increased local renal sympathetic nervous system activity and further intrarenal shunting of blood away from the glomeruli.

Laparoscopic Surgery

Laparoscopic surgery increases IAP,[49] and there have been reports of increased AKI after laparoscopic procedures. However, the incidence of AKI reported has generally been less than 3%.[50,51] Risk factors, apart from intraoperative hypotension, have been morbid obesity and prolonged operative times, and there is also an increased risk of around 1% for rhabdomyolysis.[51]

Hepatobiliary Surgery

It was recognised more than half a century ago that jaundiced patients undergoing surgery had an increased risk for death and AKI. This led to the introduction of the Child-Turcotte-Pugh scoring system to grade patients with increasing severity of chronic liver disease from A to C. Recent reports suggest a similar incidence of AKI to other forms of major surgery, with a reported AKI incidence of 7.6% in patients with a preoperative eGFR more than 60 mL/min/1.73 m^2, with the risk being greater for those with greater Model of End-Stage Liver Disease Sodium (MELD-Na) scores.[52]

Anaesthetic Management

Anaesthetic agents act on renal function, not only directly but also by affecting cardiovascular function and neuro-humeral activity, leading to reduced blood pressure and cardiac output, increased sympathetic nervous system activity and increased release of catecholamines, renin, angiotensin and vasopressin. The effects of anaesthetics on the kidney also include loss or renal autoregulation, so kidney perfusion becomes dependent on systemic blood pressure.

Most barbiturates and inhalational anaesthetic agents typically reduce renal blood flow (RBF) and GFR. There is a suggestion that volatile anaesthetic agents, such as isoflurane, may help reduce the incidence of AKI, particularly for patients undergoing cardiac surgery.[53] Opiates, including morphine and fentanyl, tend to decrease urinary flow and GFR, whereas RBF increases or decreases, depending on whether a direct or indirect measurement technique is used.[54] Spinal and epidural anaesthesia may be complicated by hypotension, and reports have suggested that epidural anaesthesia may be an independent risk factor for developing AKI.[34] The risk of hypotension will depend on intravascular volume and the quantity of intravenous fluids given.

More recent studies have suggested that the use of propofol and dexmedetomidine reduces the risk of perioperative AKI with cardiac surgery.[55] This may be due to a combination of reducing tissue oxygen requirements, free radical oxygen production, and reducing the inflammatory response to surgical stress.[56,57]

High ventilatory inflation pressures can cause lung barotrauma, with increased inflammatory changes in distant organs, including the kidney, resulting in increased AKI.[57]

Ischaemic Preconditioning

Ischaemic preconditioning is whereby creating an inflammatory reaction at one site by ischaemia, followed by a second insult, leads to less organ damage in a distant site after the second insult, compared with when there is no earlier insult. Animal experiments have repeatedly shown that preconditioning with an ischaemic insult leads to less cardiac and renal damage after a second insult. Although single-centre studies suggested that ischaemia to the arm or leg in the anaesthetic room resulted in a reduction in AKI post cardiac surgery, large prospective multicentre clinical trials have failed to demonstrate any reduction in the incidence of postoperative AKI.[58,59]

Fluid Management

High-molecular-weight dextrans and starches were reported in the 1980s and 1990s to be associated with an increased incidence of AKI after cardiac surgery and renal transplantation. This led to the development of a newer generation of lower-molecular-weight starches and gelatins. As these compounds are dissolved in 0.9% saline, questions were asked about higher concentrations of sodium and chloride, as in vivo studies in healthy individuals reported higher RBF and shorter time to start a diuresis when more physiologic solutions, such as Ringer's lactate, were administered, compared with 0.9% saline.[60]

Again, studies predominantly in patients with cardiac surgery reported an increased incidence of postoperative AKI when these lower-molecular-weight starches and gelatins were used, as compared with crystalloids. However, for any volume of starch, such as 6.0% hydroxyethyl starch (HES), a correspondingly greater volume of crystalloid was given, and as serum creatinine is a concentration, it will be affected by fluid administration; then, these studies have to be interpreted cautiously because of the confounder of a dilution factor when defining AKI as a change in creatinine concentration. The situation was then confounded by a series of studies reporting lower incidence of AKI post cardiac surgery, when HES was administered in a more physiological solution with lower sodium and chloride concentrations and added lactate, but the majority of these reports were then retracted because of technical problems with the trials.

So, although repeated administration of HES to intensive care patients is associated with increased risk of death and AKI,[61] there appears to be no substantial evidence to suggest that these colloids when used during surgery increase the risk of death or AKI.[62] Single-centre retrospective studies have reported an increase in AKI with the increasing volumes of starches used during surgery, but whether this was directly due to starch administration or whether starch administration was a result of intraoperative complications remains to be ascertained.[63] Even so, meta-analysis of currently available trials does not suggest an increased risk of AKI or death with the use of these colloids.[64]

INVESTIGATION AND MANAGEMENT

As AKI is associated with increased mortality, cases of AKI should be investigated promptly, as many will respond to simple fluid administration; however, other causes and obstructions have to be excluded (Algorithms 3.2 and 3.3). Patient examination is important to ensure that he or she has been adequately resuscitated; Table 3.6 outlines the clinical features and physiological parameter targets.

Urinary electrolytes may be helpful in determining which patients have reversible prerenal AKI and will

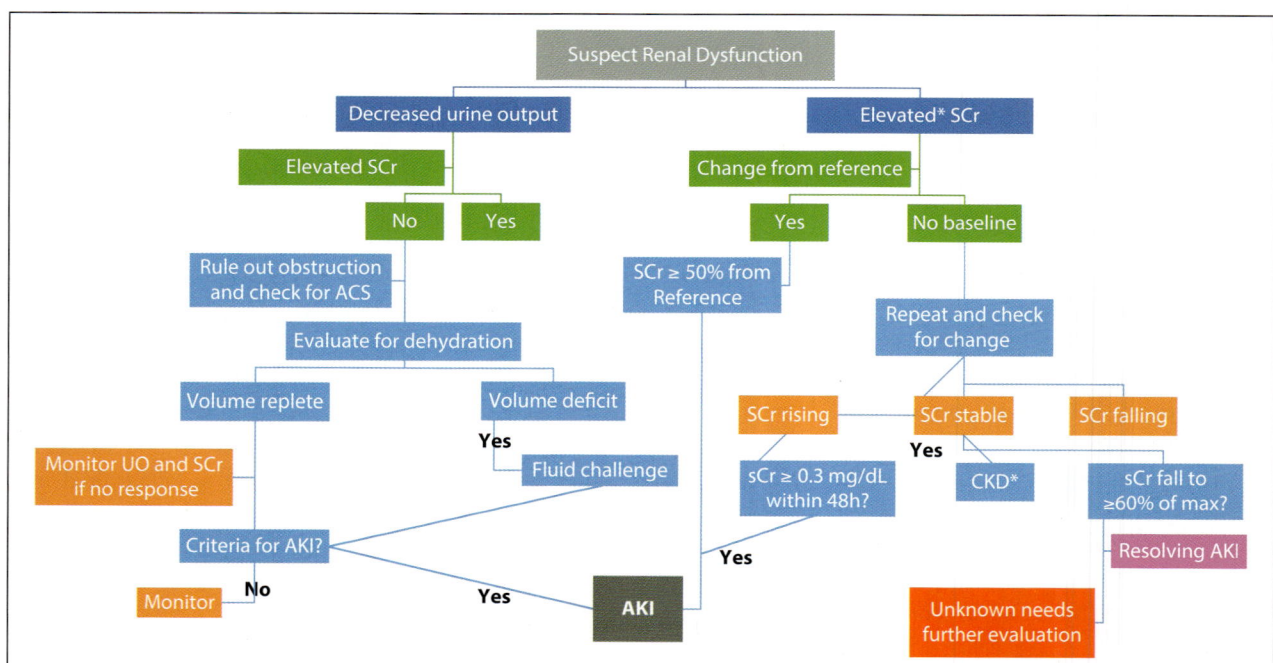

Algorithm 3.2 Algorithm to investigate changes in serum creatinine. *Baseline serum creatinine is known.

Abbreviations: ACS, acute coronary syndrome; AKI, acute kidney injury; CKD, chronic kidney disease; SCr, serum creatinine; UO, urinary output.

Courtesy: Andrew Davenport.

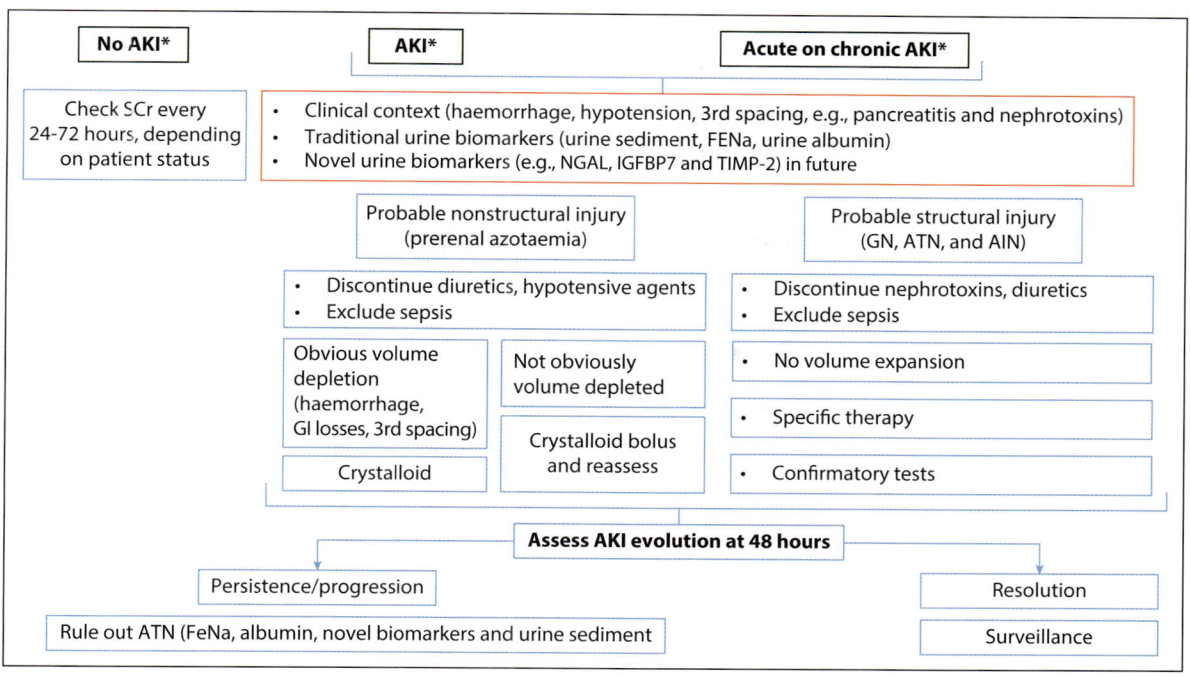

Algorithm 3.3 Algorithm to investigate a patient suspected to have acute kidney injury. *Baseline serum creatinine is known.

Abbreviations: FENa, fractional excretion of sodium; GN, glomerulonephritis; ATN, acute tubular necrosis; AIN, acute tubulo-interstitial nephritis; NGAL, neutrophil gelatinase-associated lipocalin; IGFBP7, insulin-like growth factor-binding protein 7; SCr, serum creatinine; TIMP-2, tissue inhibitor of metalloproteinase-2.

Courtesy: Andrew Davenport.

respond to fluid administration. However, urinary sodium excretion can be affected by pre-existing chronic kidney disease and prior treatment with diuretics. In those patients with prerenal AKI, the fractional excretion of sodium (FENa) is less than 1% and the fractional excretion of urea (FEUrea) is less than 35%.

Table 3.6 Clinical parameter targets to ensure that patient is appropriately fluid-resuscitated

Variable	Desired range
Mean arterial blood pressure	>65 mmHg
S_vO_2 mixed venous oxygenation	>70% sat, 4–6 kPa
$S_{cv}O_2$ central venous oxygenation	>65% sat
Arterial/venous lactate	<2 mmol/L or <2.5 mmol/L
Metabolic acidosis – base excess	±2 mmol/L
Capillary refill time/peripheral cyanosis	<2 s
Tachycardia	<100 beats/min

Reprinted with permission from: Davenport A. Renal diseases and emergencies (Table 11.8). In: Leach R, Moore K, Bell D, editors. *Oxford Desk Reference: Acute Medicine*. Oxford, UK: Oxford University Press; 2016. pp. 487–531.

FENa = (urinary sodium concentration × plasma creatinine concentration × 100)/(plasma sodium × urinary creatinine).

Normal FENa is more than 1% and the FEUrea is more than 45%. However, the FENa can be less than 1% in cases of cardiac failure, contrast nephropathy or haeme-pigment nephropathy. The FEUrea is a better discriminant of prerenal AKI than FENa, as even when patients have been given diuretics, the FEUrea will be less than 35%, whereas the FENa is often more than 2%. In addition, in established AKI, both FENa and FRUrea are elevated. In the hepatorenal syndrome, the FEUrea is low and the UNa is typically less than 10 mmol/L.

Although many patients will respond to volume replacement, it is equally important not to volume-overload a patient who cannot respond to the fluid challenge and precipitate pulmonary oedema. If arterial monitoring is available, then a 15% or greater change in the tracing between inspiration and expiration would favour volume expansion. In cases of uncertainty, small boluses of fluid should be administered and the effects monitored, and then, a decision should be made as to whether to repeat, depending on the response (Table 3.6).

The decision to start RRT is based on clinical assessment and biochemical parameters. The commonest reasons to initiate RRT in clinical practice are the correction of volume overload in an oliguric patient and hyperkalaemia, followed by correction of metabolic acidosis and elevated serum urea.

CONCLUSIONS

The introduction of consensus staging criteria for AKI has allowed the incidence of AKI after major abdominal surgery to be established, as clinical reports now use the same classifications, thus allowing comparison between studies. Although these reports show that there is major variation in the incidence of AKI both between centres in the same country and between countries, the overall incidence of AKI around 13.4% is similar to that reported for cardiac surgery. As the development of AKI is associated with increased postoperative complications, hospital stay and mortality, it is important to identify risk factors for AKI preoperatively, so that they can be addressed and risks can be minimised. Ideally, patients should be appropriately resuscitated before surgery, medications that increase the risk for developing AKI should be withdrawn, and nephrotoxin exposure should be minimised.

REFERENCES

1. Pearse RM, Moreno RP, Bauer P, et al; European Surgical Outcomes Study (EuSOS) group for the Trials groups of the European Society of Intensive Care Medicine and the European Society of Anaesthesiology. Mortality after surgery in Europe: a 7-day cohort study. *Lancet* 2012;380:1059–65.

2. Longo WE, Virgo KS, Johnson FE, et al. Risk factors for morbidity and mortality after colectomy for colon cancer. *Dis Colon Rectum* 2000;43:83–91.

3. Uchino S, Kellum JA, Bellomo R, et al; Beginning and Ending Supportive Therapy for the Kidney (BEST Kidney) Investigators. Acute renal failure in critically ill patients: a multinational, multicenter study. *JAMA* 2005;294:813–8.

4. Bihorac A, Yavas S, Subbiah S, et al. Long-term risk of mortality and acute kidney injury during hospitalization after major surgery. *Ann Surg* 2009;249:851–8.

5. Harris SK, Lewington AJ, Harrison DA, Rowan KM. Relationship between patients' outcomes and the changes in serum creatinine and urine output and RIFLE classification in a large critical care cohort database. *Kidney Int* 2015; 88:369–77.

6. Andres-Hernando A, Dursun B, Altmann C, et al. Cytokine production increases and cytokine clearance decreases in mice with bilateral nephrectomy. *Nephrol Dial Transplant* 2012;27:4339–47.

7. Li X, Hassoun HT, Santora R, Rabb H. Organ crosstalk: the role of the kidney. *Curr Opin Crit Care* 2009;15:481–7.

8. Bellomo R, Ronco C, Kellum JA, et al. Acute renal failure—definition, outcome measures, animal models, fluid therapy and information technology needs: the Second International Consensus Conference of the Acute Dialysis Quality Initiative (ADQI) Group. *Critical care* 2004;8:R204–12.

9. Mehta RL, Kellum JA, Shah SV, et al. Acute Kidney Injury Network (AKIN): report of an initiative to improve outcomes in acute kidney injury. *Critical care* 2007;11:R31.

10. Kidney Disease: Improving Global Outcomes (KDIGO). Acute Kidney Injury Work Group. *KDIGO Clinical Practice Guideline for Acute Kidney Injury* Kidney inter., suppl. 2012;2:1–138.

11. Bellomo R, Ronco C, Kellum JA, Mehta RL, Palevsky P; Acute Dialysis Quality Initiative workgroup. Acute renal failure—definition, outcome measures, animal models, fluid therapy and information technology needs: the Second International Consensus Conference of the Acute Dialysis Quality Initiative (ADQI) Group. *Crit Care* 2004;8:R204–12.

12. Bernardi MH, Schmidlin D, Ristl R, et al. Serum creatinine back-estimation in cardiac surgery patients: misclassification of AKI using existing formulae and a data-driven model. *Clin J Am Soc Nephrol* 2016;11:395–404.

13. Thongprayoon C, Cheungpasitporn W, Harrison AM, et al. The comparison of the commonly used surrogates for baseline renal function in acute kidney injury diagnosis and staging. *BMC Nephrol* 2016;17:6.

14. Nah H, Lee SG, Lee KS, Won JH, Kim HO, Kim JH. Evaluation of bilirubin interference and accuracy of six creatinine assays compared with isotope dilution-liquid chromatography mass spectrometry. *Clin Biochem* 2016;49:274–81.

15. Okusa MD, Davenport A. Reading between the (guide) lines—the KDIGO practice guideline on acute kidney injury in the individual patient. *Kidney Int* 2014;85:39–48.

16. Hoste EA, Kashani K, Gibney N, et al; 15 ADQI Consensus Group. Impact of electronic-alerting of acute kidney injury: workgroup statements from the 15(th) ADQI Consensus Conference. *Can J Kidney Health Dis* 2016;3:10.

17. Wilson FP, Shashaty M, Testani J, et al. Automated, electronic alerts for acute kidney injury: a single-blind, parallel-group, randomised controlled trial. *Lancet* 2015; 16;385:1966–74.

18. Macedo E. Urine output assessment as a clinical quality measure. *Nephron* 2015;131:252–4.

19. Kellum JA, Sileanu FE, Murugan R, Lucko N, Shaw AD, Clermont G. Classifying AKI by urine output versus serum creatinine level. *J Am Soc Nephrol* 2015;26:2231–8.

20. Macedo E, Malhotra R, Bouchard J, Wynn SK, Mehta RL. Oliguria is an early predictor of higher mortality in critically ill patients. *Kidney Int* 2011;80:760–7.

21. Ostermann M, Philips BJ, Forni LG. Clinical review: biomarkers of acute kidney injury: where are we now? *Crit Care* 2012;16:233.

22. Pajenda S, Ilhan-Mutlu A, Preusser M, Roka S, Druml W, Wagner L. NephroCheck data compared to serum creatinine in various clinical settings. *BMC Nephrol* 2015;16:206.

23. Levey AS, Coresh J, Greene T, et al; Chronic Kidney Disease Epidemiology Collaboration. Using standardized serum creatinine values in the modification of diet in renal disease study equation for estimating glomerular filtration rate. *Ann Intern Med* 2006;15;145:247–54.

24. O'Connor ME, Kirwan CJ, Pearse RM, Prowle JR. Incidence and associations of acute kidney injury after major abdominal surgery. *Intensive Care Med* 2016;42:521–30.

25. Lee EH, Kim HR, Baek SH, et al. Risk factors of postoperative acute kidney injury in patients undergoing esophageal cancer surgery. *J Cardiothorac Vasc Anesth* 2014;28:936–42.

26. Armstrong T, Welsh FK, Wells J, Chandrakumaran K, John TG, Rees M. The impact of pre-operative serum creatinine on short-term outcomes after liver resection. *HPB (Oxford)* 2009;11:622–8.

27. Coca SG, King JT Jr, Rosenthal RA, Perkal MF, Parikh CR. The duration of postoperative acute kidney injury is an additional parameter predicting long-term survival in diabetic veterans. *Kidney Int* 2010;78:926–33.

28. Correa-Gallego C, Berman A, Denis SC, et al. Renal function after low central venous pressure-assisted liver resection: assessment of 2116 cases. *HPB (Oxford)* 2015;17:258–64.

29. Kim CS, Oak CY, Kim HY, et al. Incidence, predictive factors, and clinical outcomes of acute kidney injury after gastric surgery for gastric cancer. *PLoS One* 2013; 8:e82289.

30. Teixeira C, Rosa R, Rodrigues N, et al. Acute kidney injury after major abdominal surgery: a retrospective cohort analysis. *Crit Care Res Pract* 2014;2014:132175.

31. Tomozawa A, Ishikawa S, Shiota N, Cholvisudhi P, Makita K. Perioperative risk factors for acute kidney injury after liver resection surgery: an historical cohort study. *Can J Anaesth* 2015;62:753–61.

32. Vaught A, Ozrazgat-Baslanti T, Javed A, Morgan L, Hobson CE, Bihorac A. Acute kidney injury in major gynaecological surgery: an observational study. *BJOG* 2015;122:1340–8.

33. Grams ME, Sang Y, Coresh J, et al. Acute kidney injury after major surgery: a retrospective analysis of Veterans Health Administration Data. *Am J Kidney Dis* 2016;67:872–80.

34. Kamnakamba P, Slankamenac K, Tschuor C, et al. Epidural analgesia and perioperative kidney function after major liver resection. *Br J Surg* 2015;102:805–12.

35. Chawla LS, Goldstein SL, Kellum JA, Ronco C. Renal angina: concept and development of pretest probability assessment in acute kidney injury. *Crit Care* 2015;19:93.

36. Kheterpal S, Tremper KK, Heung M, et al. Development and validation of an acute kidney injury risk index for patients undergoing general surgery: results from a national data set. *Anesthesiology* 2009;110:505–15.

37. Bell S, Dekker FW, Vadiveloo T, et al. Risk of postoperative acute kidney injury in patients undergoing orthopaedic surgery—development and validation of a risk score and effect of acute kidney injury on survival: observational cohort study. *BMJ* 2015;351:h5639. doi: 10.1136/bmj.h5639

38. Dripps RD. New classification of physical status. *Anesthesiology* 1963;24:111.

39. Liu YL, Prowle J, Licari E, Uchino S, Bellomo R. Changes in blood pressure before the development of nosocomial acute kidney injury. *Nephrol Dial Transplant* 2009;24:504–11.

40. Bell S, Davey P, Nathwani D, et al. Risk of AKI with gentamicin as surgical prophylaxis. *J Am Soc Nephrol* 2014;25:2625–32.

41. Skelding KA, Best PJ, Bartholomew BA, Lennon RJ, O'Neill WW, Rihal CS. Validation of a predictive risk score for radiocontrast-induced nephropathy following percutaneous coronary intervention. *J Invasive Cardiol* 2007;19:229–33.

42. Mehran R, Aymong ED, Nikolsky E, et al. A simple risk score for prediction of contrast-induced nephropathy after percutaneous coronary intervention: development and initial validation. *J Am Coll Cardiol* 2004;44:1393–9.

43. El-Hajjar M, Bashir I, Khan M, Min J, Torosoff M, DeLago A. Incidence of contrast-induced nephropathy in patients with chronic renal insufficiency undergoing multidetector computed tomographic angiography treated with preventive measures. *Am J Cardiol* 2008; 102:353–6.

44. Schilp J, de Blok C, Langelaan M, Spreeuwenberg P, Wagner C. Guideline adherence for identification and hydration of high-risk hospital patients for contrast-induced nephropathy. *BMC Nephrol* 2014;15:2.

45. International Conference of Experts on Intra-abdominal Hypertension and Abdominal Compartment Syndrome. I. Definitions. *Intensive Care Med* 2006;32:1722–32.

46. Malbrain ML, Deeren D, De Potter TJ. Intra-abdominal hypertension in the critically ill: it is time to pay attention. *Curr Opin Crit Care* 2005;11:156–71.

47. Roberts DJ, Ball CG, Kirkpatrick AW. Increased pressure within the abdominal compartment: intra-abdominal hypertension and the abdominal compartment syndrome. *Curr Opin Crit Care* 2016;22:174–85.

48. Kirkpatrick AW, Roberts DJ, Jaeschke R, et al. Methodological background and strategy for the 2012–2013 updated consensus definitions and clinical practice guidelines from the abdominal compartment society. *Anaesthesiol Intensive Ther* 2015;47 Spec No:s63–77.

49. Li W, Cao Z, Xia Z, et al. Acute kidney injury induced by various pneumoperitoneum pressures in a rabbit model of mild and severe hydronephrosis. *Urol Int* 2015;94:225–33.

50. Weingarten TN, Gurrieri C, McCaffrey JM, et al. Acute kidney injury following bariatric surgery. *Obes Surg* 2013;23:64–70.

51. Sharma SK, McCauley J, Cottam D, et al. Acute changes in renal function after laparoscopic gastric surgery for morbid obesity. *Surg Obes Relat Dis* 2006;2:389–92.

52. Cho E, Kim SC, Kim MG, Jo SK1, Cho WY, Kim HK. The incidence and risk factors of acute kidney injury after hepatobiliary surgery: a prospective observational study. *BMC Nephrol* 2014;15:169.

53. Kim M, Ham A, Kim JY, Brown KM, D'Agati VD, Lee HT. The volatile anaesthetic isoflurane induces ecto-5'-nucleotidase (CD73) to protect against renal ischemia and reperfusion injury. *Kidney Int* 2013;84:90–103.

54. Mercatello A. Changes in renal function induced by anaesthesia. *Ann Fr Anesth Reanim* 1990;9:507–24.

55. Luo C, Yuan D, Li X, et al. Propofol attenuated acute kidney injury after orthotopic liver transplantation via inhibiting gap junction composed of connexin 32. *Anesthesiology* 2015;122:72–86.

56. Cho JS, Shim JK, Soh S, Kim MK, Kwak YL. Perioperative dexmedetomidine reduces the incidence and severity of acute kidney injury following valvular heart surgery. *Kidney Int* 2016;89:693–700. doi: 10.1038/ki.2015.306

57. John S, Willam C. Lung and kidney failure. Pathogenesis, interactions, and therapy. *Med Klin Intensivmed Notfmed* 2015;110:452–8.

58. Hausenloy DJ, Candilio L, Evans R, et al; ERICCA Trial Investigators. Remote ischemic preconditioning and outcomes of cardiac surgery. *N Engl J Med* 2015;373: 1408–17.

59. Meybohm P, Bein B, Brosteanu O, et al; RIPHeart Study Collaborators. A multicenter trial of remote ischemic preconditioning for heart surgery. *N Engl J Med* 2015;373:1397–407.

60. Lobo DN, Awad S. Should chloride-rich crystalloids remain the mainstay of fluid resuscitation to prevent 'pre-renal' acute kidney injury?: con. *Kidney Int* 2014;86:1096–105.

61. Myburgh JA, Finfer S, Bellomo R, et al; CHEST Investigators; Australian and New Zealand Intensive Care Society Clinical Trials Group. Hydroxyethyl starch or saline for fluid resuscitation in intensive care. *N Engl J Med* 2012;367:1901–11.

62. Gillies MA, Habicher M, Jhanji S, et al. Incidence of postoperative death and acute kidney injury associated with i.v. 6% hydroxyethyl starch use: systematic review and meta-analysis. *Br J Anaesth* 2014;112:25–34.

63. Kashy BK, Podolyak A, Makarova N, Dalton JE, Sessler DI, Kurz A. Effect of hydroxyethyl starch on postoperative kidney function in patients having noncardiac surgery. *Anesthesiology* 2014;121:730–9.

64. Raiman M, Mitchell CG, Biccard BM, Rodseth RN. Comparison of hydroxyethyl starch colloids with crystalloids for surgical patients: a systematic review and meta-analysis. *Eur J Anaesthesiol* 2016;33:42–8.

4

Perioperative Haemostasis and Thrombosis Problems in Gastrointestinal Surgery

M.M. Levi

ABSTRACT

Adequate haemostasis is crucial for the surgical patients. Significant intraoperative and postoperative haemorrhage may be the result of a local problem in surgical haemostasis; alternatively, an impaired function of the coagulation system may be responsible. Adequate surgical haemostasis and sufficient working of the haemostatic system are complementary. In this chapter, we discuss contemporary views on the physiology and pathophysiology of the haemostatic system and pharmacological interventions that affect coagulation. In particular, coagulation defects leading to enhanced perioperative blood loss and situations that may increase the risk of thromboembolic complications, in particular, related to surgery of the gastrointestinal tract, are highlighted.

KEYWORDS

Coagulation, anticoagulants, fibrinolysis, perioperative bleeding, thrombosis, mesenteric vein thrombosis, portal vein thrombosis

INTRODUCTION

Haemorrhage is one of the most important complications of a surgical procedure. Severe haemorrhage during or after the operation may be due to a localised issue in surgery, such as an unsuccessful ligature, but may also be the result of an impaired coagulation system. Surgical haemostasis and a good haemostatic physiology are paired. In some situations, a patient with an insignificant coagulation defect may undergo uncomplicated surgery in the absence of any specific coagulation intervention, whereas in alternative cases, amelioration of haemostasis may be required before surgery.[1]

Clot formation, especially clots blocking the circulation (thrombosis), may result in clinically relevant problems for the patient and may have a marked effect on the postoperative recovery. Often, postoperative clots will result in venous thromboembolism. Classic manifestations entail postoperative thrombosis of the leg veins and/or pulmonary veins (pulmonary embolism). In addition,

patients that have undergone gastrointestinal operations may also develop thrombosis localised at the portal or mesenteric veins.[2] Increased risk for these types of thrombosis may be due to the underlying constitution of the patient or an enhanced (usually genetic) propensity to develop clot (thrombophilia).

Current views on the physiology of the haemostatic system, and anticoagulant and prohaemostatic interventions that affect coagulation, are subject of this chapter. In addition, situations that may carry an increased risk of perioperative thrombosis or bleeding and interventions that can be applied to overcome these complications are discussed.

CURRENT VIEWS ON THE PHYSIOLOGY OF THE COAGULATION SYSTEM IN VIVO

Normal haemostasis can be separated into three distinct mechanisms: (1) primary haemostasis, which result in the formation of a thrombocyte plug accompanied by vasoconstriction; this is the primary line of defence of the organism against haemorrhage, (2) formation of a fibrin thrombus, which is the final product when activation of various haemostatic plasma proteins occurs, eventually leading to the development of thrombin and ensuing conversion of fibrinogen to fibrin, and (3) elimination of fibrin, which is a consequence of activation of fibrinolysis.[1]

Primary Haemostasis

After disruption of the inner layer of the vessel wall, thrombocytes link to the (sub)endothelium through their membrane glycoprotein receptor Ib (adhesion). The ligand between the Ib receptor and the subendothelium is mainly circulating von Willebrand factor. During this process, thrombocytes will be activated, which leads to the expression of another surface receptor glycoprotein, that is, the IIb/IIIa receptor. Consequently, platelets may clump together via this receptor, using plasma fibrinogen as a ligand (aggregation). During the activation of thrombocytes and through several enzymatic processes, arachidonic acid (derived from the thrombocyte membrane) is transformed into various eicosanoids, including thromboxane A_2 and other prostaglandins. These factors are responsible for vasoconstriction and thereby facilitate primary haemostasis. Another result of thrombocyte activation is the occurrence of a series of proteins that are released from thrombocyte-storage organelles, such as (1) several agonists of platelet function (e.g., adenosine diphosphate [ADP] and serotonin), (2) clotting factors (e.g., von Willebrand factor and factor V), (3) heparin-binding factors (including β-thromboglobulin and platelet factor 4), and (4) factors that act as a growth factor or inflammatory mediator (such as platelet-derived growth factor [PDGF], platelet transforming growth factor-$β_1$ [platelet TGF-$β_1$], epidermal growth factor and thrombopoietin [TPO]). Importantly, the membrane of the activated thrombocyte (consisting of phospholipids) offers a superb scaffold on which the formation of thrombin and conversion of fibrinogen to fibrin may occur.[3]

Plasma Blood Coagulation

Although the plasma haemostatic system has conventionally been distinguished between an intrinsic and extrinsic part, such a separation does not occur in vivo.[4]

A schematic overview of the function of plasma coagulation in vivo is given in Algorithm 4.1. The most important pathway for activation of coagulation is through the tissue factor–factor VII route (also known as 'extrinsic system'). Tissue factor is a membrane-related glycoprotein that is separated from the circulation during normal circumstances. Tissue factor is localised at subendothelial places and becomes uncovered to the circulating blood after interruption of the endothelial lining of the vessel wall (e.g., in case of trauma). In addition, tissue factor can be exposed by endothelium or by monocytes and macrophages under the influence of specific stimuli, such as cytokines. This mechanism is responsible for the expression of tissue factor and for ensuing activation of haemostasis, which takes place in various situations such as traumatic endothelial perturbation or upon severe infection. After exposure of tissue factor to the circulation, a complex between tissue factor and plasma factor VII is formed, whereafter factor VII is activated to factor VIIa. The tissue factor–factor VIIa protein combination complexes and activates plasma factor X, converting it into factor Xa. Factor Xa subsequently converts prothrombin (factor II) into thrombin (factor IIa). This step reaction necessitates factor V as a cofactor and occurs most efficiently on a suitable phospholipid surface, which is formed by the activated thrombocyte. Another pathway for the activation of factor Xa by the tissue factor–factor VIIa combination is through the activation of factor IX. The relevance of this alternative route for activation of haemostasis is best proven by the marked bleeding tendency of patients with haemophilia, that is, a deficiency of factor VIII or IX. A third augmenting route of the haemostatic system is a consequence of the activation of factor XI by thrombin. Factor XIa can activate factor IX, leading to further generation of factor Xa and thrombin. Thrombin is the pivotal protein in the activation of haemostasis. Thrombin is not only crucial for the activation of fibrinogen into fibrin, but this enzyme is also capable of activating several haemostatic factors and cofactors, resulting in a potent positive feedback loop leading to its own formation. In addition, thrombin is a potent mediator of thrombocyte aggregation. The occurrence of cross-linked fibrin is the last step in the haemostatic cascade. Cleavage of peptides from fibrinogen by thrombin leads to the formation of fibrin monomers and, thereafter, polymers. Cross-linking of fibrin by thrombin-activated factor XIII results in further clot stability. Synthesis of virtually all haemostatic factors occurs in the liver. A number of haemostatic factors (II, VII, IX and X) necessitate vitamin K for adequate synthesis—if there is no vitamin K, inactive precursor enzymes are assembled.

Physiological Anticoagulant Mechanisms

Activation of the haemostatic system is mediated at various levels (Algorithm 4.1).[5]

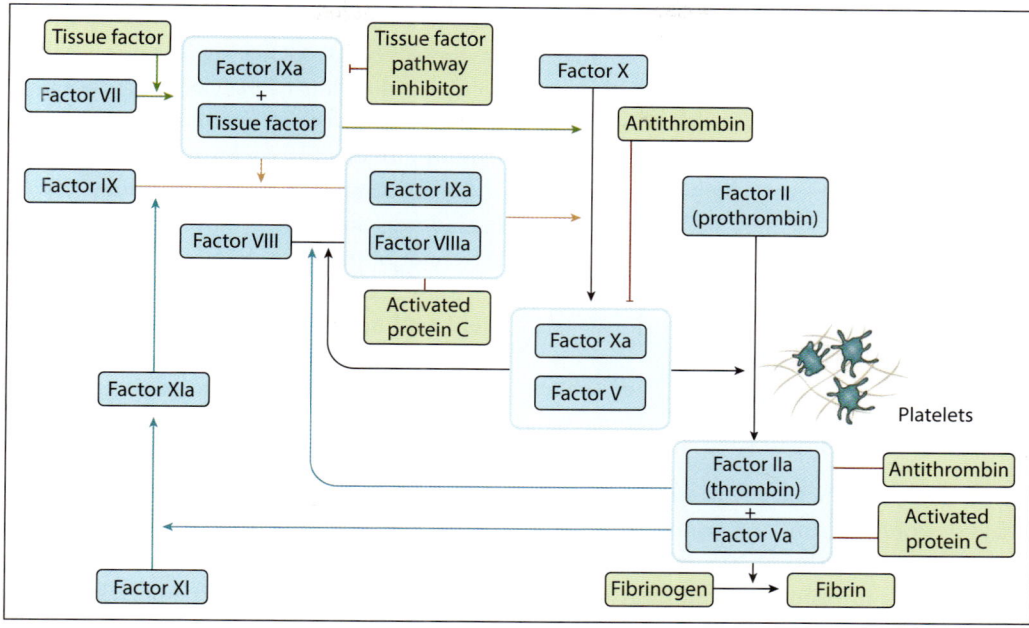

Algorithm 4.1   Schematic representation of the function of blood coagulation in vivo. The principal route of thrombin generation proceeds by the direct activation of factor X by the tissue factor–factor VIIa complex (*green arrows*). An alternative pathway is formed by the activation of factor IX by the tissue factor–factor VIIa complex and the activation of factor X by this activated factor IX (and cofactor VIII) (*orange arrows*). A third amplifying pathway consists of the thrombin-mediated activation of factor XI, which can subsequently activate factors IX and X (*blue arrows*). The points of impact of the three inhibitory systems (antithrombin III, the protein C and S system and tissue factor pathway inhibitor [TFPI], respectively) are indicated with *magenta lines*.

Attenuation of the tissue factor–factor VIIa complex is achieved by tissue factor pathway inhibitor (TFPI), an endothelial-associated enzyme inhibitor. Another anticoagulant mechanism is represented by the activated protein C system. This coagulation inhibitor, supported by its crucial cofactor protein S, proteolytically destroys the pivotal cofactors Va and VIIIa. Activated protein C is generated after activation of plasma zymogen protein C by the vessel wall-associated factor thrombomodulin bound to thrombin. Therefore, thrombin not only has a crucial position role in haemostatic activation but is also key in the attanuation of blood haemostasis. Both protein C and protein S are vitamin K-dependent coagulation enzymes. A third regulatory pathway is represented by antithrombin. This coagulation protease inhibitor forms complexes with activated clotting factors, such as thrombin and factor Xa, which cause them to lose their haemostatic activity. The inhibition of thrombin and factor Xa by antithrombin III is intensely augmented when heparin is present.

A (typically congenital) deficiency of antithrombin, protein C or protein S leads to a procoagulant situation, and patients with these defects are susceptible to thrombotic disease. This complication may particularly occur in settings with an increased risk of thrombosis, such as during immobilisation and postoperatively. A clinical condition in which there is a normal amount of protein C but a decreased sensitivity of factor Va to activated protein C is termed activated protein C resistance (APC resistance), which is the result of a point mutation in factor V (factor V Leiden). Likewise, a genetic defect in prothrombin (prothrombin 20110 mutation) leads to enhanced prothrombin activity and will also cause a procoagulant state. The prevalence of these genetic variants is about 3 to 5% in the population and may be responsible for about 30% of all idiopathic venous thromboembolism and a higher incidence of thrombosis in the gastrointestinal tract.

Endogenous Fibrinolysis

The fibrin plug plays only a provisional role and must be degraded to restore the circulation and subsequently normal tissue function. The removal of fibrin is a function of the fibrinolytic system. Fibrinolysis, mimicking the cascade mechanism of haemostasis, entails proenzyme to enzyme conversion, feedback amplification and a finely tuned regulation with various inhibitory proteins.[6]

The fibrinolytic scheme is graphically shown in Algorithm 4.1. The crucial step in the fibrinolytic pathway is the activation of the zymogen plasminogen into the active enzyme plasmin. Plasmin is capable of cleaving cross-linked fibrin, leading to the dissolution of a fibrin thrombus. Plasminogen activators, of which tissue-type plasminogen activator (tPA) and urokinase-type plasminogen activator (uPA) are most prominent, initiate the transformation of plasminogen into plasmin. Both tPA and uPA are stored in the endothelium and are released by various factors, including stress and hypoxia, as may be present upon thrombotic obstruction. Regulation of fibrinolysis takes place by plasminogen activator inhibitors (e.g., PAI-1) or by direct inhibition of plasmin, caused by the plasma protein α_2-antiplasmin.

MONITORING OF BLOOD COAGULATION

The coagulation system can be checked by various laboratory assays.[1] For adequate functioning of primary haemostasis, a thrombocyte number of 30×10^9 to 50×10^9 is required. The working of primary haemostasis may be evaluated by 'platelet function analysers'. The traditional bleeding time does not play a role in coagulation monitoring anymore because of its inconstant performance. More incisive evaluation of platelet function may be achieved by ex vivo platelet aggregation tests. However, these assays require a lot of effort and may not be broadly obtainable.

Most commonly used screening tests for plasma haemostasis are the prothrombin time (PT) and the activated partial thromboplastin time (aPTT). It is good to realise that both PT and aPTT are highly nonnatural assays and hence do not accurately mirror coagulation in vivo, but these assays are valuable to detect deficiencies of single or multiple coagulation proteins. When the screening tests are abnormal, determination of the coagulant activity of specific coagulation factors can be executed to more precisely evaluate the function of blood coagulation. In addition, the PT is used to monitor treatment with vitamin K antagonists, while the aPTT is most commonly employed to evaluate the dose of heparin anticoagulation (Table 4.1).

Table 4.1 Common causes for abnormalities in coagulation screening tests in the surgical setting and suggestions for initial further analysis

Finding	Potential cause	Further test
Thrombocytopenia	Immune thrombocytopenia	Antiplatelet antibodies, thrombopoietin
	Decreased platelet production	Complete blood cell count and bone marrow analysis
	Disseminated intravascular coagulation	aPTT, PT and fibrin degradation products
Prolonged bleeding time	von Willebrand disease or platelet defect	Platelet aggregation tests and von Willebrand factor
	Uraemia, liver failure myeloproliferative disorder, etc.	—
aPTT prolonged, PT normal	Coagulation factor deficiency (factor VIII, IX, XI or XII)	Measure specific coagulation factors
	Use of heparin	Antifactor Xa analysis
PT prolonged, aPTT normal	Coagulation factor deficiency (factor VII)	Measure coagulation factor
	Vitamin K deficiency	Measure factor VII (vitamin K-dependent) and factor
		V (vitamin K-independent) or administer vitamin K and repeat after 1–2 days
	(Mild) hepatic insufficiency	—
Both aPTT and PT prolonged	Coagulation factor deficiency (factor X, V, II or fibrinogen)	Measure specific coagulation factors
	Use of vitamin K antagonists	—
	Severe hepatic insufficiency	Measure coagulation factors
	Disseminated intravascular coagulation	Platelets, fibrin degradation products
	Loss/dilution caused by excessive bleeding/massive transfusion	—

Abbreviations: PT, prothrombin time; aPTT, activated partial thromboplastin time.

Some centres presently use point-of-care tests such as thromboelastography (TEG) to quickly deliver a global view of the haemostatic system. Regardless the practicality of these assay, they have not been adequately validated in clinical settings, and this could impede their interpretation.

CLINICAL MANAGEMENT OF HAEMOSTATIC ABNORMALITIES AND HAEMORRHAGE

Hereditary Coagulation Abnormalities

Congenital deficiencies, either in primary coagulation or in the blood haemostatic system, may result in severe haemorrhage during and after the operation. A shortcoming in primary haemostasis will cause immediate haemostatic problems, whereas an impaired plasma coagulation system may result in postoperative haemorrhage up to 1 week after the intervention, although this is not an absolute rule.

The most commonly occurring hereditary defect in platelet haemostasis is caused by a shortage of von Willebrand factor, also termed von Willebrand disease. The incidence of severe von Willebrand disease is approximately 1:25,000, but milder (heterozygous) manifestations of this disease may occur in 1 to 5 of 1,000 patients. Low levels of von Willebrand factor lead to a haemorrhagic predisposition that is variable in clinical manifestation (somewhat reliant on the plasma concentration of von Willebrand factor). von Willebrand factor is also crucial as the carrier and stabilising protein for circulating factor VIII. A deficiency of von Willebrand factor is usually accompanied by low concentrations of factor VIII and a consequent defect in blood coagulation. A typical patient with von Willebrand disease has a permanent haemorrhagic predisposition, predominantly of mucosal tissues (such as gingival or nose bleeding). Laboratory assays will show attenuated platelet function analysis and a low concentration of von Willebrand factor (and factor VIII). Management or prevention of haemorrhage in a patient that needs an invasive intervention may be based on the administration of 1-deamino-8-D-arginine vasopressin (DDAVP), which will cause a 2-fold to 3-fold enhancement of endogenous von Willebrand factor concentrations. Controlled studies have demonstrated the effectiveness and safety of DDAVP in patients with mild and moderate types of von Willebrand disease undergoing invasive interventions and operations. As an alternative, von Willebrand factor concentrates may be administered.[7]

Other hereditary abnormalities in primary coagulation are dysfunctional platelets, including the infrequently occurring absence of platelet membrane receptors (e.g., glycoprotein Ib, Bernard–Soulier syndrome and glycoprotein IIb/IIIa and Glanzmann's disease). Relatively modest series of patients have shown that an adequate amelioration of coagulant function can be derived through the administration of DDAVP, possibly together with antifibrinolytic agents.[3] If this is not enough, a platelet transfusion is an option.

Most well-known hereditary abnormalities in blood coagulation are haemophilia A and haemophilia B (low levels of factors VIII and IX, respectively). Severe haemophilia is manifested by a spontaneous haemorrhagic tendency, especially in muscles and joints. Moderate or mild haemophilia is commonly characterised by bleeding on trauma or an invasive procedure. Spontaneous haemorrhage is rare in moderate or mild haemophilia. A low level of factor XI is not so rare in some ethnic groups (e.g., Ashkenazi Jews) and presents with a haemorrhagic tendency of a variable severity. Deficiencies in all other coagulation proteins exist but are relatively infrequent.

Coagulation protein shortages may be picked up by abnormal clotting times (aPTT or PT), and further laboratory exploration will show a low concentration of the specific factor. However, these screening assays do not demonstrate a deficiency of factor XIII, which is manifested by recurrent haemorrhage after initial adequate coagulation. Management of coagulation protein deficiencies is based on infusion of coagulation factor concentrates. A patient with haemophilia undergoing a major invasive procedure need to be supplemented with coagulation factors for at least 7 to 10 days. Methodologically sound trials have demonstrated the safety and effectiveness of this approach in patients with haemophilia who underwent a major procedure. Therefore, the presence of haemophilia (or any other coagulation defect) should not be a reason to renounce a necessary surgical procedure.

Liver Insufficiency

As the liver synthesises most coagulation proteins, liver failure is associated with low concentrations of clotting factors.[8] A concomitant shortage of vitamin K, for example, due to biliary tract obstruction (see following) or as a consequence of injury to storage sites in liver disease, can also decrease concentrations of vitamin K-dependent clotting factors. When liver insufficiency occurs in combination with portal hypertension and an enlarged spleen, a significant thrombocytopenia can also occur. In patients with liver cirrhosis, defective platelet function is often present. Owing to these combined haemostatic abnormalities, patients with liver disease are at markedly high threat by perioperative haemorrhage; however, it is difficult to accurately quantitate that threat. A proper approach to these patients encompasses perioperative evaluation of the haemostatic status by assessment of platelet count, platelet function and screening coagulation tests (and potentially one or two coagulation factors). In case of a possible shortage of vitamin K, vitamin K_1 should be supplemented. Restoration of deficient levels of coagulation proteins may be realised by the infusion of plasma or prothrombin complex concentrates (PCCs). Important to note, there are some risks associated with the use of PCCs in patients with liver failure. These compounds may encompass trace concentrations of activated coagulation proteins that cannot be properly deactivated in patients with liver failure because of their low concentrations of antithrombin and reduced liver clearance. The effect of these concentrates on haemostasis persists for a few hours and may necessitate repetitive infusion of plasma. However, large volumes of plasma may evoke hepatic encephalopathy or contribute to circulatory overload. Patients with a severe low platelet count (i.e., platelets $<30 \times 10^9$ to 50×10^9/L) should be administered a platelet transfusion. Importantly, platelet transfusion may correct haemostasis only for a short while because of the rapid capture of platelets by splenomegaly. In addition, some studies have demonstrated that the infusion of DDAVP leads to an improvement of primary haemostasis, albeit that a reduction in perioperative haemorrhagic risk has not been established so far.[9]

Renal Failure

Patients with kidney failure may manifest haemostatic abnormalities and have an enhanced risk of a haemorrhagic tendency. The bleeding risk in patients with end-stage kidney failure can be ascribed to the combination of impaired platelet function. In addition, a low haematocrit in patients with impaired kidney function may contribute to the haemostatic defect; however, at present, this is less usual, as most patients are regularly supplemented with erythropoietin.[10] Prospective studies have demonstrated the effectiveness and safety of DDAVP in uraemic patients that undergo surgery or invasive procedures such as kidney biopsy. When a proper correction of coagulation cannot be attained, transfusion of platelets can be combined with DDAVP treatment. Additional interventions encompass the normalisation of red blood cells (through transfusion) and haemodialysis, which has been demonstrated to (partially) normalise primary haemostasis.

Vitamin K Deficiency

Vitamin K is crucial for the synthesis of several coagulation proteins (factors II, VII, IX and X), and a shortage in vitamin K levels leads to low plasma concentrations of these factors.[11]

Vitamin K in food is a fat-soluble agent, which is absorbed in the gastrointestinal tract. In addition, vitamin K is produced by microorganisms that are present in the small intestine and colon. Consequently, important reasons for vitamin K shortage are insufficient dietary intake (which may also occur in patients who are not properly administered vitamin K during parenteral feeding), deficient intestinal adsorption (e.g., in case of biliary obstruction) and insufficiency of storage sites in case of hepatic failure. Vitamin K shortage will lead to the prolongation of global clotting assay, especially the prothrombin time. A definitive diagnosis may be done by assaying both a vitamin K-dependent and a vitamin K-independent clotting factor. A more hands-on approach could be to supplement vitamin K and to evaluate the effect on the PT, which should be normalised within a day. Vitamin K_1 (often 5–10 mg) can be given orally and parenterally, but oral administration is evidently not sufficient in case of adsorption problems. Intravenous treatment is preferred over intramuscular administration (beware of muscle bleeds after intramuscular injections in patients with deficiencies of coagulation factors) but has been reported to cause adverse responses. When instantaneous normalisation of vitamin K-dependent coagulation proteins is necessary, the infusion of PCC will at once correct the defect.

Immune Thrombocytopenia and Other Immune Coagulation Disorders

Immune thrombocytopenia (immune thrombocytopenic purpura [ITP]) is due to autoantibodies, commonly aimed at platelet surface receptors. Enhanced thrombocyte destruction and clearance by the reticuloendothelial system may result in an enlarged spleen. In most severe situations, platelet count may be reduced to 10×10^9/L, and autoantibodies to platelets are invariably present in the blood. Usually, patients with ITP have a higher haemorrhagic risk, and clinical studies have demonstrated that a platelet count of less than 50×10^9/L increases the risk of perioperative haemorrhage.[12] Administration of intravenous immunoglobulin may cause a swift but relatively short-lasting amelioration of the platelet count and hence may be feasible when a nonelective large invasive intervention is required. Platelet transfusion may result in the generation of new antiplatelet antibodies and should be executed only in emergency settings. The risk of major haemorrhage in patients with ITP is relatively low on an adequate preoperative preparation.

The occurrence of autoantibodies to a coagulation protein (most commonly factor VIII) results in an uncommon but perilous situation.[13] These coagulation protein inhibitors may occur not only in patients treated for a hereditary coagulation protein deficiency with coagulation factor transfusion but also in patients with an earlier uncompromised haemostatic system ('acquired haemophilia'). Acquired haemophilia may develop in the framework of a lymphoproliferative or other immune disease, after giving birth or as a reaction to certain pharmaceutical agents. This disease manifests as a severe spontaneous haemorrhagic tendency and is related to significant morbidity and a high mortality from haemorrhage. Laboratory analysis will show a prolongation of conventional clotting assays that are not normalised after incubation with normal plasma. A final diagnosis can be ascertained by analysing the specific coagulation factors and by quantifying the inhibitory antibody. Management includes (high doses of) coagulation protein concentrate, activated PCCs or recombinant factor VIIa. The treatment of this defect is complex and should be executed in a specialised hospital.

Other Conditions Associated with Coagulation Abnormalities

Several other situations that may present with haemostatic dysfunction encompass myeloproliferative or lymphoproliferative diseases, in combination with defective primary coagulation, due to a combination of low platelet count and impaired platelet function. Oncology patients may manifest a variety of haemostatic disorders caused by impaired primary haemostasis, low-grade disseminated intravascular coagulation (DIC) or overactive fibrinolysis.

HOW TO IDENTIFY PATIENTS AT RISK FOR HAEMORRHAGE

The fundament for appreciation of a clinically important haemostatic defect is the patient's history, which should include questions specifically related to previous invasive procedures, haemorrhage after trauma and complications after tooth extraction.[1]

A possible hereditary haemostatic defect might be picked up on the basis of a history of lifelong haemorrhagic complications after minor trauma or interventions and a haemorrhagic tendency in family members. In addition, the questions should particularly emphasise the use of agents that may affect coagulation. Physical examination may reveal abnormal haematomas, petechiae or an enlarged spleen, all of which could indicate the presence of abnormal haemostasis. Several studies have demonstrated

that routine clotting analysis for most surgical interventions is useless in case of a negative medical history and normal physical examination. Potential exemptions are anticipated extensive surgery or interventions that pose a great challenge to a competent coagulation system. Laboratory analysis for preoperative screening in patients with signs or symptoms of a heightened haemorrhagic tendency includes a platelet count, aPTT and PT. If a defect in primary haemostasis is assumed, platelet function analysis and measurement of von Willebrand factor concentration are required. If these assays are normal but a very high suspicion of a haemorrhagic tendency pertains, analysis of factor XIII and α-2-antiplasmin can be executed. If any of these screening assays are abnormal, additional analysis is important.

RISK OF THE PREOPERATIVE USE OF ANTICOAGULANT AGENTS FOR PERIOPERATIVE HAEMORRHAGIC COMPLICATIONS

Anticoagulant and antiplatelet pharmaceuticals are crucial in the primary management and subsequent prevention of cardiovascular disorders and venous thrombosis. An increasing number of patients scheduled for a surgical intervention will use aspirin or any other antiplatelet agents or oral anticoagulants.

Several studies have evaluated whether preoperative administration of aspirin causes an enhanced risk of perioperative haemorrhage.[14] For large surgical interventions, most studies show that the preoperative administration of aspirin leads to an increased perioperative blood loss, a larger need for transfusion of red cells and other blood products, prolonged operation duration and a slightly increased requirement for reoperation due to excessive postoperative haemorrhage. Specifically, a controlled study in patients on relatively high dose of aspirin preoperatively showed markedly increased bleeding and an estimated odds ratio for reintervention of 1.8 in comparison with nonusers of aspirin. Nevertheless, more recent studies demonstrated that more commonly used lower doses of preoperative aspirin (80–100 mg daily), though associated with enhanced perioperative haemorrhage, were not associated with more transfusion needs, increased need for reoperation because of bleeding or a longer duration of hospitalisation. Importantly, interruption of aspirin or other antiplatelet agents may precipitate a perioperative arterial thrombotic event, such as acute coronary syndrome and ischaemic cerebrovascular disease. There is abundant literature that suggests that most interventions in patients on aspirin can be executed safely without interruption or any other specific haemostatic intervention. In addition, several studies have demonstrated that the preoperative ingestion of other nonsteroidal anti-inflammatory drugs (NSAIDs) does not cause enhanced perioperative haemorrhage.[14]

Concerning the preoperative use of oral anticoagulants, earlier trials demonstrated a high risk of enhanced perioperative haemorrhage, especially in case of major interventions. Recent clinical studies showed that interventions can be safely carried out at low levels of anticoagulation (international normalised ratio [INR] <1.5).[15] The dose of vitamin K antagonists should be markedly tempered preoperatively to attain these levels. Similar strategies are to be followed for the new-generation direct oral anticoagulants (DOACs) such as dabigatran, rivaroxaban and apixaban. These drugs cannot be monitored by INR and could better be interrupted altogether 1 or 2 days before surgery. The indication for oral anticoagulant treatment should always be taken into account. Interruption of anticoagulant treatment for recent venous thrombosis or pulmonary embolism may render the patient at an increased risk of recurrence in the postoperative period.

Similarly, in patients with mechanical heart valves (in particular in combination with heart arrhythmias such as atrial fibrillation), interruption of anticoagulant treatment should be prevented or kept as short as possible. This can be done by cessation of oral anticoagulation and simultaneous instalment of intravenous unfractionated heparin or subcutaneous low-molecular-weight heparin. Briefly before the intervention, heparin may be interrupted and can be reinitiated at 6 to 12 hours postoperatively.[16] In patients with recent venous thrombosis or pulmonary embolism, temporary cessation of anticoagulation and concurrent insertion of an inferior caval filter to avert pulmonary embolism could be a viable strategy. For nonelective interventions, a quick (12–24 hours) reversal of vitamin K antagonist therapy may be realised by the administration of 10 mg of vitamin K. This administration should be sustained for 3 to 5 days, reliant on the half-life of the type of coumarin used. If required, instantaneous and full restoration of coagulation may be achieved by the infusion of PCC, both for vitamin K antagonists and for DOACs.

The preoperative administration of preventive (low-molecular-weight) heparin for the prophylaxis of postoperative venous thrombosis or pulmonary embolism does not result in an increased risk of intraoperative and postoperative haemorrhage in a large series of randomised controlled studies.[17]

In patients who receive therapeutic doses of heparin, cessation of heparin will lead to an almost complete restoration of coagulation in approximately 3 to 4 hours. If immediate reversal of heparin is required (e.g., in case of serious haemorrhage), this may be achieved by the administration of protamine.

MANAGEMENT OF PERIOPERATIVE BLOOD LOSS BY PHARMACOLOGICAL INTERVENTIONS

Perioperative haemorrhage may be due to failed surgical haemostasis or impaired coagulation. In fact, both causes may contribute to bleeding in various complex settings. Regardless of whether a proper haemostatic function is the most crucial aetiology of increased blood loss, prohaemostatic measures may be advantageous to manage excessive haemorrhage and downstream complications.[7] This management strategy has been broadly studied in settings such as major liver surgery and transplantation. Clinical studies have shown that in particular in this type of surgery, the efficacy and safety of these strategies were successful. There is a lot of discussion on whether any advantageous effects of management strategies to prevent massive perioperative haemorrhage might be counterbalanced by a possibly detrimental net procoagulant situation, which might lead to graft occlusion and complications characterised by thrombosis.[18]

Major surgical liver interventions, such as orthotopic liver transplantation, can be accompanied by excessive perioperative haemorrhage. Impaired synthesis of coagulation factors by the failing liver, a pre-existing low platelet count in combination with thrombocytopathy and reduced clearance of activated coagulation and fibrinolytic proteins during the anhepatic phase may all contribute to this complication. A small series of randomised controlled studies demonstrated that the infusion of either aprotinin or antifibrinolytic lysine analogues (e.g., tranexamic acid) caused a reduction of perioperative haemorrhage and the need for transfusion.[19] At present, however, newer surgical techniques of liver transplantation have been developed and widely introduced; these techniques have rendered the requirement for prohaemostatic measures during this operation questionable. Hence, the precise place of prohaemostatic interventions in extensive liver interventions needs to be established.

MANAGEMENT OF POSTOPERATIVE HAEMORRHAGE

A crucial theme in the setting of a patient who has massive blood loss during or after an invasive procedure is the assessment of whether the haemorrhage is due to a systemic coagulation defect or a local problem, for example, caused by insufficient surgical haemostasis. This differential diagnosis can, in some situations, be complex if there are no obvious signs of a systemic haemorrhagic tendency (haemorrhage from various locations at the same time or at insertion sites of intravascular cannules). In every case of abnormal haemorrhage, global clotting assays (aPTT and PT) and platelet count should be quickly performed. If these assays report abnormal results, treatment with replacement of deficient coagulation factors or platelets should be initiated. Only when there is satisfactory interruption of bleeding, this supportive strategy should not postpone the decision to reoperate if there is suspicion of a insufficient local surgical haemostasis.

General haemostatic defects in patients who present with major haemorrhage and who have a pre-existing normal haemostatic system are usually due to two distinct mechanisms: (1) insufficiently compensated loss of platelets and coagulation proteins due to haemorrhage and dilution on substantial transfusion of blood cells and plasma, and (2) ongoing depletion of platelets and coagulation proteins consumed in the process of DIC (see **Disseminated Intravascular Coagulation**).[20] Patients with severe haemorrhage may need massive fluid replacement to maintain a proper circulation, and this is usually carried out by employing crystalloids, colloids, dextrans or starch solutions. It has been shown that these synthetic plasma volume expanders, when used in volumes over 1 L/h may lead to an impairment of primary haemostasis (mostly due to interference with von Willebrand factor function) and decreased fibrin formation (due to dilution). This effect has been observed for dextrans and gelatin-based synthetic volume expanders.[21] Therefore, the unbalanced administration of these agents may cause a worsening of haemostatic function and may exacerbate haemorrhage. Hence, if there is a requirement for substantial expansion of circulating volume in patients with haemorrhage, the application of these compounds should be paired with infusion of plasma.

Infusion of large amounts of red cells without simultaneous administration of platelets and coagulation proteins may result in a systemic dilution coagulopathy, which can be easily assessed by a decrease in platelet count to about 50×10^9 to 100×10^9/L and abnormal global clotting assays (aPTT and PT). In absence of hard evidence, it is often suggested that for every 2 to 3 units of red cells administered, one unit of plasma should be transfused.[22] If there are no other reasons that may cause a haemostatic defect, this strategy will yield a (near) normalisation of clotting times. A slightly more conservative approach may be applied to address dilutional thrombocytopenia. Clinical studies did not show an advantage of prophylactic platelet transfusion in

patients with massive red cell transfusion (>12 units of red cells). Nevertheless, retrospective studies demonstrated that in patients with haemorrhagic complications and a platelet count of less than 50×10^9/L, platelet transfusion is useful.

Although there is no evidence from clinical trials to support such treatment, pharmacotherapeutic interventions to improve haemostasis may, in some exceptional cases, be contemplated. These interventions may consist of antifibrinolytic strategies, such as the administration of ε-aminocaproic acid, tranexamic acid or aprotinin. The administration of recombinant factor VIIa has shown impressive effects in patients with excessive bleeding in a small series of case reports, but the safety and efficacy of this approach require further study.[23]

DISSEMINATED INTRAVASCULAR COAGULATION

Disseminated intravascular coagulation is not uncommon in surgical patients, as it is a common complication of several conditions that are present in these patients, including severe infection, major trauma and malignant disease.[24] Disseminated intravascular coagulation is not a disease in itself and should be regarded as a syndrome, secondary to an underlying condition (Table 4.2). It is caused by a systemic activation of blood coagulation, deposition of fibrin in small- and mid-sized vessels and thrombotic obstruction that may occur in various organs and thereby may contribute to multiorgan dysfunction. Simultaneously, the ongoing consumption of coagulation factors and thrombocytes may cause significant haemorrhagic complications.[20] Severe haemorrhage in the setting of DIC is hard to manage in surgical patients or during the early postoperative period.

Table 4.2 Underlying surgical diseases causing acute or chronic disseminated intravascular coagulation

Septicaemia/infections
Polytrauma
Malignancies
Aortic aneurysm
Brain injury
Extended liver surgery
Extracorporeal circulation
Thermal injury/hypothermia
Fat embolism
Peritoneovenous shunt
Massive transfusion

No single laboratory assay will ascertain a conclusive diagnosis of DIC. Nevertheless, this diagnosis can be made reliably by considering the present of an underlying disease known to be associated with DIC and by a combination of laboratory tests. Usually, DIC can be diagnosed using markers of advanced consumption of coagulation factors and platelets, that is, prolonged clotting times (aPTT and PT) in combination with thrombocytopenia, together with a test that detects the degradation of cross-linked fibrin (fibrin degradation products or D-dimers). It is important to realise that a single measurement is usually not sufficient, and repeated assays may yield more useful insight. Since a few years, a simple scoring algorithm for DIC, based on readily available laboratory assays, has been developed and has been validated in several clinical studies.[25]

A number of topics surrounding the most appropriate treatment of patients with DIC remain debatable. The fundament of DIC management is the precise and vigorous management of the underlying condition. In some situation, coagulopathy will fully resolve within hours after the proper and effective treatment of the underlying disease. However, there are many alternative settings, such as most cases of sepsis and associated systemic inflammatory response, in which DIC may sustain for several days, even after adequate treatment has been done. In these settings, supportive treatment aimed at coagulopathy may be required. Infusion of coagulation proteins or platelets may be effective, especially if haemorrhage persists. In addition, pharmacological interventions targeted at the cessation of ongoing thrombin generation may have a useful effect. There is no sound evidence supporting the administration of therapeutic doses of heparin as routine therapy in patients with DIC. Exceptional patients who present with overt signs of extensive fibrin deposition such as purpura fulminans, acral ischaemia and venous thromboembolism may warrant heparin anticoagulation. Low (prophylactic) dose of (low-molecular-weight) heparin is effective as prophylaxis for venous thromboembolism and is generally not associated with an enhanced risk of bleeding complications.[26]

PROPHYLAXIS OF PERIOPERATIVE VENOUS THROMBOEMBOLISM

Venous thrombosis and pulmonary embolism are frequently occurring postoperative complications. Apart from the intervention itself, several acquired and inherited factors may account for the occurrence of venous thromboembolism.[27] Increasing age is a prominent risk for venous thrombosis (population attributable risk >90%),

but simultaneous comorbidities, such as malignant disease and inflammation, are also significant factors. All these causes add on, which means that the risk of venous thromboembolism surges when multiple risk factors are present.

Effective prevention against venous thromboembolism can be achieved even for patients at the highest risk. Use of pharmacological prevention is more efficacious, precluding mortality and morbidity, owing to thrombosis or pulmonary embolism, than is the management of the disease once it has been diagnosed. Evidence-based guidelines for prophylaxis are reviewed in other publications. In summary, prevention with administration of subcutaneous low dose of (low-molecular-weight) heparin virtually completely protects against venous thromboembolism and leads to only a very small increment in the risk of major bleeding. At present, the most significant risk for venous thromboembolism in surgical patients is the incorrect disregard of proper thromboprophylaxis. Multidimensional actions, including checklists, computerised alerts and stickers on patient files, are capable of enhancing the prescription of adequate prophylaxis against thrombosis in immobilised surgical patients. In addition, there is proof that application of thrombotic risk assessment on hospitalisation is helpful for eliminating venous thromboembolism-related mortality and readmission with venous thrombosis or pulmonary embolism.

THROMBOSIS IN THE GASTROINTESTINAL TRACT

Abdominal vein thrombosis is an infrequent but potentially life-threatening form of venous thrombosis. It mainly involves the mesenteric veins, portal veins and hepatic veins (Budd–Chiari syndrome).[2,28] Recently, a number of large studies have investigated the underlying aetiological factors in these thrombotic conditions. Both inherited and acquired risk factors for thrombosis are often observed in these patients. Factor V Leiden mutation is frequently found in patients with Budd–Chiari syndrome and the prothrombin 10120 gene variant, as well as JAK-2 mutations are observed more frequently in patients with portal vein thrombosis. In patients with hepatic vein thrombosis, the prevalence of factor V Leiden mutation ranges between 7 and 32%, which resembles the percentage in patients with deep vein thrombosis. Case–control studies showed only a 2-fold risk of portal vein thrombosis in factor V Leiden carriers.[13] Factor V Leiden mutation in patients with portal vein thrombosis ranged between 3 and 9%.[2] However, factor V Leiden carriers have a 4- to

11-fold increased risk of Budd–Chiari syndrome. On the contrary, the prothrombin G20210A gene variant is more frequently found in portal vein thrombosis than in hepatic vein thrombosis, with prevalence ranging from 3 to 8% in the latter situation. A recent study reported a 4-fold to 5-fold increase in the incidence of portal vein thrombosis in carriers of the prothrombin 20210 gene, whereas the risk of hepatic vein thrombosis is increased roughly 2-fold. So far, the mechanism behind the differential effect of the various gene mutations and the prevalence of abdominal vein thrombosis remains to be elucidated. Lupus anticoagulant and other manifestations of antiphospholipid antibodies may cause an increased propensity for mesenteric vein thrombosis and portal vein thrombosis. The prevalence of these antibodies in patients with venous thrombosis in the gastrointestinal tract has been projected to be approximately 5 to 15%. The relevance as a risk factor is hard to definitively establish, as antiphospholipid antibodies are detected in patients with chronic liver disease without thrombosis as well. Chronic myeloproliferative diseases, mostly polycythaemia vera and essential thrombocythaemia, are frequently found conditions in 30 to 40% of patients with venous thrombosis in the gastrointestinal tract.[29] Remarkably, many patients presenting with abdominal vein thrombosis have multiple risk factors: in almost half of the patients, two prothrombotic factors, and in more than 15%, even three prothrombotic factors are detected. As patients with abdominal vein thrombosis have a relatively high recurrence risk, sustained antithrombotic treatment is often required.

Local factors that increase the risk of Budd–Chiari syndrome are, for example, the presence of malignant disease, and the occurrence of masses such as cysts and abscesses that compress or infiltrate into the venous system. Alternatively, portal vein thrombosis is frequently seen as a complication of chronic liver failure or hepatobiliary malignant disease. Other local settings that contribute to the risk of portal vein thrombosis are surgery near the portal vein and abdominal infections or inflammation, with or without in combination with other thrombophilic conditions. However, it is important to emphasise that virtually all studies on underlying factors for abdominal vein thrombosis consisted of selected patient series and were relatively small. In the largest multicentre European study (En-Vie study), 163 consecutive patients with Budd-Chiari thrombosis and 105 patients with nonmalignant, noncirrhotic portal vein thrombosis and an extensive analysis for underlying factors showed the presence of prothrombotic conditions in 84% and

42%, respectively.[2] Several of these underlying factors are acknowledged risk factors for venous thrombosis of the extremities as well, but a substantial number of prothrombotic conditions were more specific for venous thrombosis in the abdominal tract.

The cornerstone in the management of abdominal vein thrombosis is the instantaneous initiation of antithrombotic treatment, usually with (low-molecular-weight) heparin, followed by long-term use of oral anticoagulants.[30]

In Budd–Chiari syndrome, therapy for undetermined duration is justified in view of the seriousness of the disease. In patients with acute portal vein thrombosis, antithrombotic treatment is given for 3 to 6 months, but contingent on the underlying condition, this therapy is continued indefinitely. The duration of antithrombotic treatment is much reliant on the risk of thrombosis recurrence and the assessment of the risk of bleeding complications. A limited number of trials have investigated the risk of recurrent portal vein thrombosis. One study evaluated the outcome of portal vein thrombosis in a cohort of 136 patients, of whom 84 patients were taking antithrombotic agents. A recurrence rate of 5.5 per 100 person-years was demonstrated for all types of thrombosis and an underlying thrombophilic condition was demonstrated to be an independent risk factor for recurrent thrombosis. In another trial with a median follow-up of more than 3 years in 121 patients with thrombosis of the gastrointestinal tract that were not on anticoagulant treatment, the recurrence rate was 10.5%. Nearly 75% of these recurrent thromboses were located at gastrointestinal sites. The majority of these patients had a chronic myeloproliferative condition. In the analysis of 120 patients with portal vein thrombosis, recurrence was detected in 4%, 8% and 27% of the patients after a follow-up of 1, 5 and 10 years, respectively.[31]

Again, prothrombotic conditions were highly prevalent in the recurrence group. Patients with abdominal vein thrombosis have, besides their high thrombotic risk, an increased risk of haemorrhage. As patients with portal vein obstruction may commonly manifest variceal haemorrhage, endoscopic interventions may be necessary to prevent or treat bleeding. In two relatively large series of patients with gastrointestinal thrombosis, bleeding rates after 3- and 5-year follow-up were 15% and 46%, respectively. Hence, it is not easy to provide standard guidelines on the duration of antithrombotic therapy in patients with mesenteric and portal vein thrombosis, and management should be individualised. It has been advocated to administer long-term antithrombotic treatment to only those patients with a persistent thrombophilic risk factors, such as factor V Leiden mutation and prothrombin 20210 mutation. In patients with a chronic myeloproliferative disease, antithrombotic therapy should also be prescribed indefinitely, in addition to proper haematological treatment aiming at the restoration of normal blood cell counts. Additional therapeutic strategies for venous thrombosis in the gastrointestinal tract, employing invasive procedures or stents, are experimental and awaiting further evidence, indicated for very specific cases only.

CONCLUSIONS

Proper function of the coagulation system is important for patients undergoing major surgery. Adequate function of the haemostatic system relies on correct platelet–vessel wall interaction, sufficient concentrations of coagulation factors and accurate interaction between those proteins, as well as intact function of endogenous anticoagulant pathways and fibrinolysis. Insufficient function of the haemostatic system may result in enhanced perioperative blood loss, which may be managed by adequate monitoring and prohaemostatic interventions. In addition, some specific circumstances surrounding surgery of the gastrointestinal tract may increase the risk of hypercoagulable states and thromboembolic complications.

REFERENCES

1. Levi M, Seligsohn U, Kaushansky, K. Classification, clinical manifestations, and evaluation of disorders of hemostasis. In: Kaushansky K, et al. *Williams Hematology* 9th ed. New York, NY: McGraw and Hill; 2015.

2. Leebeek FW, Smalberg JH, Janssen HL. Prothrombotic disorders in abdominal vein thrombosis. *Neth J Med* 2012;70:400–5.

3. Versteeg HH, Heemskerk JW, Levi M, Reitsma PH. New fundamentals in hemostasis. *Physiol Rev* 2013;93: 327–58.

4. Davie EW. Biochemical and molecular aspects of the coagulation cascade. *Thrombosis Haemostasis* 1995;74: 1–6.

5. Esmon CT. Coagulation inhibitors in inflammation. *Biochem Soc Trans* 2005;33:401–5.

6. Collen D. On the regulation and control of fibrinolysis. Edward Kowalski Memorial Lecture. *Thrombosis Haemostasis* 1980;43:77–89.

7. Mannucci PM, Levi M. Prevention and treatment of major blood loss. *N Engl J Med* 2007;356:2301–11.

8. Lisman T, Caldwell SH, Burroughs AK, et al. Hemostasis and thrombosis in patients with liver disease: the ups and downs. *J Hepatol* 2010;53:362–71.

9. Agnelli G, Parise P, Levi M, Cosmi B, Nenci GG. Effects of desmopressin on hemostasis in patients with liver cirrhosis. *Haemostasis* 1995;25:241–7.

10. Mannucci PM, Remuzzi G, Pusinri F, et al. De-amino-8-D-arginine vasopressin shortens the bleeding time in uremia. *N Engl J Med* 1983;308:8–12.

11. Ansell J, Hirsh J, Hylek E, Jacobson A, Crowther M, Palareti G. Pharmacology and management of the vitamin K antagonists*. *Chest* 2008;133:160S–98S.

12. Schipperus M, Fijnheer R. New therapeutic options for immune thrombocytopenia. *Neth J Med* 2011;69: 480–5.

13. Hay CR, Negrier C, Ludlam CA. The treatment of bleeding in acquired haemophilia with recombinant factor VIIa: a multicentre study. *Thromb Haemost* 1997;78: 1463–7.

14. Levi M, van der Poll T. Hemostasis and coagulation. In: Norton JA, Bollinger, R.A, Chang AE, Lowry SF, editors. *Surgery: Scientific Basis and Current Practice* New York, NY: Springer-Verlag; 2001.

15. Kearon C, Hirsh J. Management of anticoagulation before and after elective surgery. *N Engl J Med* 1997;336: 1506–11.

16. Douketis JD, Berger PB, Dunn AS, et al. The perioperative management of antithrombotic therapy: American College of Chest Physicians Evidence-Based Clinical Practice Guidelines (8th Edition). *Chest* 2008;133: 299S–339S.

17. Nurmohamed MT, Rosendaal FR, Buller HR, et al. Low molecular weight heparin versus standard heparin in general and orthopaedic surgery: a meta-analysis. *Lancet* 1992;340:152–6.

18. Levi M, Levy JH, Andersen HF, Truloff D. Safety of recombinant activated factor VII in randomized clinical trials. *N Engl J Med* 2010;363:1791–800.

19. Levi M, Cromheecke ME, de Jonge E, Prins MH, de Mol B, Briet E, et al. Pharmacological strategies to decrease excessive blood loss in surgery: a meta-analysis of clinically relevant endpoints [see comments]. *Lancet* 1999;354:1940–7.

20. Levi M, ten Cate H. Disseminated intravascular coagulation. *N Engl J Med* 1999;341:586–92.

21. de Jonge E, Levi M. Effects of different plasma substitutes on blood coagulation: a comparative review. *Crit Care Med* 2001;29:1261–7.

22. Hambleton J, Leung LL, Levi M. Coagulation: consultative hemostasis. *Hematology Am Soc Hematol Educ Program* 2002:335–52.

23. Levi M, Vink R, de Jonge E. Management of bleeding disorders by prohemostatic therapy. *Int J Hematol* 2002;76: 139–44.

24. Levi M, Seligsohn U. Disseminated intravascular coagulation. In: Kaushansky K, Lichtman M, Beutler E, Kipps T, Prchal J, Seligsohn U, editors. *Williams Hematology*. Philadelphia, PA: McGraw Hill; 2010.

25. Levi M, Toh CH, Thachil J, Watson HG. Guidelines for the diagnosis and management of disseminated intravascular coagulation. British Committee for Standards in Haematology. *Br J Haematol* 2009;145:24–33.

26. Cook D, Attia J, Weaver B, McDonald E, Meade M, Crowther M. Venous thromboembolic disease: an observational study in medical-surgical intensive care unit patients. *J Crit Care* 2000;15:127–32.

27. Levi M, Middeldorp S. Inherited thrombophilia. In: Young NS, Gerson SL, High KA, editors. *Clinical Hematology*. New York, NY: Mosby; 2003. pp. 867–80.

28. Hoekstra J, Janssen HL. Vascular liver disorders (I): diagnosis, treatment and prognosis of Budd-Chiari syndrome. *Neth J Med* 2008;66:334–9.

29. Barbui T, Finazzi G, Falanga A. Myeloproliferative neoplasms and thrombosis. *Blood* 2013;122:2176–84.

30. Schoots IG, Koffeman GI, Legemate DA, Levi M, Van Gulik TM. Systematic review of survival after acute mesenteric ischaemia according to disease aetiology. *Br J Surg* 2004;91:17–27.

31. Hoekstra J, Janssen HL. Vascular liver disorders (II): portal vein thrombosis. *Neth J Med* 2009;67:46–53.

5

Strategy of Preoperative and Postoperative Nutritional Support

E.M.H. (Lisbeth) Mathus-Vliegen

ABSTRACT

During the first visit of a patient referred for elective surgery, the nutritional assessment is often neglected. Patients should be identified as being at nutritional risk by adequate instruments. The Nutritional Risk Screening-2002 has been validated for use in surgical patients. In malnourished patients, the operation should be postponed in order to allow for a 7- to 10-day nutritional rehabilitation period. Preoperative fasting should be avoided. Preoperative carbohydrate loading mitigates the insulin resistance provoked by the insult of surgery. During the operation, measures should be taken that favour a rapid recovery of the gastrointestinal tract postoperatively. In addition, the need of an enteral access should be considered. In the postoperative period, patients should resume their normal food intake or the intake of oral supplements within 24 hours. Parenteral nutrition is indicated only when oral/enteral feeding is contraindicated or not tolerated. Adequate perioperative nutrition has convincingly shown to improve clinical outcome in patients undergoing major gastrointestinal surgery.

KEYWORDS

Malnutrition, nutrition, enteral nutrition, parenteral nutrition, carbohydrate loading, immunonutrition, insulin resistance, ERAS

INTRODUCTION

During the first referral for elective surgery, attention is given to surgical planning, cardiopulmonary risk stratification and assessment of the severity of surgical insult.[1] The risks of infectious complications, the duration of hospitalisation, the possibility of anatomical alterations after surgery and, herewith, the associated potential need of placement of an enteral access are discussed with the patient. In this first consultation, nutritional assessment of the patient is often neglected. Many, mostly retrospective, studies in the period 2008 to 2012 have characterised the relationship between preoperative nutritional status, risk of malnutrition and postoperative outcomes.[2–7] They confirm previous observations that disease-related malnutrition is associated with increased mortality, morbidity, length of hospital stay (LOHS), greater risks of readmission and institutionalisation and higher hospital costs. Yet, it is difficult to isolate the putative contribution of malnutrition in the poor clinical outcome or its association with poor outcome when the disease clearly affects the nutritional status.[2] As the population ages and fattens, special consideration should be given to the elderly with frailty and/or sarcopenia and to the obese who despite a considerable fat store may be at risk of depleted muscle mass and function (sarcopenic obesity).

NUTRITIONAL STATUS: MALNUTRITION

The definition of malnutrition, defined by the European Society of Parenteral and Enteral Nutrition (ESPEN) in 2006 as a state of nutrition in which a deficiency or excess (or imbalance) of energy, protein and other nutrients causes measurable adverse effects on tissue/ body form (body shape, size and composition) and function and clinical outcome, also included imbalanced and excess nutrient intakes and thus overweight and obesity.[8] These states of malnutrition are less prominent in the more recent ESPEN definition of 2015, where malnutrition due to starvation, disease or ageing is defined as a state resulting from the lack of intake or uptake of nutrition, leading to altered body composition (decreased fat-free mass [FFM]) and body cell mass, resulting in diminished physical and mental functions and impaired clinical outcome from diseases.[9] Many factors contribute to malnutrition and should be particularly considered in patients presenting with gastrointestinal (GI) diseases for surgery (Table 5.1).

As a consequence, the prevalence of malnutrition on admission is considerable and is present in 14 to 87% of the surgical patients (average 40–50%).[2–7,10] Two-thirds of patients lose weight during hospitalisation.

Even patients with colorectal cancer, traditionally not considered to be at risk of malnutrition, were malnourished in 20% of cases, and half of the 132 patients were losing weight.[11] It should be noted that diagnostic criteria for malnutrition vary across studies and include the amount of food intake, body weight loss, body mass index (BMI), biochemical parameters (albumin and prealbumin), assessment questionnaires and bioimpedance analysis (BIA), which quantifies fat and lean body mass (LBM).

Ideally, patients at risk of malnutrition and thus at risk of developing complications should be identified before surgery and specific (nutritional) therapy should be provided.[10] This signifies that malnutrition has to be diagnosed, and ESPEN 2015 has operationalised this by first defining the criteria of being at risk of malnutrition by any validated risk-screening tool.[9] It suggested the use of Nutritional Risk Screening (NRS-2002) in hospitals,

Table 5.1 Factors contributing to malnutrition in patients presenting with gastrointestinal diseases for surgery

1.	Decreased oral intake	
	a.	By the disease anorexia, by complaints after food intake or inability to eat (obstruction)
	b.	By deficiencies impairing taste and smell, such as zinc deficiency
	c.	Iatrogenic malnutrition by restriction of food, such as restriction of energy, protein, lactose or dietary fibre
2.	Maldigestion	
	a.	Impaired secretion of gastric acid, pepsin and intrinsic factor by the stomach
	b.	Impaired bile secretion
	c.	Impaired pancreatic juice secretion
3.	Malabsorption	
	a.	Decreased absorbing mucosal surface because of disease or treatment of a disease, surgery or enteroenteric fistula
	b.	Small intestinal bacterial overgrowth (SIBO)
	c.	Diminished bile acid pool because of disease, surgery or SIBO
4.	Increased losses	
	a.	Protein-losing enteropathy
	b.	Steatorrhoea
	c.	Blood loss
	d.	Intestinal losses of fluid, electrolytes, minerals and trace elements
5.	Increased needs	
	a.	Increased needs by active inflammation (fever, inflammation and infection) or catabolic illnesses (cancer or cancer treatment)
	b.	Increased needs for tissue repair, wound healing and growth
	c.	Increased needs induced by medication
6.	Interactions of medication and nutrition	
	a.	Bile acid binders with fat-soluble vitamins
	b.	Corticosteroids with calcium, corticosteroids with glucose intolerance, increased lipolysis and protein catabolism
	c.	Methotrexate or sulphasalazine with folate

the Mini Nutritional Assessment (MNA) in the elderly and the Malnutrition Universal Screening Tool (MUST) in the community setting. It also unanimously gave two alternatives:

- Alternative 1: BMI <18.5 Kg/m^2 (with a complementary suggestion for relevant cut-off values according to age; see under Alternative 2).
- Alternative 2: Unintentional weight loss >10% indefinite of time, or >5% over the last 3 months, combined with either:
  - BMI <20 Kg/m^2 if <70 years of age, or <22 Kg/m^2 if ≥70 years of age, *or*
  - Fat-free mass index <15 Kg/m^2 in women and <17 Kg/m^2 in men.

Ethnic variability in BMI may need to be considered. In Asian countries, BMI values had to be adopted with categories of no risk when BMI ≥18.5 Kg/m^2, moderate risk when BMI is 16.0 Kg/m^2 to 18.4 Kg/m^2 and severe risk when BMI ≤16.0 Kg/m^2.[5,12] The current 2015 ESPEN statement provides malnutrition criteria independent of aetiology. Others prefer to apply aetiology-driven criteria, arguing that malnutrition and underlying disease are inextricably interwoven.

If someone is defined as being 'at risk' of malnutrition or malnourished by screening tools, nutritional assessment should follow by defining body composition and function by measuring BMI, FFM, muscle strength and functional tests.

Screening tools for detecting malnutrition have been designed. The prognostic capabilities of each of these screening scores were reviewed in a recent publication.[13] The most valuable and the only truly validated tool for nutritional screening of surgical patients is the NRS-2002, which is based on weight loss, reduced food intake and BMI, as well as on the severity of disease.[14] If one of these criteria is present, a more extensive list follows, assessing impaired nutritional status; the disease itself, because of increased nutritional needs; and age (+1 point for age ≥70 years). The score has a range of 0 to 7, and patients are considered at nutritional risk when NRS-2002 score is ≥3. Other scores used in surgery are the Reilly's Nutritional Risk Screening (NRS)[15], which assesses weight loss, BMI, appetite, ability to eat and retain food and a disease factor (range: 0–15, being at nutritional risk when score is ≥4) and the Nutritional Risk Index (NRI)[2], an equation that uses recent weight loss and serum albumin. The MUST rates current BMI and percentage weight loss in the last 3 to 6 months between 0 and 2 and gives one point for the acute disease effect with no or little intake for at least 5 days (range: 0–5, being at risk when score is ≥2).[16]

Schiesser et al, using NRS, NRI and BIA in patients admitted for elective GI surgery, found the Reilly's NRS to best predict the development of infectious complications.[3] In Schwegler's study, the NRS-2002 predicted morbidity but not mortality, whereas the opposite was true for Reilly's NRS.[4] Guo et al found that in patients with gastric cancer, an NRS-2002 score ≥3 predicted morbidity and length of stay (LOS).[5] Ho et al used the Chinese version of the MUST in 946 GI surgery patients. The MUST independently predicted 30- and 60-day mortality, LOHS and medical complications. Although the amount of time required to calculate a score for each patient may have restricted the widespread use of the NRS-2002—which, however, may be done by nurses—Guo et al reported that no more than 10 minutes were needed for the assessment of each patient.[5,17] Lower food intake before hospital admission (<50% of normal) was the only nutrition-related variable in the NRS-2002 that was associated with postoperative mortality and morbidity, suggesting that simplification of scoring might be feasible.[7] Almeida et al looked for a valid, feasible and easy screening score for use in surgical patients.[10] They tested the capacity of BMI, recent percentage weight loss, NSR-2002, MUST and NRI in identifying patients at nutritional risk. The MUST, NSR-2002 and weight loss ≥5% in the previous 6 months performed the best.

Not only the risk of malnutrition but also underlying pathophysiological processes should be taken into consideration, such as the cachexia-anorexia status mostly in cancer patients and frailty and sarcopenia present in frail, old and obese patients. Moreover, preoperative fasting, surgery and injury initiate a series of reactions causing catabolism.[18] Insulin resistance is a key feature of the metabolic response to surgical stress and is closely related to surgical complications and postoperative delayed recovery and leads to prolonged LOHS and fatigue.[18]

PATHOPHYSIOLOGY OF SURGICAL STRESS AND EFFECTS OF FASTING

The metabolic response to surgery is mainly characterised by an increase in metabolic rate, a negative nitrogen balance, increased gluconeogenesis and increased synthesis of acute-phase proteins, most of which can be explained by a reduced insulin sensitivity, with the key clinical features of hyperglycaemia and loss of body protein.[18–22] Insulin has several metabolic functions such as the stimulation of glucose uptake in the periphery, glucose oxidation and glycogen formation, especially in muscle, and triglyceride uptake in fat cells, mediated by lipoprotein lipase.[20–22] Insulin inhibits lipolysis in adipose tissue and suppresses the release of free fatty acids (FFAs) from fat. It inhibits hepatic gluconeogenesis from glycerol, glucogenic amino acids such as alanine and glutamine, lactate and pyruvate. It also inhibits renal gluconeogenesis from glutamine. However, its major effect is the suppression of protein breakdown, especially in peripheral tissues. It stimulates protein synthesis selectively, for instance, albumin synthesis in the liver.

So, the insulin resistance state as a key feature of injury ensures the production and delivery of endogenous substrates (glucose and FFAs) to glucose-dependent tissues such as the brain, heart, immune system, nerves, renal medulla, bone marrow and healing wounds.[20,21] Insulin-dependent tissues such as skeletal muscle change from glucose to fat as their source of energy. So, initially, the insulin resistance may be essential for survival.[22] However, the reduced insulin sensitivity has also counterproductive consequences, such as hyperglycaemia because of increased endogenous glucose production, decreased peripheral glucose uptake and glycogen formation, which may result in dehydration, weight loss, poor wound healing and increased infectious complications. Resistance to the anabolic actions of insulin, such as minimising protein breakdown, may result in increased nitrogen loss, reduction in LBM and poor recovery. Reduced LBM not only decreases muscle strength along with impaired cardiorespiratory function and impaired mobilisation but also delays wound healing and compromises immune function.[18]

The degree of reduced insulin sensitivity is determined by the type and technique of surgery, being greater with increasing magnitude of surgery and with open versus laparoscopic surgery.[22] The reduced impact of laparoscopic procedures is possibly mediated through the reduction of tissue trauma and mitigation of the inflammatory response. After open cholecystectomy, insulin sensitivity does not normalise within 9 days, and normalisation appears to take approximately 3 weeks.[22]

Most of the impairment of insulin function can be explained by the stress-induced increased secretion of counter-regulatory hormones with metabolic effects by inhibiting insulin secretion and/or by opposing its peripheral action, such as glucagon (promoting glycogenolysis and hepatic gluconeogenesis), cortisol (stimulating breakdown of structural proteins in peripheral tissues and hepatic gluconeogenesis) and catecholamines (promoting glycogenolysis, hepatic gluconeogenesis and lipolysis).[18,23] Inflammatory mediators such as cytokines (tumour necrosis factor-α, interleukin [IL]-1, IL-2 and IL-6) may also be involved in the development of postoperative insulin resistance.[18,23]

Prolonged fasting, hypocaloric intake and immobilisation can induce an insulin-resistance state. To provide energy during fasting, carbohydrates stored as glycogen in liver and muscle are mobilised in a low-insulin and high-glucagon environment, and after an overnight fast, hepatic glycogen is reduced by half. Prolonged fasting leads to muscle protein breakdown and lipolysis, thereby providing substrates for gluconeogenesis and ketosis. During a 22-hour fast, gluconeogenesis accounts for approximately 65% of total glucose production.[24] The negative effects of starvation are not simply due to starvation per se but due to starving of the gut.[21]

So, the combination of surgical injury and fasting may amplify postoperative insulin resistance, depletion of carbohydrate stores, consumption of LBM and changes in metabolism from an anabolic to a catabolic state. Malnutrition further aggravates the unfavourable condition.

OTHER PATHOPHYSIOLOGICAL PROCESSES

Cachexia is a complex metabolic syndrome associated with underlying illness, mostly in cancer patients; wherein it induces proteolysis and lipolysis due to tumour-derived proteins and proinflammatory cytokines.[23,25] A prominent clinical feature of cachexia is weight loss. Diagnostic criteria consist of weight loss or a BMI <20.0 Kg/m^2 *plus* three of the following: decreased muscle strength, fatigue, anorexia or poor appetite, low fat-free muscle index and abnormal biochemistry (increased inflammatory markers, anaemia and/or low serum albumin).[23,25,26]

Frailty is defined as a clinical syndrome in which three or more of the following criteria are present: unintentional weight loss, self-reported exhaustion, weakness (hand-grip strength), slow walking speed and low physical activity.[27] In a prefrail condition, one or two criteria are present.

Sarcopenia is a condition characterised by loss of muscle mass and muscle strength.[26,27] As mentioned above, during metabolic stress, muscle protein is rapidly mobilised in order to provide amino acids to the immune system, liver and gut. The sarcopenic person has a decreased availability of such protein depots and is thus at an increased risk during the insult of surgery. Sarcopenia is primarily a disease of the elderly, but it may also be associated with other conditions such as neurodegenerative and endocrine diseases.[27] Obesity is a metabolic, low-grade inflammatory disease of excess and ill-distributed fat, defined by a BMI >30 Kg/m^2. Sarcopenic obesity is defined by an excess of fat mass, combined with depleted LBM and function.

NUTRITION

Increasing evidence is accumulating that nutritional support may improve clinical outcome in patients undergoing major GI surgery.[28] Already in the previous century, the Veterans Affairs Preoperative Parenteral Nutrition in Surgical Patients study stressed the importance of artificial feeding but only in the most severely malnourished patients. The observation that severely malnourished, catabolic patients benefitted most from supplemental nutrition may be explained by the fact that these patients experience a more profound shift from the fasted to the fed state with preoperative feeding, with preservation of glycogen stores, decreased insulin resistance and establishment of a more anabolic milieu before going into surgery.[18,29] Preoperative carbohydrate loading may, in fact, work by this same mechanism. Postoperative nutrition aims at maintaining nutritional status in the catabolic period after surgery, with the purpose of enhancing postoperative recovery and maintaining muscle, immune and cognitive functions.

It is important to realise that the available data have to be placed in the context with other recent innovations in surgical management, such as immunonutrition, designed to improve immune function, and Enhanced Recovery after Surgery (ERAS) protocols, a multimodal perioperative care programme designed to accelerate postoperative recovery, reduce complication rates and achieve an early discharge.

Preoperative Nutrition in the Days before Surgery

According to the ESPEN guidelines for surgical patients, dating back to 2006, malnourished patients or patients at risk of malnutrition should receive preoperative nutrition for 7 to 10 days, even if the operation had to be postponed.[30] At that time, the risk of malnutrition was defined by an NRS-2002 score ≥ 3 or the presence of at least one of the following criteria: weight loss of 10 to 15% within 6 months, BMI <18.5 Kg/m^2, Subjective Global Assessment grade C and serum albumin <30 g/L with no evidence of hepatic or renal dysfunction.[30,31] In addition, the North American Surgical Nutrition Summit has defined patients at nutritional risk by a decreased recent oral intake; BMI <18.5 Kg/m^2 or >40 Kg/m^2; actual body weight <90% of the ideal body weight (IBW) or a weight loss of >5% in 1 month, 7.5% in 3 months and 10% in 6 months.[32] They advise to postpone surgery not only to address poor nutrition but also to achieve an HbA1c <7.5% and to attempt smoking cessation or weight loss in those with BMI >35 Kg/m^2. This concept of prehabilitation, a short-course optimisation

before surgery, which might also include exercise and protein supplementation, had beneficial effects on functional recovery after surgery.[33]

The primary goal of nutrition is to prepare the patient metabolically for the stress of surgery, to optimise nutrient delivery and to attenuate protein wasting. However, nutrition will fail to produce an anabolic state. It is, therefore, also very unlikely that a chronic condition of underfeeding that has lasted for several weeks or months can be reversed by 1 week of nutritional support. Preoperative nutrition might work through a reduction of postoperative insulin resistance, as has been investigated extensively for preoperative carbohydrate loading. It may also support the malnourished patient with enough substrate to cover the requirements after surgery. This concept therefore explains why in appropriate patients as little as 5 to 7 days of nutrition intervention can affect outcomes.[18] As a general rule, patients have a caloric need of 25 Kcal/Kg and a protein need of 1.5 to 2 g/Kg.[1,34] In the past, the main focus was energy, now it is protein.[34]

Two options are available for artificial feeding:

- Parenteral nutrition (PN), where the intravenous route via large veins is used to deliver highly osmolar solutions of amino acids, dextrose and lipids, supplemented with vitamins, minerals and trace elements.
- Enteral nutrition (EN), where via a tube or via percutaneous access, adequately balanced solution can be administered into the GI tract, which can be completely predigested as in the case of elemental nutrition, partly digested as in the case of oligopeptide-, semi-elemental feeds and undigested as in the case of polymeric solutions.

The oral or enteral route is clearly preferred over the parenteral route. Oral nutrition or EN combats the starvation of the gut and has proven to be successful in blunting the metabolic response after injury and improving protein kinetics.[18,21] It also supports the structure and function of the gut; stimulates peristalsis, blood flow and the release of GI hormones and bile salts and inhibits colonisation by pathogens.[35] Oral and enteral food may support the immune system by IgA and T helper 2 cells and regulate inflammation and oxidative stress by fermentation products such as butyrate.[35] Both options have their complications (Tables 5.2 and 5.3). An excellent report by the North American Surgical Nutrition Summit summarises the role of PN in an era dominated by ERAS components that focus on a greater utilisation of the gut for feeding, feeding closer to the time of surgery, avoiding preoperative bowel preparation and the use of nasogastric tubes and promoting or maintaining gut motility.[36]

Table 5.2   Complications associated with total parenteral nutrition

Catheter insertion-related	Catheter-related	Metabolic
Arterial puncture	Thrombosis	Hyperglycaemia/hypoglycaemia
Pneumothorax	Catheter-site infection	Ketoacidosis
Haemothorax	Septic phlebitis	Azotaemia
Air embolism	Bloodstream infection	Hyperosmolar state
Thoracic duct injury		Electrolyte imbalance
Catheter malposition		Hypertriglyceridaemia
		Metabolic acidosis
		Refeeding syndrome
		Hepatic dysfunction/steatosis
		Fluid overload
		Coagulopathy
		Fat overload syndrome
		Hypercapnia

Modified from: Abunnaja S, Cuviello A, Sanchez JA. Enteral and parenteral nutrition in the perioperative period: state of the art. *Nutrients* 2013;5:608–23 and published with permission.

Table 5.3   Complications associated with enteral nutrition

Mechanical	Gastrointestinal	Metabolic
Aspiration	Nausea/vomiting	Hyperglycaemia/hypoglycaemia
Tube malposition	Diarrhoea/constipation	Electrolyte imbalance
Tube clogging	Malabsorption/maldigestion	Early satiety
		Dehydration
		Refeeding syndrome

Modified from: Abunnaja S, Cuviello A, Sanchez JA. Enteral and parenteral nutrition in the perioperative period: state of the art. *Nutrients* 2013;5:608–23 and published with permission.

Parenteral nutrition should be restricted to circumstances where EN is not feasible, such as intestinal obstruction, ischaemia and acute peritonitis, or where EN is relatively contraindicated, such as multiple fistulas with high output, severe malabsorption, short bowel syndrome, severe shock with impaired splanchnic perfusion and fulminant sepsis.[36]

Conventional Nutritional Interventions in Surgical Patients

Nutritional interventions have the potential to offset some of the excessive losses and deficiencies but can also result in undesired consequences if delivered at the wrong time, in the wrong form or by the wrong way, as shown recently in the acute phase of critical illness.[37] Nutrition goals, at the most basic level, should be to provide caloric and nitrogenous support for wound healing and to avoid excessive loss of LBM.[29] It should be realised that there are only a few studies that compare EN with standard therapy and about 80% of the studies compare immunonutrition with standard therapy.[1]

Oral or enteral nutrition

In a meta-analysis, Burden et al investigated postoperative complications and LOHS as primary outcome in studies that started with supplemental feeding 10 days before surgery in malnourished patients.[38] Thirteen trials were evaluated. Seven studies investigated immunomodulating formula (IMF) and reported a decrease in infectious complications and LOHS. Three studies with PN were rather old and applied hyperalimentation without strict glucose control. They showed a decreased overall complication rate but not so for the infectious complications, which favoured the control group. Two studies with EN and three studies with oral nutrient supplements (ONS) did not show benefits in the primary outcomes.

A very recent meta-analysis by Zhong et al included 15 randomised controlled trials (RCTs); it assessed the effect of nutritional support on clinical outcomes in malnourished surgical patients, 10 trials in GI cancer, 3 trials in patients with mixed surgery, and 2 trials in patients with cardiac surgery and head and neck cancer surgery.[39] Nine studies reported on standard nutrition support and six reported on immunonutrition support. Compared with the control group, nutritional support was more effective in decreasing the incidence of infectious and noninfectious complications and shortening the LOHS. Moreover, the incidence of infectious complications in the immunonutrition group was significantly lower than that in the standard nutrition group, without any difference in the incidence of noninfectious complications. There were no significant differences in hospital costs and postoperative mortality between the groups.

A large prospective cohort study of 1,085 patients investigated the effect of preoperative nutritional support.[40] Patients deemed to be at nutrition risk (NRS-2002 score ≥3) were randomised to nutrition intervention versus no nutritional support (standard of care). Adequate nutritional support was defined by a minimum of 7 days of PN or EN and a minimum of 3 days of PN or EN after surgery. Preoperative nutrition intervention in the high-risk group (NRS-2002 of at least 5, n = 120, 11% of patients) decreased postoperative complications by 50% and reduced the postoperative hospital stay significantly by 4 days. Adequate nutritional support was obtained in 36% of patients. Of the 392 patients with an NRS score of 3 to 4, the complication rate and the postoperative hospital stay were similar to those in the standard care group. Very few patients with malnutrition (NRS-2002 score ≥3) achieved goal support with enteral formulas, without the use of supplemental PN. Seventy-three percent of those patients achieved goal caloric intake with the use of PN. So, in both high- and low-risk patients receiving the same interventions, only the high-risk group benefitted in outcome. One study that evaluated preoperative supplementation with standard oral supplement versus control nutrition demonstrated less postoperative weight loss and fewer minor complications with preoperative supplementation.[41] Gastrointestinal intolerance, anorexia, noncompliance and other factors may have minimised any potential benefit, as total caloric intake was minimally improved with the addition of the oral supplements.

Parenteral nutrition

Parenteral feeding should be used only in those severely malnourished patients who cannot be fed enterally.[36,42] One of the first meta-analysis of 33 RCTs included 13 studies involving patients with GI cancer, thought to be at least moderately malnourished.[43] Patients who received preoperative PN had 10% fewer postoperative complications than the control group with no specialised nutrition therapy. A total of five meta-analyses have been published, and no effect on postoperative mortality was seen.[21] Most of the studies provided PN for at least 7 days or longer, and this led to the recommendation that to achieve a clinical benefit from PN, therapy should be provided for at least 7 days before surgery, as no benefit was noticed when PN lasted less than 5 days.[43] With delivery of PN to the severely malnourished patient, the development of the refeeding syndrome, with its associated hypokalaemia and hypophosphataemia, is a concern. These electrolyte imbalances are particularly dangerous in the perioperative period. Starting total parenteral nutrition (TPN) at least 7 days before surgery allows time to address any electrolyte disturbances that may occur.

Immunonutrition in Surgical Patients

Immunonutrition or immunomodulating formulas (IMFs) are hydrolysed peptide-based protein-rich formulas that include some combination of fish oils, including eicosapentaenoic acid and docosahexaenoic acid, arginine, nucleic acids and antioxidants (vitamins A and C, zinc and selenium).[44] There are two studies that used glutamine instead of RNA.[45] Immunomodulating formulas as such are not designed to provide nutritional support but to improve immune function, explaining why benefits from the provision of IMFs have also been demonstrated in well-nourished cohorts.[29,44] This also implies that there are physiological benefits to (pharmacological) nutritional intervention, not necessarily associated with improvements in anthropometric measurements but associated with improved immune, respiratory and cardiac functions, along with improved wound healing and mobility.[29,44] Biochemical effects of these formulas include increased cell membrane stability, improved GI mucosal integrity, enhanced cell-mediated immune responses, attenuation of the inflammatory response to stress and improved blood flow to poorly vascularised and ischaemic tissues.[29,44]

Both glutamine and arginine can be considered conditionally essential in catabolic stress states and serious illness. Avenell et al performed a meta-analysis on parenteral and enteral glutamine supplementations.[46] They found a significant reduction in infections in patients who were given glutamine-containing parenteral solutions after surgery. Higher doses of glutamine appeared more effective. However, a strong warning against the use of high glutamine doses (0.35 g/Kg parenterally or 30 g/day enterally) in the critically ill came from the REducing Deaths due to OXidative Stress (the REDOX study), which showed a higher mortality with early provision of glutamine and antioxidants.[47] Enteral glutamine postoperatively did not show beneficial effects.[46] Perioperative parenteral glutamine supplementation was recently investigated in a meta-analysis of 16 studies, which showed a decrease in postoperative infections, shorter LOHS and improved nitrogen balance.[48]

A large meta-analysis of perioperative use of arginine-containing formulations identified a major reduction in infectious complications and LOHS.[49] Concern has been raised that supplemental arginine, when given to septic patients, particularly nonsurgical septic patients, may result in elevated nitrate and nitrite levels, potential damage of mitochondria by the metabolite peroxynitrite, exaggerated vasodilation, haemodynamic instability and worsening outcomes in sepsis.[44] However, patients with sepsis and surgical trauma may regulate arginine metabolism differently.[50,51] Arginine levels are lower and arginase activity is higher in patients after surgical trauma compared with sepsis. Nitric oxide is elevated in sepsis and decreased after surgical trauma. Because metabolism of arginine differs in surgical versus nonsurgical patients, the effects of arginine supplementation in these patients is also likely to differ. Many recent studies have demonstrated that supplemental arginine can be delivered to septic patients with no ill effects.

A meta-analysis of fish-oil-enriched PN with standard PN demonstrated positive effects on LOHS and postoperative infections.[52] Marik and Zaloga investigated the impact of immunonutrition supplemented with arginine, fish oil or both on the clinical outcomes of high-risk patients undergoing elective (mainly GI) surgery in 21 trials.[50] They demonstrated that the ability of immunonutrition to reduce infectious complications appears to require administration of both arginine and fish oil, explained by the fact that fish oil acts synergistically with arginine by inhibiting arginase in correcting the arginine-deficiency state.[50,51]

Over the past 20 years, nine meta-analyses, including a large number of randomised clinical trials, have consistently reported that perioperative immunonutrition is associated with a substantial reduction in both infectious complications and LOHS, regardless of the patient's baseline nutritional status. These results have been found in patients electively operated for both upper and lower GI tract disease. There is some evidence that the beneficial effects of immunomodulating therapy may be most pronounced in patients undergoing higher-risk GI surgery, where the potential for postoperative critical illness and metabolic stress may be higher.[29] Most of the studies gave IMFs at home orally for 5 to 7 days before surgery and/ or after operation through a nasojejunal tube for 7 days.[53]

Some meta-analyses reported the prevalence of malnutrition (26% in Cerantola et al's study and 40%

in Osland et al's study).[54,55] Zhong et al included only malnourished surgical patients, and whereas nutritional support in general significantly decreased infectious and noninfectious complications and reduced LOHS when compared with controls, immune support was superior in reducing the incidence of infectious complications than standard nutrition support.[39] Others included only those series where isoenergetic, isonitrogenous standard enteral formulas were given to the control group.[54] Osland et al noted that 6 of the 14 studies (42%) used intervention products that contained between 20 and 46% more protein and/or up to 600 Kcal (20%) more energy than control formulations.[55] Few studies and meta-analysis quantified the amount of immune nutrition actually received. In addition, most of the preoperative trials were not balanced with appropriate isocaloric and isonitrogenous control solutions.

Some meta-analyses also investigated the impact of timing of IMF administration.[45,54,55] The meta-analysis by Osland et al reported statistically significant reductions in infectious complications and LOS with perioperative and postoperative administrations of arginine-dominant IMFs (>9 g arginine/L).[55] Perioperative administration was also associated with a statistically significant reduction in anastomotic dehiscence, whereas a reduction in noninfective complications was demonstrated with postoperative administration. Only preoperative administration demonstrated no notable advantage over standard nutrition provision in any of the clinical outcomes assessed and confirmed the findings of Cerantola et al of no reduction of LOHS by preoperative IMF.[54] Experimental and clinical works have suggested that it may take 3 to 5 days before the manifestation of benefits of IMFs.[51] Similarly, it may be conceivable that the cessation of IMFs on the day of surgery may result in subtherapeutic or declining levels of circulating immunonutrients in the immediate postoperative period at a time when their action may be most valuable. Within the new anaesthesia guidelines, it might be feasible to give these solutions up to 6 hours before the operation.

Song et al conducted a Bayesian network meta-analysis (NMA), realising that traditional head-to-head meta-analyses can analyse the comparison of only two individual interventions and cannot compare more than two treatments (preoperative, perioperative and postoperative interventions) simultaneously.[56] A total of 27 RCTs on immunonutrition in selective surgery for resectable GI malignancy were incorporated. Pair-wise meta-analyses suggested that preoperative, postoperative and perioperative IMFs reduced the incidence of postoperative infectious complications compared with standard EN. Moreover, perioperative IMFs reduced the incidence of postoperative noninfectious complications, and perioperative and postoperative IMFs also shortened the length of postoperative hospitalisation. Network meta-analysis found, by ranking all alternatives, that perioperative IMFs was the best option for managing patients who underwent selective surgery for GI cancer. The impact of IMFs on hospital costs has been studied in GI cancer surgery in Germany, Italy and the United States. These trials, together with a very recent study from Switzerland, demonstrated that IMFs are a cost-effective and cost-saving intervention.[57]

The ESPEN and Society of Critical Care Medicine (SCCM)/American Society for Parenteral and Enteral Nutrition (ASPEN) guidelines support the use of immune-enhancing diets in patients with mild to moderate sepsis.[58,59] However, both advise against the use of immune-enhancing diets in patients with severe sepsis. The Canadian Clinical Practice Guidelines (CCPG) maintain that arginine-supplemented immune-enhancing diets should not be used for critically ill patients (especially with sepsis).[60] The SCCM/ASPEN guidelines propose that at least 50 to 65% of goal energy requirements should be delivered to receive optimal therapeutic benefit from immune-modulating formulas. The ESPEN guidelines maintain that critically ill ICU patients who do not tolerate >700 mL of EN per day should not receive immune-enhancing diets. The North American Surgical Nutrition Summit advises to start 500 to 1000 mL/d of enteral nutrition 5 to 7 days preoperatively and to continue in the postoperative period.[32] It is unclear what should be done in elective surgery patients who develop systemic infections while being on immune formulations. In the studies cited in the meta-analysis of Marik and Zaloga, infected patients remained in their study group for the duration of the study, apparently without ill effects.[50]

Nutrition on the Day of Surgery

The old dogma of keeping patient on nil per mouth from midnight till the operation because of fear of aspiration during intubation has been replaced by a more liberal approach of allowing the intake of clear fluids until 2 hours, solid foods until 6 hours and fatty foods until 8 hours before the operation in many anaesthesiologist guidelines worldwide. These are based on a meta-analysis showing that fasting in patients from midnight neither reduced gastric content nor raised the pH of gastric fluid, compared with patients allowed free intake of clear fluids until 2 hours before anaesthesia for surgery.[61] It also did not affect the prevalence of complications. Obese (and even morbidly obese) patients have been reported to have the same gastric-emptying characteristics as lean patients. Patients with uncomplicated type 2 diabetes mellitus have been reported to have normal gastric emptying, whereas those with polyneuropathy may have delayed gastric emptying (DGE) of solids, with no conclusive data as to emptying of fluids.

Although the preoperative intake of clear fluids up to 2 hours before surgery resulted in reduced thirst, hunger and a dry mouth preoperatively and decreased nausea and vomiting postoperatively, it did not go far enough in optimising patient's condition. Ljungqvist et al were the first to recognise that in animals, responses to stress are different in the fasted as opposite to the fed state and that preoperative glucose infusion at a rate of 5 mg/Kg/min reduced the postoperative insulin resistance and increased hepatic glycogen content in men.[62] This high glucose concentration dose was needed in order to achieve an insulin response equivalent to the response by a normal meal. Patients were in a state of hyperinsulinaemia and normoglycaemia before the operation, reminiscent of a normal fed state.[62–64] The need of a hypertonic 20% glucose solution to avoid fluid overload and the need for access to large veins stimulated the search for an oral fluid supplement, being safe for oral administration before surgery and being capable of inducing a meal-simulating endogenous insulin release (plasma concentrations of 60 mU/mL).[62] Firstly, factors defining the rate of gastric emptying and thus, indirectly determining the risk of aspiration and its safety had to be considered. Volume, carbohydrate content, osmolality, pH and temperature of the drink determine the rate of gastric emptying. A 12.5% solution of complex carbohydrates (i.e., maltodextrins) with an osmolality of 290 mOsmol/Kg and a pH of 5.0 that appeared to be safe was developed (Nutricia preOp©, Nutricia, Zoetermeer, the Netherlands).[63] Gastric emptying was complete within 120 minutes (mean 90 minutes) after intake, even in anxious patients. Secondly, beneficial effects had to be demonstrated by inducing an endogenous insulin response, and three studies, two in elective total hip replacement patients and one in elective colorectal surgery, showed a significantly less reduction in insulin sensitivity when compared with patients on a placebo drink.[63,64] The postoperative insulin resistance was reduced by ≈50%. The beneficial changes were due to less reduction in insulin sensitivity in peripheral tissues, with a lesser reduction in glucose oxidation and nonoxidative glucose disposal, suggesting a better activation of glucose transport and glycogen synthase.

It should be stressed that carbohydrate drinks have to be given before the onset of stress and not at the moment of the stressed state, which is feasible in case of elective surgical procedures but not in emergency situations. So, at the time of surgery, patients are in an anabolic rather than a catabolic state, with loaded glycogen stores and an empty stomach. Mainly glucose homeostasis has been investigated. Data on the effects of insulin on protein and fat metabolism are sparse.[22,63] Three studies investigated the nitrogen-sparing effect of insulin. Insulin was not proven to have any effect on muscle protein synthesis, but the anabolic effect of insulin is likely to be exerted by minimising protein breakdown and a better maintenance of LBM.[63, 64]

The practice generally involves the consumption of 100 g carbohydrates in 800 mL the night before surgery and 50 g in 400 mL 2 hours before surgery. Data from RCTs indicated an accelerated recovery in patients receiving preoperative carbohydrate loading, and data from two meta-analyses demonstrated an overall 0.3-day shorter LOHS, with a decrease of 1.66 day[65] and 1 day[66] in patients undergoing major open abdominal surgery. The Cochrane meta-analysis found no effect at all when the six adequately blinded studies were analysed.[65] The Awad et al's meta-analysis found no effect when laparoscopic and minor surgeries (expected hospital stay ≤2 days) or orthopaedic surgery were investigated, procedures known to be associated with minimal development of insulin resistance and with low complication rates.[66] Since no differences in complication rates have been observed between control and carbohydrate treated groups, presumably the improved recovery after surgery with decreased postoperative protein catabolism and reduced loss of muscle mass may be responsible for the shorter LOHS. No increases in complications and aspiration pneumonitis were seen.

Data on the safety and clinical benefit of preoperative carbohydrate in patients with diabetes are limited to one study with 35 patients and patients with factors that increase the risk of gastric aspiration such as pregnancy; obesity; history of metabolic disorders, including diabetes; American Association of Anesthesiologists (ASA) grade >2 and GI disorders were excluded from the trial. Several products are available, quite different in costs per patient per surgery: Nutricia preOp© (Nutricia, Zoetermeer, the Netherlands) £21.00; Roosvicee Vruchtenmix (Heinz, Zeist, the Netherlands) £1.39; Vitajoule™ (Vitaflo, Liverpool, UK) £1.13; and Aminoleban® EN (Otsuka Pharmaceutical, Tokyo, Japan), a mixture of carbohydrates and branched-chain amino acids, £40.00 per patient per surgery.[65] Sports drinks do not have enough carbohydrates for an adequate effect (sports drinks contain 6–7% carbohydrates).

Actions to Promote Postoperative Physiological Function

Enhanced Recovery after Surgery, previously named fast-track surgery of fast-track rehabilitation, is a multimodal approach that integrates many components with the aim to maintain physiological function, to minimise the stress of major surgery and to enhance earlier recovery.[67] It challenges two conventional concepts: the concept that a stress response to surgery is inevitable and untreatable and the concept that postoperative rest should benefit both the patients and their GI tract.[67] New insights with high levels of evidence resulted in the replacement of old dogmas, such as preoperative bowel cleansing, fasting from midnight, routine postoperative gastric tube insertion, postoperative bed rest and resumption of food intake only after return of bowel movements, by new ones. Avoiding preoperative fasting, pain control, early mobilisation, immediate restart of food intake and measures to combat postoperative nausea and vomiting are some of the new rules. Measures taken to enable an early return of GI function and gastric emptying include the preoperative carbohydrate loading, the omission of bowel preparation, the early removal of nasogastric tubes and drips, the strict perioperative fluid management to avoid fluid overload, strict glycaemic control (<10 mmol/L), the avoidance of opiates, epidural anaesthesia, the use of laxatives and a multimodal approach to prevent and treat postoperative nausea and vomiting. The use of chewing gum has a positive effect on reducing the time to first bowel movement.[68] An early resumption of oral food intake after surgery (oral fluids 2 hours postsurgery and a total of >800 mL on the day of the operation) and going out of bed for 2 hours on the day of surgery are also important components. Nygren et al showed that in a large prospective series, an oral diet after colorectal resection within an ERAS protocol can be substantial (≈1200 Kcal daily from the first day after surgery), but in itself, it cannot prevent postoperative weight loss (by ≈3 Kg on postoperative day 28).[69] Recently, guidelines related to ERAS in colon surgery, rectal/pelvic surgery and pancreatoduodenectomy have been updated or newly established.[70–72] Enhanced Recovery after Surgery reported a seemingly normal nutritional status in colon surgery patients and in >93% of patients scheduled for a pancreatoduodenectomy, thus obviating the need of preoperative nutrition supplementation.[70,72] The latter was contested by Bozzetti and Mariani, who reported a high prevalence of malnutrition (and consequently of postoperative complications) in 28 to 74% of patients with pancreatic cancer.[73] They showed that within classes of malnourished patients with cancer undergoing pancreatectomy, complications were progressively reduced by shifting from standard isotonic infusions to PN, to standard EN and finally to immunonutrition.[74] They also noticed a consistent gap between the recommended and the effective start of oral fluid and solid feedings postoperatively and opposed against the discouragement of the use of nasogastric/jejunal tubes or a needle-catheter jejunostomy by the ERAS guidelines.[73]

Nutrition after Surgery

Oral or Enteral Feeding

Martindale et al touched the sore spot in their analysis of why it is such a problem to get EN started.[17] Several factors contribute to this delay, such as a poor understanding of the potential benefits of early feeding, poor understanding of postoperative ileus, the waiting for flatus or signs of bowel activity, the concern for complications (most of all being the fear of anastomotic dehiscence and bowel ischaemia and aspiration), the lack of skills for enteral tube placement, the fear of possible need for reoperative intervention and the perception of inability to feed when patients are on vasopressors or have an open abdomen. A meta-analysis by Lewis et al showed that keeping patients nil by mouth is pointless.[75] This study compared feeding within 24 hours (six studies directly into the small bowel and five studies with oral feeds) with nil per mouth and demonstrated a significantly decreased rate of infections (with the largest reduction in wound infections), a decreased LOHS and a trend for reduced anastomotic dehiscence with early feeding. However, a 27% increased risk of vomiting and a 21% increased risk of nasogastric tube positioning have to be taken into consideration. A more recent meta-analysis by the same authors demonstrated a significant reduction in mortality, a trend towards reduced LOHS and no benefit or harm related to anastomotic dehiscence.[76] In 2011, updated 2006 Cochrane review on feeding early, within 24 hours after colorectal surgery (eight studies with feeding via a jejunostomy and six studies with feeding orally), versus later commencement of feeding found only trends of a reduced complication rate and a 1-day shorter LOHS.[77] The meta-analysis by Osland et al, which included 15 studies, reported a 45% decrease in morbidity, with no increase in anastomotic leaks.[78] Nowadays, normal oral food or enteral tube feeding should be started within 24 hours.

In the ERAS protocol, normal food is advised 4 hours after colorectal surgery and within 1 day after gastrectomy.

A large study in 317 malnourished patients with proven cancer and scheduled for elective surgery randomised patients to receive either enteral feeding via a jejunostomy or via the parenteral route the morning after surgery.[79] The study was unique as isonitrogenous, isocaloric feeds were given in both groups (27 Kcal/Kg, 1.4 g amino acids/Kg) and blood glucose levels were strictly monitored to remain below 8.3 mmol/L. Enteral nutrition significantly reduced postoperative (infectious) complications and the LOHS, but PN was better tolerated as GI side effects were 2.5 times more frequent in the enterally fed group; 9% of enterally fed patients needed to switch over to PN.

For a variety of reasons, many patients do not meet their nutritional needs postoperatively. A nutritional sip supplement of 400 mL (600 Kcal, 24 g protein) to increase postoperative intake may be helpful.[80] It reduced postoperative weight loss by 55% compared with the no-supplement group with improved anthropometric measures. Chest and wound infections and antibiotic usage were significantly reduced.[80] Similarly, patients undergoing lower GI tract surgery were randomised to receive or not receive nutritional supplements preoperatively for 15 days or postoperatively for 4 weeks.[41] Patients receiving supplements received an additional 540 Kcal preoperatively and an additional 315 Kcal postoperatively. Those receiving supplements both pre- and postoperatively and those receiving supplements postoperatively had less weight loss and fewer minor complications. The clinical benefits were not impressive but could be explained by a preoperative adequate nutritional status and a high preoperative intake of 1,900 Kcal/day.[41] The implementation of early oral nutrition in the setting of ERAS was investigated in 26 hospitals.[81] Comparison of 1,126 pre-ERAS patients, with 861 ERAS patients undergoing colorectal surgery, demonstrated a 3-day earlier implementation of oral food in ERAS patients and the intake of normal food by 65% in contrast to 7% of pre-ERAS patients. Nausea and vomiting occurred in 21%.

Parenteral Feeding

Postoperative parenteral feeding is indicated in undernourished patients who are unable to receive or tolerate adequate amounts of EN as well as in patients with postoperative complications impairing normal GI function, who are unable to receive adequate oral nutrition or EN for at least 7 days.[28,30,32,36] In a 1997 meta-analysis of 33 RCTs involving more than 2500 surgery patients, the benefit of PN was lost if it was first initiated in the postoperative period: in comparison with the control group, the use of PN was associated with a 10% increase in overall complication.[43] This was confirmed by a meta-analysis from 2001, which reported a 23% reduction in infectious complication in the control group without nutrition support compared with the postoperative parenterally fed group.[82]

Bozetti et al randomised malnourished patients with a ≥10% weight loss to 10 days of preoperative and 9 days of postoperative PN (35 Kcal/Kg, 1.6 g protein/Kg) versus a control group not receiving preoperative nutrition but fed postoperatively with a hypocaloric parenteral solution, adequate in nitrogen content (940 Kcal, 85 g protein).[83] Parenteral nutrition given for 10 days preoperatively and continued postoperatively reduced the complication rate by one-third and prevented mortality in the severely malnourished cancer patients.[83]

Despite being heavily criticised because of the inadequate composition of the parenteral solution, the Early Parenteral Nutrition Completing Enteral Nutrition in Adults Critically Ill Patients (EPaNIC) study by Casear et al demonstrated that in a subgroup of 517 patients in whom EN was contraindicated because of bowel discontinuity, the early initiation of PN at 2 days resulted in higher infectious complicates and less probability to be discharged alive than when started later, after 8 days.[37] All the above-mentioned findings resulted in a recommendation by the North American Surgical Nutrition Summit experts to not initiate PN before 5 to 7 days postoperatively and to initiate PN only if the duration is anticipated to be longer than 7 days.[32,36] In patients on PN preoperatively, because of malnutrition and inability to be fed enterally, PN has to be stopped 2 to 3 hours before surgery and restarted on the morning after surgery.[32] In the postoperative setting, permissive underfeeding, that is, intentional underfeeding with PN (80% of caloric requirements, i.e., 15–20 Kcal/Kg), might be an alternative to full caloric parenteral support, as it reduced infectious complications and LOHS.[84]

Supplemental Parenteral Nutrition to Enteral Nutrition in Patients Not Meeting Nutritional Needs

Early initiation of oral or enteral feeding postoperatively may result in problems of tolerance.[75] Supplemental PN might then be indicated. A meta-analysis of five studies in 2003 did not show any benefit of supplemental PN.[60] The already-mentioned EPaNIC study in more than 4,600 elective surgical patients provides the evidence that supplemental PN added in the first

week to hypocaloric EN showed tremendous adverse effects in patients with moderate surgical stress.[37] In a subgroup of patients with greater disease severity, significant adverse effects of early supplemental PN were seen on LOHS, multiorgan failure and mortality, when compared with late supplemental PN.[85]

SPECIFIC CONDITIONS

As the population ages and fattens, most of the surgical patients will be elderly and/or obese and thus be more at risk of adverse outcomes because of frailty or sarcopenia. In this context, the concept of prehabilitation is extremely valuable, but it will take 4 to 6 weeks.[17,32,33,86]

Elderly

As mentioned earlier, the MNA is the screening list used in the elderly.[87] The first part is a screening form with questions about food intake, weight loss, mobility, disease or physical stress, neuropsychological problems and BMI. When less than 11 of the 14 points are scored, the full MNA has to be filled out. Apart from malnutrition, sarcopenia and frailty can be present, which disturb early mobilisation and rehabilitation after surgery. In addition to negative impacts of sarcopenia on short-term operative outcomes, long-term risks of adverse events, associated with sarcopenia, are also evident, with 1.6 to 3 times higher 3-year mortality after pancreatic resection, liver transplantation and resection of colorectal liver metastasis.[88] Progressive resistance training and nutrient modifications such as (whey) protein supplements with or without added leucine and vitamin D, either alone or in combination, are well-established interventions to reverse sarcopenia.[89] The recommended dietary allowance (RDA) for protein of 0.8 g/Kg/d is clearly insufficient in aged individuals, for whom a protein allowance of 1.25 to 1.5 g/Kg is more advisable. A very recent meta-analysis investigated the role of added protein or amino acid supplements in people 60 years and older who received 6 weeks or more of resistance training. The nine RCTs showed a gain in fat-free mass, which was not associated with changes in muscle mass or muscle strength, when compared with control groups undergoing only resistance training.[90] Three studies quantified the protein supplementation to body mass of patients with 0.3 to 0.8 g/Kg/d extra protein (mean: 0.46 g/Kg/d). The others provided mean amount of proteins of 20.7 (range: 6–40) g/d. Study quality was low, and the authors suggested improvements to maximise the gains in muscle mass and strength by providing enough energy to support the building of muscle mass and by timing the protein ingestion close to the performance of resistance exercise. Physical activity is medicine for older adults, and probably, as such, it is difficult to be surpassed by nutrition.[91]

Oral nutritional supplements were investigated in two meta-analyses in elderly patients with hip fracture. The first mentioned that the evidence was too weak to draw definite conclusions about ONS for elderly patients with hip fracture, whether surgery was performed or not.[92] The second focussed on hip surgery and found positive effects on the serum total protein, a significantly decreased number of complications and significant decreases in wound, respiratory and urinary tract infections.[93]

Obesity

Almeida et al found that 30% of GI surgical patients were overweight or obese.[10] A median involuntary weight loss of 7 Kg was found in 70% patients, of whom 25% were still classified as being overweight or obese. Of those patients classified by the NRI as being at risk, 61% were overweight or obese.[10] Obese patients pose unique problems for surgeons, not only because of their pre-existing obesity-associated comorbidities but also because of a greater likelihood to develop postoperative complications such as wound dehiscence, nosocomial infections, respiratory complications and delayed cardiac recuperation.

There exists a profound misunderstanding that obese patients have plenty of 'energy storage' in their fat mass, and aggressive nutrition intervention is not needed.[32,86,94,95] However, many of (morbidly) obese surgical patients have sarcopenic obesity, and 15 to 20% are deficient in at least one micronutrient and are thus at risk of further loss of LBM through gluconeogenesis and micronutrient deficiency during times of acute stress.[18,29,86] Permissive underfeeding is intentional underfeeding. Patients receive 60 to 70% of their caloric requirements while receiving protein provision that meets or exceeds their requirements, with the intention to maintain LBM. Two meta-analysis investigated permissive underfeeding.[84,96] Owais et al showed improved outcome and reduced morbidity in critically ill patients but noted clinical heterogeneity in the eight RCTs and also warned that underfeeding occurred by default rather than by intention.[96] Jiang et al evaluated five RCTs, with four RCTs dealing with GI surgical patients.[84] Intentional underfeeding with PN in the postoperative setting reduced infection by 40% and LOHS by 2.5 days, compared with full caloric provision at goal. Albeit the evidence upon which the recommendation is based is weak, suggested caloric requirements for obese patients are 22 to 25 Kcal/Kg IBW (or 11–14 Kcal/Kg actual body weight) per day, with 2 g protein/Kg IBW at BMI 30 to 40 Kg/m^2 and 2.5 g protein/Kg IBW at BMI ≥40 Kg/m^2 per day.[59,94,95] A retrospective study of hypocaloric high-protein enteral tube feeding according to these recommendations appeared to be effective and safe.[97] For bariatric surgery patients, a clinical practice guideline has recently been published.[98]

SPECIFIC SURGICAL PROCEDURES

There are two surgical procedures, that is, oesophagectomy and pancreatoduodenectomy, where the surgery is based on preoperative data, experience and predictors of postoperative complications, and need of neoadjuvant therapy has to decide on establishing a route for feeding, such as a jejunostomy.

Oesophagectomy

Early enteral feeding after oesophagectomy can be given orally, via a jejunostomy or via a nasojejunal tube. However, the best feeding route is as yet unclear. A systematic review, including 17 eligible studies on early oral intake (3 studies), nasojejunal tube feeding (1 study) or jejunostomy (13 studies), is not helpful in the right decision making.[99] Early oral intake (vs. tube feed or nil per os) did not result in an increased incidence of anastomotic leakage or pneumonia. Length of hospital stay was significantly shorter. Comparison of nasojejunal tube with jejunostomy feeding showed similar outcomes and tube-related complications were found in 29% and 38%, respectively. Dislocation in about one-fifth to one-third of patients is the most frequently reported complication of tubes. Jejunostomy tubes (JTs) not only had minor complications such as entry site infection and leakage but also had major complications resulting in reoperation in 0 to 2.9% and a mortality in up to 0.5% patients. Poor attainment of nutritional needs in studies that reported intake and weight changes is very disappointing.

Pancreatoduodenectomy

Few studies have focussed on the relation between oral nutrition or EN and postoperative complications such as DGE, postoperative pancreatic fistula (POPF) and postpancreatic haemorrhage (PPH). In 2006, Goonetilleke and Siriwardena addressed the role of routine perioperative nutritional support by EN or PN after pancreatoduodenectomy (PD).[100] They showed that early postoperative PN was not associated with improved outcomes, whereas the administration of postoperative EN resulted in decreased infectious complications. A recent meta-analysis by Shen et al evaluated the safety and efficacy of early EN after PD.[101] Enteral nutrition did not increase the rate of DGE. It appeared safe and well-tolerated, even if it did not reveal any advantages in terms of POPF, PPH, LOS and infectious complications. A systematic review of five feeding routes after pancreatoduodenectomy, with LOHS as the primary outcome, also investigated normal oral nutrition.[102] Fifteen studies and 3474 patients were included: 2210 patients on oral diet, 424 on PN and the remainder on EN via a nasojejunal feeding tube (NJT, 165), gastrojejunostomy tube (GJT, 52) or a JT (623). Length of hospital stay was shortest, 15 days, in the oral-diet and GJT groups, followed by 19 days in the JT group, 20 days in the TPN group and 25 days in the NJT group. Normal solid food was taken after 6 days in the oral-diet group. However, also a higher incidence of vomiting was reported in one study (29.2% in the oral-diet vs. 10% in the enterally fed group), whereas 29.4% of patients in the oral-diet group in another study needed TPN at some point in their hospital stay because of complications such as DGE. Tube-related problems, addressed in two studies, showed blockage and dislodgement in 30.6% of all NJT, GJT and JT together. The review concluded that oral nutrition may be considered the preferred strategy after PD, without evidence to support routine enteral or parenteral feeding. However, one should realise that LOHS is influenced by many other factors and that oral feeding might be a 'function test' of the GI tract and, as such, characterising a group with having a more favourable outcome.

CONCLUSIONS

During the first visit of a patient referred for elective surgery, attention is given to surgical planning, cardiopulmonary risk stratification and assessment of the severity of the surgical insult with its associated risks of infectious morbidity and duration of hospitalisation. Though mandatory, nutritional assessment of surgical patients is often neglected. Patients should be identified as being at nutritional risk by adequate instruments. The NRS-2002 has been validated for use in surgical patients. Malnourished patients have a significantly higher morbidity and mortality, a longer LOHS and increased hospital costs. Special attention should be paid to the elderly and obese patient.

In malnourished patients planned to undergo major GI surgery, the operation should be postponed in order to allow for a 7- to 10-day nutritional rehabilitation period of oral supplemental nutrition or EN—and, by exception, PN—though not with the intention to completely reverse the malnutrition status. Parenteral nutrition for a period of at least 7 to 10 days is indicated when oral or enteral feeding is contraindicated or not tolerated. Preoperatively, oral immunonutrition is of benefit in cancer patients, both in well-nourished patients and in patients at nutritional risk.

Prolonged fasting should be avoided, and a carbohydrate drink 2 hours before the operation should be advised. During the operation, measures should be taken that favour a rapid recovery of the GI tract postoperatively. In addition, the need of an enteral access should be considered.

In the postoperative period, patients should resume their normal oral intake or the intake of oral supplements within 24 hours. In malnourished patients, EN should be instituted immediately after surgery. Parenteral nutrition is indicated in severely malnourished patients who cannot tolerate enteral feeding. It is indicated after 7 days of trial of EN in patients with impaired GI function after postoperative complications.

Adequate perioperative nutrition has convincingly shown to improve clinical outcome in patients undergoing major GI surgery. This knowledge is also embedded in the ERAS guidelines. Thus, there is ample evidence that adequate nutrition support should be integrated in the general care of the surgical patient.

REFERENCES

1. Miller KR, Wischmeyer PE, Taylor B, McClave SA. An evidence-based approach to perioperative nutrition support in the elective surgery patient. *JPEN J Parenter Enteral Nutr* 2013;37:39S–50S.

2. Schiesser M, Müller S, Kirchhoff P, Breitenstein S, Schäfer M, Clavien P-A. Assessment of a novel screening score for nutritional risk in predicting complications in gastrointestinal surgery. *Clin Nutr* 2008;27:565–70.

3. Schiesser M, Kirchhoff P, Müller S, Schäfer M, Clavien P-A. The correlation of nutrition risk index, nutrition risk score, and bioimpedance analysis with postoperative complications in patients undergoing gastrointestinal surgery. *Surgery* 2009;145:519–26.

4. Schwegler I, von Holzen A, Gutzwiller J-P, Schlumpf R, Mühlebach S, Stanga Z. Nutritional risk is a clinical predictor of postoperative mortality and morbidity in surgery for colorectal cancer. *Brit J Surg* 2010;97:92–7.

5. Guo W, Ou G, Li X, Huang J, Liu J, Wei H. Screening of the nutritional risk of patients with gastric carcinoma before operation by NRS 2002 and its relationship with postoperative results. *J Gastroenterol Hepatol* 2010; 25:800–3.

6. Awad A, Lobo DN. What's new in perioperative nutritional support? *Curr Opin Anesthesiol* 2011;24:339–348.

7. Kuppinger D, Hartl WH, Bertok M, et al. Nutritional screening for risk prediction in patients scheduled for abdominal operations. *Brit J Surg* 2012;99:728–37.

8. Lochs H, Allison SP, Meier R, et al. Introductory to the ESPEN Guidelines on enteral nutrition: terminology, definitions and general topics. *Clin Nutr* 2006;25:180–6.

9. Cederholm T, Bosaeus I, Barazzoni R, et al. Diagnostic criteria for malnutrition. An ESPEN Consensus Statement. *Clin Nutr* 2015;34:335–40.

10. Almeida AI, Correia M, Camilo M, Ravasco P. Nutritional risk screening in surgery: Valid, feasible, easy! *Clin Nutr* 2012;31:206–11.

11. Burden ST, Hill J, Shaffer JL, Todd C. Nutritional status of preoperative colorectal cancer patients. *J Hum Nutr Diet* 2010;23:402–7.

12. Ho JWC, Wu AHW, Lee MWK, et al. Malnutrition risk predicts surgical outcomes in patients undergoing gastrointestinal operations: results of a prospective study. *Clin Nutr* 2015;34:679–84.

13. Mueller C, Compher C, Ellen DM; the American Society for Parenteral and Enteral Nutrition (A.S.P.E.N.) Board of Directors. A.S.P.E.N. clinical guidelines: nutrition screening, assessment, and intervention in adults. *JPEN J Parenter Enteral Nutr* 2011;35:16–24.

14. Kondrup J, Rasmussen HH, Hamberg O, Stanga Z. Nutritional risk screening (NRS 2002): a new method based on an analysis of controlled clinical trials. *Clin Nutr* 2003;22:321–36.

15. Reilly HM, Martineau JK, Moran A, Kennedy H. Nutritional screening evaluation and implementation of a simple Nutrition Risk Score. *Clin Nutr* 1995;14:269–73.

16. Elia M. *Screening for Malnutrition: A Multidisciplinary Responsibility. Development and Use of the Malnutrition Universal Screening Tool ("MUST") For Adults.* Malnutrition Advisory Group (MAG), a standing committee of BAPEN. Redditch, Worcestershire, U.K.: BAPEN; 2003. ISBN: 1899467 70 X.

17. Martindale RG, McClave SA, Taylor B, Lawson CM. Perioperative nutrition: what Is the current landscape? *J Parenter Enteral Nutr* 2013;37:5S–20S.

18. Thomas Schricker, Ralph Lattermann. Perioperative catabolism. *Can J Anaesth* 2015;62:182–93.

19. Abunnaja S, Andrea Cuviello A, Sanchez JA. Enteral and parenteral nutrition in the perioperative period: State of the Art. *Nutrients* 2013;5:608–23.

20. Thorell A, Nygren J, Ljungqvist O. Insulin resistance: a marker of surgical stress. *Curr Opin Clin Nutr Metab Care* 1999;2:69–78.

21. Bozetti F. Peri-operative nutritional management. *Proc Nutr Soc* 2011;70:305–10.

22. Ljungqvist O, Nygren J, Thorell A. Insulin resistance and elective surgery. *Surgery* 2000;128:757–60.

23. Guirao X. Impact of inflammatory reaction on intermediary metabolism and nutrition status. *Nutrition* 2002;18:949–52.

24. Rothman DL, Magnusson I, Katz LD, Shulman RG, Shulman GI. Quantitation of hepatic glycogenolysis and gluconeogenesis in fasting humans with 13C NMR. *Science* 1991;254:573–6.

25. Evans WJ, Morley JE, Argiles J, et al. Cachexia: a new definition. *Clin Nutr* 2008;27:793–9.

26. Muscaritoli M, Anker SD, Argile J, et al. Consensus definition of sarcopenia, cachexia and pre-cachexia: Joint document elaborated by Special Interest Groups (SIG) "cachexia-anorexia in chronic wasting diseases" and "nutrition in geriatrics". *Clin Nutr* 2010;29:154–9.

27. Fried LP, Tangen CM, Walston J, et al. Frailty in older adults: evidence for a phenotype. *J Gerontol Med Sci* 2001;56A:M146–56.

28. Braga M, Ljungqvist O, Soeters P, Fearon K, Weimann A, Bozzetti F. ESPEN guidelines on parenteral nutrition: surgery. *Clin Nutr* 2009;28:378–86.

29. Evans DC, Martindale RG, Kiraly LN, Jones CM. Nutrition optimization prior to surgery. *Nutr Clin Pract* 2014;29:10–21.

30. Weimann A, Braga M, Harsanyi L, et al. ESPEN guidelines on enteral nutrition: surgery including organ transplantation. *Clin Nutr* 2006;25:224–44.

31. Kondrup J, Allison SP, Elia M, Vellas B, Plauth M. ESPEN guidelines for nutrition screening 2002. *Clin Nutr* 2003;22:415–21.

32. McClave SA, Kozar R, Martindale RG, et al. Summary points and consensus recommendations from the North American Surgical Nutrition Summit. *JPEN J Parenter Enteral Nutr* 2013;37:99S–105S.

33. Li C, Carli F, Lee L, et al. Impact of a trimodal prehabilitation program on functional recovery after colorectal cancer surgery: a pilot study. *Surg Endosc* 2013;27:1072–82.

34. Martindale RG, McClave SA, Taylor B, Lawson CM. Perioperative nutrition: what is the current landscape? *JPEN J Parenter Enteral Nutr* 2013;37:5S–20S.

35. McClave SA, Heyland DK. The physiologic response and associated clinical benefits from provision of early enteral nutrition. *Nutr Clin Pract* 2009;24:305–15.

36. McClave SA, Martindale R, Taylor B, Gramlich L. Appropriate use of parenteral nutrition through the perioperative period. *JPEN J Parenter Enteral Nutr* 2013;37:73S–82S.

37. Casaer MP, Mesotten D, Hermans G, et al. Early versus late parenteral nutrition in critically ill adults. *N Engl J Med* 2011;365:506–17.

38. Burden S, Todd C, Hill J, Lal S. Pre-operative nutrition support in patients undergoing gastrointestinal surgery. *Cochrane Data System Rev* 2012;11:CD008879.

39. Zhong J-X, Kang K, Shu X-L. Effect of nutritional support on clinical outcomes in perioperative malnourished patients: a meta-analysis. *Asia Pac J Clin Nutr* 2015;24:367–78.

40. Jie B, Jiang Z-M, Nolan MT, Zhu S-N, Yu K, Kondrup J. Impact of preoperative nutritional support on clinical outcome in abdominal surgical patients at nutritional risk. *Nutrition* 2012;28:1022–7.

41. Smedley F, Bowling T, James M, et al. Randomized clinical trial of the effects of preoperative and postoperative oral nutritional supplements on clinical course and cost of care. *Brit J Surg* 2004;91:983–90.

42. ASPEN Board of Directors and the Clinical Guidelines Task Force. Guidelines for the use of parenteral and enteral nutrition in adult and pediatric patients. *J Parenter Enteral Nutr* 2002;26:1SA–138SA.

43. Klein S, Kinney J, Jeejeebhoy K, et al. Nutrition support in clinical practice: review of published data and recommendations for future research directions. Summary of a conference sponsored by the National Institutes of Health, American Society for Parenteral and Enteral Nutrition, and American Society for Clinical Nutrition. *Am J Clin Nutr* 1997;66:683–706.

44. Mizock. Immunonutrition and critical illness: an update. *Nutrition* 2010;26:701–7.

45. Zhang Y, Gu Y, Guo T, Li Y, Cai H. Perioperative immunonutrition for gastrointestinal cancer: a systematic review of randomized controlled trials. *Surg Oncol* 2012; 21:e87–95.

46. Avenell A. Current evidence and ongoing trials on the use of glutamine in critically-ill patients and patients undergoing surgery. *Proc Nutr Soc* 2009;68:261–8.

47. Heyland D, Muscedere J, Wischmeyer PE, et al. A Randomized trial of glutamine and antioxidants in critically ill patients. *N Engl J Med* 2013;368:1489–97.

48. Yue C, Tian W, Wang W, et al. The impact of perioperative glutamine-supplemented parenteral nutrition on outcomes of patients undergoing abdominal surgery: a meta-analysis of randomized clinical trials. *Amer Surg* 2013;79: 506–13.

49. Drover JW, Dhaliwal R, Weitzel L, Wischmeyer PE, Ochoa JB, Heyland DK. Perioperative use of arginine-supplemented diets: a systematic review of the evidence. *J Am Coll Surg* 2011;212:385–399.

50. Marik PE, Zaloga GP. Immunonutrition in high-risk surgical patients: a systematic review and analysis of the literature. *J Parenter Enteral Nutr* 2010;34:378–86.

51. Mizock BA, Sriram K. Perioperative immunonutrition. *Expert Rev Clin Immunol* 2011;7:1–3.

52. Li N-N, Zhou Y, Qin X-P, et al. Does intravenous fish oil benefit patients post-surgery? A meta-analysis of randomised controlled trials. *Clin Nutr* 2014;33:226–39.

53. Braga M. Perioperative immunonutrition and gut function. *Curr Opin Clin Nutr Metab Care* 2012;15:485–8.

54. Cerantola Y, Hübner M, Grass F, Demartines N, Schäfer M. Immunonutrition in gastrointestinal surgery. *Brit J Surg* 2011;98:37–48.

55. Osland E, Hossain B, Khan S, Memon MA. Effect of timing of pharmaconutrition (immunonutrition) administration on outcomes of elective surgery for gastrointestinal malignancies: a systematic review and meta-analysis. *J Parenter Enteral Nutr* 2014; 38:53–69.

56. Song G-M, Tian X, Zhang L, et al. Immunonutrition support for patients undergoing surgery for gastrointestinal malignancy: preoperative, postoperative, or perioperative? A Bayesian network meta-analysis of randomized controlled trials. *Medicine* 2015;94:e1225.

57. Chevrou-Séverac H, Pinget C, Cerantola Y, Demartines N, Wasserfallen J-B, Schäfer M. Cost-effectiveness analysis of immune-modulating nutritional support for gastrointestinal cancer patients. *Clin Nutr* 2014;33: 649–54.

58. Kreymann KG, Berger MM, Deutz NEP, et al. ESPEN guidelines on enteral nutrition: intensive care. *Clin Nutr* 2006;26:210–23.

59. Martindale RG, McClave SA, Vanek VW, et al. Guidelines for the provision and assessment of nutrition support therapy in the adult critically ill patient: Society of Critical Care Medicine and American Society for Parenteral and Enteral Nutrition: executive summary. *Crit Care Med* 2009; 37:1757–61.

60. Heyland DK, Dhaliwal R, Drover JW, Gramlich L, Dodek P; Canadian Critical Care Clinical Practice Guidelines Committee. Canadian practice guidelines for nutrition support in mechanically ventilated, critically ill adult patients. *J Parenter Enteral Nutr* 2003;27:355–73.

61. Brady MC, Kinn S, Stuart P, Ness V. Preoperative fasting for adults to prevent perioperative complications. *Cochrane Data Syst Rev* 2003;4:CD004423. Updated 2010.

62. Ljungqvist O, Thorell A, Gutniak M, Häggmark T, Efendic S. Glucose infusion instead of ppreoperative fasting redcued postoprative insulin resistance. *J Am Coll Surg* 1994;178:329–36.

63. Ljungqvist O, Nygren J, Hausel J, Thorell A. Preoperative nutrition therapy—novel developments. *Scand J Nutr* 2000; 44:3–7.

64. Nygren J. The metabolic effects of fasting and surgery. *Best Pract Red Clin Anaesthesiol* 2006;20:429–38.

65. Smith MD, McCall J, Plank L, Herbison GP, Soop M, Nygren J. Preoperative carbohydrate treatment for enhancing recovery after elective surgery. *Cochrane Data Syst Rev* 2014;8:CD009161.

66. Awad S, Varadhan KK, Ljungqvist O, Lobo DN. A meta-analysis of randomised controlled trials on preoperative oral carbohydrate treatment in elective surgery. *Clin Nutr* 2013;32:34–44.

67. Fearon KCH, Ljungqvist O, Von Meyenfeldt M, et al. Enhanced recovery after surgery: A consensus review of clinical care for patients undergoing colonic resection. *Clin Nutr* 2005;24:466–77.

68. Fitzgerald JE, Ahmed I. Systematic review and meta-analysis of chewing-gum therapy in the reduction of postoperative paralytic ileus following gastrointestinal surgery. *World J Surg* 2009;33:2557–66.

69. Nygren J, Soop M, Thorell A, Hausel J, Ljungqvist O. An enhanced-recovery protocol improves outcome after colorectal resection already during the first year: a single-center

experience in 168 consecutive patients. *Dis Colon Rectum* 2009;52:978–85.

70. Gustafsson UO, Scott MJ, Schwenk W, et al. Guidelines for perioperative care in elective colonic surgery: Enhanced Recovery After Surgery (ERAS) Society recommendations. *Clin Nutr* 2012;31:783–800.

71. Nygren J, Thacker J, Carli F, et al. Guidelines for perioperative care in elective rectal/pelvic surgery: Enhanced Recovery After Surgery (ERAS) Society recommendations. *Clin Nutr* 2012;31:801–16.

72. Lassen K, Coolsen MME, Slim K, et al. Guidelines for perioperative care for pancreaticoduodenectomy: Enhanced Recovery After Surgery (ERAS®) Society recommendations. *Clin Nutr* 2012;31:817–30.

73. Bozzetti F, Mariani L. Perioperative nutritional support of patients undergoing pancreatic surgery in the age of ERAS. *Nutrition* 2014;30:1267–71.

74. Bozzetti F, Gianotti L, Braga M, Di Carlo V, Mariani L. Postoperative complications in gastrointestinal cancer patients: the joint role of the nutritional status and the nutritional support. *Clin Nutr* 2007;26:698–709.

75. Lewis SJ, Egger M, Sylvester PA, Thomas S. Early enteral feeding versus "nil by mouth" after gastrointestinal surgery: systematic review and meta-analysis of controlled trials. *BMJ* 2001;323:773–6.

76. Lewis SJ, Andersen HK, Steve Thomas S. Early enteral nutrition within 24 h of intestinal surgery versus later commencement of feeding: A systematic review and meta-analysis. *J Gastrointest Surg* 2009;13:569–75.

77. Andersen HK, Lewis SJ, Thomas S. Early enteral nutrition within 24h of colorectal surgery versus later commencement of feeding for postoperative complications. *Cochrane Data Syst Rev* 2006;4:CD004080. Updated 2011.

78. Osland E, Yunus RM, Khan S, Memon MA. Early versus traditional postoperative feeding in patients undergoing resectional gastrointestinal surgery: a meta-analysis. *JPEN J Parenter Enteral Nutr* 2011;35:483–7.

79. Bozzetti F, Braga M, Gianotti L, Gavazzi C, Mariani L. Postoperative enteral versus parenteral nutrition in malnourished patients with gastrointestinal cancer: a randomised multicentre trial. *Lancet* 2001;358:1487–92.

80. Beattie AH, Prach AT Baxter JP, Pennington CR. A randomised controlled trial evaluating the use of enteral nutritional supplements postoperatively in malnourished surgical patients. *Gut* 2000;46:813–8.

81. Maessen JCM, Hoff C, Jottard K, et al. To eat or not to eat: Facilitating early oral intake after elective colonic surgery in the Netherlands. *Clin Nutr* 2009;28:29–33.

82. Braunschweig CL, Levy P, Sheean PM, Wang X. Enteral compared with parenteral nutrition: a meta-analysis. *Am J Clin Nutr* 2001;74:534–42.

83. Bozzetti F, Gavazzi C, Miceli R, et al. Perioperative total parenteral nutrition in malnourished, gastrointestinal cancer patients: a randomized, clinical trial. *J Parenter Enteral Nutr* 2000;24:7–14.

84. Jiang H, Sun MW, Hefright B, Chen W, Lu CD, Zeng J. Efficacy of hypocaloric parenteral nutrition for surgical patients: a systematic review and meta-analysis. *Clin Nutr* 2011;30:730–7.

85. Casaer MP, Wilmer A, Hermans G, Wouters PJ, Mesotten D, Van den Berghe G. Role of disease and macronutrient dose in the randomized controlled EPaNIC trial: a post hoc analysis. *Am J Respir Crit Care Med* 2013;187:247–55.

86. Cullen A, Ferguson A. Perioperative management of the severely obese patient: a selective pathophysiological review. *Can J Anaesth* 2012;59:974–96.

87. Vellas B, Guigoz Y, Garry PJ, et al. The Mini Nutritional Assessment (MNA) and its use in grading the nutritional state of elderly patients. *Nutrition* 1999;15:116–22.

88. Fujita T. Perioperative strategy for severe nutritional risk-related frail patients. *J Am Coll Surg* 2015;220:977–9.

89. Malarafina V, Uriz-Otano F, Iniesta R, Gil-Guerrero L. Effectiveness of nutritional supplementation on muscle mass in treatment of sarcopenia in old age: a systematic review. *J Am Med Dir Assoc* 2013;14:10–7.

90. Finger D, Reistenbach Goltz F, et al. Effects of protein supplementation in older adults undergoing resistance training: a systematic review. *Sports Med* 2015;45:245–55.

91. Taylor D. Physical activity is medicine for older aldults. *Postgrad Med J* 2014;90:26–32.

92. Avenell A, Handoll HHG. Nutritional supplementation for hip fracture aftercare in older people (review). *Cochrane Data Syst Rev* 2010;1:CD001880.

93. Liu M, Yang J, Yu X, et al. The role of perioperative oral nutritional supplementation in elderly patients after hip surgery. *Clin Intervent Aging* 2015;10:849–58.

94. McClave SA, Kushner R, Van Way CW, et al. Nutrition therapy of the severely obese, critically ill patient: summation of conclusions and recommendations. *J Parenter Enteral Nutr* 2011;35:88S–96S.

95. Kaafarani HMA, Shikora SA. Nutritional support of the obese and critically ill obese patient. *Surg Clin N Am* 2011;91:837–55.

96. Owais AE, Bumby RF, MacFie J. Review article: permissive underfeeding in short-term nutritional support. *Aliment Pharmacol Ther* 2010;32:628–36.

97. Dickerson RN, Boschert KJ, Kudsk KA, Brown RO. Hypocaloric enteral tube feeding in critically ill obese patients. *Nutrition* 2002;18:241–6.

98. Mechanick JI, Youdim A, Jones DB, et al. Clinical practice guidelines for the perioperative nutritional, metabolic, and nonsurgical support of the bariatric surgery patient—2013 update: cosponsored by American Association of Clinical Endocrinologists, the Obesity Society, and American Society for Metabolic & Bariatric Surgery. *Obesity* 2013;21:S1–S25.

99. Weijs TJ, Berkelmans GHK, Nieuwenhuijzen GAP, et al. Routes for early enteral nutrition after esophagectomy. A systematic review. *Clin Nutr* 2015;34:1–6.

100. Goonetilleke KS, Siriwardena AK. Systematic review of peri-operative nutritional supplementation in patients undergoing pancreaticoduodenectomy. *JOP* 2006; 7:5–13.

101. Shen Y, Jin W. Early enteral nutrition after pancreatoduodenectomy: a meta-analysis of randomized controlled trials. *Langenbecks Arch Surg* 2013;398:817–23.

102. Gerritsen A, Besselink MGH, Gouma DJ, Steenhagen E, Borel Rinkes IHM, Molenaar IQ. Systematic review of five feeding routes after pancreatoduodenectomy. *Brit J Surg* 2013;100:589–98.

6

Severe Surgical Sepsis and Peritonitis after Gastrointestinal Surgery: Pathophysiology, Clinical Signs and Treatment

P.B. Soeters

ABSTRACT

Abdominal sepsis arising spontaneously or after abdominal surgery is responsible for substantial morbidity and mortality. Prevention of these complications not only depends on technical skills but also on surgical strategy and perioperative nonsurgical treatment. Optimal diagnostic skills are required. When should immediate intervention be performed and when is there still time for diagnostic procedures? These procedures could establish the origin of sepsis, facilitating treatment with minimal-invasive techniques or guiding the surgical approach. Treatment should also depend on a risk analysis (nutritional assessment, including inflammatory activity and functional capacities) to tailor the extent of surgery to healing capacity. In elective surgery, this capacity should be optimised, improving nutritional state, muscle and organ function and haemoglobin levels and stopping smoking and steroids, if possible. After surgery, clinical signs, laboratory results and fluid balance indicate whether patient is recovering well or whether reintervention is required. Leaking anastomoses should be diagnosed early and treated urgently following similar principles as in acute abdominal infection. Postoperative sepsis often heralds the development of enterocutaneous fistulas and may lead to abdominal wall and skin dehiscence and exposure of the fistula(s) in open wounds. Their treatment requires setting priorities for treatment (especially sepsis) and adherence to a time frame (SOWATS protocol). In this chapter, pathophysiology and clinical signs of all these elements will be discussed in detail, including prevention and treatment of acute or postoperative peritonitis and sepsis, as well as their sequelae such as enterocutaneous fistulas.

KEYWORDS

Surgical sepsis, sepsis, peritonitis, inflammation, malnutrition, nutritional assessment, enterocutaneous fistula, albumin, fat-free mass, body composition, pathophysiology, clinical signs, SOWATS protocol, cognitive function, immune function, muscle function, postoperative infection

INTRODUCTION

In this chapter, factors determining immediate postoperative surgical outcome will be described. Especially, infectious complications are the most frequent and most feared complications after surgery. Prevention of these complications does not only depend on technical skills but also on other more holistic aspects of treatment. Similarly, management of patients that present with acute abdominal infections should, besides surgical technique, include nonsurgical treatment aspects to achieve optimal results. These aspects play crucial roles in the healing process before, during and after surgery.

Acute abdominal infections require optimal diagnostic skills. Is acute intervention necessary, should computed tomographic (CT) scanning always be performed, can the septic focus be treated with minimal-invasive radiology or ultrasound-guided techniques, is there room for a conservative approach—all are factors that should be considered. In addition, both in acute and in postoperative infections, a risk analysis or nutritional assessment should have been performed to decide whether surgical treatment can be aggressive (for instance, creating anastomoses and extensive regional surgery for malignancies) or defensive (damage control: for instance, drainage and temporary stomata after resection of a perforated segment of bowel).

In elective surgery, there is time to optimise the condition of the patient in several ways and it is crucial to do this to improve the outcome.

After operation, the time course of normal and abnormal healing will be described and indicated, and which signals should lead to intervention and how to intervene will also be discussed. Especially, the management of leaking anastomoses and intestinal fistulas as well as the adequacy of early source control will be emphasised.

PREOPERATIVE MANAGEMENT

In this section, we will describe the risk analysis and methods to improve the preoperative condition of the patient.

Risk Analysis

Nutritional Assessment

Modern methods to assess nutritional state include an estimate of function, indicating whether the patient can generate a healthy healing response. This should give guidance whether the patient will successfully heal from major surgery with anastomoses or requires a less elaborate operation, without taking the risk of performing extensive oncologic surgery or multiple anastomoses.

Malnutrition is defined by some as 'a subacute or chronic state of nutrition, in which a combination of varying degrees of undernutrition (negative nutrient balance) and inflammatory activity has led to changes in body composition and diminished function and clinical outcome'[1–3] (Table 6.1). Others leave out inflammation, which leads to a heated debate between national and international nutritional and metabolic societies. [2,4] Regardless of the definition, it is crucial to assess inflammation, while analysing risk of treatment, in view of interfering with an adequate immune response after surgery. Consequently, nutrient balance, body composition,

Table 6.1 Nutritional assessment defines function, body composition and causes of dysfunction (undernutrition and inflammation)

Nutritional assessment/risk analysis	
Undernutrition	**Inflammation**

Decreases FFM/muscle mass/FM
Decreases function
  Wound, bone, anastomotic healing
  Immune function
  Muscle force/endurance, ADL
  Cognition
When nutritional intake is inadequate, dysfunction depends on the degree of undernutrition and takes longer to develop than in the presence of inflammation. (significant when loss > 10% BW)
	Causes catabolism in peripheral tissues (muscle, bone, skin)
	Decreases function
	  Wound, bone, anastomotic healing
	  Muscle force/endurance, ADL
	  Immune function (second hit)
	  Cognition
	*Dysfunction occurs even when nutritional intake is adequate
	Infectious inflammation increases risk more than noninfectious inflammation*

Laboratory values	**Laboratory values**
Hb slowly decreasing Na normal CRP low Albumin normal Creatinine low Leucocytes normal unless cachectic	Hb quickly decreasing Na low unless Na administered CRP elevated Albumin decreased (dysfunction significant when <35 g/L) Creatinine elevated Leucocytes elevated unless hypodynamic sepsis: leucopenia with left shift
Body composition	**Body composition**
Slowly decreasing fat-free mass, normal water content FM decreases BW decreases slowly	Rapidly decreasing FFM solids Positive fluid balance, leading to increased water content FM only decreases when nutritional intake is insufficient BW may not decrease due to increased water content: oedema

Abbreviations: ADL, activities of daily living; FFM, fat-free mass; FM, fat mass; BW, body weight; CRP, C-reactive protein; Hb, Haemoglobin; BW, body weight; Na, Sodium.

inflammatory activity, and muscle, immune and cognitive function should be assessed. There has always been much resistance against the measurement of body composition, requiring much time or sophisticated equipment. However, activation of a function available in the software of modern CT and magnetic resonance imaging (MRI) can achieve a rather precise impression of body composition.[5] In view of CTs or MRIs performed almost routinely before major abdominal surgery, this would furnish a measure of body composition. Specifically, fat-free mass is of interest, as it determines to a major extent nutritional state and health.

Pre-existing inflammatory activity is equally important as undernutrition and is a cause of diminished fat-free mass and dysfunction. It causes a deficient immune and healing response to an additional trauma, which is well known as the phenomenon of the 'second hit,' already described by Moore,[6] who was one of the founding fathers of surgical metabolism. The second hit phenomenon was modelled at a later stage.[7,8] The notion implies that when a patient is in an inflammatory state due to recent shock, trauma or infectious or noninfectious illnesses, the capacity to generate a renewed adequate host response is compromised. Not only is immune function diminished but also muscle force and cognition.

All this knowledge should be taken into account when treating, for instance, old and frail patients. Treatment should be right the first time, because when (infectious) complications occur, patients cannot be weaned from the respirator, owing to further deterioration of their ability to perform muscle work. Even after clean uncomplicated surgery, the response to a second challenge (trauma, operation and infection) is weakened.[9]

Surgery also increases the virulence of *Pseudomonas aeruginosa* and possibly other microorganisms.[10] The group of Alverdy has done much research, elucidating mechanisms.[11] Bacteria are apparently able to sense the host's stress and then can upregulate their virulence. If possible, infection should be treated before performing surgery. When this is impossible and immediate surgery must be performed, it should be defensive, removing the septic focus, without performing hazardous anastomoses (*see* **Operation**). In this chapter, we will refer repeatedly to the dysfunctional state caused by the combined actions of 'undernutrition and inflammation'.

At the bedside or in the outpatient clinic, a few specifically selected questions and one 'test' may already obtain a fair impression of the condition of the patient:

- Did you lose weight?
- Can you climb stairs? Do you shop yourself? Do you practice sports? How is your memory? Do you still practice your hobbies?
- Give me a firm handshake.

Anaemia

Many patients with abdominal cancer, cardiovascular disease or benign inflammatory disease have anaemia, which may have different causes. Low-grade long-standing inflammation and malnutrition may suppress bone marrow activity. Anaemia has been found to be strongly correlated with hypoalbuminaemia and may be caused by depression of the bone marrow by chronic inflammation, without exception, leading to low plasma albumin levels.[12] Consequently, the anaemia of malnutrition can be caused by overall depletion, specific deficiencies (iron and folic acid) and inflammation. Another cause of anaemia is blood loss, often accompanying benign or malignant conditions in the abdomen. Morphological classification based on mean corpuscular volume is due to these different coinciding causes, generally difficult to accurately define the pathogenesis of anaemia in the elderly.[13] In recent decades, transfusions (especially with whole blood or blood older than 3 weeks) to normalise haemoglobin (Hb) levels before operation have become unpopular in view of negative effects on the immune response[14] and increased risk to develop postoperative complications.[15,16] According to the 2012 guidelines 'Surviving Sepsis Campaign', a transfusion indication exists at an Hb levels less than 4.4 mmol/L (1B recommendation). In case of cardiovascular instability or a central-venous saturation (ScvO$_2$) < 70%, an Hb level of at least 6 mmol/L is aimed for.[17] Preoperative anaemia as an independent risk factor has been well established.[18] Similarly, oral iron supplementation does not appear to be beneficial, but intravenous iron supplementation may increase Hb levels, especially when anaemia is caused by iron deficiency related to bleeding or lack of intake.[19] At present, in some institutions, studies are performed to assess the potential benefit of intravenous iron before elective operations, hopefully increasing Hb concentrations.

Intoxication

Smoking and substantial alcohol intake increase infectious complications and mortality after surgery,[7,20] although in plastic surgery, smokers tend to have thinner and smaller scars but with lower tensile strength. Both addictions cause mild but chronic inflammation, which may explain a lower healing tendency after the 'second hit' of the operation. It is neither clearly proven nor refuted that discontinuing smoking for a month or longer diminishes the risk of infectious complications and mortality.

Although it was known since decades that nonsteroidal anti-inflammatory drugs (NSAIDs) increase the risk to develop heart failure, renal dysfunction and gastrointestinal

(GI) ulcer formation with all their sequelae,[21] it becomes apparent that especially the nonspecific NSAIDs rather than the specific Cox-2 inhibitors increase the likelihood of developing anastomotic breakdown and disturbed wound healing.[22] Large prospective randomised studies should answer the question which drugs effectively treat pain, without interfering with anastomotic and wound healing. The adage not to use opioids in view of their depressing effect on intestinal motility and ventilation should be weighed against these harmful effects of NSAIDs. Epidural anaesthesia during and after operation may effectively treat pain, but which metabolic effects are caused is not very well investigated. Cardiovascular instability is a risk that should especially be taken into account in patients with cardiac pump failure using NSAIDs and receiving epidural anaesthesia.

Many patients are operated while on steroids. Operation can be successful, but when complications develop, they are often diagnosed late because of the mitigation of symptoms of infection. This threatens to delay intervention and increase mortality. Steroids should, therefore, preferably be discontinued at least a month before operation, if possible. Nevertheless, steroids must be resumed shortly before and some days after operation, depending on whether adrenal function has not yet recovered.

Neoadjuvant chemotherapy is advocated and applied in colonic and other types of GI surgery. Care should be taken to exclude patients that are frail, which, by definition, includes low functional capacity. They lose even more fat-free mass while on chemotherapy before operation.

Cardiorespiratory Comorbidity

Patients with severe cardiorespiratory comorbidity generally will also prove to be malnourished, especially characterised by decreased muscle mass and muscle function. Patients with cardiac failure are prone not to survive infectious complications after surgery because of their inability to generate a hyperdynamic circulation required to meet requirements during sepsis. Similarly, patients with chronic obstructive pulmonary disease (COPD) Global Initiative for Chronic Obstructive Lung Disease (GOLD) grade 2 to 3 have the risk to develop ventilatory and respiratory failure when complications arise after abdominal surgery. In the presence of abdominal sepsis, compression atelectasis in the lower lung fields leads to shunting requiring increased cardiac output, and extravascular fluid overload will diminish alveolar diffusion capacity. Any major abdominal operation obligatorily leads to loss of muscle mass, diminishing muscle strength. In addition, muscle function is decreased by the septic state, even when muscle mass was adequate before the septic episode. Therefore, patients with bad lungs are difficult to wean from the respirator, are prone to develop ventilator-associated pneumonias (VAPs) and have a high risk to die once complications occur.

Consequently, severe cardiorespiratory failure should urge to perform defensive surgery with lesser dissection and less risky anastomoses.

Liver Failure

Child–Pugh score of 2 to 3 or a Model for End-Stage Liver Disease (MELD) score above 15 increases the complication risk in true liver failure several fold.[23] The liver is the most important immune organ, harbouring immune cells, producing acute phase proteins, clotting factors and a multitude of other proteins, with important roles in host defence, and it plays an important role in intermediary metabolism. Therefore, surgery should be defensive or not performed at all.

Renal Failure

Patients with chronic renal failure are generally malnourished, often suffer from low-grade inflammation and cardiovascular disease and are prone to develop postoperative complications.[24] Defensive surgery is indicated.

Disease, Organ Failure and Inflammation

Any disease and isolated or generalised organ failure are inflammatory conditions. Although it may be advisable to separately assess the presence of severe organ failure, its presence will also be reflected in the activation of acute-phase proteins such as C-reactive protein (CRP), albumin, procalcitonin and others.

Preoperative Preparation

Indications for Elective Surgery

Self-evidently indications for elective surgery should follow well-accepted surgical guidelines. In the presence of a clear indication, the risk to develop complications after surgery should be taken into account (*see* **Risk Analysis**). In the presence of an increased risk, a defensive approach might be followed and less extensive surgery should be performed. In surgery, it is well accepted not to institute full treatment (for instance, neoadjuvant chemotherapy, extensive surgery and adjuvant chemotherapy) but only institute treatment that is aimed to prevent immediate threats or to address complaints to improve quality of life, despite knowing that life expectancy may be shorter than if full treatment was performed and survived. In frail old (and sometimes young) patients, one may decide to refrain from surgical treatment and to institute other types of palliative treatment. Precise guidelines are difficult to establish, but cachexia (low fat-free mass and fat mass) and sarcopenia (low fat-free mass), combined with inflammation, are associated with a strongly elevated risk of treatment failure and may therefore lead to refrainment from surgery.

Preparation for Elective Surgery

In the absence of severe infection/inflammation, patients with malignancies and severe undernutrition benefit from preoperative nutritional support. Depending on the accessibility of the gut, this may consist of enteral supplements, tube feeding or parenteral nutritional support. In the presence of body weight loss of 5 Kg in 3 months or 10 Kg in 6 months, even 7 to 10 days of preoperative nutritional support benefits clinical outcome, despite the fact that, in this short period, changes in body composition have not been demonstrated.[25,26] Some evidence suggests that even in well-nourished patients, perioperative administration of 'immunonutrition', consisting of an enteral supplement with extra arginine, omega-3 fatty acids and RNA, has beneficial effects on postoperative infectious complications.[27] However, after several prospective, randomised, controlled trials (PRCTs) and meta-analyses, there is no convincing conclusion possible.[28] In patients that have lost more than 10% of their body weight (especially fat-free mass), longer courses of nutritional support might be instituted, provided that there is no acute severe infection with major systemic effects, which would require urgent intervention (for more detail, see Chapter 5).

When possible, other risk factors should be dealt with. A healthy lifestyle is recommendable and should especially include physical rehabilitation. Smoking and steroids should be stopped, preferably a month before operation (see **Preoperative Management, Intoxication**). In case of cardiorespiratory illness, ensuring cardiac recompensation and pulmonary rehabilitation is necessary. Beta-blockers are indicated only in patients with unstable angina pectoris. They have negative effects in patients without coronary insufficiency but with cardiomyopathy and pump failure,[29] possibly due to the interference with the necessity to increase cardiac output to meet increased metabolic demand while undergoing surgical trauma.[30]

Indications for Emergency Surgery

The approach to emergency surgery has substantially changed. Until two decades ago, medical history, physical examination, simple laboratory tests (Hb, leucocyte count, sedimentation rate, electrolytes, renal function, liver enzymes and urinary sediment), upright abdominal X-ray and chest X-ray were employed to diagnose an 'acute abdomen' and formed the basis to decide whether acute intervention was indicated. All aspects of abdominal examination, including inspection, auscultation, percussion, palpation and a rectal examination, were generally diligently executed in adults. On the basis of this examination, a decision was made whether acute intervention was necessary. In case of doubt, the examination was repeated 6 to 12 hours later and, generally, a definitive decision was taken whether to intervene acutely or not.

This approach has changed considerably. In many parts of the world, it is rare to perform surgery without sophisticated radiological examination. Ultrasound is used when an appendicitis or biliary problem is suspected. Alternatively, a CT scan is performed using enteral and parenteral contrast, enhancing the visibility of the intestinal lumen, the vasculature, abscesses and free gas outside the GI tract. The availability of these imaging techniques has greatly improved preoperative diagnosis. However, it has also increased the dependency on these techniques and hesitation to intervene acutely, even when clinical signs are severe and distinct. A balance should be found between the severity of the clinical findings and the desirability to confirm or establish a precise diagnosis, also guiding whether, and if so how, to intervene. Owing to uncertainty regarding a precise diagnosis, intervention is sometimes delayed for a day or days, leading to an increase in the severity of sepsis, deterioration of the condition of the patient and worse outcome.

Another important factor leading to this delay is that the radiological examination (for instance, CT scan) has diagnostic limitations. The first phase of ischaemia cannot be detected by CT scan. The conclusion 'no signs of ischaemia' of the radiologist, therefore, does not exclude the presence of ischaemic bowel, and this should be indicated in the report. Another concern is that in severely depleted patients, contrast enhancement of infected fluid collections is absent or diminished due to compromised immune function.

A short history of severe sickness; abdominal guarding; rare high-pitched bowel sounds in addition to leucocytosis, low albumin, low sodium, elevated levels of CRP and lactate; and cardiorespiratory instability may urge to perform acute surgery, laparoscopic or open, depending on the technical expertise of the attending surgeon. In case of a disease course of a week or longer, with signs of inflammation but in a stable cardiorespiratory condition and only localised abdominal guarding, more extensive diagnostic procedures can be performed, because the infectious disease process appears to be localised and not have led to organ failure. In case of localised abscesses without generalised peritonitis (appendicitis and diverticulitis), radiological drainage can be performed first, in case of diverticulitis, sometimes but not necessarily, followed by elective resection at a later stage, when infection has subsided.[31,32] The worst form of generalised sepsis presents in frail patients or in patients that have gone through a long course of infectious disease leading to severe depletion. It is characterised by somnolence or delirium at presentation, muscle weakness, marginal blood pressure, oliguria, hypothermia, leucopenia (with left shift), low Hb, very low plasma albumin and hyponatraemia, reflecting a hypodynamic form of sepsis. The prognosis of these patients is bad and early intervention is required, or one should consider not to institute surgery at all.

An often neglected cause of postponement of acute intervention is the inclination to ascribe infectious symptoms to easier-to-treat conditions. This occurs especially when patients are admitted to nonsurgical departments. Even when abdominal complaints prevail, pneumonia or urinary tract infections are often considered and treated as primary causes of the septic state. Pulmonary opacities on chest X-ray may arise from infectious processes below the diaphragm because of atelectasis and pleural effusions and are sometimes mistakenly interpreted as pneumonia. Modest leucocyturia may be caused by bladder catheters. Antibiotics are generally not effective in severe abdominal infection and may play a beneficial role only in mild cases of acute appendicitis or diverticulitis or temporarily in obstructive infectious cholangitis or obstructive pyelitis or pyelonephritis.

Acute (mechanical) small bowel obstruction of unknown pathogenesis should urge to acutely intervene to prevent the rapid occurrence of peritonitis due to increased permeability of the distended small bowel, even in the absence of macroscopic perforations. In this situation, hyperosmolar cathartics enterally administered and contrast enhancement by intravenous and enteral contrast may decrease the integrity of the distended small bowel.

OPERATION

Elective Operation

Elective operations in severely undernourished patients with low functional capacity but without significant

inflammation may still fail to overcome major surgery, when complications arise. Their condition will further deteriorate even when all elements of the protocol and all criteria of oncological surgery are followed.

Consequently, surgery may be less extensive. Critical anastomoses should not be performed, or they should be protected by temporary diverting stomata, even when this requires additional surgery after full-recovery months later. Neoadjuvant chemotherapy and radiotherapy may be omitted, because they will further deteriorate the clinical condition of a frail patient and lead to surgical treatment failure, complications and mortality. Surgical treatment may be palliative, for instance, relieving obstruction. Alternatively, treatment should be restricted to nonsurgical forms of palliative therapy. In younger patients in good condition, more risk can be taken, because even when, in rare cases, infectious complications occur (anastomotic breakdown and abscess formation), in the majority of cases, these patients survive a septic episode when properly managed. The advantage of this more risky approach in healthy individuals is that the majority needs to undergo only one operative procedure.

Findings during elective operation also dictate the type of procedure to be performed. Abdominal spread of tumour or opening of the GI tract and contamination of the intra-abdominal cavity with intestinal contents should lead to tailoring the extent and art of the operation to the risk to develop infectious complications (*see also* **Emergency Operation**).

Emergency Operation

In acute abdominal sepsis, leading to a symptomatology suggesting generalised peritonitis, measures should be taken quickly to improve the cardiovascular and respiratory conditions of the patient and subsequently to intervene without delay. Early intervention has been proven to increase the chances of cure.[33] Theoretically, rapid intervention within the proinflammatory phase of wound healing leads to an optimal host response, whereas after 3 days, an anti-inflammatory response may already be active, explaining compromised healing due to a 'second hit' situation. Computed tomographic scanning is diagnostic only when enteral and parenteral contrasts are administered, which not only delay the intervention but are, in addition to causing renal damage, potentially also stressful for the intestine because of the hyperosmolarity of the contrast medium. There are several stages of contamination that correlate with the risk of surgical site infection. The Hinchey stages have been found to predict morbidity and mortality and are based on the

Table 6.2   Hinchey classification[59] and modified classification[60] adapted from Klarenbeek et al[61]

Hinchey classification		Modified Hinchey classification	
I	Pericolic abscess or phlegmon	I	Pericolic abscess
II	Pelvic, intra-abdominal or retroperitoneal abscess	IIa	Distant abscess amendable to percutaneous drainage
		IIb	Complex abscess associated with fistula
III	Generalised purulent peritonitis	III	Generalised purulent peritonitis
IV	Generalised faecal peritonitis	IV	Faecal peritonitis

Adapted from: Klarenbeek BR, de Korte N, van der Peet DL, Cuesta MA. Review of current classifications for diverticular disease and a translation into clinical practice. *Int J Colorectal Dis* 2012;27:207–14.

degree of infection found at operation[34] (Table 6.2). In a generalised purulent or faecal peritonitis, primary anastomoses are generally dissuaded, but the condition of the patient should also be considered. The extent and risk of the operation should be tailored to the extent of contamination and to the ability of the patient to generate an adequate healing response. The Mannheim Peritonitis Index combines the severity of abdominal infection and aspects of organ function and therefore furnishes a more complete risk analysis[33,35] (Tables 6.3 and 6.4). In the risk factor analysis, intervention later than 24 hours after the beginning of symptoms was independently associated with an increase in complications and mortality.

It is important to achieve control of the infectious focus. Localised abscesses are preferably treated by local (radiological or surgical) drainage, in some cases requiring definitive surgery at a later stage but with less risk and higher probability of complete healing. Even when, inadvertently, acute laparotomy is performed and, during operation, an inflammatory mass is found surrounding an abscess, for instance, in Crohn's disease, primary drainage can be preferable. The primary diseased Crohn's segment, leading to perforation and abscess formation, is the basis of the perforation and is often short, and when trying to dissect the inflammatory mass, lacerations of the covering healthy bowel may occur, also leading to resection of healthy bowel. When inflammatory bowel disease is not involved, preservation of as much bowel as possible is less urgent, because there may be a one-time problem. In small bowel obstruction of longer duration, a primary anastomosis may be hazardous when the bowel is severely distended. Temporary stomata may be advisable when patients are in bad condition.

Reoperative Surgery

After operations or drainage procedures for abdominal sepsis, ileus, and ischaemia and in situations with an open abdomen (with or without fistulas) due to abdominal

Table 6.3   The Mannheim peritonitis index[33]

Risk factor	Weighing if present
Age > 50 years	5
Female sex	5
Organ failure*	7
Malignancy	4
Preoperative duration of peritonitis >24 hours	4
Origin of sepsis, not colonic	4
Diffuse generalised peritonitis	6
Exudate	
Clear	0
Cloudy, purulent	6
Faecal	12

*For definitions of organ failure, see Table 6.4.

Adapted from: Linder MM, Wacha H, Feldmann U, Wesch G, Streifensand RA, Gundlach E. The Mannheim peritonitis index. An instrument for the intraoperative prognosis of peritonitis. *Chirurg* 1987;58:84–92.

compartment syndrome or abdominal wall dehiscence, reoperative surgery is often required at a later stage. Diseased bowel must be resected, fistulas or temporary stomata closed and intestinal continuity restored. Similarly, in the presence of an open abdomen, abdominal wall closure must be achieved. If sepsis is absent or adequately treated, a definitive operation is required, which can be performed when the patient is in a good condition.

As few anastomoses as possible should be made, even when this requires sacrificing 10 or 15 cm of small bowel, provided that the remaining length of the bowel is adequate and the patient is not suffering from Crohn's disease. In our opinion, end-to-end anastomoses should be made to limit the length of the suture lines. This makes it easier to bury the anastomoses under healthy bowel, lateral abdominal wall or transverse colon and omentum,

Table 6.4   Definitions of organ failure used in computing the Mannheim peritonitis index[33]

Kidney	Creatinine level >177 µmol/L Urea level >167 mmol/L Oliguria <20 mL/h
Lung	P_{O2} <50 mmHg P_{CO2} <50 mmHg
Shock (definition according to Shoemaker)	Hypodynamic or hyperdynamic
Intestinal obstruction (only if profound)	Paralysis >24 hours or complete mechanical ileus

Adapted from: Linder MM, Wacha H, Feldmann U, Wesch G, Streifensand RA, Gundlach E. The Mannheim peritonitis index. An instrument for the intraoperative prognosis of peritonitis. *Chirurg* 1987;58:84–92.

so that even in case of abdominal dehiscence, anastomoses are not exposed to the air. Anastomoses should not be positioned adjacent to damaged tissue (for instance, after radiotherapy), because for adequate healing, a healthy matrix surrounding the anastomosis supports adequate healing. This is important because in this situation and when they are exposed, as in an open wound, anastomoses dehisce in the majority of cases.

Very often, parts of the abdominal wall are lost or the volume of the abdominal content is increased due to inflammatory oedema, so that primary closure of the abdominal wall requires much tension. This may lead to increased intra-abdominal pressure, increasing the likelihood of abdominal wall dehiscence or requiring open-abdomen treatment. In this situation, we have, in most cases, preferred not to try to close the abdominal wall but to employ a 'semi-open abdomen' technique using three layers of Vicryl® mesh, bridging the defect in the abdominal wall fascia. Before applying the mesh, also in this situation, care is taken to cover the bowel with omentum and especially to bury suture lines under the remaining abdominal wall or healthy intestine, as explained in the preceding paragraph. When the (absorbable) sutures attaching the mesh to the fascia are torn or have cut through fascia layers, preferably healthy bowel should be exposed, covered by omentum or transverse colon. Vicryl® mesh is less likely to damage underlying bowel and when more layers are used, this often forms a dense fibrotic sheath, strong enough to prevent bulging of the abdominal content when straining, standing or changing from a lying to a sitting position. While employing this technique, primary closure of the skin is often possible when the skin is mobilised. Tension on the cutaneous suture line can be relieved by adhesive plaster drawn in transverse direction across the bandage on the wound under moderate tension and fixed on both sides of the wound on skin-protective base plates generally consisting of pectin or other organic not erosive material.

Some authors in this situation recommend to apply component-separation methods (Ramirez techniques).[36,37] We have applied this technique only in rare situations, where the restorative operation was of minor magnitude, the patient was in excellent shape and no infection was present or no spilling of intestinal contents had occurred. Similar criteria are adhered to in patients with large abdominal wall hernias.

Surgical Experience

Surgical technique should be adequate. Studies of different types of operation revealed risk factors for infectious complications after surgery via multivariate analyses. The outcome after surgery did not differ when residents or licensed surgeons had performed the operation, provided the operation was performed under supervision of an experienced surgeon.[38] It appears that surgical strategy and decision making have a decisive influence on outcome. A critical volume of the specific type of surgery under study, performed in the institution, is another factor that determines outcome.

POSTOPERATIVE MANAGEMENT

In the last decade, much attention has been payed to the challenging dogmas existing in perioperative care. The so-called ERAS program (enhanced recovery after surgery) has rationalised measures that have been taken since a century.[39] Fasting before surgery is shortened, and it is recommended to use glucose drinks the night before and 2 hours before surgery to diminish glucose resistance. Patients are encouraged to resume eating and mobilise early after operation. Opiates are minimised so as to not diminish intestinal motility, and epidural anaesthesia is recommended. Drains, stomach tubes and bladder catheters are removed early after operation in the recovery room or not given at all. Altogether, these measures are intended to remove unnecessary stress and to limit the stress/inflammatory response after operation to the part that is required for healing.[39] This program has made life after operation more agreeable and led to shortened hospital stay and decreased associated costs. However, no influence on postoperative infectious complications and mortality has been demonstrated.[40] In the same study, it was found that laparoscopic surgery was associated with fewer infectious complications.

The stress response inevitably leads to increased permeability and increased capillary escape of fluid into the interstitium (Table 6.5). As a consequence, during and immediately after major surgery, substantial infusion of balanced salt solutions in combination with no electrolyte containing fluids is required, leading to weight gain due to accumulation of 5 to 10 L of fluid, which is lost after operation, when inflammatory activity abates.[41] Efforts to diminish the infused volume during and in the first 2 days after surgery have led to a decrease in the amount of fluid accumulating and subsequent weight gain and oedema formation. Nonetheless, in general, after major surgery, a minimal positive fluid balance of 4 to 5 L is necessary to maintain cardiovascular stability and urine production. It is claimed that measures to limit a positive fluid balance to not more than 5 L improve GI motility.[42]

Time Course of Septic Complications after Operation (Table 6.5)

Zero to Two Days after Operation

The stress/inflammatory response after surgery requires, in addition to adaptive changes in metabolism, activation of the cardiorespiratory system, leading to increased cardiac output, increased respiration and ventilation, modest hyperthermia and pain. Pain relief is necessary to ensure deep breathing to prevent atelectasis in the lower lung fields. How to deal with pain is becoming more and more uncertain. Use of opiates has been minimised because of their inhibitory effects on intestinal motility. On the other hand, it has become increasingly clear that NSAIDs inhibit the healing response, interfere with cardiac and renal functions, lead to GI ulceration and compromise anastomotic healing. Cox-2 inhibitors may have less deleterious effects.[21,22,43] Although postoperative epidural anaesthesia minimises the use of opiates, it delays mobilisation of the patient.

Immediate postoperative infectious complications are difficult to differentiate from the normal postoperative metabolic response (Table 6.5). In general, the infectious response is more severe, including higher fever, cardiovascular instability and increased respiratory rates due to hypoxia, leading to hypocapnia. Increased parenteral fluids and electrolytes are required to maintain intravascular volume, blood pressure and urinary output. These septic symptoms are generally caused by leakage from accidental perforation, laceration or anastomotic breakdown. Bowel ischaemia may also present with severe symptoms of instability and organ failure and is frequently associated with severe hyperlactataemia (>4 mmol). Immediate postoperative anastomotic breakdown is generally considered to result from technical errors or inadvertent lacerations made during surgery. Loss of liquid stools into the abdominal cavity (small bowel) causes more severe symptoms due to easier spread and possibly due to the presence of enzymes and bile than the loss of more solid stools from the large bowel. In severe cases with cardiorespiratory instability, immediate relaparotomy or relaparoscopy may be indicated to prevent further spread of leakage, which might lead to generalised peritonitis. When the symptoms are less severe, diagnostic procedures may be performed, but when confirmed, reintervention may be necessary when major leakage, accompanied by clear signs of sepsis, is present. Minor leakage generally causes less severe symptoms and may heal due to walling off of the site of perforation/leakage. Percutaneous CT or ultrasound-guided drainage may be effective in these cases. Such patients receive, without exception, broad-spectrum antibiotics, but their efficacy is not well established. There are exceptions to the rule that minor leakage causes minor symptoms. In rare cases, minor leakage may lead to a fulminant septic course and mortality. Possibly, this is related to single nuclear polymorphisms, for instance, of the tumour necrosis factor-α (TNF-α) gene, increasing the inflammatory response above normal requirements.[44]

Two to Three Days after Operation

In this phase, after operation, the tipping point should be reached, changing from a positive to negative fluid balance, because the inflammation-induced capillary escape of fluid and electrolytes into the interstitial space reverses to a decrease in volume of this compartment, owing to the return of fluid into the intravascular space. The excess intravascular fluid must be excreted by the kidney, which requires good cardiac and renal function. Patients with failure of these organs may develop cardiac failure and should receive diuretics or temporary renal replacement therapy. Altogether, the total extracellular space decreases in size, leading to increases in plasma electrolytes, albumin and others.[45] Delay or absence of the tipping point and clinical deterioration of the patient should also, at this stage, lead to rapid further diagnosis and, in case of surgical complications, lead to reintervention.

Table 6.5 Schematic representation of commonly occurring postoperative changes in clinical state, body composition, laboratory values and blood gas values. The difference in normal healing and a continuous septic course consists of an unrelenting progression of inflammation-induced capillary leakage, leading to fluid accumulation and hypoalbuminaemia and related disorders. This is accompanied by a rapid loss of cell mass solids (muscle, skin and bone), cognitive immune and muscular disturbances and increased mortality risk

Postoperative day	Day 1 Uncomplicated	Day 2–3 Uncomplicated	Day 4–6 Uncomplicated	Day 40 Uncomplicated	*Day 1 Complicated*	*Day 2–3 Complicated*	*Day 4–6 Complicated*
Clinical state							
Cardiovascular	5–7 L↑	6–8 L↑↑	1–3 L↑	1–3 L↓	7–10 L↑	10–12 L	12–14 L↑
Cognition	↓↓↓	↓↓	↓	Normal	↓↓↓	↓↓↓	↓↓↓↓
Strength	↓↓↓	↓↓	↓↓	↓	↓↓↓	↓↓↓	↓↓↓↓
Body composition							
Body weight	↑↑	↑↑↑	↑	↓	↑↑↑	↑↑↑	↑↑↑
Fat-free mass	↑↑	↑↑↑	↑↑	↓	↑↑↑	↑↑↑	↑↑↑
Fat-free mass solids	↓	↓↓	↓↓↓	↑	↓↓	↓↓↓	↓↓↓↓
Total fluids	↑↑	↑↑↑	↓	↓↓	↑↑↑	↑↑↑	↑↑↑
Laboratory values							
Plasma albumin	↓↓	↓↓↓	↓↓	↓-Normal	↓↓	↓↓↓↓	↓↓↓↓↓
C-reactive protein%	↑↑	↑↑	↑↑↑=	Normal	↑↑	↑↑↑	↑↑↑↑
Na+	↓↓	↓	↓	Normal	↓↓	↓↓↓	↓↓↓
Leucocytes*	↑	↑	↑-N	Normal	↑↑↑	↑↑↑	↑↑↑
Difference	Left shift	Normal	Normal	Normal	Left shift	Left shift	Left shift
Zn@	↓↓	↓↓↓	↓↓	Normal	↓↓	↓↓↓↓	↓↓↓↓
Fe#	↓↓	↓↓↓	↓↓		↓↓↓	↓↓↓↓	↓↓↓↓
Transferrin#	↓↓	↓↓↓	↓↓	Normal	↓↓	↓↓↓↓	↓↓↓↓
Fe-binding capacity#	↓↓	↓↓↓	↓↓	Normal	↓↓	↓↓↓	↓↓↓
Lactate, mmol$	1.5–2.5	1.5–2.5	1.5–2.5	<1.0	2.5 or >	2.5 or >	2.5 or >
Blood gas							
pO$_2$	↓-N	↓-N	Normal	Normal	↓	↓↓	↓↓↓
pCO$_2$	↓-N	↓-N	Normal	Normal	↓-N	↓	↓↓ - ↑↑
pH&	↑-N	↑-N	Normal	Normal	↑-N	Varying	Varying

%C-reactive protein increases within a day after trauma and to higher levels when infection is superimposed. After a few days, it is not an accurate quantitative reflection of the severity of infection.

*Leucocytes are generally increased after trauma and further increase as a consequence of infection, accompanied by a left shift. In frail patients, a hypodynamic form of sepsis can develop, including neutropaenia with left shift, hypothermia and somnolence. This state constitutes a high mortality risk.

@Zinc levels drop parallel with albumin levels, because Zn is largely bound to albumin.

#Iron drops because its binding protein transferrin, to which iron is bound, is a negative acute-phase protein, decreasing after stress/trauma/infection.

$Lactate levels are slightly elevated after trauma and increase even more in hyperdynamic inflammatory (septic) states to between 2.5 mmol and 4 mmol. Only after true shock periods or in the presence of organ ischaemia, higher levels are attained.

&pH is variable in these conditions and may range from respiratory alkalosis due to hyperventilation in hypoxia or pain, metabolic acidosis after shock periods and renal failure or respiratory acidosis due to muscle weakness or opiate use. Combinations may lead to normal pH (for instance, metabolic acidosis compensated by hyperventilation, leading to hypocapnia).

When bowel function has not recovered completely, abdominal distention may lead to atelectasis of the lower lung fields, which is often falsely interpreted as pneumonia. Similarly, leucocyturia may erroneously suggest the presence of a urinary infection (*see also* **Indications for Emergency Surgery**).

Three to Six Days after Operation

Clear symptoms of infectious intra-abdominal problems generally present in this period (Table 6.5). These include pain, abdominal distension, no or high-pitched bowel sounds, paradoxical diarrhoea or no stools, fever and, in old and depleted patients, hypothermia, cardiorespiratory instability and laboratory signs of inflammation. Diarrhoea may often be erroneously interpreted as improvement of motility. Stagnant bowel leads to mucosal inflammation, interfering with adequate resorption of water, electrolytes and nutrients, leading to a liquid stool, more or less passively moving distally and often foul-smelling.

There are also cognitive symptoms such as somnolence, confusion, inactivity and depression. Delirium may occur almost always, indicating that there is a serious physical problem. Patients with no earlier cardiovascular symptoms may develop atrial fibrillation, an ominous sign potentially heralding an abdominal or other complication or resulting from hypovolaemia. Wound dehiscence and spontaneous drainage of serosanguinous fluid or pus are additional symptoms that increase the likelihood that an anastomotic leak, perforation or bowel ischaemia has occurred.

At this stage, a relaparotomy or relaparoscopy can still be performed and should be done as early as possible to shorten the period of severe catabolism and deterioration of the physical condition, which would especially be catastrophic in frail patients. It is crucial to deal adequately with the infectious focus, and the primary goal is to allow the patient to survive. Stages of abdominal infection[34] and the condition of the patient (*see* **Preoperative Management, Risk Analysis**) should dictate the surgical procedure. In the presence of a generalised faecal peritonitis, anastomoses should not be constructed in view of the high risk of a leakage. When less severe infectious activity is encountered, reanastomosis can be performed in a patient in good condition with only mild general symptoms of inflammation and most parts of the abdomen not clearly secondarily infected. A proximal diverting stoma may be considered also depending on the local and general conditions and the time elapsed since the primary operation. The longer after primary surgery, the less likely the healing of a reanastomosis. In older frail patients or younger patient in bad condition, defensive surgery should be performed. In high-risk patients, resection and diversion (proximal stoma and distal mucous fistula) or exteriorisation of the leaking bowel segment should be considered.

Seven to Fourteen Days after Operation

Abscesses are the main cause of abdominal sepsis in this period. This time period has allowed surrounding tissues to cover a laceration or an anastomotic leak, resulting in an abscess. This does not happen in patients who are severely malnourished or on steroids. In recent decades, radiology has allowed precise detection of these abscesses and drainage via CT or ultrasound-guided puncture techniques. Very small abscesses may not always require drainage, but larger abscesses (>5 cm diameter) generally do, depending on the severity of clinical and local symptoms of infection and sepsis. True sepsis should be treated aggressively. Reintervention in this period is hazardous because of the relative inaccessibility of the abdomen. Bowel loops stick to each other in such a way that dissection is fraught with lacerations due to the difficulty of developing cleavage planes. Only after 6 weeks do these adhesions mature and the bowel becomes less oedematous and more solid, allowing dissection, without afflicting additional harm (renewed lacerations, inadvertent perforations, etc.). If abscesses cannot be drained radiologically, small surgical incisions may allow drainage. When these abscesses originate from a perforation or anastomotic leak, drainage can lead to the formulation of a fistula, which may require definitive surgery at a later stage or which may close spontaneously, depending on the anatomy of the defect in the bowel (*see* **Management of Bowel Fistulas, Timing of Surgery**).

Multilocular abscesses can develop when free peritoneal fluid is secondarily infected, initiated by a primary abscess at the site of a bowel defect in the bowel or a haematoma. In rare cases, patients in bad condition develop abscesses after operation, without a clear primary focus. Treatment of multiple abscesses poses an enormous radiological and surgical challenge. A multidisciplinary approach is sometimes required, combining radiological and (local) surgical techniques. Local pelvic abscesses after low anterior resection can often be treated transanastomotically or transrectally, in case of extensive abscess formation combined with a diverting proximal double-barrel colostomy. Diverting ileostomies have been popular, and meta-analyses have been published, suggesting that ileostomies produce stools earlier than colostomies and lead to fewer wound infections.[46,47] Mortality does not differ. We have a slight preference for transversostomies because of internal herniation around an ileostomy in a few cases requiring reoperation and bad experiences with passage after reanastomosing ileostomies. Admittedly, transversostomies are associated with more skin infections and sometimes develop low-output faecal fistulas, which, however, generally close spontaneously.

Analysis of secretions from wounds or obtained with puncture can provide information regarding the origin and underlying cause. Recognition of food components clearly represent an intestinal origin. Microbiological investigation reveals the presence of infection. Clinical chemical analysis of the components of abdominal fluid can help establish the diagnosis (Table 6.6). Small bowel content always contains bilirubin, amylase, very low levels of albumin and sodium. Bile does, however, contain little amylase, whereas pancreatic juice does contain little bilirubin. Ascites or serous collections contain substantial concentrations of albumin but lower than plasma level; when infected or in cases of malignant ascites, albumin levels approach plasma levels. In some cases, measurement of triglycerides, lymphocytes (chyle) or creatinine and urea (in urine) may establish the diagnosis. Microbiology and, in suspected cases of malignancy, cytology can be helpful.

Is the Septic Focus Adequately Controlled?

It is important to deal adequately with the septic focus, which may be difficult when causes cannot be eliminated or perforations cannot be exteriorised or defunctionalised by constructing deviating stomata. Hematomas, debris and necrotic or nonviable tissue should be removed. The earlier and the more thorough the intervention performed after occurrence of an acute infection, substantial bleeding or ischaemic intestinal event, the better the prognosis. In case of uncertainty regarding clearance of the primary inflammatory event, planned relaparotomy may be an option but has become less popular in recent decades. In case of bowel ischaemia and necrosis, recurrence is frequent because of ischaemia developing proximally or/and distally of the initially ischaemic bowel segment. Clinical improvement, including improvement of organ function, decreased fluid requirements, decreasing plasma lactate and increasing albumin levels are reliable parameters, indicating that treatment has eliminated the septic focus or the ischaemic bowel section and that reintervention is not required (Table 6.5). Mortality, related to bowel ischaemia, amounts to 50%, which may be explained by accompanying liver ischaemia, apparent when plasma lactate and transaminase levels rise precipitously and hypoglycaemia develops. Relaparotomy can be performed relatively safely only in the first week after the first intervention (see **Three to Seven Days after Operation**).

Management of Bowel Fistulas

Pathogenesis of Bowel Fistulas

Fistulas arise from perforation or laceration of the bowel and from anastomotic dehiscence, generally leading to a septic episode, with abscess formation. Drainage of the abscess may lead to formation of a fistula, defined as a connection from the perforated site of the bowel via drainage to the skin or to another hollow organ. Spontaneous fistulae occur in inflammatory bowel diseases (diverticulitis and Crohn's disease), radiation enteritis or cancer. Surgical fistulae occur due to inadvertent injury of the bowel or from anastomoses performed during surgery or other interventions. Most spontaneous fistulae have a low output but have a limited tendency to heal spontaneously. In contradistinction, postoperative fistulae may heal spontaneously when treated well and depending on the size of the primary intestinal defect, the quality of the bowel at the site of the fistula and the passage distal to the fistula. High-output fistulae of the proximal small bowel may lead to insufficient absorption of food, thus

Table 6.6 The origin of abdominal secretions, as derived from their relative composition: ↑ = high concentration; ↓ = low concentration; ↑↑ is very high concentration approaching plasma concentration

Origin	Bilirubin	Pancreases	Albumin	Triglycerides	Microscopy
Bile	↑	↓	↓	↓	Negative unless infected
Pancreatic juice	↓	↑	↑	↓	Negative unless infected
Small bowel content	↑	↑	↓	↓ or ↑	Fibre
Ascites not infected	↓	↓	↑	↓	Leucocytes ↓
Ascites infected	↓	↓	↑↑	↓	Leucocytes ↑
Ascites malignant	↓	↓	↑	↓	Cytology +
Chyle	↓	↓	↑	↑	Lymphocytes ↑

requiring artificial nutrition. Colonic fistulae generally have a low output and have less impact on nutritional state and absorption of food.

Management of Bowel Fistulas (SOWATS Protocol)[48]

The management priorities that should be followed when treating intestinal fistulas are described below (Table 6.7).

Sepsis treatment

The first priority of treatment is to control sepsis, which is generally the starting point of fistula formation. An adequate immune and healing response is possible only when sepsis is adequately controlled. Diagnostic and treatment techniques have been described in the section **Indications for Emergency Surgery**.

Optimisation of the nutritional state

As soon as sepsis has been treated and when organ functions (heart, lungs and kidney) are optimised, the nutritional state should be improved, generally starting after a few days. At present, 'collateral' evidence suggests that in previously well-nourished individuals, in the acute

Table 6.7   Schematic representation of priorities and time frame for the treatment of complex enterocutaneous fistulas (SOWATS protocol)[48]

Phases of fistula treatment	Actions	Time frame

Sepsis treatment	Septic focus localised
	  CT scanning/ultrasound
	  Guided puncture techniques if focus localised
	  Small incisions when focus localised
	Generalised peritonitis with cardiorespiratory instability
	  Urgent laparotomy/laparoscopy (ultrasound may take a little time)
		Urgent
		Within 24 hours

Optimisation of nutritional state	Parenteral nutrition when:
	  high output small bowel fistula
	  25% of RDA of enteral formula feeding if wound care allows ≥ combinations
	Physiotherapy when stable
		After 3–7 days, depending on previous nutritional state

Wound care	Fistulas in open wounds
	  Suction drainage of effluent fistula (dedicated specialised nursing required)
	  Skin protection with bags and base plates
	  Saline rinsing and sump suction in open abdominal wound
	Fistulas with surrounding skin
	  Treated as stomata with skin-protecting base plates
		Immediately after commencement of fistula

Anatomy diagnostics	CT scan of abdomen (contrast enhancement)
	  Fistulography with iodine-containing contrast
	  Small bowel follows through with iodine-containing contrast
	  Assess patency distal to the fistula (antegrade when lateral fistula; retrograde when no connection, with bowel distal to the fistula)
		After minimal 3–4 weeks, when patient is stable

Timing of definitive surgery	When patient in good condition: Alert, strong, active and eager to be operated (no oedema and spontaneously normal Hb and albumin)	After minimal 6–12 weeks

Surgical management	Operate defensively
	  Take care not to damage the bowel; dissect full length of bowel
	  Create end-to-end anastomoses
	  Cover with healthy surrounding tissue
	  Make sure that after eventual wound dehiscence, anastomoses are not exposed to the air
	  Employ semiopen technique for wound closure (see text)
		Do not hurry
		Operations with fistulae exposed in open wounds take on average 5–6 hours

Abbreviations: CT, computed tomography; Hb, haemoglobin; RDA, recommnded daily allowance.

phase of sepsis or critical illness, nutritional support may be delayed up to a week. This has recently been supported by findings in critically ill children admitted to the paediatric intensive care.[49] Severely depleted patients are an exception in view of the possibility that they will be able to generate an adequate host response only when nourished well.

Despite the fistula, enteral nutrition is not strictly prohibited. In case of proximal small bowel fistulae, fistula output may be high, precluding exclusive reliance on enteral nutritional intake. In this case, complete or partial parenteral nutrition is warranted. Some enteral nutrition can still be administered to expose the proximal bowel to nutrients, which may improve intestinal integrity. Surgical fistulas may heal spontaneously when the fistula is lateral and occupies only a quarter or less of the circumference of the fistula, when there is no distal obstruction and the bowel at the site of the fistula is of good quality, allowing adequate passage of bowel contents. Fistulas arising from cancer or radiation do not close spontaneously, whereas Crohn's disease fistulas often close but will generally recur when enteral intake is resumed.[50]

Wound care

Wound care is difficult, especially in fistulas in open wounds. The goals are to keep the wounds dry and to prevent stasis of bowel content in the wound. Rinsing with physiological saline and using sump drainage and protecting the surrounding skin with pectin base plates can help limit further laceration of the skin. Vacuum treatment of wounds in our opinion is safe only if the intestine is not exposed in the wound and when covered with omentum or Vicryl® mesh. In case of high-output fistulas located in the middle of an abdominal dehiscence, sump drainage may help keep wounds dry and allow them to granulate and epithelialise adequately. The principle of the sump drain is that negative pressure to drain bowel effluent builds up only when effluent is present. Fistulas presenting in open wounds close only rarely, if at all. When wounds become infected, granulation tissue and newly epithelialised surfaces are damaged and often slough off. Along similar pathophysiological lines, anastomoses do not heal.

Anatomy of the fistula

When the patient is stable and functionally improving, the anatomy of the fistula and the remaining bowel should be carefully defined by CT scanning (Table 6.6). Often, ingestion of contrast in the fistula, anally or proximally with a tube, with the tip located at the ligament of Treitz, may establish the location of the fistula as well

the quality of the intestine distal to the fistula. Injection of iodine-containing contrast in the fistula can give an impression of the art of the origin of the fistula (small lateral, or originating from most of the circumference of the bowel), which will give information regarding the likelihood that the fistula will close spontaneously. The art of the fistula should be defined before the operation, and this can safely be performed 3 to 4 weeks after its development. When it is likely that the fistula can heal spontaneously, nutritional intake proximal to the fistula is generally restricted but not totally stopped. Fistulas heal rarely after 4 to 6 weeks. Alternatively, patients can be nourished enterally with limited amounts of formula feeds, even when this will increase fistula output somewhat but only if output can be collected adequately without harming the wound.

Timing of surgery

In most nonclosing fistulas, a definitive operation is ultimately required if fistula output is high, leading to insufficient food uptake. One should wait at least 6 weeks after its occurrence, before embarking upon a restorative operation.[48,51] By this time, adhesions mature and can be safely dissected. Some centres recommend to wait 3 months, and this would lead to an even better condition of the patient, but home artificial nutrition is not available everywhere and continued hospitalisation is very expensive. Laboratory parameters to follow are Hb, albumin, leucocyte count and differentiation, electrolytes, trace elements and vitamins (Table 6.5). Albumin levels very accurately reflect inflammation, and rising values indicate improvement and shrinkage of interstitial volume (drying up) as a consequence of a decrease in capillary escape of fluid, electrolytes, immune cells and proteins.[41] This also explains why patients lose weight but become stronger and accumulate fat-free mass solids, despite a decrease in fat-free mass volume. Clinically, patients become more active, take more interest in their surroundings and remember better what they have read or heard. They should receive physiotherapy as soon as possible after dealing with sepsis. At all stages of treatment, the patient should be informed in detail. When the initial sepsis has been adequately treated and the presence of a high-output fistula is apparent, patients should know that definitive treatment will be minimally 6 weeks postponed and that their collaboration (exercise) is needed.

Surgical technique

Care should be taken not to cause additional damage to the bowel. Dissection should be slow and careful and speed should decelerate when 'almost there'—the moment when most renewed lacerations are made. In most cases, the complete length of the bowel should be dissected and it should be ascertained that there is no distal obstruction (*see further* **Reoperative Surgery**).

Treatment of Metabolic Disorders

High-output small bowel fistulas or short bowel often lead to fatty liver and intrahepatic cholestasis. When long-standing, superimposed inflammatory changes can occur in the liver, ultimately resulting in fibrosis, cirrhosis and liver failure, especially in young children. At present, more is known about how to prevent these complications. Two major reasons underlie the inability of the liver to excrete bile in case of substantial loss of bile from the proximal bowel. One reason is that the distal small intestine is not exposed to bile and other secreta. It is now known that the integrity of the small bowel requires activation of bile acid receptors (for instance, the FXR receptor) by bile.[52,53] If this does not occur, the intestine exhibits inflammatory changes, even aggravated by decreased motility, leading to bacterial overgrowth. Proof for these mechanisms comes from the observation that when proximal effluent, collected from the high-output small bowel fistula, is infused in the distal defunctionalised small bowel segments, cholestasis and fatty liver improve[54] (Figure 6.1). At present, bile acid receptor activators are developed but not yet available for clinical use. An additional advantage of this practice is that re-establishing the enterohepatic cycling of bile acids and increasing the bile acid pool improve fat absorption in the proximal small bowel and prevent electrolyte losses. More recently, it has been shown that the liver also contains bile acid receptors, which when stimulated by

bile acids mediate insulin sensitivity and metabolism of carbohydrates and lipids.[55]

In the last decade, it has also been demonstrated that enteral fat improves the integrity of the intestine by stimulating vagal pathways and making macrophages in the gut less responsive to bacterial influences.[56] Parenteral fat may, however, increase the lipid content of the liver and lead to cholestasis. Even modest signs of cholestasis and hyperlipaemia (alkaline phosphatase, γ-glutamyl(33)-transpeptidase and hypertriglyceridaemia > 3.5 mmol) should be an indication to diminish the fat content of the parenteral nutrition mix.[57,58]

Patients with high-output fistulas often develop dehydration, become thirsty and increase fluid intake. Water without electrolytes will be rendered isotonic by secreting electrolytes into the lumen, 'desalting' the patient when these electrolytes cannot be reabsorbed further distally in the small bowel. Drinks should, therefore, contain isotonic electrolytes (Na, K, Ca, Mg, Cl and P) and glucose and should be limited to not more than 2 L/d.

CONCLUSIONS

Successful treatment of severe sepsis due to peritonitis and its prevention does not only depend on surgical 'cutting' skills but also on noncutting management. There is no one superior way of preventing or dealing with abdominal sepsis. In this chapter, principles are outlined that should be adhered to, in order to achieve optimal results, but weighing the capacity of the patient to heal well against the metabolic burden of treatment will probably be an estimate rather than a precise calculation.

Nonetheless, the surgeon should try to tailor the extent of surgery to the ability of the patient to heal well. It is crucial to deal with the primary infectious focus early but, at the same time, to prevent secondary complications and mortality. In elective cases without (major) pre-existing infectious inflammation, preoperative refeeding and rehabilitating patients by physical exercise have been shown to improve outcome, especially by limiting postoperative infectious complications.

In acute intra-abdominal infections, rapid diagnosis and intervention are essential to make effective use of 'the window of opportunity', when the physical condition of the patient has not yet substantially deteriorated. Antibiotics have a limited effect and should not lull the surgeon to sleep, postponing acute intervention. In severe peritonitis, constructing anastomoses is hazardous and surgery should be restricted to 'damage control'. On the other hand, when sepsis is effectively treated and fistula or stomas remain, nutritional support, physical exercise

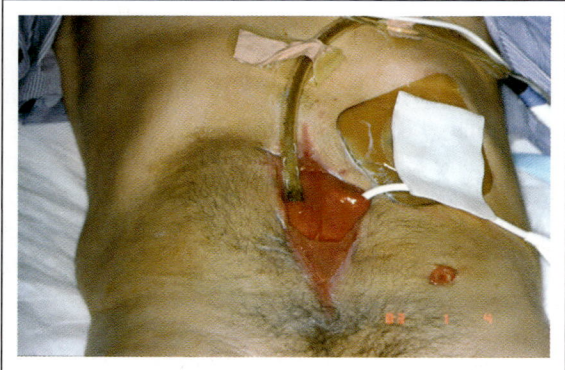

Figure 6.1 Reinfusion of the effluent from a high-output proximal jejunal fistula into the defunctionalised distal small bowel.[54] The fistula presents as a double-barrel jejunostomy.
Courtesy: Peter B. Soeters.

and wound care should be optimal. Restorative surgery should be delayed at least 6 weeks and preferably longer to allow the patient to recover and the abdomen to become accessible again. Only when muscle, immune and cognitive functions are restored, adequate healing is likely. This is possible only when inflammatory activity has subsided. This can be judged on clinical grounds at the bed side and by simple laboratory parameters such as a rise in Hb and albumin and a decrease in CRP and leucocyte counts.

A holistic approach is required to achieve optimal results. Knowledge should be acquired to deal adequately with the many metabolic and clinical challenges posed by patients with abdominal infectious catastrophe. There should be one experienced captain on the ship.

REFERENCES

1. Soeters PB, Reijven PL, van Bokhorst-de van der Schueren MA, et al. A rational approach to nutritional assessment. *Clin Nutr* 2008;27:706–16.
2. Jensen GL. Global leadership conversation: addressing malnutrition. *J Parenter Enteral Nutr* 2016;40:455–7.
3. Jensen GL, Mirtallo J, Compher C, et al. Adult starvation and disease-related malnutrition: a proposal for etiology-based diagnosis in the clinical practice setting from the International Consensus Guideline Committee. *Clin Nutr* 2010;29:151–3.
4. Cederholm T, Bosaeus I, Barazzoni R, et al. Diagnostic criteria for malnutrition—an ESPEN Consensus Statement. *Clin Nutr* 2015;34:335–40.
5. Lodewick TM, van Nijnatten TJ, van Dam RM, et al. Are sarcopenia, obesity and sarcopenic obesity predictive of outcome in patients with colorectal liver metastases? *HPB* 2015;17:438–46.
6. Moore FA, Moore EE, Read RA. Postinjury multiple organ failure: role of extrathoracic injury and sepsis in adult respiratory distress syndrome. *New Horiz* 1993;1:538–49.
7. Kasperk R, Philipps B, Vahrmeyer M, Willis S, Schumpelick V. Risk factors for anastomosis dehiscence after very deep colorectal and coloanal anastomosis. *Chirurg* 2000;71:1365–9.
8. Murphy TJ, Paterson HM, Kriynovich S, et al. Linking the "two-hit" response following injury to enhanced TLR4 reactivity. *J Leukoc Biol* 2005;77:16–23.
9. Kaneko A, Kido T, Yamamoto M, et al. Intestinal anastomosis surgery with no septic shock primes for a dysregulatory response to a second stimulus. *J Surg Res* 2006;134:215–22.
10. Wu LR, Zaborina O, Zaborin A, et al. Surgical injury and metabolic stress enhance the virulence of the human opportunistic pathogen Pseudomonas aeruginosa. *Surg Infect (Larchmt)* 2005;6:185–95.
11. Wu L, Estrada O, Zaborina O, et al. Recognition of host immune activation by Pseudomonas aeruginosa. *Science* 2005;309:774–7.
12. Rohrig G, Becker I, Polidori MC, Schulz RJ, Noreik M. Association of anemia and hypoalbuminemia in German geriatric inpatients: relationship to nutritional status and comprehensive geriatric assessment. *Z Gerontol Geriatr* 2015;48:619–24.
13. Bach V, Schruckmayer G, Sam I, Kemmler G, Stauder R. Prevalence and possible causes of anemia in the elderly: a cross-sectional analysis of a large European university hospital cohort. *Clin Interv Aging* 2014;9:1187–96.
14. Tartter PI. Immunologic effects of blood transfusion. *Immunol Invest* 1995;24:277–88.
15. Golub R, Golub RW, Cantu R, Jr., Stein HD. A multivariate analysis of factors contributing to leakage of intestinal anastomoses. *J Am Coll Surg* 1997;184:364–72.
16. Mynster T, Nielsen HJ. The impact of storage time of transfused blood on postoperative infectious complications in rectal cancer surgery. Danish RANX05 Colorectal Cancer Study Group. *Scand J Gastroenterol* 2000;35:212–7.
17. Dellinger RP, Levy MM, Rhodes A, et al. Surviving sepsis campaign: international guidelines for management of severe sepsis and septic shock: 2012. *Crit Care Med* 2013;41:580–637.
18. Leichtle SW, Mouawad NJ, Lampman R, Singal B, Cleary RK. Does preoperative anemia adversely affect colon and rectal surgery outcomes? *J Am Coll Surg* 2011;212:187–94.
19. Munoz M, Gomez-Ramirez S, Martin-Montanez E, Auerbach M. Perioperative anemia management in colorectal cancer patients: a pragmatic approach. *World J Gastroenterol* 2014;20:1972–85.
20. Sorensen LT, Jorgensen T, Kirkeby LT, Skovdal J, Vennits B, Wille-Jorgensen P. Smoking and alcohol abuse are major risk factors for anastomotic leakage in colorectal surgery. *Br J Surg* 1999;86:927–31.
21. Coxib, traditional NTC, Bhala N, Emberson J, et al. Vascular and upper gastrointestinal effects of non-steroidal anti-inflammatory drugs: meta-analyses of individual participant data from randomised trials. *Lancet* 2013;382:769–79.
22. Gorissen KJ, Benning D, Berghmans T, et al. Risk of anastomotic leakage with non-steroidal anti-inflammatory drugs in colorectal surgery. *Br J Surg* 2012;99:721–7.
23. Rai R, Nagral S, Nagral A. Surgery in a patient with liver disease. *J Clin Exp Hepatol* 2012;2:238–46.
24. Iannuzzi JC, Deeb AP, Rickles AS, Sharma A, Fleming FJ, Monson JR. Recognizing risk: bowel resection in the chronic renal failure population. *J Gastrointest Surg* 2013;17:188–94.
25. Bozzetti F, Gavazzi C, Miceli R, et al. Perioperative total parenteral nutrition in malnourished, gastrointestinal cancer patients: a randomized, clinical trial. *J Parenter Enteral Nutr* 2000;24:7–14.

26. Windsor JA, Hill GL. Weight loss with physiologic impairment. A basic indicator of surgical risk. *Ann Surg* 1988;207:290–6.

27. Gianotti L, Braga M, Fortis C, et al. A prospective, randomized clinical trial on perioperative feeding with an arginine-, omega-3 fatty acid-, and RNA-enriched enteral diet: effect on host response and nutritional status. *J Parenter Enteral Nutr* 1999;23:314–20.

28. Hegazi RA, Hustead DS, Evans DC. Preoperative standard oral nutrition supplements vs immunonutrition: results of a systematic review and meta-analysis. *J Am Coll Surg* 2014;219:1078–87.

29. Morris AM, Regenbogen SE, Hardiman KM, Hendren S. Sigmoid diverticulitis: a systematic review. *JAMA* 2014;311:287–97.

30. Devereaux PJ, Yang H, Yusuf S, et al. Effects of extended-release metoprolol succinate in patients undergoing non-cardiac surgery (POISE trial): a randomised controlled trial. *Lancet* 2008;371:1839–47.

31. Alverdy JC, Chi HS, Selivanov V, Morris J, Sheldon GF. The effect of route of nutrient administration on the secretory immune system. *Curr Surg* 1985;42:10–3.

32. Humes D, Spiller RC. Colonic diverticular disease: medical treatments for acute diverticulitis. *BMJ Clin Evid* 2016;2016:0405.

33. Linder MM, Wacha H, Feldmann U, Wesch G, Streifensand RA, Gundlach E. The Mannheim peritonitis index. An instrument for the intraoperative prognosis of peritonitis. *Chirurg* 1987;58:84–92.

34. Schilling MK, Maurer CA, Kollmar O, Buchler MW. Primary vs. secondary anastomosis after sigmoid colon resection for perforated diverticulitis (Hinchey Stage III and IV): a prospective outcome and cost analysis. *Dis Colon Rectum* 2001;44:699–703; discussion 5.

35. Schirrmacher E, Seifert J. The Mannheim Peritonitis Index. Its reliability for the assessment of prognosis in peritonitis patients. *Fortschr Med* 1988;106:454–6.

36. Ramirez OM, Ruas E, Dellon AL. "Components separation" method for closure of abdominal-wall defects: an anatomic and clinical study. *Plast Reconstr Surg* 1990;86:519–26.

37. Beck DE, Cohen Z, Fleshman JW, Kaufman HS, van Goor H, Wolff BG. A prospective, randomized, multicenter, controlled study of the safety of Seprafilm adhesion barrier in abdominopelvic surgery of the intestine. *Dis Colon Rectum* 2003;46:1310–9.

38. Singh KK, Aitken RJ. Outcome in patients with colorectal cancer managed by surgical trainees. *Br J Surg* 1999;86:1332–6.

39. Fearon KC, Ljungqvist O, Von Meyenfeldt M, et al. Enhanced recovery after surgery: a consensus review of clinical care for patients undergoing colonic resection. *Clin Nutr* 2005;24:466–77.

40. Spanjersberg WR, van Sambeeck JD, Bremers A, Rosman C, van Laarhoven CJ. Systematic review and meta-analysis for laparoscopic versus open colon surgery with or without an ERAS programme. *Surg Endosc* 2015;29:3443–53.

41. Fleck A, Raines G, Hawker F, et al. Increased vascular permeability: a major cause of hypoalbuminaemia in disease and injury. *Lancet* 1985;1:781–4.

42. Lobo DN, Bostock KA, Neal KR, Perkins AC, Rowlands BJ, Allison SP. Effect of salt and water balance on recovery of gastrointestinal function after elective colonic resection: a randomised controlled trial. *Lancet* 2002;359:1812–8.

43. Ungprasert P, Cheungpasitporn W, Crowson CS, Matteson EL. Individual non-steroidal anti-inflammatory drugs and risk of acute kidney injury: a systematic review and meta-analysis of observational studies. European journal of internal medicine. 2015;26:285–91.

44. Soeters PB, Grimble RF. Dangers and benefits of the cytokine mediated response to injury and infection. *Clin Nutr* 2009;28:583–96.

45. Soeters PB. Rationale for albumin infusions. *Curr Opin Clin Nutr Metab Care* 2009;12:258–64.

46. Chen TA. Loop ileostomy or loop colostomy: which one is better for fecal diversion? *Int J Colorectal Dis* 2012;27:131–2.

47. Lin ZL, Yu WK, Shi JL, Chen QY, Tan SJ, Li N. Temporary decompression in critically ill patients: retrospective comparison of ileostomy and colostomy. *Hepatogastroenterology* 2014;61:647–51.

48. Visschers RG, Olde Damink SW, Winkens B, Soeters PB, van Gemert WG. Treatment strategies in 135 consecutive patients with enterocutaneous fistulas. *World J Surg* 2008;32:445–53.

49. Fivez T, Kerklaan D, Mesotten D, et al. Early versus late parenteral nutrition in critically ill children. *N Engl J Med* 2016;374:1111–22.

50. Gouma DJ, von Meyenfeldt MF, Rouflart M, Soeters PB. Preoperative total parenteral nutrition (TPN) in severe Crohn's disease. *Surgery* 1988;103:648–52.

51. Visschers RG, van Gemert WG, Winkens B, Soeters PB, Olde Damink SW. Guided treatment improves outcome of patients with enterocutaneous fistulas. *World J Surg* 2012;36:2341–8.

52. Makishima M, Okamoto AY, Repa JJ, et al. Identification of a nuclear receptor for bile acids. *Science* 1999;284:1362–5.

53. Modica S, Petruzzelli M, Bellafante E, et al. Selective activation of nuclear bile acid receptor FXR in the intestine protects mice against cholestasis. *Gastroenterology* 2012;142:355–65.e1–4.

54. Rinsema W, Gouma DJ, von Meyenfeldt MF, Soeters PB. Reinfusion of secretions from high-output proximal stomas or fistulas. *Surg Gynecol Obstet* 1988;167:372–6.

55. Lefebvre P, Cariou B, Lien F, Kuipers F, Staels B. Role of bile acids and bile acid receptors in metabolic regulation. *Physiol Rev* 2009;89:147–91.

56. Luyer MD, Greve JW, Hadfoune M, Jacobs JA, Dejong CH, Buurman WA. Nutritional stimulation of cholecystokinin

receptors inhibits inflammation via the vagus nerve. *J Exp Med* 2005;202:1023–9.

57. Colomb V, Jobert-Giraud A, Lacaille F, Goulet O, Fournet JC, Ricour C. Role of lipid emulsions in cholestasis associated with long-term parenteral nutrition in children. *J Parenter Enteral Nutr* 2000;24:345–50.

58. Visschers RG, Olde Damink SW, Gehlen JM, Winkens B, Soeters PB, van Gemert WG. Treatment of hypertriglyceridemia in patients receiving parenteral nutrition. *J Parenter Enteral Nutr* 2011;35:610–5.

59. Hinchey EJ, Schaal PG, Richards GK. Treatment of perforated diverticular disease of the colon. *Adv Surg* 1978;12:85–109.

60. Sher ME, Agachan F, Bortul M, Nogueras JJ, Weiss EG, Wexner SD. Laparoscopic surgery for diverticulitis. *Surg Endosc* 1997;11:264–27.

61. Klarenbeek BR, de Korte N, van der Peet DL, Cuesta MA. Review of current classifications for diverticular disease and a translation into clinical practice. *Int J Colorectal Dis* 2012;27:207–14.

7

The Role of Antibiotics in Prevention and Management of Infections after Gastrointestinal Surgery

T. Mulder, J.A.J.W. Kluytmans and M.J.M. Bonten

ABSTRACT

Gastrointestinal surgery may be complicated by postoperative infections. Most infections occur at the surgical site, and others include hospital-acquired pneumonia, urinary tract infections or catheter-related bloodstream infections. Despite the improvement in infection control and the advances in surgical techniques, postoperative infections remain a substantial cause of morbidity, prolonged hospitalisation and readmission after gastrointestinal surgery. Consequently, these infections are associated with an increase in mortality and higher healthcare costs. Adequate antimicrobial management and prevention measures are required to reduce the disease burden. This chapter provides an overview of the most common postoperative infectious complications of gastrointestinal surgery, as well as an in-depth analysis of surgical site infections, including pathogenesis and risk factors. Furthermore, determinants of adequate antimicrobial treatment and different strategies for antimicrobial prophylaxis for prevention and management of postoperative infections are discussed.

KEYWORDS

Hospital-acquired infections, postoperative infections, surgical site infections, antibiotic prophylaxis, antimicrobial management.

INTRODUCTION

The human digestive tract is colonised by an unimaginable number of microorganisms that form a complex community called the gastrointestinal microbiome. These microorganisms normally reside in symbiosis with the human host and may serve an important function in metabolic processes, such as fermentation of undigested carbohydrates or the production of vitamins and hormones. Furthermore, the microbiome plays an important role in the protection against potentially pathogenic microorganisms (PPM), which can cause disease.[1] This protective effect is called colonisation resistance. Disturbance of the microbiome may lower the colonisation resistance, which puts the host at a higher risk for the development of disease. This disturbance can emerge from ageing or underlying chronic disease, from iatrogenic factors such as antibiotics, immune-suppressive agents and indwelling devices, or from surgery, which disturbs the natural protective barriers.[2]

Hospital-acquired infections (HAIs) are frequent complications during hospitalisation.[3] These infections have been reported in 8% of all patients, but incidences are even higher in patients who have undergone surgery. The risk of developing HAIs after surgery is multifactorial. Surgical intervention, the manipulation of organs that are highly colonised with microorganisms or the introduction of nonhuman implants or indwelling devices can facilitate introduction of PPMs to several body sites. Combined with a temporary depression of the immune response after surgery, ideal circumstances for infections are conceived.[4]

Surgical site infections (SSIs) account for nearly a third of all HAIs after surgery.[5] The reported incidences vary between surgical procedures; however, SSIs are particularly common after gastrointestinal surgery. Approximately 20% of all patients undergoing gastrointestinal surgery will develop an SSI within 1 month after the procedure. Besides SSIs, surgical patients are also at the risk of developing other postoperative infections such as urinary tract infections, pneumonia and bloodstream infections.

Postoperative infections often complicate recovery. Therefore, these infections are associated with an extension of hospital stay and an increased morbidity and mortality.[6,7] Furthermore, the attributable costs after SSIs are estimated to range from $3,000 to $29,000, depending on the type of surgical procedure, the infecting pathogen and area of the world.[6]

SURGICAL SITE INFECTIONS

Definition and Risk Factors of Surgical Site Infections

Surgical site infections are the most common HAIs diagnosed in surgical patients. According to the criteria that have been established by the Centers for Disease Control and Prevention, SSIs are defined as wound infections that develop within 30 days after the surgical procedure or within 90 days after the procedure, when prosthetic materials are implanted. These criteria are used internationally for diagnosing SSIs and for surveillance measures. SSIs are often localised at the primary incision site, but these infections may also extend into deeper anatomical structures (Figure 7.1).

In order to develop infection prevention measures, it is important to understand the pathogenesis and to identify factors that increase the risk of SSIs. Microbial contamination of the surgical site is a necessary precursor of SSI.[7] For SSIs after gastrointestinal surgery, the most likely source of pathogens is the endogenous microflora of the gastrointestinal tract. When the gastrointestinal tract is opened during surgery, the microorganisms have the potential to contaminate the surgical site and the surrounding tissues. The microorganisms that are part of the intestinal microbiota are therefore often cultured as the causative pathogens of SSIs as well.

Several risk factors that are independently associated with the development of SSIs have been identified (Table 7.1). The chance of developing an SSI also depends on whether the surgical procedure is considered to be clean, clean-

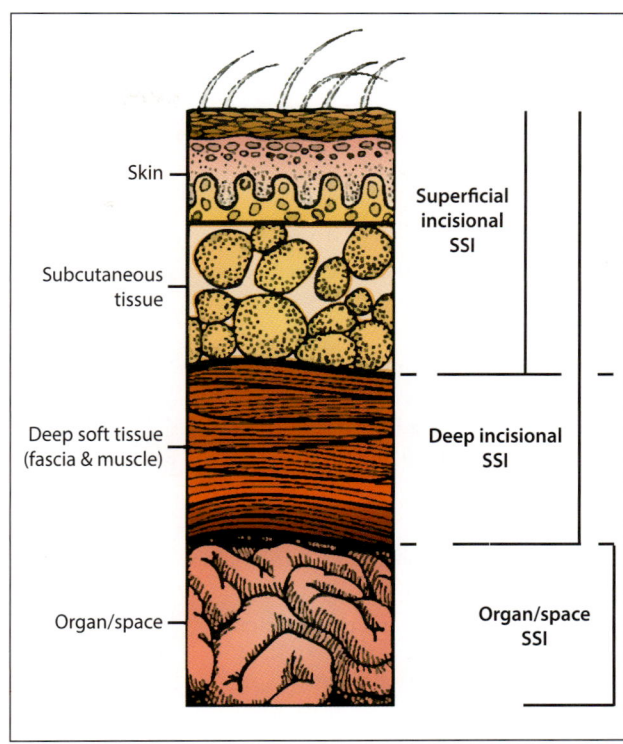

Figure 7.1 Classification of surgical site infections (SSIs).

Reproduced with permission from: Horan TC, Gaynes RP, Martone WJ, Jarvis WR, Emori TG. CDC definitions of nosocomial surgical site infections, 1992: a modification of CDC definitions of surgical wound infections. *Am J Infect Control* 1992;20:271–4.

contaminated, contaminated or dirty (Table 7.2).[8,9] Improvements in the sterilisation of surgical instruments, surgical techniques and operation room ventilation, as well as in glycaemic regulation and thermoregulation during surgery have led to a decrease in SSIs in the past decades. The use of antibiotic prophylaxis before or during surgery has also contributed greatly to the reduction of SSIs. Yet, all these measures that have made surgery safer have also allowed the use of more advanced surgical techniques, even in older patients as well as patients suffering from more severe underlying illnesses.

Gastrointestinal surgical procedures are mainly categorised as clean-contaminated procedures and are consequently associated with substantial SSI rates. Therefore, adequate antimicrobial prophylaxis during these procedures is warranted. To provide appropriate antimicrobial coverage, knowledge of the most common microorganisms associated with SSIs after gastrointestinal procedures is essential. An overview of the microbiology of SSIs as well as the rationale and establishment of adequate surgical antimicrobial prophylaxis will be provided in the following sections.

Table 7.1 Patient- and surgery-related risk factors for development of surgery site infections

Patient-related	Surgery-related
Extremes of age	Duration of surgery
Diabetes mellitus	Preoperative shaving
Smoking	Use of antimicrobial prophylaxis
Obesity	Inadequate sterilisation of surgical instruments
Immune suppression	Surgical drains
Colonisation with pathogenic microorganisms	Surgical technique (open vs. laparoscopic)
(e.g., *Staphylococcus aureus*)	Prosthetic or foreign implants
Poor nutritional status	Length of surgical scrub
Infections at other (nonsurgical) sites	Skin antisepsis
Recent surgery	Inadequate perioperative in glycaemic control
Duration of preoperative hospitalisation	Inadequate perioperative thermosregulation
Severity of underlying illness(es)	

Adapted from: Mangram AJ, Horan TC, Pearson ML, Silver LC, William R. Guideline for prevention of surgical site infection. *Bull Am Coll Surg* 2000;85:23–9.
Owens CD, Stoessel K. Surgical site infections: epidemiology, microbiology and prevention. *J Hosp Infect [Internet]* 2008;70:3–10.

Table 7.2 Surgical wound classification

Wound	Definition	Risk of infection	Examples
Class I			
Clean	Nontraumatic wound without signs of inflammation. The respiratory, alimentary, genital or uninfected urinary tracts are not entered. The wound is primarily closed and, if necessary, drained with closed drainage.	<2%	Neurosurgical procedures Endocrine surgery Eye surgery Orthopaedic procedures Vascular prostheses Skin procedures (e.g., mastectomy, lumpectomy and lipoma)
Class II			
Clean–contaminated	Wound in which the respiratory, alimentary, genital or urinary tracts are entered under controlled conditions, without significant spillage. Nontraumatic wounds, with a minor break in technique.	5–15%	Thoracic procedures Gastrointestinal procedures, including laparoscopy, colonoscopy and gastroscopy Urological procedures Nose/oropharynx procedures Gynaecological procedures
Class III			
Contaminated	Open, fresh traumatic wound from a clean source or operative wound, with a major break in sterile technique or gross spillage from the gastrointestinal tract. Incisions encountering nonpurulent inflammation.	15–30%	Gross spillage, e.g., from bowel resections with peritonitis Open fractures >4 hours
Class IV			
Dirty/infected	Old traumatic wounds with retained devitalised tissue and that involving existing clinical infection or perforated viscera. This definition suggests that the organisms causing postoperative infection were present in the operative field before the operation.	>30%	Bowel resection with perforation, sinus infection, pelvic abscess, infected pilonidal cysts Wound debridement

Adapted from: Mangram AJ, Horan TC, Pearson ML, Silver LC, William R. Guideline for prevention of surgical site infection. *Bull Am Coll Surg* 2000;85:23–9.
Zinn J, Swofford V. Quality-improvement initiative: classifying and documenting surgical wounds. *Wound Care Advis* 2014;3:32–8.

Microbiology of Surgical Site Infections

Surgical site infections are often caused by microorganisms that are part of the commensal microbiota of the patient.[10] Consequently, superficial SSIs that develop after most types of surgery are often caused by bacteria that colonise the skin, such as coagulase-negative staphylococci (CONS) and *Staphylococcus aureus*. Particularly for SSIs after gastrointestinal surgery, the most likely reservoir of the causative pathogens is the endogenous microflora of the gastrointestinal tract.[11] Since the microbial composition differs between the different parts of the gastrointestinal tract, the microbiology of SSIs associated with different types of procedures also varies.[5,11–14] The microbiology of SSIs after surgery of the upper digestive tract (gastric, pancreatic and hepatobiliary procedures) is comparable to lower gastrointestinal interventions (appendectomy and colorectal surgery). *Staphylococcus aureus* and CONS are cultured more often from SSIs of the upper gastrointestinal tract, whereas SSIs after procedures on the lower gastrointestinal tract are more often caused by Enterobacteriaceae and *Bacteroides* spp. Besides a comparison between the upper and lower gastrointestinal tract procedures, several studies have investigated the organ-specific spectrum of pathogens (Table 7.3).

Oesophageal Procedures

Data on pathogens associated with SSIs after oesophagus surgery are limited. One study evaluated SSIs after these procedures in 12 patients.[12] The microorganisms that were isolated in most patients were CONS, *Pseudomonas aeruginosa* and *Bacteroides* spp.

Gastroduodenal Procedures

The reported incidences of SSIs after gastroduodenal surgery have ranged from 3 to 10%.[15] Enterobacteriaceae, anaerobic bacteria, enterococci and staphylococci are the most common pathogens associated with SSIs after these procedures.[14] In addition, *Candida* infections also contribute to SSI development. *Candida* species are occasional residents of the intestinal microbiome in some patients but will not result in infections in most individuals. *Candida* colonisation rates are increased in patients suffering from chronic gastrointestinal disease such as inflammatory bowel disease and ulcer disease.[16] Although SSIs caused by *Candida* species may occur more frequently in these patients, there are limited data on SSIs in this specific subgroup.

Table 7.3   Microorganisms associated with surgical site infections after gastrointestinal surgery

Surgical procedure	Pathogens				
	Bacteria				Fungi
	Gram-positive		Gram-negative		
	Aerobic cocci	Anaerobes	Facultative anaerobic bacilli	Anaerobes	
Oesophageal surgery	CONS *S. aureus* *Streptococcus* spp.		*P. aeruginosa*	*Bacteroides* spp.	
Gastroduodenal surgery	CONS *Enterococcus* spp.		Enterobacteriaceae*	*Bacteroides* spp.	*Candida* spp.
Biliary and pancreatic surgery	CONS *S. aureus* *Enterococcus* spp.	*Clostridium* spp.	*P. aeruginosa* Enterobacteriaceae*	*B. fragilis*	*C. albicans* *C. glabrata*
Appendectomy	*Enterococcus* spp. *S. aureus*		Enterobacteriaceae*	*B. fragilis*	
Surgery of the small intestines	*Enterococcus* spp. *S. aureus*		Enterobacteriaceae*	*B. fragilis*	
Colorectal surgery	*Enterococcus* spp. *S. aureus*		Enterobacteriaceae*	*B. fragilis*	

*Enterobacteriaceae is a family of facultative anaerobe gram-negative bacteria. Predominant intestinal genera are *Escherichia coli*, *Klebsiella* spp., *Enterobacter* spp. and *Proteus* spp.

Abbreviations: *B. fragilis*: Bacteroides fragilis; *C. albicans*: Candida albicans; *C. glabrata*: Candida glabrata; CONS: coagulase-negative *Staphylococci*; *P. aeruginosa*: Pseudomonas aeruginosa; *S. aureus*: Staphylococcus aureus.

Biliary and Pancreatic Procedures

The overall risk of development of SSIs in biliary surgery is approximately 10%.[12,17] In these procedures, not only the general risk factors but also bile contamination plays an important role in the development of infections. Bile ducts are usually sterile but may be colonised by *Escherichia coli* (and other Enterobacteriaceae) or staphylococcal species, for example, due to cholecystitis and bile duct obstruction. When the bile ducts are colonised before surgery, SSIs are often polymicrobial and are predominantly caused by enterococci, *E. coli*, *P. aeruginosa*, CONS, *Candida* spp. and *Clostridium* species.[17,18]

The pathogens associated with SSIs after pancreatic surgery are similar. However, *Klebsiella* spp. and *Candida albicans* infections may be more common after these procedures.[12]

Appendectomy

Postoperative SSIs are estimated to develop in about 5% of the patients who have undergone an appendectomy for appendicitis.[19] The predominant microorganisms associated with acute appendicitis are similar to those associated with SSIs after appendectomy; *E. coli*, *Klebsiella* spp., *Enterobacter* spp., anaerobes and *Enterococcus* spp.[20] Acute appendicitis can be either classified as uncomplicated (i.e., inflamed appendix) or complicated appendicitis. In the latter, the appendix is perforated or gangrenous. Preoperative prophylaxis to prevent infectious complications therefore only applies to the first category. This will be discussed in the following section on antimicrobial prophylaxis.

Surgery on the Small Intestines and Colorectal Procedures

Surgical site infections affect 10 to 20% of all patients who undergo colorectal surgery. Enterobacteriaceae, *Enterococcus* spp. and *Bacteroides* spp. are the most common pathogens causing SSIs after these procedures.[21] The predominant pathogens isolated from SSIs after small intestine surgery are similar.

Antimicrobial Management of Surgical Site Infections

Antimicrobial treatment is not always indicated in the treatment of SSIs. Minor superficial infections often respond to drainage of pus by opening the surgical wound. However, for deep infections, drainage may need to be supplemented with adjunctive antibiotic treatment. Optimal empirical therapy needs to be based on the local antibiotic susceptibility pattern of the microorganisms associated with SSIs, which includes gram-negative bacilli and anaerobes in almost all circumstances for patients undergoing gastrointestinal surgery. Empirical treatment may be adapted when culture results are available (e.g., when multiresistant microorganisms are cultured). For effective antimicrobial treatment of individual and future patients, it is, therefore, essential to obtain cultures from the infected sites, whenever possible.

OTHER POSTOPERATIVE INFECTIONS AFTER GASTROINTESTINAL SURGERY

Hospital-Acquired Pneumonia

Hospital-acquired pneumonia (HAP) is the most frequently diagnosed HAI in the intensive care unit (ICU) because of impaired local defence mechanisms in the upper respiratory tract and increased risk of aspiration in critically ill and intubated patients. Surgical patients are also at risk of developing HAP during their postoperative hospital stay because of the risk of aspiration of gastric contents during or shortly after surgery. This risk is further enhanced by the use of sedatives, which impair the pharyngeal reflex, and because of intubation for several hours.[4] Microorganisms from the upper digestive tract, such as *S. aureus*, *P. aeruginosa*, *E. coli* and *Klebsiella* spp., can therefore migrate into the respiratory tract.

The clinical diagnosis of HAP is based on the presence of at least two clinical indicators of infection such as cough, fever and leucocytosis, combined with a new or progressive pulmonary infiltrate on the chest radiograph.[22] Furthermore, sputum or blood cultures should be taken to guide empirical treatment. Broad-spectrum antibiotics are usually administered empirically but should be de-escalated after obtaining the results of clinical cultures.

Catheter-Associated Urinary Tract Infections

Urinary tract infections are common among hospitalised patients and are associated with indwelling bladder catheters in 80% of the cases.[4] During surgery, bladder function is impaired and catheters are inserted to prevent urinary retention. These catheters can serve as a port of entry for microorganisms to enter the urinary tract. Furthermore, the materials used for catheters can facilitate biofilm formation, creating a firm breeding ground for bacteria.

Catheter-associated urinary tract infections (CAUTIs) are defined as urinary tract infections in patients with a urine catheter in place for at least 2 days. Although these infections are associated with less morbidity and mortality compared with other HAIs, they can lead to bacteraemia and death when they remain untreated. Microorganisms that are often associated with CAUTIs usually originate from the digestive tract; these include *E. coli*, *Enterococcus* spp. and *Klebsiella* spp. In addition, *Candida* spp. can be isolated in patients that have received broad-spectrum antibiotics.[4]

The initial management of CAUTIs should include removal or replacement of the urine catheter. Broad-spectrum antibiotics should be initiated empirically, based on the local susceptibility pattern of pathogens involved with de-escalation based on culture results.

Catheter-Related Bloodstream Infections

Catheter-related bloodstream infections account for approximately 5% of all HAIs and are associated with high mortality rates.[23] Infections are often a result of indwelling venous catheters that penetrate the skin and allow introduction and migration of skin flora into the bloodstream. Most cases of hospital-acquired bacteraemia are therefore caused by common skin flora such as CONS, *S. aureus* (including methicillin-resistant *S. aureus* [MRSA]) and *Candida* spp.[23]

Catheter-related bloodstream infections should be suspected in patients with intravascular catheters that develop clinical or laboratory signs of systemic infection. The exit sites of indwelling intravascular catheters should be inspected to identify local inflammation, Moreover, two sets of blood cultures should be taken before initiation of antibiotic treatment.

The initial management of the infection should start with removal or change of the intravenous catheter. In the case of a bloodstream infection with CONS, catheter removal without the administration of antibiotics is often sufficient for treating the infection.[24]

In bloodstream infections caused by other pathogens, antibiotic treatment is almost always indicated.

Antibiotic treatment will depend on the isolated pathogen, on the severity of the clinical disease and on potential risk factors (e.g., immunosuppression and pre-existent colonisation with multiresistant bacteria) and should cover the most likely pathogens if culture results are not available. Empirical coverage of gram-negative bacilli can be provided with fourth-generation cephalosporins, beta-lactam antibiotics or carbapenems. The choice of antimicrobials and the duration of the antibiotic treatment should be based on the antimicrobial susceptibility patterns. Catheter-associated bloodstream infections that are caused by *S. aureus* should be treated for at least 14 days.

Empirical antifungal treatment is not generally recommended in patients with catheter-related bloodstream infections. However, administration of echinocandins or fluconazole can be considered in patients with a high risk of developing *Candida* bacteraemia such as patients in the ICU, those who have undergone abdominal surgery, those who develop anastomotic leakage and those who have known *Candida* colonisation.[24]

ANTIBIOTIC PROPHYLAXIS FOR GASTROINTESTINAL SURGERY

Antibiotic prophylaxis is one of the most important measures to prevent SSIs. The concept of this prophylaxis is to kill microorganisms that are seeded to the surgical site during the procedure, consequently lowering the risk of SSIs. The antibiotics in the prophylaxis should cover the most common pathogens associated with SSIs at the lowest cost and the lowest toxicity, for the shortest treatment duration as possible. Perioperative intravenous prophylaxis is the international standard of care during gastrointestinal surgery, but novel, additional antimicrobial strategies have been proposed to further reduce incidence of SSIs.

With the introduction of perioperative intravenous antibiotic prophylaxis for patients undergoing gastrointestinal surgery, the incidence of abdominal SSIs has decreased. In a systematic review of 26 randomised trials published in 1981, perioperative intravenous antimicrobial prophylaxis was, compared with placebo or no antimicrobial treatment during surgery, associated with an absolute risk reduction of 14% (from 36% without to 22% with antibiotic prophylaxis).[25] Since then, withholding antibiotic prophylaxis from patients is no longer considered ethical.[21] Recent guidelines for gastrointestinal surgery therefore consider the use of antimicrobial prophylaxis to be imperative.

Antimicrobial prophylaxis can be provided in several ways, differing in route of administration, duration of treatment and the use of antimicrobial agents. Since the predominant pathogens causing SSI throughout the gastrointestinal tract are comparable, antibiotic prophylaxis providing coverage against enteric gram-negative bacilli and anaerobes (e.g., *Bacteroides fragilis*), as well as gram-positive streptococci, has yielded the best results in randomised studies.[8]

Prophylactic Strategies

Perioperative Antibiotic Prophylaxis

Perioperative antibiotic prophylaxis is defined as antibiotic treatment before and during the surgical procedure. Intravenous application of antibiotics is most widely practiced in gastrointestinal surgery.

After gastrointestinal surgery, wounds are classified as clean-contaminated or contaminated, and antibiotics for prophylaxis should be based on this classification and the pathogens associated with these interventions. Adequate perioperative antimicrobial prophylaxis is based on four principles to maximise the benefits.[7] Firstly, to use antibiotics for those procedures in which their use has been demonstrated to reduce SSI rates. Secondly, an antimicrobial agent must be safe, inexpensive and have a bactericidal effect in vitro for the most probable pathogens of SSI. Thirdly, the timing of infusion of the initial dose of antimicrobial agents should reach a bactericidal concentration in serum and tissues at the time of incision. International guidelines recommend that the first dose is administered within 60 to 30 minutes before the surgical procedure.[26,27] Fourthly, therapeutic serum and tissue levels should be maintained throughout surgery and until at most a few hours after closure of the surgical wound in the operation room. This implicates additional intraoperative antibiotic dosing during prolonged surgical procedures or for antimicrobials with short half-lives.[26] For instance, when a surgical procedure exceeds three times the half-life of the antimicrobial agent, administration of an additional dose is strongly recommended.[27] This is also recommended in case of excessive blood loss during surgery (>1.500 mL). Prophylaxis exceeding 24 hours is strongly discouraged, as this will unnecessarily affect the nonpathogenic microflora, increasing the risk of selection of antimicrobial resistance or *Clostridium difficile* infections (CDI), and may lead to antimicrobial toxicity and unnecessary expense.[8]

An overview of the antimicrobial agents is provided in Tables 7.4 and 7.5. A single dose of first- or second-generation cephalosporins is often the first choice for several surgical interventions. Most generations of cephalosporins cover a variety of gram-negative and gram-positive species. They are reasonably safe and have predictable pharmacokinetics, with a relatively long half-life. Cefazolin, a first-generation cephalosporin, is used internationally as a first-choice antimicrobial for gastrointestinal surgery prophylaxis. Cefazolin covers the most common facultative anaerobic species (Enterobacteriaceae), streptococcal species and some species of *Staphylococcus*. Anaerobes and *Enterococcus* spp. are not affected by cefazolin. Second-choice antimicrobials can be beta-lactams (e.g., ampicillin–sulbactam and amoxicillin–clavulanic acid) or cephalosporins belonging to the second or third generation. Because anaerobic activity is limited for most cephalosporins, European guidelines often recommend addition of metronidazole for gastrointestinal

surgery.[27] Penicillins such as ampicillin or amoxicillin combined with a beta-lactamase inhibitor are advised as an alternative to cephalosporins but not if these antibiotics are frequently used in other patient groups. Cefoxitin, a second-generation cephalosporin, also covers both aerobic and anaerobic species. However, it is not the first treatment of choice because of a short half-life and relatively high costs.

The routine use of vancomycin is not recommended during abdominal surgical procedures, but may be an acceptable antimicrobial prophylaxis in the case of known colonisation with MRSA or when a cluster of SSIs caused by MRSA has been detected in an institution.[7] In these cases, vancomycin is added to the standard of a first- or second-generation cephalosporin with activity against gram-negative organisms. Colonisation with other (multi-) resistant microorganisms should be evaluated per patient and prophylactic treatment should be individualised.

Table 7.4 Recommended doses of antimicrobials used as surgical prophylaxis

Antimicrobial	Usual dose (adults)*	Redosing interval in hours
Intravenous prophylaxis		
Ampicillin-sulbactam	3 g (2 g/1 g)	2
Cefazolin	<120 Kg: 2 g, >120 Kg: 3 g	4
Cefoxitin	2 g	2
Cefotetan	2 g	6
Clindamycin	900 mg	6
Metronidazole	500 mg	–
Vancomycin	15 mg/Kg	–
*Oral prophylaxis***		
Neomycin	1 g	–
Erythromycin base	1 g	–
Metronidazole	1 g	–

*Recommended doses are based on adults with normal liver and kidney functions.
**Oral prophylaxis is used in colorectal procedures and is administered in combination with mechanical bowel preparation.

Adapted from: Bratzler DW, Houck PM. Antimicrobial prophylaxis for surgery: An advisory statement from the National Surgical Infection Prevention Project. *Am J Surg* 2005;189:395–404.
Van Kasteren ME, Gyssens IC, Kullberg BJ, Bruining HA, Stobbering EE, Goris RJ. Optimizing antibiotics policy in the Netherlands. V. SWAB guidelines for perioperative antibiotic prophylaxis. Foundation Antibiotics Policy Team. *Ned Tijdschr Geneeskd [Internet]* 2000;144:2049–55.

Table 7.5 Recommended antimicrobial prophylaxis for gastrointestinal procedures

Procedure	Recommended antimicrobials[*]	Alternative antimicrobials
Esophageal surgery	Cefazolin	Vancomycin
Gastroduodenal surgery	Cefazolin	Clindamycin Vancomycin + aminoglycoside
Biliary tract and pancreatic surgery		
Open procedure	Cefazolin	Cefoxitin Cefotetan Ampicillin-sulbactam Clindamycin
Laparoscopic procedure – Low risk[**]	No prophylaxis	No prophylaxis
– High risk[**]	Cefazolin	Cefoxitin Cefotetan Ampicillin-sulbactam Clindamycin
Appendectomy[***]	Cefazolin + metronidazole	Cefoxitin Cefotetan Clindamycin + aminoglycoside
Small intestine surgery		
Not obstructed	Cefazolin	Cefoxitin Cefotetan
Obstructed	Cefazolin + metronidazole	Cefoxitin Cefotetan
Colorectal surgery		
Intravenous prophylaxis	Cefazolin + metronidazole	Cefoxitin Cefotetan Ampicillin-sulbactam Clindamycin Vancomycin + aminoglycoside
Oral prophylaxis	Neomycin + erythromycin base	Neomycin + metronidazole

[*]In patients known to be colonised with methicillin-resistant *Staphylococcus aureus*, a single perioperative dose of vancomycin is recommended.
[**]High-risk procedures include emergency procedures, age >70 years, ASA classification >3, acute cholecystitis, immunosuppression, pregnancy and insertion of nonhuman tissue implants.
[***]Appendectomy without complicated (i.e., perforated) appendicitis.
Adapted from: Bratzler DW, Houck PM. Antimicrobial prophylaxis for surgery: An advisory statement from the National Surgical Infection Prevention Project. *Am J Surg* 2005;189:395–404.
Van Kasteren ME, Gyssens IC, Kullberg BJ, Bruining HA, Stobberingh EE, Goris RJ. Optimizing antibiotics policy in the Netherlands. V. SWAB guidelines for perioperative antibiotic prophylaxis. Foundation Antibiotics Policy Team. *Ned Tijdschr Geneeskd [Internet]* 2000;144:2049–55.

Preoperative Oral Antibiotic Prophylaxis

During the past decades, preoperative oral administration of antibiotics has been a popular prophylactic strategy in the United States, specifically for colorectal surgery. Oral prophylaxis usually contains neomycin combined with erythromycin or metronidazole and is administered 1 to 2 days before surgery.[26]

Several studies have evaluated the effect of oral prophylaxis combined with the abovementioned perioperative intravenous prophylaxis on the development of SSIs. In a recent meta-analysis, the combination of oral and intravenous prophylaxis was superior to intravenous prophylaxis, resulting in a relative risk of developing SSI of 0.55 (95% confidence interval [CI]: 0.41–0.74).[21]

The use of oral preoperative antimicrobial prophylaxis is invariably combined with mechanical bowel preparation. The rationale of this preparation is to clean the colon before the procedure, reducing the risk of perioperative contamination of the abdominal cavity with faeces. Along with the mechanical preparation, often a polyethylene glycol solution, antibiotics are administered orally. Until recently, mechanical bowel preparation was the standard of care before colorectal surgery. However, recent systematic reviews concluded that the use of mechanical bowel preparation should be omitted before colorectal surgery, because it had no overall beneficial effect and because of the fact that it causes substantial discomfort for the patient. The use of mechanical bowel preparation is nowadays considered to be controversial and has therefore been abandoned from guidelines.[28,29]

The use of selective decontamination has been proposed as another oral preoperative prophylactic treatment for gastrointestinal surgery. Other than the neomycin/erythromycin prophylaxis used in bowel preparations, the use of nonabsorbable, selectively decontaminating antibiotics has been investigated in the past decades as prophylaxis in gastrointestinal surgery.[30–32]

The underlying hypothesis is that infections caused by endogenous PPMs occur due to loss of colonisation resistance in the digestive tract. The latter results from the use of systemic antibiotics, disrupting the assumed protective anaerobic gut flora, which then facilitates overgrowth of gram-negative bacilli. Maintaining colonisation resistance should decrease the risk of infections with these gram-negative bacilli. This should be realised by using antibiotics that have a selective activity against PPMs but not against anaerobes.

The use of selective decontamination as an infection-prevention strategy was first described in neutropenic patients[33] and was subsequently introduced in ICU patients in 1984 by Stoutenbeek et al.[34] Patients in the ICU are highly susceptible to infections with gram-negative bacilli, aerobes and yeasts, due to severe underlying illness, the use of mechanical ventilation and the use of other indwelling devices. This strategy, introduced as selective decontamination of the digestive tract (SDD) is nowadays the standard of care in ICUs in several countries across Europe.

The antimicrobials used in SDD are nonabsorbable antibiotics, which implies that the antibiotics do not enter the systemic circulation after oral ingestion and therefore remain restricted to the lumen of the digestive tract. This provides direct killing of PPMs, with low risks of systemic side effects of antibiotics.

The classical SDD treatment consists of colistin (polymyxin E), tobramycin and amphotericin B and is applied four times daily. Colistin is used in the treatment of gram-negative infections with *Acinetobacter* spp., Enterobacteriaceae such as *Klebsiella* spp., *E. coli* and

P. aeruginosa. Tobramycin has a strong bactericidal effect against a broad spectrum of aerobic gram-negative microorganisms, such as *Pseudomonas* spp., *Enterobacter* spp. and *E. coli*, and specific gram-positive staphylococcus species such as *S. aureus*. Amphotericin B is administered to prevent infections with *Candida* species. The effects of SDD, when used as surgical prophylaxis on the occurrence of SSI, have been determined in several studies in the past decades. SDD was associated with significant reductions in the incidence of SSIs, pneumonia and urinary tract infections.[31] However, because of the heterogeneity between studies, the before-mentioned association with mechanical bowel preparation and the limited availability of results from randomised and double-blinded studies, the true effects of preoperative antibiotic prophylaxis on postoperative infectious outcomes remain unknown, precluding firm recommendations regarding the timing of treatment and choice of antimicrobial agents.

Topical Administration of Gentamicin-Containing Collagen

Application of gentamicin-containing collagen implants (GCCI) provides high local concentrations of gentamicin without systemic absorption, thus avoiding potential systemic side effects such as nephrotoxicity. Besides an antibiotic effect, the GCCI may also stimulate wound healing by improving epithelialisation and granulation and help with local haemostasis. Gentamicin has a clinical efficacy against gram-positive microorganisms such as *S. aureus* and CONS and also covers gram-negative bacilli that are typically associated with gastrointestinal procedures.[35] In a systemic review of 13 clinical studies evaluating local application of GCCI in gastrointestinal surgery, most reported reduced incidences of SSI and accelerated wound healing compared with standard prophylaxis.[36] There was, however, substantial heterogeneity between studies, and large randomised controlled trials (RCTs) of high quality will be necessary to quantify the effect of GCCI for future recommendations.

Antimicrobial-Coated Sutures

Surgical site infections may also be prevented by using antimicrobial-coated sutures. The rationale of this strategy is to prevent microbial colonisation of the sutures, reducing the risk of developing infections of the surgical incision. In a recent meta-analysis of 15 RCTs with 4,800 patients, the use of triclosan-coated sutures, compared with non-coated sutures, was associated with a reduced SSI incidence (relative risk: 0.67; 95% CI: 0.54–0.84; p < 0.00053).[37] Although it was not possible to evaluate the effect of triclosan-coated sutures specifically during abdominal surgery, more recently, a large multicentre RCT of 1224 patients undergoing elective midline abdominal laparotomy, which was not included in the meta-analysis, failed to confirm these results (odds ratio: 0.91; 95% CI: 0.66–1.25; p = 0.64).[38] Although promising, the effect of antimicrobial sutures in gastrointestinal surgery is still unclear.

Risks and Side Effects of Antimicrobial Prophylaxis

The beneficial effects of surgical antimicrobial prophylaxis are substantial. However, the routine use of antibiotic prophylaxis is not without any consequences and should therefore be administered with caution. Besides the risk of developing antibiotic-related diarrhoea or allergic reactions, one should be aware of other potential adverse events that may develop because of antibiotic treatment.

Clostridium difficile Infection

Clostridium difficile infections are important healthcare-associated infections and account for 20 to 30% of cases of antibiotic-related diarrhoea. The risk of CDI is multifactorial and is increased in patients that have undergone gastrointestinal surgery as well as after administration of antimicrobials. The use of first- or third-generation cephalosporins, for example, when applied as perioperative prophylaxis, is the greatest contributing factor for developing CDI.

Clostridium difficile is a gram-positive spore-forming bacterium that produces toxins. Toxin release often causes infectious diarrhoea, which may progress to severe life-threatening infection of the colon. Predisposing signs and symptoms are new-onset diarrhoea (>3 unformed stools in 24 or fewer consecutive hours), abdominal pain and fever.[39] When these symptoms develop in patients after gastrointestinal surgery or in any other situation where antibiotics have been administered, CDI must be considered. The diagnosis can be confirmed by detection of *C. difficile* toxins in the faeces.

As soon as CDI is suspected, infection prevention measures should be taken to prevent further spread of the infection to other hospitalised patients. General contact precautions such as transfer of the patient to a private room and the use of gloves and gowns must be undertaken for the duration of diarrhoea. Hand hygiene should be performed with soap instead of alcohol-based products, since *C. difficile* spores are highly resistant to killing by alcohol.[39]

Antibiotic treatment should be discontinued when the diagnosis is confirmed, and antimicrobials that cover *C. difficile* should be initiated, depending on the severity of the infection. For mild CDI, metronidazole is the treatment of first choice. When signs of systemic toxicity develop, CDI is considered a severe infection and treatment with vancomycin is indicated.[40]

Antimicrobial Resistance

Any antibiotic use, including prophylactic use, is associated with selection of antimicrobial resistance. Prolonged administration of antibiotics therefore facilitates selection of bacteria harbouring resistance genes. In consequence, guidelines for perioperative antimicrobial prophylaxis discourage to extend the prophylaxis postoperatively for more than 24 hours.

CONCLUSIONS

Patients who undergo gastrointestinal surgery are at substantial risk of developing postoperative hospital-acquired infections such as surgical site infections, hospital-acquired pneumonia, urinary tract infections and catheter-related bloodstream infections. Adequate antimicrobial management and prevention measures are important strategies in order to reduce the burden of these infections. The choice of antimicrobials is dependent on the type of the surgical procedure and the local pathogen-susceptibility patterns. With the exception of patients that show signs of infection, antimicrobial prophylaxis should be discontinued after the surgical procedure.

REFERENCES

1. Gerritsen J, Smidt H, Rijkers GT, De Vos WM. Intestinal microbiota in human health and disease: the impact of probiotics. *Genes Nutr* 2011;6:209–40.

2. Lapthorne S, Bines JE, Fouhy F, et al. Changes in the colon microbiota and intestinal cytokine gene expression following minimal intestinal surgery. *World J Gastroenterol* 2015;21:4150–8.

3. Kirchhoff P, Clavien P-A, Hahnloser D. Complications in colorectal surgery: risk factors and preventive strategies. *Patient Saf Surg* [Internet] 2010;4:5. Accessed on 1 Feb 2016. Available from: http://www.pubmedcentral.nih.gov/articlerender.fcgi?artid=2852382&tool=pmcentrez&rendertype=abstract.

4. Hedrick TL, Smith PW, Gazoni LM, Sawyer RG. The appropriate use of antibiotics in surgery: a review of surgical infections. *Curr Probl Surg* 2007;44:635–75.

5. Najjar PA, Smink DS. Prophylactic Antibiotics and Prevention of Surgical Site Infections. *Surg Clin North Am* [Internet] 2015;95:269–83. Accessed on 28 Oct 2015. Available from: http://linkinghub.elsevier.com/retrieve/pii/S0039610914002138.

6. Anderson DJ, Podgorny K, Berríos-Torres SI, et al. Strategies to prevent surgical site infections in acute care hospitals:

2014 update. *Infect Control Hosp Epidemiol* [Internet] 2014;35:605–27. Accessed on 5 Mar 2016. Available from: http://www.ncbi.nlm.nih.gov/pubmed/24799638.

7. Mangram AJ, Horan TC, Pearson ML, Silver LC, William R. Guideline for prevention of surgical site infection. *Bull Am Coll Surg* 2000;85:23–9.

8. Enzler MJ, Berbari E, Osmon DR. Antimicrobial prophylaxis in adults. *Mayo Clin Proc* [Internet] 2011;86:686–701. Accessed on 19 Feb 2016. Available from: http://dx.doi.org/10.4065/mcp.2011.0012.

9. Zinn J, Swofford V. Quality-improvement initiative: classifying and documenting surgical wounds. *Wound Care Advis* 2014;3:32–8.

10. Ramcharan AA, Heijer CDJ Den, Smeets EEJ, et al. Microbiology of surgical site infections after gastrointestinal surgery in the south region of The Netherlands. *Future Microbiol* 2014;9:291–8.

11. Múñez E, Ramos A, Álvarez De Espejo T, Vaqué J, Castedo E, Martínez-Hernández J, et al. Etiología de las infecciones del sitio quirúrgico en pacientes intervenidos de cirugía cardiaca. *Cir Cardiovasc* 2013;20:139–43.

12. Jannasch O, Kelch B, Adolf D, Tammer I, Lodes U, Weiss G, et al. Nosocomial infections and microbiologic spectrum after major elective surgery of the pancreas, liver, stomach, and esophagus. *Surg Infect (Larchmt)* [Internet] 2015;16:338–45. Accessed on 18 Feb 2016. Available from: http://www.ncbi.nlm.nih.gov/pubmed/26046248.

13. Misteli H, Widmer AF, Rosenthal R, Oertli D, Marti WR, Weber WP. Spectrum of pathogens in surgical site infections at a Swiss university hospital. *Swiss Med Wkly* 2011;140:2–5.

14. Owens CD, Stoessel K. Surgical site infections: epidemiology, microbiology and prevention. *J Hosp Infect* [Internet] 2008;70:3–10. Accessed on 28 Oct 2015. Available from: www.sciencedirect.com.

15. Jeong SJ, Hea Won A, Jae Kyung Kim HC, et al. Incidence and risk factors for surgical site infection after gastric surgery: a multicenter prospective cohort study. *Infect Chemother* 2013;45:422–30.

16. Kumamoto CA. Inflammation and gastrointestinal Candida colonization. *Curr Opin Microbiol* 2011;14:386–91.

17. Herzog T, Belyaev O, Akkuzu R, Holling J, Uhl W, Chromik AM. The Impact of Bile Duct Cultures on Surgical Site Infections in Pancreatic Surgery. *Surg Infect (Larchmt)* [Internet] 2015;16:443–9. Accessed on 18 Feb 2016. Available from: http://ovidsp.ovid.com/ovidweb.cgi?T=JS&CSC=Y&NEWS=N&PAGE=fulltext&D=emed13&AN=2015227600\nhttp://sfx.ucl.ac.uk/sfx_local?sid=OVID:embase&id=pmid:&id=doi:10.1089/sur.2014.104&issn=1096-2964&isbn=&volume=16&issue=4&spage=443&pages=443-449&date=2015&title=.

18. Wittmann DH, Condon RE. Prophylaxis of postoperative infections. Infection [Internet]. 1991;19:S337–44.

19. Wu W-T, Tai F-C, Wang P-C, Tsai M-L. Surgical site infection and timing of prophylactic antibiotics for appendectomy. *Surg Infect (Larchmt)* [Internet] 2014;15:781–5. Accessed on 18 Feb 2016. Available from: http://www.ncbi.nlm.nih.gov/pubmed/25401521.

20. Andersen BR, Kallehave FL, Andersen HK. Antibiotics versus placebo for prevention of postoperative infection after appendicectomy. *Cochrane Database Syst Rev* 2005;3:CD001439.

21. Nelson RL, Glenny AM, Song F. Antimicrobial prophylaxis for colorectal surgery. *Cochrane Database Syst Rev* [Internet] 2009;1:CD001181. Accessed on 28 Oct 2015. Available from: http://www.thecochranelibrary.com.

22. American Thoracic Society. Guidelines for the Management of Adults with Hospital-acquired, Ventilator-associated, and Healthcare-associated Pneumonia. *Am J Respir Crit Care Med* 2005;171:388–416.

23. World Health Organization. *Prevention of Hospital-Acquired Infections.* Geneva, Switzerland: World Health Organization. 2002;72.

24. Gyssens IC, Bax HI, Schippers EF, et al; Dutch Working Party on Antibiotic Policy (SWAB). SWAB guidelines for antibacterial therapy of adult patients with sepsis. *SWAB richtlijn Sepsis* 2010. Available from: http://www.swab.nl/swab/cms3.nsf/uploads/65FB380648516FF2C125780F002C39E2/$FILE/swab_sepsis_guideline_december_2010.pdf.

25. Baum ML, Anish DS, Chalmers TC, Sacks HS, Smith H, Fagerstrom RM. A survey of clinical trials of antibiotic prophylaxis in colon surgery: evidence against further use of no-treatment controls. *N Engl J Med* 1981;305:795–9.

26. Bratzler DW, Houck PM. Antimicrobial prophylaxis for surgery: An advisory statement from the National Surgical Infection Prevention Project. *Am J Surg* 2005;189:395–404.

27. Van Kasteren ME, Gyssens IC, Kullberg BJ, Bruining HA, Stobberingh EE, Goris RJ. [Optimizing antibiotics policy in the Netherlands. V. SWAB guidelines for perioperative antibiotic prophylaxis. Foundation Antibiotics Policy Team]. *Ned Tijdschr Geneeskd* [Internet] 2000;144:2049–55. Accessed on 29 Oct 2015. Available from: http://ovidsp.ovid.com/ovidweb.cgi?T=JS&CSC=Y&NEWS=N&PAGE=fulltext&D=med4&AN=11072507.

28. Slim K, Vicaut E, Launay-Savary M-V, Contant C, Chipponi J. Updated systematic review and meta-analysis of randomized clinical trials on the role of mechanical bowel preparation before colorectal surgery. *Ann Surg* [Internet] 2009;249:203–9. Accessed on 29 Oct 2015. Available from: http://www.ncbi.nlm.nih.gov/pubmed/19212171.

29. Güenaga KF, Matos D, Wille-Jørgensen P. Mechanical bowel preparation for elective colorectal surgery. *Cochrane*

Accessed on 23 Feb 2016. Available from: http://link.springer.com/10.1007/BF01715775.

Database of Systematic Reviews 2011;9:CD001544. doi: 10.1002/14651858.CD001544.pub4.

30. Taylor EW, Lindsay G. Selective decontamination of the colon before elective colorectal. *World J Surg* 1994;18: 926–32.

31. Roos D, Dijksman LM, Oudemans-van Straaten HM, de Wit LT, Gouma DJ, Gerhards MF. Randomized clinical trial of perioperative selective decontamination of the digestive tract versus placebo in elective gastrointestinal surgery. *Br J Surg* [Internet] 2011;98:1365–72. Accessed on 28 Oct 2015. Available from: http://www.ncbi.nlm.nih.gov/pubmed/21751181.

32. Tetteroo GWM, Castelein A, Tilanus HW, Ince C, Bruining HA, Wagenvoort JHT. Selective decontamination to reduce gram-negative colonisation and infections after oesophageal resection. *Lancet* 1990;335:704–7.

33. Rodriguez V, Bodey GP, Freireich EJ, et al. Randomized trial of protected environment – prophylactic antibiotics in 145 adults with acute leukemia. *Medicine* (Baltimore) 1978;57:253–66.

34. Stoutenbeek CP, van Saene HK, Miranda DR, Zandstra DF. The effect of selective decontamination of the digestive tract on colonisation and infection rate in multiple trauma patients. *Intensive Care Med* 1984;10:185–92.

35. Chang WK, Srinivasa S, Maccormick AD, Hill AG. Gentamicin-collagen implants to reduce surgical site infection: systematic review and meta-analysis of Randomized Trials. *Ann Surg* [Internet] 2013;258:59–65. Accessed on 23 Feb 2016. Available from: http://www.ncbi.nlm.nih.gov/pubmed/23486193.

36. De Bruin AFJ, Gosselink MP, van der Harst E. Local application of gentamicin-containing collagen implant in the prophylaxis of surgical site infection following gastrointestinal surgery. *Int J Surg* [Internet] 2012;10:S21–7. Accessed on 5 Feb 2016. Available from: http://dx.doi.org/10.1016/j.ijsu.2012.05.014.

37. Daoud FC, Edmiston CE, Leaper D. Meta-analysis of prevention of surgical site infections following incision closure with triclosan-coated sutures: robustness to new evidence. *Surg Infect (Larchmt)* [Internet] 2014;15:165–81. Accessed on 22 Mar 2016. Available from: http://www.pubmedcentral.nih.gov/articlerender.fcgi?artid=4063374&tool=pmcentrez&rendertype=abstract.

38. Diener MK, Knebel P, Kieser M, et al. Effectiveness of triclosan-coated PDS Plus versus uncoated PDS II sutures for prevention of surgical site infection after abdominal wall closure: the randomised controlled PROUD trial. *Lancet (London, England)* [Internet] 2014 [cited 2016 Mar 22];384:142–52. Available from: http://www.thelancet.com/article/S0140673614602385/fulltext.

39. Xu S, Huang H, Li G. Clinical practice guidelines for Clostridium difficile infection in adults: 2010 update by the Society for Healthcare Epidemiology of America (SHEA) and the infectious diseases society of America (IDSA). *Chinese J Infect Chemother* 2011;11:426–7.

40. Bos JC, Schultsz C, Vandenbroucke-Grauls CMJ, Prins PSJM. Optimaliseren van het antibioticabeleid in Nederland. IX. SWAB-richtlijn voor antimicrobiële therapie bij acute infectieuze diarree. *Ned Tijdschr Geneeskd* 2006;150: 1116–22.

Part II

General Institutional Issues in the Management of Gastrointestinal Complications

8

Management of Complications of Gastrointestinal Surgeries in the Limited-Resource Setting

N.P. Raykar, N. Roy, M.U. Khajanchi and S.S. Nagral

ABSTRACT

The purpose of this chapter is to share best practices and workarounds employed by surgeons to treat complications of gastrointestinal surgery in the lowest-resource areas of the world. People still die at home from untreated acute abdominal conditions, as they have no access to surgery. The low-resource settings have a different surgical burden of disease, poor baseline of health due to the interaction of poverty and disease and a critical shortage of surgical providers. The challenges of care provision in this setting include the lack of diagnostic investigations, imaging, nutrition, blood and intensive care facilities. The innovative and indigenous strategies used by remarkable surgeons in low-resource settings, for specific gastrointestinal surgical complications, are described.

KEYWORDS

Low-resource, poverty, surgical burden, access to surgery, district hospital, global surgery

INTRODUCTION

A 2015 study from the University of Toronto showed that better access to first-level hospitals in India may have prevented almost two-thirds of the estimated 72,000 deaths from acute abdominal emergencies in 2010.[1] The authors mapped hospital locations and reviewed healthcare quality in over 3800 of 4064 postal codes and found that mortality from abdominal conditions increased with increasing distance from surgical care. Populations living farther than 100 Km were at the highest risk. Not surprisingly, only 21% of the 72,000 deaths from acute abdominal conditions occurred in hospitals. However, the study's most important finding may be that simple access to a hospital is insufficient. Only staffed and functional health facilities actually lowered mortality.

However, the challenge of accessing a staffed and functional surgical facility is not trivial. The Lancet Commission on Global Surgery estimates that at least 5 billion people lack access to safe and affordable and timely surgical and anaesthetic care.[2] The reasons are multifactorial and include that almost 75% of the global population lives in areas with less than 40 surgeons, anaesthetists and obstetricians (SAOs) per 100,000, the threshold below which health outcomes tend to be poor across populations.[3] Nonetheless, in these settings, surgery still occurs and the burden of providing safe, affordable and high-quality care rests on the relative few people who provide it. Surgeons in busy rural private clinics in South Asia report performing in the range of 1000 to 2000 procedures annually (Figure 8.1).[4]

Although a thorough description of the 'low-resource setting' follows, its definition for the purpose of this chapter will consist of settings where its surgical facilities lack intensive care units, ventilators, endoscopic

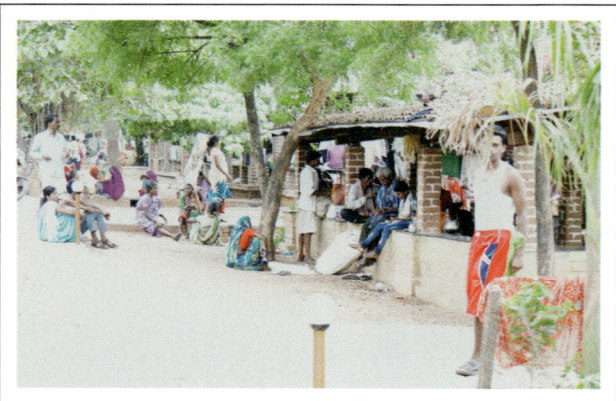

Figure 8.1 Desperate for surgical care. Patients wait patiently outside the Jan Swasthya Sahyog (JSS) Hospital in Chhattisgarh, India, the only free-care hospital providing surgery in its region. Patients travel from a total of five states to visit the clinic.

Courtesy: Nakul P. Raykar, Nobhojit Roy, Monty U. Khajanchi and Sanjay S. Nagral.

retrograde cholangiopancreatography (ERCP), computed tomography (CT), expensive but staple therapeutics such as total parenteral nutrition (TPN), a safe blood supply and an easy access to daily laboratory investigations.

This chapter is based on a review of the existing literature; direct communications with rural surgeons across limited-resource settings in South Asia, Asia-Pacific and sub-Saharan Africa; and the experience of the authors working in these settings across urban and rural landscapes.[5,6] We focus on how complex surgical care is delivered in these settings, starting with a granular inspection of how care delivery in low-resource settings can differ from better-resourced areas of the world. We will follow with an overview of diagnostic and management approaches to specific complications adapted for low-resource settings.

HOW LOW-RESOURCE SETTINGS ARE DIFFERENT

Three broad categories separate the lower-resource setting from its higher-resourced counterparts: variations in disease epidemiology, access and affordability of care for its patients and availability of the workforce and tools necessary for diagnosis and treatment.

Differences in Disease Burden

The surgical disease burden in low-resource settings represents conditions ranging from infectious disease to cancer and includes common conditions not typically considered 'surgical'.[7,8] For example, only 9% of all preventable deaths from surgical conditions in low- and middle-income countries (LMICs) could be treated with care that addresses four common conditions in the high-resource world: appendicitis, gallbladder or biliary ductal disease, hernia, and paralytic ileus or bowel obstruction.[9] Injuries, on the other hand, account for almost three-quarters of disease burden, whereas maternal conditions requiring surgery (e.g., obstructed labour) account for approximately 15%.

Importantly, traditionally, 'medical' diagnoses such as that of gastritis, cellulitis, *Salmonella typhi* and tuberculosis (TB) infection often have dramatic surgical manifestations without appropriate medical therapy. Sickle-cell disease, for example, is prevalent in certain tribal populations in South Asia and sub-Saharan Africa and often presents with abdominal crisis. Intestinal perforation will manifest in up to a third of those infected with *Salmonella* and, in some series, as high as 60%.[10] Intestinal TB presents in up to a third of patients with TB and is another common cause of intestinal perforation, stricture and fistula formation throughout the gastrointestinal (GI) tract (Figure 8.2).[11]

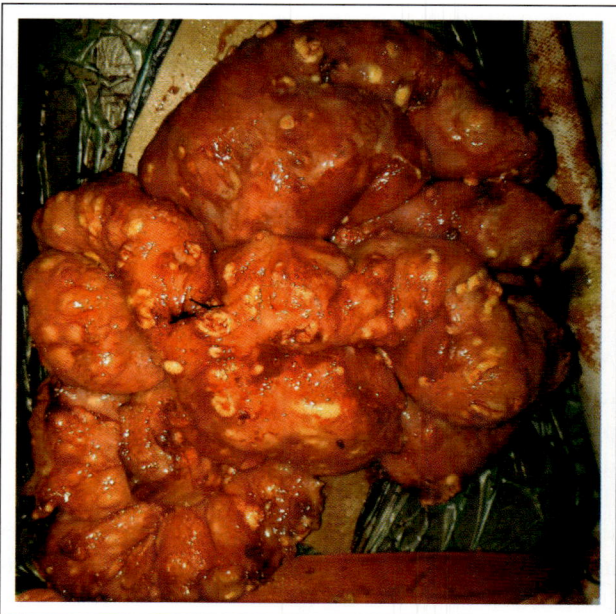

Figure 8.2 Different disease burdens and different challenges. Here, abdominal tuberculosis has ravaged the small intestine, leading to perforative peritonitis. Poor nutrition leads to weakened immunity and increased susceptibility to many infectious processes, including tuberculosis. Unfortunately, this needs to be considered in the management of these patients.

Courtesy: Nakul P. Raykar, Nobhojit Roy, Monty U. Khajanchi and Sanjay S. Nagral.

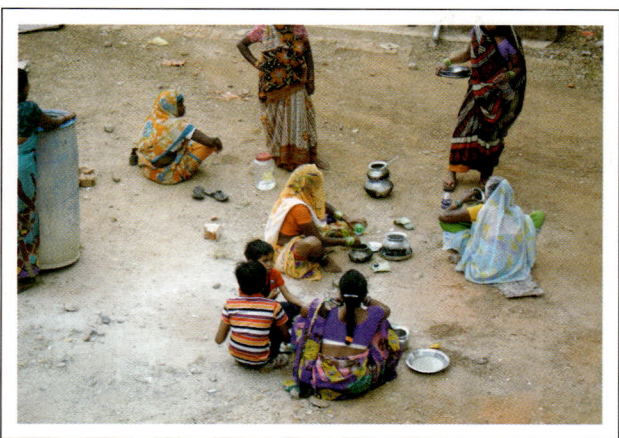

Figure 8.3 Poverty, hospitals and sustanance. Women gather around the grounds at the Jan Swasthya Sahyog (JSS) hospital to cook dinner. Given extremely low affordability, patients and families who have long hospital stays will opt to bring their own food and cook at the hospital. The hospital provides open-range stoves to help facilitate.

Courtesy: Nakul P. Raykar, Nobhojit Roy, Monty U. Khajanchi and Sanjay S. Nagral.

As expected, there is variation in disease burden across low-resource settings.[9] Sub-Saharan Africa, for example, has a high burden of preventable deaths from appendicitis, with over 14,000 deaths per year, almost seven times that of South Asia. Over 21,000 people are estimated to die yearly from gallbladder and biliary disease in the Asia Pacific region, a disease with a substantial but lower estimated prevalence in other regions. Hernias represent a smaller number of deaths—only about 14,000 across all LMICs—but account for a staggering 120,000 combined years of death and disability (disability-adjusted life years [DALYs]) in South Asia. Small bowel obstruction and/or paralytic ileus impact sub-Saharan Africa and South Asia nearly equally, with a combined total of 40,997 deaths per year.

Differences in Patient Demographics, Accessibility and Trust

The complex cross links between poverty and disease affect how patients interact with the health system. Patients have few financial resources when it comes to affording care (Figure 8.3). The Lancet Commission on Global Surgery used World Bank data on population income levels and hospitalisation costs in Zambia for surgical procedures and found that 94% of the Zambian population would be at risk of an impoverishing expense from a caesarean delivery or laparotomy.[15] In some parts of rural India, just a few

hundred rupees of unexpected medical expenditure can push a family into poverty.[12]

Worsening the situation, hundreds of kilometres separate communities and hospitals, and no organised transportation mechanisms exist in between them.[12] The hospitals that do exist are understaffed and underfunded, common problems that are not lost on patients who recognise that the likelihood of receiving care may not be worth the effort of getting there.[13] In a study of 1000 patients at a rural Indian hospital, 92% reported word of mouth in the community, which played a significant role in determining whether and where to seek care.[14] In settings where a hospital is dogged by infrastructure or workforce deficits, patients will choose further expectant waiting, herbal remedies or to see an informal provider (traditional healer) in the community first.

Finally, population baseline health is poor, affected by years of chronic poverty, malnutrition and poor access to the healthcare system.[16,17] The mean haemoglobin and weight in the Indian population, skewed by a large proportion the world's extremely poor, is 10.6 g/dL and 48 Kg, respectively.[18] Patients who are mal- and undernourished on presentation are predisposed to infection, compromised wound healing and delayed postoperative recovery.

Differences in Provider Resources

Providers in these settings also face a variety of challenges, ranging from shortages in workforce, equipment and supplies to deficient hospital infrastructure. A World Health Organization (WHO) database on infrastructure in surgical hospitals found that almost one-third did not have reliable electricity and a quarter did not have reliable or clean running water.[3] In a setting where service contracts from manufacturers are rare, more than half of district hospitals in sub-Saharan Africa lacked a functional anaesthesia machine and 70% were without a pulse oximeter.

Access to laboratory tests was dependent on the availability of specific reagents. Therefore, a complete blood count was usually available, but serum chemistries and liver function tests (LFTs) were scarcer. Coagulation profiles were the least likely to be available. Microbiology and pathology laboratories were generally unavailable. When testing was available, it was likely to be expensive.

This is also true for magnetic resonance imaging (MRI), CT scan, advanced fluoroscopy, ERCP and interventional radiology. Although CT and MRI may be more commonplace in urban areas, providers note that scheduling and routine equipment malfunction overwhelmed the likelihood of receiving a timely test. A provider in a large urban hospital in sub-Saharan Africa noted that he was offered a 2-week wait time for an emergency CT scan. The vast majority of hospitals in these settings are without a formal critical care unit, ventilator capacity, monitoring equipment and dedicated intensivists or nursing.[1] Most surgeons note difficulty in accessing blood products for their patients, when needed.

Finally, workforce deficits were the norm. Most specialised clinicians opted to work in urban tertiary centres or to migrate to higher-paying jobs in richer countries. Anaesthesiologists, likewise, are difficult to employ full time in rural areas and may be hired by surgeons on a part-time, per-case basis. The closest anaesthesiologist, however, may be hours away, and the story is the same for nurses, technicians and other support staff.

STRATEGIES TO MITIGATE DEFICITS

Providers have developed strategies to mitigate these deficits. Firstly, providers strive to achieve a broad skillset to treat a wide variety of surgical conditions. General surgeons are multiskilled and are able to provide the basics of thoracic surgery, endoscopy, urology, obstetrics, ENT and orthopaedics.[4] Without a qualified anaesthesia provider for general anaesthesia, many surgeons report relying on spinal anaesthesia for most of their procedures, including laparotomies, and training support staff for its safe delivery. Some surgeons have even adapted procedures such as laparoscopic appendectomy and cholecystectomy to be performed under spinal anaesthesia without an anaesthesiologist. In 'gasless laparoscopy',[22] abdominal insufflation is replaced with manual elevation of the abdominal wall and, without the discomfort and diminished venous return caused by abdominal insufflation, surgeons can perform the procedure under spinal anaesthesia[23] (Figure 8.4).

Another notable innovation to remedy the workforce deficit is the training and employment of community members or nonphysicians in specific surgical, anaesthetic, nursing or other technical tasks. This is known as 'task-sharing', and in the surgical arena, this extends to utilisation of providers formally trained in alternative systems of medicine as surgical assistants or even primary surgeons under supervision.[24]

To overcome care provision obstacles from deficient infrastructure, many surgeons reported that they have invested in standby generators with dedicated lines to the operating suite as well as low- or no-power options such as pump-operated suction machines and battery and manual

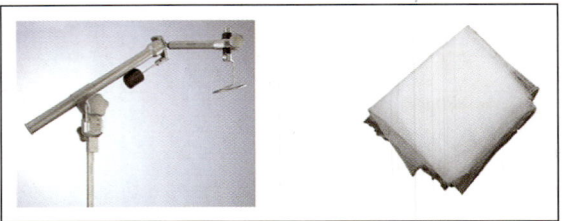

Figure 8.4 Innovation for the low-resource setting. Surgeons and patients in low-resource settings rely on innovation to make care affordable. On the left, the 'Abdo-Lift' (www.endogyn.com) allows for manual elevation of the abdominal wall, facilitating laparoscopic surgery without abdominal insufflation. On the right, a stack of cloths used for mosquito bed nets. Surgeons in low-resource settings across the world, particularly in South Asia and Africa, have been using sterilised mosquito net as a substitute for expensive, commercial hernia mesh for decades. A recent Lofgren et al's article published in the *New England Journal of Medicine* confirmed equivalency of outcomes.

Courtesy: Nakul P. Raykar, Nobhojit Roy, Monty U. Khajanchi and Sanjay S. Nagral

backup anaesthesia machines and ventilators.[25,26] Rather than depending on municipality-supplied water, providers build large water tanks or use water well systems and employ reverse-osmosis water purification.[19] Oxygen concentrators replace oxygen cylinders that are subject to the whims of the supply chain. Single-use instruments are reused after sterilisation. Even used gloves are meticulously cleaned and reused or double up as incentive spirometers for perioperative chest physiotherapy.[27]

Providers across sub-Saharan Africa, South Asia and Asia Pacific noted that commercial preparations of enteral nutrition were frequently replaced with low-cost preparations of the following: 'home-made' peanut butter, sometimes using Plumpy'Nut®, a preparation originally designed for malnourished children; hard-boiled eggs; a combination of avocados and milk; sosoma porridge combined with over-the-counter multivitamins and fortified milk-based protein-rich mixes. Since TPN was unavailable or prohibitively expensive by most accounts, providers noted an early reliance on surgical solutions such as gastric tubes or jejunostomy tubes for maintaining postoperative enteral nutrition, when possible.

If a coagulopathy was suspected, providers suggested that the best test was to place a drop of blood in a plain test tube and manually observe its clotting time. One provider from the Asia-Pacific region noted that laboratory tests often incurred out-of-pocket expense not covered under universal health-coverage schemes and, as a result, stressed the need for prudence in ordering laboratory testing. In some situations, clinicians without access to on-site laboratories would make clever use of public transportation systems to send samples to neighbouring centres for same-day analysis and return.[27]

The absence of a wide array of imaging options has forced clinicians to master the available option. Ultrasound has emerged as the most important imaging tool for the low-resource surgeon, and surgeons tend to do their own ultrasound examinations and interpretations. This comes with the added advantage of being able to attempt interventions such as inserting tubes into fluid collections or abscess cavities under ultrasound guidance.

To work around the absence of ventilators, hospital staff will bag-ventilate a patient, as needed, and alternate in these responsibilities with the patient's family members. Vasopressor support is generally available in the form of epinephrine and dopamine. Blood pressure monitoring while on vasopressor support is generally in the form of periodic manual blood pressure measurement with a standard cuff.

To address blood needs, surgeons reported the use of 'walking blood banks', adapted from the military, where community members are prescreened for transfusion-transmissible illness (TTI) and identified as potential donors.[28] When an urgent need for blood arises, these community members are called upon for rapid donation. Blood is tested for the major TTIs by using rapid test assays and is transfused immediately. Alternatively, in situations where blood banks exist but require replacement donation, these individuals are directed to donate to the blood bank in exchange for release of prescreened and tested blood to patients in need.

However, hospital-based interventions are insufficient to remedy the community-level challenges mentioned earlier. Many surgeons hold health education, diagnostic and treatment camps in surrounding communities and with informal providers. These help diminish concerns about accessibility and quality of care and, by bringing diagnosis and treatment to the community, can reduce the costs of receiving care.[3,5] In addition, by leveraging mobile phone technology, even the poorest communities can follow up by messaging photographs of wound status and physical condition instead of expensive trips back to the hospital.[21]

SPECIFIC GASTROINTESTINAL SURGERY COMPLICATIONS AND LOW-RESOURCE MANAGEMENT STRATEGIES

It is little surprise that differences in management will be required to treat the complications encountered in the low-resource setting. Here, we highlight differences amongst the major categories of GI complications.

Enteric Leak

Clinicians we interviewed stressed on the reliance on clinical examination over laboratory investigations and imaging with a low threshold for operative re-exploration in patients suspected of having an enteric leak. Ultrasound would be the primary imaging modality to define fluid collections in the abdomen. Ultimately, in the face of persistent uncertainty, laparoscopy (where available) or laparotomy is the diagnostic and therapeutic modality of choice. Surgeons were more accepting of a negative exploration (and its attendant morbidity) in the young and fit, while reserving imaging and draining collections in moribund and older patients.

Intraoperatively, providers are faced with the critical decision of a primary resection with reanastamosis or a bowel diversion (a diverting loop ostomy or, in the case of the distal bowel and rectum, an endostomy with a Hartmann's pouch). Although a bowel diversion is recognised to be the 'safer' option, some providers described ostomy creation as a 'last resort', because of poor stoma management options.

Stoma Management

Managing an ostomy in a limited-resource setting is challenging. Affordability of ostomy supplies is limited. There is a high rate of societal stigma. There are no dedicated stoma care nurses. The humidity, heat and inability of most patients to remain in cool or air-conditioned climates make the adherence of ostomy appliances to the skin tenuous. Some local companies produce stoma supplies at a fraction of the cost of commercial brands available in the high-income world.[29] To make them even more affordable, providers replace commercial, disposable ostomy supplies with local alternatives (Figure 8.5). Some describe affixing plastic bags to a ring, whereas others use fabric lined with plastic sheeting (saran wrap or plastic bags). To enhance skin care and adhesion, providers use layers of aluminium paint and a paste made of egg whites. To help with patient acceptance and their relatives, patients are often offered extended stays in the hospital, instead of being sent home.

However, formal colostomy supplies, even if domestically produced, are still too expensive for many or simply unavailable. In these cases, providers use a cloth soaked in oil to cover the stoma, a cloth wrapped circumferentially around the stoma to provide some padding and additional clothing, tied loosely around the abdomen, to hold the stoma (surrounding cloth) and the oil-soaked cloth in

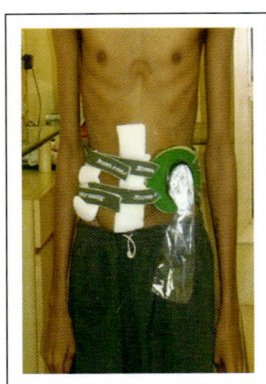

Figure 8.5 Low-resource alternatives. Surgical manufacturers exist in low-resource settings, and some supplies are available at significantly reduced cost as compared with those in high-income countries. Unfortunately, these are often still too expensive for the poor.

Courtesy: Nakul P. Raykar, Nobhojit Roy, Monty U. Khajanchi and Sanjay S. Nagral

place. A loose wrap allows a small reservoir for stool, and all the clothing can be washed and reused.

Enterocutaneous Fistula

Treatment of an enterocutaneous fistula would initially focus on quantifying fistula output. High-output, proximal fistulas are much more complicated to manage than low-output fistulas in the distal GI tract. Electrolytes (if available and affordable) will be obtained as frequently as possible but rarely sooner than once every other day and with a particular focus on repletion of sodium and potassium. In high-output fistulas and where options for adequate nutritional support are limited, operative therapy is necessary. In the operating theatre, the bowel would first be evaluated for distal obstruction. Then, one of several options exist. For proximal fistulas, a distal enteral feeding tube could be placed for nutritional access and conservative therapy pursued once again. For mid and distal fistulas, a proximal diversion may be necessary, in addition to any potential resection that may be performed based on clinician judgement. With matured fistulas, or those with multiple openings, some providers report routine attempt and success with fistuloclysis, where Foley catheters are inserted into existing fistulas as a means of enteral feeding[30] (Figure 8.6).

Nutrition

Maintaining adequate nutrition is a major challenge, a common reason why patients with enteric fistulae fare

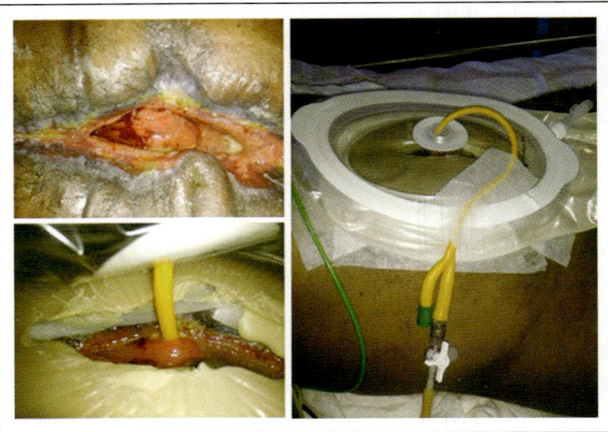

Figure 8.6 Creative workarounds for a small bowel fistula. Providers here were dealing with a small bowel fistula, likely from the proximal ileum. Without parenteral nutrition, providers opted to provide fistuloclysis with a Foley catheter inserted into the fistula and balloon inflated to 15 cc to prevent reflux. A feeding pump was used with the Foley catheter for 4 weeks to ensure continuous feed, without tube clogging.

Courtesy: Nakul P. Raykar, Nobhojit Roy, Monty U. Khajanchi and Sanjay S. Nagral.

poorly, with mortality rates reaching up to 25%.[31,32] Total parenteral nutrition is near unavailable or prohibitively expensive, not to mention the workforce shortfalls for the placement and management of central venous catheters. In some urban centres, there is an increasing trend towards using peripheral parenteral nutrition. For lower-resourced areas, 100 mL of 25% dextrose solution five to eight times a day can supply a carbohydrate calorie intake of at least 500 to 800 Kcal. Many providers report that they must default to enteral nutrition, despite its drawbacks in the management of fistulae. A combination of homemade oral rehydration solution, eggs and chicken soup is given to maintain electrolytes and protein. Efforts to decrease effluent volume such as loperamide, codeine, tincture of opium and high-dose proton-pump inhibitors (PPIs) may be employed and are mostly available.[33] Somatostatin and octreotide may be useful adjuncts to decrease fistula output but are usually prohibitively expensive.

Bleeding—Upper Gastrointestinal Tract

Gastric bleeds are unfortunately very common in low-resource settings, especially in patients with complicated hospital course and surgical history. It can originate from several sources, including stress gastritis, variceal disease and gastric ulceration, especially in the absence of PPIs. Alternatively, bleeding can originate from a fresh anastomotic site. Less likely, the source could be from a new primary site. Haematemesis, haematochezia and melaena are important clinical signs.

Insertion of a nasogastric tube is an important first step, as presence of fresh blood helps confirm the diagnosis of an intraluminal bleeding from an upper GI source. Endoscopy may be attempted, where available, but surgeons who perform endoscopies frequently note that disposables such as clips and glue are often unavailable. Therefore, its role is generally limited to diagnosis and minor therapeutic attempts through injection of epinephrine. Gastric lavage of vasopressin or noradrenalin (8 mg) in 200 to 400 mL ice-cold saline is often attempted for 2 hours. Similarly, a Sengstaken–Blakemore tube is still used for temporary control.

However, ultimately, surgery is likely the first and only line of definitive therapy. Given the difficulty in accessing a safe and affordable blood supply, neither clinicians nor their patients can afford the risk of additional bleeding in favour of lesser interventions. In the operating room, a gastric ulcer will be repaired by simply oversewing the ulcer. Given the high prevalence and undertreatment for *Helicobacter pylori* infection, it is prudent to follow up with its treatment. In the case of a perforated duodenal ulcer, a primary repair with omental patch, abdomen wash out and drain placement is the procedure of choice.[34] If the bleeding is from an anastomotic site, proximal gastrotomy above the anastomotic line and underrunning of the anastomotic site bleeder, resection and reanastomosis and simple packing are the top options.

Bleeding—Presacral

Providers have developed a variety of indigenous strategies to control presacral bleeding. Some note the use of presterilised thumbtacks, whereas others describe rectus abdominus muscle welding. In this technique, a small piece of muscle from the rectus abdominus is put over the presacral bleeding areas and cauterised at high energy (100 Hz), effectively 'welding' the bleeding site.[35]

Small Bowel Obstruction

The initial management of small bowel obstruction is fairly similar in the lowest-resource settings with nasogastric tubes and intravenous (i.v.) fluids. Where available, serial supine plain X-rays are obtained to confirm diagnosis and evaluate proximal versus distal obstruction. What differs, however, is the aetiology of small bowel obstruction. Unlike in the West, where postoperative adhesions are the most common cause of small bowel obstruction and

abdominal TB is a strong contender in TB-endemic parts of the world.[36] In settings where the prevalence of HIV is high, large mesenteric lymph nodes are likely to be caused by TB or lymphoma. Infection diagnosis and therapy, then, are a core component of the initial evaluation when these conditions are encountered.

The limited-resource setting warrants a significant reliance on serial abdominal examinations and clinical signs. Worsening distention, focal tenderness, or generalised abdominal guarding must be actively anticipated, given the potential for perforation in patients with abdominal TB. Most practitioners note that in the absence of white blood cell count and CT imaging, identifying ischaemic complications early on physical examination is unreliable. Some take the presence of a mild fever as a warrant for an operation. In the absence of fever or deterioration, many providers will still move to an early laparotomy within a maximum of 48 hours after presentation, with most recommending it within 24 hours.

Hepatobiliary—Choledocholithiasis

Although choledocholithiasis is not traditionally classified as a complication of GI surgery, it does require manipulation of the bile duct, which can lead to either purposeful or inadvertent injury to the common bile duct (CBD). Managing CBD injury is a scenario that presents challenges even in the high-income environment. Low-resource management differs in several important ways. Firstly, whereas ultrasound and laboratory investigations, including LFTs, may be available, additional diagnostics generally are not available. Further, there are few options for referral for complex disease. The primary surgeon must be able to handle complex biliary disease, including residual duct stones. Some centres, depending on proximity, will refer the patient for CBD clearing and stenting with ERCP.

In the more common situation of unavailability of ERCP, where laparoscopy is available, centres will opt for a laparoscopic cholecystectomy with intraoperative CBD exploration and pickup or basket retrieval of stones in the duct, followed by cholangiogram to confirm removal of all stones. However, advanced laparoscopic equipment, such as a formal choledochoscope, is unlikely to be available.

In the absence of laparoscopy, the removal of CBD stones in the open approach will use similar techniques after cholecystectomy, including access to the CBD through the cystic duct, flushing with saline, using a Foley catheter in the fashion of Fogarty catheter to sweep the duct and use of stone-extraction forceps (Desjardins). Crossover surgical skills from urology and gastroenterology allow practitioners to substitute with a paediatric gastroscope or a rigid cystoscope in open procedures. If successful with stone extraction, closure will likely include leaving a t-tube for access to the biliary system and consistent drainage as well as to a subhepatic drain (Figure 8.7).

In the event that a stone is too large for extraction, requiring incision of the CBD, several options exist. Firstly, primary closure of the duct over a t-tube is the preferred route for patients with sufficiently large ducts (generally at least 1.5 cm in diameter). A choledochoduodenostomy is another option, but a leak of duodenal secretions is associated with significant morbidity and mortality. If the duct diameter is too small or if there is insufficient length for an anastomosis, the safe default is with a hepaticojejunostomy, which can take advantage of even a minimally dilated system by using the confluence of the common duct with the left duct. If a hepaticojejunostomy anastomotic leak ensues, it is generally a benign leak that most often heals on its own. T-tubes are frequently left in place by using the shortest path to assist with postoperative drainage and monitoring. Where t-tubes are unavailable, a Foley catheter with the end split into two halves can serve as a substitute. This workaround yields the added benefit of starting with a sterilised material, ready for insertion into the CBD.

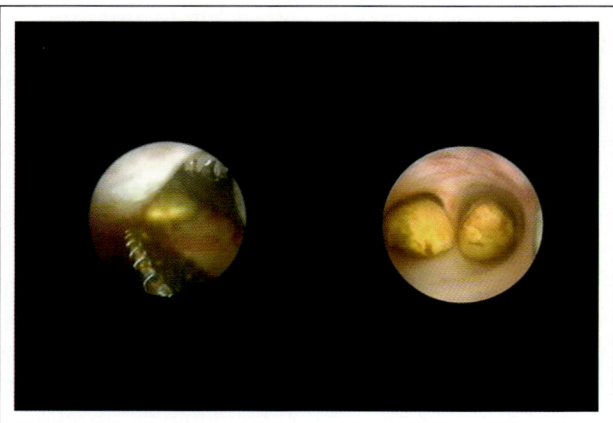

Figure 8.7 Nobody said it was easy. Images from a paediatric cystoscope during a common bile duct exploration. Given the expense of formal choledochoscopes, practitioners often substitute paediatric cystoscopes or paediatric gastroscopes to perform common bile duct explorations. As can be seen, the images are less than ideal but functional and, when available, often obviate the need for more extensive open common bile ductal exploration.

Courtesy: Nakul P. Raykar, Nobhojit Roy, Monty U. Khajanchi and Sanjay S. Nagral.

Pancreas

In the high-income world, there is increasing pressure to perform pancreatic resections in high-volume units, as morbidity and mortality from complications is high and management can need multidisciplinary backup.[37] Such an approach is not feasible in low-resource settings. High-volume centres would be hundreds, if not thousands, of kilometres away. Instead, surgeons will have to manage the complications conservatively or struggle to shift the patient to the nearest centre that resembles a high-volume unit. Pancreatic surgeries remain the most unaffordable of the GI surgeries and with variable outcomes. As such, patients and providers often opt for a palliative triple surgical bypass of the obstruction, which involves an anastomosis between the stomach and jejunum (gastrojejunostomy), between biliary system and jejunum (choledocho-/hepatico-/cholecystojejunostomy) and a Roux-en-Y loop to prevent reflux of food into the biliary tree (jejunojejunostomy). The complications arising here are daunting because of three separate anastomosis but can still be managed by using the techniques described above.

Colorectal

A resection for low- to mid-rectal cancers is challenging in low-resource settings with poor instrumentation and nonavailability of circular staplers. Many surgeons would rather do an abdominoperineal resection if the tumour-free margin cannot be dissected or if the surgeon feels that the pelvic anastomosis will not be possible. Complications of rectal surgeries other than anastomotic leaks, fistulaes and presacral bleeding, as discussed above, are intraoperative ureteric and bladder injuries and postoperative pelvic collections and perineal sinuses. Open urological repair with ureteric stenting is performed.

Severely symptomatic anorectal conditions (fistula-in-ano, haemorrhoids, perirectal abscesses and anal fissure) are usually treated with excision and/or lateral sphincterotomy under regional anaesthesia. There are options of injection sclerotherapy and rubber band ligation for haemorrhoids, but because of limited opportunity for repeat visits, access to ointments and medicines and late presentation, surgeons are usually inclined towards early surgery. In India, a 'kshara sutra' seton, a cotton seton medicated with herbal medicines, is a low-cost, locally derived method for treating fistulas-in-ano.[38] The main complications of these conditions include postoperative bleeding, incontinence, recurrence of fistulas and perianal pain. Reactionary bleeding would be dealt with by resuturing the bleeder. Secondary bleeding would be dealt with mostly by conservative means, if not by a

Foley's balloon tamponade. Incontinence after anal procedures would be managed conservatively by anal tone exercises for a period of 6 to 12 weeks.

Strangulated Hernias

Bowel resection is required in a surprisingly large number of hernias—as high as 33% in data from West Africa—as they present in strangulated states and in a younger population with indirect hernias, in which case only few present for elective resection.[39] Hydrocele post surgery is common because of endemic filarial infections. The postabdominal surgery ventral (incisional) hernias are expensive surgeries, as the polypropylene meshes are expensive. Low-resource surgeons have been vindicated by a growing evidence that has shown that the use of meshes made of sterilised mosquito nets—a standard practice of rural surgeons for years—is equivalent to prohibitively expensive commercial meshes[20] (Figure 8.4).

Abdominal Trauma

Injuries account for the highest burden of disease requiring surgical expertise. Agriculture, transport and assault by animals or people are the likely mechanisms for abdominal trauma. Bleeding, bowel perforations and splenic ruptures are the common concerns. Trauma patients typically have a delayed arrival, and they are likely to be haemodynamically unstable, with significant blood loss and in early sepsis. Surgery for the traumatic abdomen, in the setting of poor blood availability, is to follow the principles of damage control, contain contamination and control bleeding. An emergency laparotomy, initiated by clinical and ultrasound examinations or a diagnostic peritoneal aspiration, is carried out under ketamine or spinal anaesthesia. Complications in these settings include missed bowel, vascular and diaphragmatic injuries and a stormy postoperative period. Strategies include linen tape ligation and bowel exteriorisation to prevent continuing intra-abdominal spillage.[40] Difficult closures of the abdomen, owing to bowel or abdominal wall oedema, is now possible with the use of plastic adhesive sheets and low-cost vacuum suction-closure devices, which would allow a temporary closure and an early relook. The late complications include sepsis, multiorgan systemic failure and intra-abdominal collections, and these are managed with the limitations discussed.[40]

A Note on Rarer or Missed Complications

Despite the pressure to provide a broad range of services for their patients because of the known challenges of accessing care, providers recognise the need to 'draw the line' somewhere and to weigh poor patient prognosis against the local capacity to provide care. Few surgeons in the most limited resource of settings will attempt curative resections for advanced oesophageal, gastric, pancreatic and colorectal cancers. Instead, surgeons are more likely to offer palliative bypass procedures. As such, we did not frequently encounter oesophageal anastomotic leaks, mediastinitis and pancreatic or colorectal fistulas as common GI complications in these settings. Nonetheless, there were some notable variations in preferences as to when these procedures are performed. For example, when surgeons in LMIC settings perform oesophagectomy for cancer, the favoured approach is to perform a total oesophaectomy via the transhiatal procedure. This obviates the need for opening the thorax as well and shifts the anastomosis to the neck, avoiding the deadly and difficult-to-manage complication of mediastinitis. Pancreatic pseudocysts would usually be treated with a cystogastrostomy, open or laparoscopic, depending on availability. Few would have the capability to pursue it through endoscopic means.

In addition, of note, there are likely complications that occur commonly but are rarely diagnosed in these settings either because of a lack of diagnostics or because of a lack of treatment options to respond to such diagnoses. These may include pulmonary embolism, deep vein thrombosis, coagulopathies, acute-respiratory distress syndrome, disseminated intravascular coagulopathy, acid–base disorders and chronic nutritional losses.

CONCLUSIONS

Gastrointestinal surgery in low-resource settings is prone to complications from an extensive and varied disease burden, poor population health, widespread poverty, and limitation in facility resources. Nonetheless, *despite* these challenges, our colleagues in some of the world's poorest places try to provide their patients with safe, affordable access to surgical care, when needed, by working endlessly, year round, without locum cover or professional backup. In doing so, they have had to weigh the realities of care provision in their settings against the 'ideal' management strategies reflected in most textbooks. We hope this chapter provided some insight into their world, their work and the difficult decisions they must make on a daily basis. We further hope that it encourages colleagues and policymakers to recognise the immense contributions of these heroic individuals and promote policies that support their work.

ACKNOWLEDGEMENTS

We would like to thank all those providers who live and breathe this work every day and whose commitment to their patients and their communities is reflected in their selfless service. There are several such individuals whom we would like to acknowledge, who shared their wisdom from working in these settings and made significant contributions towards generating the content for this chapter (country of experience is listed in parenthesis): Dr. Amul Pawaskar (India), Dr. Herman Lonee (Sierra Leone), Dr. J Gnanaraj (India), Dr. Nandakumar Menon (India), Dr. Raman Kataria (India), Dr. Arun Murari (Fiji), Dr. Håkon Angell Bolkan (Sierra Leone), Dr. Evans Chinkoyo (Zambia), Dr. V. G. Mehendale (India), Dr. Glenn Guest (East Timor), Dr. Daniel van Leerdam (Sierra Leone), Dr. Jose Florencio F. Lapena Jr. (the Philippines), Dr. Andreas Wladis (Uganda), Dr. Robert Riviello (Rwanda), Dr. Ramlal P Prajapati (India), Dr. Martin Smith (South Africa), Dr. Ainhoa Costas-Chavarri (Rwanda), Dr. Arturo E. Mendoza, Jr (the Phillipines) and Dr. Lesley Hunt (Sierra Leone).

REFERENCES

1. Dare A, Ng-Kamstra J, Patra J. Deaths from acute abdominal conditions and geographical access to surgical care in India: a nationally representative spatial analysis. *Lancet Glob Health* 2015;3:e646–53.

2. Alkire BC, Raykar NP, Shrime MG, et al. Global access to surgical care: a modelling study. *Lancet Glob Health* 2015; 3:e316–23.

3. Meara JG, Leather AJM, Hagander L, et al. Global Surgery 2030: Evidence and solutions for achieving health, welfare, and economic development. *Lancet* 2015;386:569–624. doi: 10.1016/S0140-6736(15)60160-X.

4. Harris JD, Hosford CC, Sticca RP. A comprehensive analysis of surgical procedures in rural surgery practices. *Am J Surg* 2010;200:820–6. doi: 10.1016/j.amjsurg.2010.07.029.

5. Gnanaraj J. What happens next? Review of patients referred for further surgical treatment from rural/mission hospitals. *Chrismed J Heal Res* 2015;2:303–7.

6. King M, Bewes P, Cairns J, Thornton J. *Primary Surgery. Vol. 1: Non-Trauma.* Canada: Oxford University Press; 1990.

7. Stewart B, Khanduri P, McCord C, Ohene-Yeboah M, et al. Global disease burden of conditions requiring emergency surgery. *Br J Surg* 2014;101:e9–22. doi: 10.1002/bjs.9329.

8. Rose J, Weiser T, Hider P, Wilson L. Estimated need for surgery worldwide based on prevalence of diseases: a modelling strategy for the WHO Global Health Estimate. *Lancet Glob Health* 2015;3:S13–20.

9. Bickler SW, Weiser TG, Kassebaum N, et al. Global burden of surgical conditions. In: Debas HT, Donkor P, Gawande A, Jamison DT, Kruk ME, Mock CN, editors. *Essential Surgery: Disease Control Priorities.* 4th ed (Vol. 1). Washington, DC: The International Bank for Reconstruction and Development/The World Bank; 2015. p. 19.

10. Ugochukwu AI, Amu OC, Nzegwu MA. Ileal perforation due to typhoid fever – review of operative management and outcome in an urban centre in Nigeria. *Int J Surg* 2013;11:218–22.

11. Debi U, Ravisankar V, Prasad KK, Sinha SK, Sharma AK. Abdominal tuberculosis of the gastrointestinal tract: revisited. *World J Gastroenterol* 2014;20:14831–40.

12. Raykar N, Yorlets R, Liu C. A qualitative study exploring contextual challenges to surgical care provision in 21 LMICs. *Lancet* 2015;385:S15.

13. Aleksandrowicz L, Malhotra V, Dikshit R, et al. Performance criteria for verbal autopsy-based systems to estimate national causes of death: development and application to the Indian Million Death Study. *BMC Med* 2014;12:21. doi: 10.1186/1741-7015-12-21.

14. Gnanaraj J. What Rural Surgical Patients Say. *Bull Assoc Rural Surg India* 2006;1:4–6.

15. Meara J. Lancet Commission London Launch. Zambia Surgical System Profile; 2015.

16. Schaible UE, Kaufmann SHE. Malnutrition and infection: complex mechanisms and global impacts. *PLoS Med* 2007; 4:e115.

17. World Health Organization, Deptartment of Nutrition for Health and Development. *Nutrition for Health and Development : A Global Agenda for Combating Malnutrition.* Geneva, Switzerland: World Health Organization; 2000.

18. Sciences II for P. National Family Health Survey India. Raw Dataset; 2006.

19. Oluyombo A. Rising to the challenge of rural surgery. Interview by Les Olson. *Bull World Health Organ* 2010; 88:331–2.

20. Löfgren J, Nordin P, Ibingira C, Matovu A, Galiwango E, Wladis A. A randomized trial of low-cost mesh in groin hernia repair. *N Engl J Med* 2016;374:146–53. doi: 10.1056/NEJMoa1505126.

21. Augestad KM, Lindsetmo RO. Overcoming distance: video-conferencing as a clinical and educational tool among surgeons. *World J Surg* 2009;33:1356–65.

22. Koivusalo AM, Kellokumpu I, Lindgren L. Gasless laparoscopic cholecystectomy: comparison of postoperative recovery with conventional technique. *Br J Anaesth* 1996;77:576–80.

23. Chu K, Rosseel P, Gielis P, Ford N. Surgical task shifting in sub-Saharan Africa. *PLoS Med* 2009;6:e1000078.

24. Beard J, Oresanya L, Akoko L. Surgical task-shifting in a low-resource setting: outcomes after major surgery performed by nonphysician clinicians in Tanzania. *World J Surg* 2014;38:1398–404.

25. Gradian Health Systems. Universal Anaesthesia Machine (UAM). [accessed: 2016 March 29]. Available from: http://www.gradianhealth.org/universal-anaesthesia-machine/.

26. Alibaba.com. Newmon Anesthesia Ventilator. [accessed: 2016 March 29]. Available from: http://lifesupportsystems.

trustpass.alibaba.com/product/106473443-101225900/Newmon_Anesthesia_Ventilator.html.

27. Sethuraman K, Tirupathi D, Raykar N, Awasthy P. Surgical care for low-income, rural populations: an alternative delivery model from Jan Swasthya Sahyog, India. *Lancet Comm Glob Surg Teach Cases* 2015;1:27.

28. Hrezo R, Clark J. The walking blood bank: an alternative blood supply in military mass casualties. *Disaster Manag Response* 2003;1:19–22.

29. Romsons. Colo Bag®. [accessed: 2016 March 30]. Available from: http://www.romsons.com/domestic/products/8_COLO_BAG.html.

30. Pflug AM, Utiyama EM, Fontes B, Faro M, Rasslan S. Continuous reinfusion of succus entericus associated with fistuloclysis in the management of a complex jejunal fistula on the abdominal wall. *Int J Surg Case Rep* 2013;4:716–8.

31. Adotey JM. External intestinal fistulae in Port Harcourt. *West Afr J Med* 1995;14:97–100.

32. Dodiyi-Manuel A, Igwe PO. Enterocutaneous fistula in University of Port Harcourt Teaching Hospital. *Niger J Med* 2013;22:93–6.

33. Monson JR, Weiser MR. Sabiston Textbook of Surgery, the biological basis of modern surgical practice. *Dis Colon Rectum* 2008;51:1154.

34. Garyali R. Experience with duodenal ulcer perforations in a district level rural hospital: a study over a period of four years. *Bull Assoc Rural Surg India* 2005;2:8–11.

35. Wolff BG, Fleshman JW. *The ASCRS Textbook of Colon and Rectal Surgery*. Vol. 2. New York, NY: Springer; 2007. doi: 10.1007/s10350-008-9229-0.

36. Chalya PL, McHembe MD, Mshana SE, Rambau P, Jaka H, Mabula JB. Tuberculous bowel obstruction at a university teaching hospital in Northwestern Tanzania: a surgical experience with 118 cases. *World J Emerg Surg* 2013;8:12. doi: 10.1186/1749-7922-8-12.

37. Gouma D, Geenen R, van Gulik TM, et al. Rates of complications and death after pancreaticoduodenectomy: risk factors and the impact of hospital volume. *Ann Surg* 2000;232:786–95.

38. Dutta G, Bain J, Ray AK, Dey S, Das N, Das B. Comparing Ksharasutra (Ayurvedic Seton) and open fistulotomy in the management of fistula-in-ano. *J Nat Sci Biol Med* 2015;6:406.

39. McConkey SJ. Case series of acute abdominal surgery in rural Sierra Leone. *World J Surg* 2002;26:509–13. doi: 10.1007/s00268-001-0258-2.

40. Meara JG, McClain CD, Rogers Jr SO, Mooney DP. *Global Surgery and Anesthesia Manual: Providing Care in Resource-limited Settings*. Baco Raton, FL: CRC Press; 2015.

9

Impact of Centralisation, Assessment of Surgical Quality and Outcome

J.A.M.G. Tol and D.J. Gouma

ABSTRACT

This chapter provides an overview of the development and impact of centralisation of low-volume complicated gastrointestinal surgery. It is about the ongoing discussion on surgery in local community hospitals versus far-abroad high-volume hospitals, and reluctance of surgeons to accept these changes. The chapter analyses the effect of volume, both surgeon and hospital, on mortality rate and other outcome parameters such as improvement of R0 resection, receiving chemotherapy, survival and, more recently, the patient-related outcome measurement and patient-reported experience measures. Furthermore, there is a discussion on the impact of volume versus the framework of the hospital setting in terms of aspects of the hospital processes and structures such as availability of intensive care units, of interventional radiology for 24/7 and of a multidisciplinary supportive team during patient selection and preoperative screening, as well as the impact of this team in the management of complications. The basic aspect is transparency and, therefore, the use of clear, well-accepted definitions and grading systems of complications and other outcome parameters as suggested, for example, by the Clavien-Dindo classification, the National Surgical Quality Improvement Program and the International Consortium for Health Outcomes Measurement, have been summarised in more detail in other chapters.

KEYWORDS

Centralisation, gastrointestinal surgery, surgical quality, low-volume surgery, hospital volume, surgical mortality, PROMS, patient-related outcome measurement, PREMS, patient-reported experience measures, MDT, multidisciplinary team, hospital structure/process

INTRODUCTION

Gastrointestinal (GI) surgery is one of the largest specialisations all over the world. Whether it is performed in a small peripheral hospital or in a large volume tertiary centre, every surgical department will be challenged by not only a wide variety of diseases, evolving sophisticated diagnostic tests and treatment guidelines but also the occurrence of a wide variety of complications.

Hospital volume and surgical volume have been reported to play an important role in reducing mortality. In achieving the best care for all patients, we are usually dependent on expert opinions and (clinical) research.

However, surgical quality and outcomes depend on a range of variables; access to experienced staff, available resources, patient characteristics, hospital structures and facilities such as an intensive care unit; and an additional multidisciplinary supportive team. In this chapter, the history of the hospital volume discussion, influence of centralisation and the important role of a multidisciplinary approach on the traditional outcome measurements of morbidity and mortality as well as the impact of these aspects on patient-related outcome measurements such as patient-reported outcome measures (PROMs) and patient-reported experience measures (PREMs) will be discussed.

THE START OF THE PROCESS OF CENTRALISATION

The hypothesis 'practice makes perfect' was originally proposed by Luft et al as long ago as 1979.[1] However, the process of centralisation started only in the early 90s, with two studies from the United States (Maryland and New York regions) clearly demonstrating a difference in mortality after pancreatic resection between low- (<5) and high-volume (>25) centres.[2,3] The landmark paper on this subject, and start of the worldwide discussion on the potential effect of high-volume centres thereafter, came from Birkmeyer et al; this paper entitled 'volume and surgical mortality in the United States' was published in the *New England Journal of Medicine (NEJM)* in 2002 and showed the effect of centralisation on mortality for many different surgical procedures.[4,5] However, the authors also pointed out that centralisation could interfere with the continuity of care, since many aspects of postoperative care would be left to local physicians who were not involved with the actual operation. This might lead to underuse of surgery in rural areas and also have an impact on the financial viability of hospitals and their ability to retain surgeons.[6] It is remarkable that, recently, there was a case vignette about 'A Man Who Needs Complex Surgery' in the *NEJM*, again covering the same issues from the past, and articulated questions with a choice between[7]:

- Recommend surgery at the local community hospital
- Recommend surgery at the high-volume hospital in the city

Therefore, this is still an ongoing discussion, despite an undeniable effect of volume, of both surgeon and hospital on postoperative outcomes, for many different complicated GI procedures. Because of data that are easily extracted and compared between different hospitals, nearly all of these studies show similar results: high volume is associated with lower mortality rates.

The Impact of Centralisation and Evaluation of This Process Within the Surgical Community in One Country

This part is an example of how difficult it is to start centralisation, research this subject and implement it in one country, in this case, the Netherlands. The pros and cons and the reaction of patients and healthcare professionals have probably been similar in other countries. It will provide some insight into what has happened over 20 years from the introduction of the process of centralisation until today.

Similar to the United States, centralisation in the Netherlands also started in the 90s, and the first evaluation over 1994 to 1995, which included 428 patients after pancreatoduodenectomy (PD) (in a country with a maximal distance of 200 Km), showed the mortality rate of 16% in hospitals performing less than five PDs per year, compared with the mortality rate of 1.5% in hospitals performing 25 or more PDs per year.[8] It was suggested that surgeons should, as a first step, at least monitor their own quality control/outcome and decide whether it was justified to continue pancreatic surgery. Most surgeons did not agree with the conclusion and suggested that the paper was promoting action for a change in referral pattern to the hospital of the authors who were situated in the Amsterdam Medical Center (AMC). The second evaluation over a longer 5-year period (1994–1998) showed similar results.[9] The generally used explanation among opponents was that the time to implement the self-monitoring strategy was too short to detect a change in mortality or referral pattern, and surgeons could start the so-called networks in management of complications only if given enough time. In 2005, a new systematic review also clearly showed an association between improved outcomes after pancreatic surgery when performed in a high-volume hospital.[10] Despite spreading this message nationally and internationally to support the ongoing plea for centralisation, there was still reluctance to refer such patients to large tertiary hospitals. This was clearly shown in the evaluation of a 10-year period (1994–2004), in which no change was reported in postoperative mortality rates (Figure 9.1) and referral pattern (Figure 9.2).[9,10] Pancreatic resections were still being performed in as many as 46 hospitals in the Netherlands, a very small country, with an area of only 40,000 Km^2, despite many presentations and discussion (Figure 9.2).[10]

Shortly afterwards, in 2004, the Dutch Health Council called for a registration of volume and outcome, and the Dutch Health Care Inspectorate (IGZ) decided that 11 procedures per year (starting with oesophagectomy) should be the minimum to continue this type of surgery. The impact of the nationwide regulation for centralisation using the volume restriction by the government was clearly shown in the next analysis from 2004 to 2009, showing only 5% of procedures performed in low-volume centres, that is, those with less than five procedures per year, and a reduction of overall mortality from 10 to 5% (Figure 9.3).[11]

Eventually, the Dutch surgical community took it upon themselves in 2005 to set the criteria for pancreatic surgery centres to a minimum of 20 procedures per year. This led to an extension of cooperation between hospitals for low-volume surgery and helped create networks to be able to stay

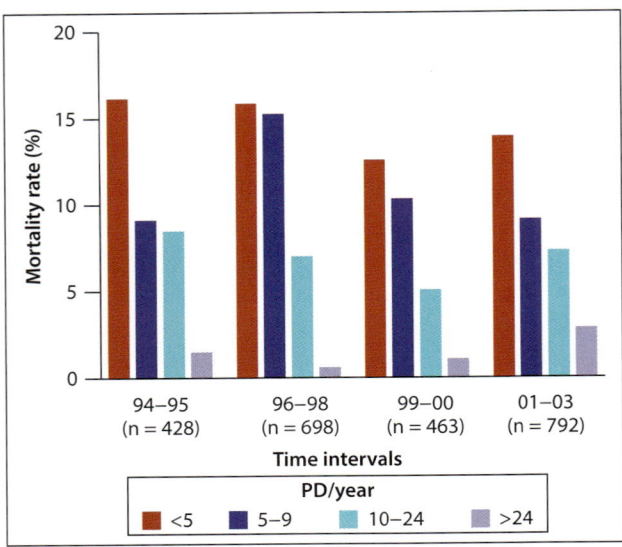

Figure 9.1 Hospital mortality in the four volume categories at the different time intervals (1994 to 1995, 1996 to 1998, 1999 to 2000 and 2001 to 2003).

Abbreviation: PD, pancreatoduodenectomy.

Reprinted with permission from: van Heek NT, Kuhlmann KF, Scholten RJ, et al. Hospital volume and mortality after pancreatic resection: a systematic review and an evaluation of intervention in the Netherlands. *Ann Surg* 2005;242:781–8, discussion 788–90.

involved. Finally, pancreatic surgeons, gastroenterologists and medical oncologists started working together via the Dutch Pancreatic Cancer Group (DPCG) as part of the Dutch Institute for Clinical Auditing (DICA).

The DICA was started by medical professionals to measure aspects of the quality of care provided in different hospitals. This organisation ensures a transparent and valid method of clinical registration, controlling this to enable physicians to perform quality research and compare outcomes between different hospitals.[12] Currently, the DICA controls many registrations containing outcomes in most GI surgical diseases (*see* Chapter 14).

This process of centralisation will vary greatly between countries, but generally, surgeons themselves are not capable of leading the implementation and solving all upcoming problems. In the United Kingdom, for example, the government decided more directly to select one centre per 3 to 4 million inhabitants for pancreatic cancer and per 1 to 2 million for oesophageal surgery, but no clear move towards centralisation has been reported after analysing their data 5 years after the decision of implementing this policy.[13] However, a recent survey in 2014 showed that patients suffering from oesophageal or gastric cancer are all discussed at multidisciplinary team (MDT) meetings and care services are more centralised now compared with data published in 2007, with improved survival reported in patients undergoing curative surgery.[14] On the other hand, centralisation in countries with small populations cannot adhere to the volume cut reported in most of such outcome studies. Beenen et al compared data on oesophageal resection in New Zealand with the available literature.[15] Their outcomes were similar to what was seen in high-volume centres. In case of centralisation, maybe only one high-volume centre would be started,

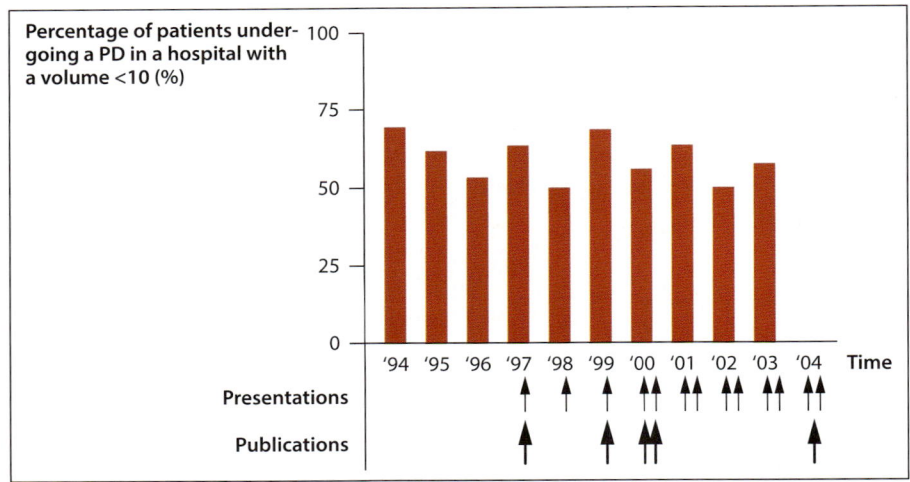

Figure 9.2 Referral pattern to hospitals performing less than 10 PDs per year over a 10-year period (1994–2004). The arrows indicate the interventions by means of national or international presentations and publications.

Abbreviation: PD, pancreatoduodenectomy.

Reprinted with permission from: van Heek NT, Kuhlmann KF, Scholten RJ, et al. Hospital volume and mortality after pancreatic resection: a systematic review and an evaluation of intervention in the Netherlands. *Ann Surg* 2005;242:781–8, discussion 788–90.

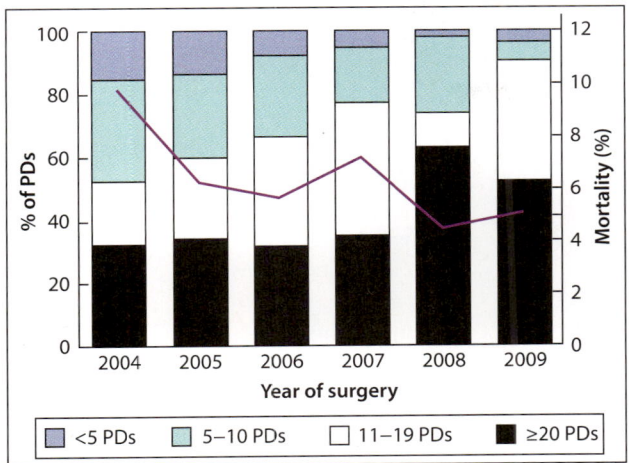

Figure 9.3 Percentage of pancreatoduodenectomies (PDs) performed in each hospital volume category (bar graph) and overall annual PD-associated in-hospital mortality during 2004 to 2009 (line graph).[11]

Reprinted with permission from: de Wilde RF, Besselink MG, van der Tweel I, et al. Impact of nationwide centralization of pancreaticoduodenectomy on hospital mortality. *Br J Surg* 2012;99:404–10.

which would burden most patients with travelling, and postoperative care would almost certainly be given in regional hospitals. This study is an example of how one might tackle centralisation in low-population-density regions and to what extent care can be centralised.

Effect of Centralisation

Centralisation has resulted in reduced postoperative mortality, the primary and most important short-term outcome in many studies. A few years ago, we analysed all systematic reviews, including four meta-analyses, describing the effect of hospital and/or surgeon volume on mortality.[16] The majority of reviews (>90%) showed a lower mortality in high-volume hospitals. This volume–outcome relationship was found in different GI procedures: oesophageal, gastric, liver and pancreatic surgery (Tables 9.1, 9.2, 9.3 and 9.4; all cited from Tol et al[16]).

The results on oesophageal cancer were recently confirmed by another review.[17] They also demonstrated better long-term survival in high-volume hospitals, with hazard ratio (HR) = 0.82 and 95% confidence interval (CI): 0.75–0.90, derived from 16 studies. A new study on major liver surgery including 23,107 patients showed the same association between high-volume hospitals and surgeons and lower hospital costs, shorter length of stay and a longer survival when analysed with propensity score matching.[18] A population-based study from England

retrieved data from the National Health Service (NHS) database and analysed surgeon volume. They stated that 'mortality after resections for oesophageal, gastric, and pancreatic cancer falls as surgeon volume rises up to 30 cases'; however, no threshold could be demonstrated.[19] A recent meta-analysis on volume and outcome after pancreatic surgery included almost 60,000 patients, with high heterogeneity (I = 63%); the overall pooled odds ratio for mortality was 2.37 (95% CI: 1.95–2.88), in favour of the high-volume hospitals.[20]

Other Endpoints of Outcome

Gooiker et al in 2014 showed an increased resection rate after centralisation of pancreatic cancer surgery, and high-volume centres had significantly better survival rates.[21] Several variables could account for this improved survival. High-volume hospitals generally have high-volume surgeons. If 'practice makes perfect', it could be that high-volume, experienced surgeons report lower complication rates or better outcomes after surgery in terms of resections margins. Onete et al also reviewed data from low- and high-volume hospitals, n < 20 or n > 20, respectively. A higher R0 resection rate was seen in the high-volume group and a higher percentage of patients had T3 and T4 tumours. The impact on survival was not assessed.[22]

Centralisation not only affects outcomes after surgery; recently, a few studies reported the association with the likelihood of undergoing surgery, in general, and also the outcome in high-volume hospitals for metastatic malignancy.[23,24] In the first study, 8,141 patients were diagnosed with nonmetastasised pancreatic cancer. Of those, 2712 patients were diagnosed in one of the 19 pancreatic centres performing more than 20 resections per year (group 1) and 5429 patients were diagnosed in one of the 74 nonpancreatic centre with less than 20 resections per year (group 2). They found that 52.4% of group 1 had only exploratory laparotomy compared with 31.4% of group 2. A pancreatectomy was performed in over 40% of the surgically explored patients in group 1 and in 25% of patients in group 2 who underwent an exploration (p < 0.001). Patients diagnosed in a pancreatic centre (>20 resections/year) had a higher chance of undergoing surgery than those in a nonpancreatic centre (<20 resections/year); odds ratio 2.21 (95% CI: 1.98–2.47) (Figure 9.4).[23] The centre of diagnosis was not associated with improved survival. Another study reported the survival after palliative chemotherapy in patients with metastatic pancreatic cancer, in which 24% of 5385 patients received palliative chemotherapy. However, this study did find an association

Table 9.1 Studies describing the association between volume and mortality after oesophageal surgery[16]

Author and year of publication	Studies with adjusted data and significant results	Cut-off high and low volume+	Results: association between volume and mortality*
Halm, 2002	3/3	Variable Low volume: 5–10 High volume: 11–200	Median absolute difference in mortality between LVH and HVH: 12%
Metzger, 2004	13/13	Very low volume: <5 Low volume: >5 Medium volume: >10 High volume: >20	Difference in median mortality rates: Very low volume: 18% Low volume: 13.8% Medium volume: 11% High volume: 4.9%; OR: 0.43; CI: 0.31–0.58
Killeen, 2005	9/10	Variable Low volume: 3–32 High volume: 8–60	NNT to prevent 1 death: 7–9
Gruen, 2009	21/26$	Low volume: 1–4# High volume: >13	First study on the effect of volume on mortality: HVS: OR 0.6; CI: 0.36–0.99 Second study: HVS: OR: 1.8; CI: 1.13–2.87 HVH: OR: 1.67; CI: 1.02–2.73
Markar, 2012	6/9	Variable Low volume: 1–22 High volume: 4–81	In-hospital mortality is increased in LVH compared with HVH; OR: 0.29; CI: 0.16–0.53

+Resections per year.   *Odds ratio, 95% confidence interval. $Two studies used for adjusted mortality risk.   #Based on one study.

Abbreviations: CI, confidence interval; HVH, high-volume hospital; HVS, high-volume surgeon; LVH, low-volume hospital; LVS, low-volume surgeon; NNT, number needed to treat; OR, odds ratio.

Reprinted with permission from: Tol JA, van Gulik TM, Busch OR, Gouma DJ. Centralization of highly complex low-volume procedures in upper gastrointestinal surgery. A summary of systematic reviews and meta-analyses. *Dig Surg* 2012;29:374–83.

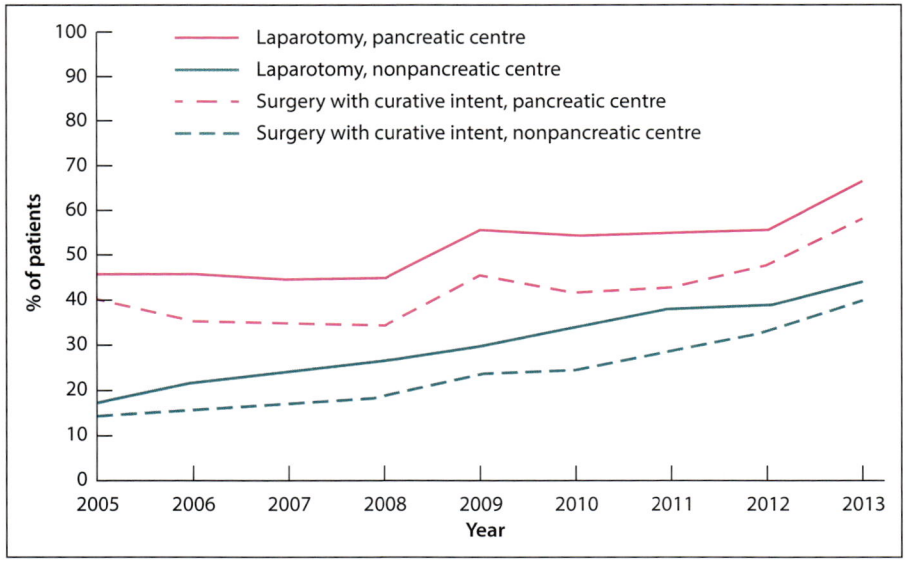

Figure 9.4   Treatment of M0 pancreatic cancer by centre of diagnosis in the Netherlands, 2005 to 2013.[23]

Reprinted with permission from: Bakens MJ, van Gestel YR, Bongers M, et al. Hospital of diagnosis and likelihood of surgical treatment for pancreatic cancer. *Br J Surg* 2015;102:1670–5.

Table 9.2 Studies describing the association between volume, mortality and survival after gastric surgery[16]

Author and year of publication	Studies with adjusted data and significant results	Cut-off high and low volume+	Results: association between volume and mortality*
Halm, 2002	2/3	Variable Low volume: 5–15 High volume: 15–201	Median absolute difference in mortality between: LVH and HVH: 6.5% LVS and HVS: 4%
Killeen, 2005	3/5	Variable Low volume: 5–26 High volume: 9–67	Mortality reduction of 1–6% NNT to prevent 1 death: 20–100 patients
Gruen, 2009	14/20$	Low volume: 1–54# High volume: 55–496	First study: Effect of volume on mortality: HVS: OR: 0.59; CI: 0.32–1.07 Effect of volume on survival: HVH: HR: 0.93; CI: 0.89–0.98 Second study: Hospital volume low–high: 11.3–3.7%; p < 0.001 Surgeon volume low–high: 12.3–3.2%; p < 0.001

+Resections per year. *OR = Odds ratio, 95% confidence interval. $Two studies used for adjusted mortality risk. #Based on one study.

Abbreviations: CI, confidence interval; HR, hazard ratio; HVH, high-volume hospital; HVS, high-volume surgeon; LVH, low-volume hospital; LVS, low-volume surgeon; NNT, number needed to treat; OR, odds ratio.

Reprinted with permission from: Tol JA, van Gulik TM, Busch OR, Gouma DJ. Centralization of highly complex low-volume procedures in upper gastrointestinal surgery. A summary of systematic reviews and meta-analyses. *Dig Surg* 2012;29:374–83.

between the centre of diagnosis and survival; HR = 0.74 (95% CI: 0.66–0.83). Patients who were being treated with chemotherapy in a high-volume treatment centre also had an improved survival; HR 0.76 (95% CI: 0.67–0.87).[24]

Although not everyone is convinced of the benefit of centralisation, Varagunam et al analysed the association between the outcome and volume for three elective procedures using postoperative complications and PROMs. No significant benefits were reported between high- and low-volume hospitals.[25] The discussion generally always will include the lack of proper real-time adequate risk adjustment. The, probably, much stronger association between the quality of hospital's structures and processes and good-quality outcome of care based on

Table 9.3 Studies describing the association between volume and mortality after liver surgery[16]

Author and year of publication	Studies with adjusted data and significant results	Cut-off high and low volume+	Results: association between volume and mortality*
Garcea, 2009	5/10	Variable Low volume: 1–60 High volume: 10–201	Mortality rate, HVH: 1.5–9.4% Mortality rate, LVH: 5.8–22.7%
Gruen, 2009	11/11	Variable# Low volume: 1–5 High volume: >34	Effect of volume on mortality: OR = 0.77 (CI: 0.72–0.83)$ NNT of 11

+Resections per year. *Odds ratio, 95% confidence interval. #Based on 10 studies. $Based on nonadjusted data.

Abbreviations: CI, confidence interval; HVH, high-volume hospital; LVH, low-volume hospital; NNT, number needed to treat; OR, odds ratio.

Reprinted with permission from: Tol JA, van Gulik TM, Busch OR, Gouma DJ. Centralization of highly complex low-volume procedures in upper gastrointestinal surgery. A summary of systematic reviews and meta-analyses. *Dig Surg* 2012;29:374–83.

Table 9.4 Studies describing the association between volume and mortality after pancreatic surgery[16]

Author and year of publication	Studies with adjusted data and significant results	Cut-off high and low volume+	Results: association between volume and mortality*
Dudley, 2000	1/8	Low volume: 1–6$	1/year: OR = 5.00; CI: 2.54–9.84 5–6/year: OR = 3.08; CI: 1.66–5.70
Gruen, 2009	23/30#	Low volume: 1–3$ High volume: 4–13	First study on the effect of volume on mortality: HVH: OR = 1.1; CI: 0.54–2.59 HVS: OR = 0.9; 0.31–2.37 Second study: HVH: OR = 2.34; CI: 1.38–3.99 HVS: OR = 2.31; CI: 1.43–3.72
Gooijker, 2011	9/14	Variable Low volume: 1–5 High volume: 7–89	Pooled data: Effect of volume on mortality: HVH: OR = 0.32; CI: 0.16–0.64 HVS: OR = 0.46, CI: 0.17–1.26

+Resections per year. *Odds ratio, 95% confidence interval. $Based on one study. #Two studies used for adjusted mortality risk.

Abbreviations: CI, confidence interval; HVH, high-volume hospital; HVS, high-volume surgeon; LVH, low-volume hospital; LVS, low-volume surgeon; OR, odds ratio.

Reprinted with permission from: Tol JA, van Gulik TM, Busch OR, Gouma DJ. Centralization of highly complex low-volume procedures in upper gastrointestinal surgery. A summary of systematic reviews and meta-analyses. *Dig Surg* 2012;29:374–83.

PROMs is hard to analyse, since these measures are often subjective, nonbinary or lacking. However, one can only assume that better quality of care does not solely depend on volume.[26]

Centralisation also has disadvantages such as increased waiting lists, especially in countries where funding is limited and expansion of the high-volume centres to adhere to the higher demand of complex GI surgery is difficult.

Considering the volume levels, it was recently shown that in high-volume hospitals for pancreatic surgery in the more-than-40-resections-per-year category, significantly more patients received adjuvant chemotherapy and had more than 10 lymph nodes retrieved compared with lower-volume categories.[27] Therefore, the optimal volume plateau for pancreatic surgery has yet to be determined. Although the standard of more than 40 patients is derived from a country with a much lower population than other countries, the actual adequate volume for centralisation is not clear.[6] One study even reported differences between the high-volume centres within Europe, even though no clear explanation could be given.[28]

Sullivan et al recently published an extensive analysis on the current and upcoming problems and changes we have to address in order to give patients the necessary high-quality care that is accessible, affordable and coordinated among providers and services.[29] Providing this care can be accomplished by addressing a few cornerstones: finance, guidelines and further development.[29]

Finance

Quality cannot be warranted without new investments; lack of investments will mostly effect the low- and middle-income countries.[30] The international funds might regulate this, and at the country level, we should prevent most funds being allocated to major hospitals by regulating the national financing plans. So far, it is often seen that major centres have relatively major resources, whereas small hospitals in rural areas have very limited resources to maintain basic surgical care. Structured help and guidance in investing in surgical cancer care, especially in low- and middle-income countries, are essential and can guide governments and stakeholders in making the right decision. This can apply to different types of care, from research to road infrastructure, and can be financed through tax earnings or health insurance.

Guidelines

By introducing guidelines and setting up criteria, which should be met when treating patients with certain diseases, an overall spread of continuous and uniform care can be generated. The quality given in high-volume hospitals by, for example, having multidisciplinary team meetings and follow-ups with patients, will then also be reproduced in the rural hospitals once these criteria are captured in protocols and guidelines. Video or conference calls can enable these meetings. Furthermore, pre- and postoperative care can be protocoled based on the best available evidence and local practice. In this way, local physicians can adhere to the standards that were set and, in case of a lack of expertise, know what treatment is appropriate.

Development

While developing around the high-volume centres and initiating referral from rural areas to major hospitals, overall improvement of quality of care can be achieved by improving care not only in the low-medium volume hospitals but also in the high-volume hospitals. This needs an individual look at what is best and what is feasible. Open surgery at the rural hospitals can have excellent outcomes when compared with the more expensive laparoscopic surgery performed at the high-volume centres. Both hospitals need different sorts of development within their surgical department to achieve a better quality of care. For instant, in China, super centres have been created to adhere to the high demand of care, since 70% of their population is based in rural areas. Development in infrastructure and geographic knowledge is, in these circumstances, very important. Countries should perform epidemiological studies to study their population needs and create guidelines.

In some countries, most cancer-related surgery is performed in general hospitals. In order to organise a system of centralisation without losing quality of care elsewhere, the framework depicted in Algorithm 9.1 is an example of how expertise and resources in major high-volume and tertiary centres can upgrade the quality of care and still maintain the same standard of care in peripheral hospitals.[29] It is a conceptual framework showing how the downside of centralisation can be attacked.

In order to initiate centralisation, it is important that hospitals and departments are already familiar with treating larger numbers of patients in a multidisciplinary setting. Furthermore, these high-volume or specialised centres should be available for a certain number of patients per region, and one has to address patients living in remote areas in order to prevent or decrease long waiting lists. Another currently frequently used option is to establish a partnership between low- and high-volume centres. A study by Ravaioli et al in 2014 showed decreased mortality rates and similar morbidity rates in low-volume centres compared with their collaborating high-volume centres.[31] In addition, partnership of hospitals located close to each other might result in better outcomes. Two high-volume hospitals decided to centralise care for patients with pancreatic cancer. After centralisation, the 2-year survival rate was 55% compared with 39% seen

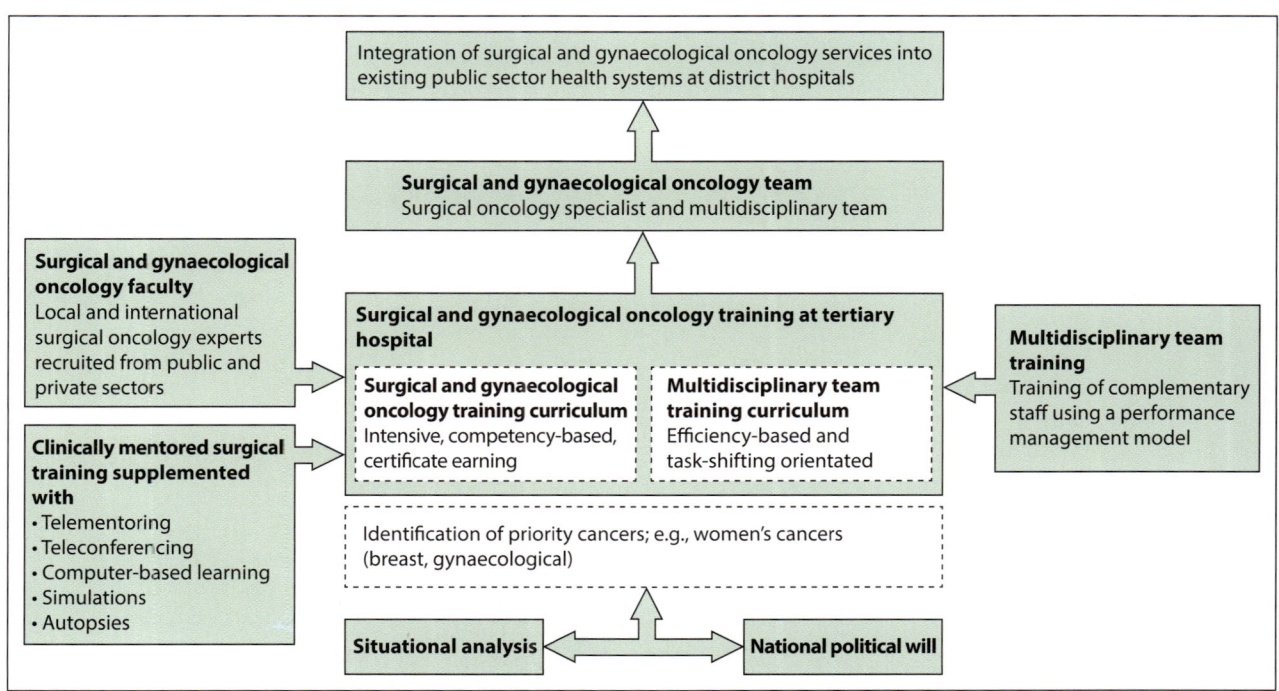

Algorithm 9.1   Conceptual framework for scaling up surgical and gynaecological cancer services in resource-limited settings.[29]

Reprinted with permission from: Sullivan R, Alatise OI, Anderson BO, et al. Global cancer surgery: delivering safe, affordable, and timely cancer surgery. *Lancet Oncol* 2015;16:1193–224.

in the previous years (HR = 0.5; 95% CI: 0.34–0.73).[32] A network between major hospitals and rural centres is one way of creating a safety net for patients who cannot reach the high-volume hospitals. Overall improvement of quality of care can only be achieved by improving care in low-, medium- and high-volume hospitals.

VOLUME VERSUS HOSPITAL RESOURCE ASPECTS RELATED TO THE PROCESS OF CARE

When analysing outcome in patients receiving complex surgery and perioperative care, high-volume hospitals and surgeons are associated with low mortality rates, as summarised above.[16] Beside this volume item, other aspects of care such as hospital structures and the local adapted processes of care are important factors responsible for the outcome and quality of care, as already extensively reported by Birkmeyer and Dimick.[33] According to their conceptual model, the association between different aspects of the hospital structure, the processes in the hospital and outcomes become visible, as shown in Algorithm 9.2.[33,34] The different categories of outcomes have been expanded in this model to depict which processes are associated with the occurrence of complications and recovery after surgery.

Hospital structures, facilities and availability such as fully equipped operating rooms; intensive care unit; interventional radiology and endoscopy; specialised surgeons, anaesthesiologists, microbiologists and nursing

staff; and the high quality of every discipline are a prerequisite for quality of care. Not only the surgical procedure but also other processes involving patient selection and screening as well as prevention and treatment of complications will directly influence the outcomes when not executed adequately.[33,35,36] However, these correlations are difficult to quantify, resulting in limited data demonstrating any effect of these different factors on patient outcomes.

Several studies have shown the importance and additional value of a multidisciplinary team. Pawlik et al have performed a study in which a multidisciplinary team reviewed patients referred to their clinic. The clinical stage of disease was altered in 18.7% of patients, leading to changes in therapeutic recommendations.[37]

An extensive study published by Ghaferi et al described nicely the association between inadequate management or detection of complications and high mortality rates.[38] Hospitals reporting low and high mortality rates after surgery, ranging from 3.5 to 6.9%, according to hospital quintile of mortality, were compared. Patients' characteristics did not differ between those hospitals, and the overall and major complication rates were not different. However, the death rate in patients with major complications was 21.4% in very-high-mortality hospitals and 12.5% in very-low-mortality hospitals.[38] The facilities and opportunity to adequately diagnose and manage major complications proved to be responsible for these differences in mortality. Complications were not recognised, recognised too late or treated too late, which

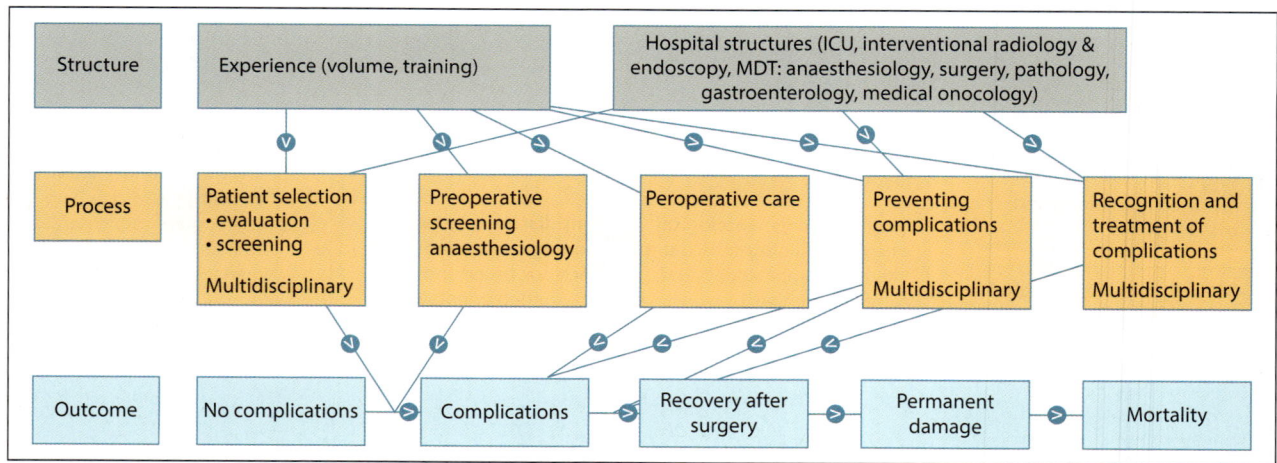

Algorithm 9.2   Association between hospital structure, process and outcome after surgery[34] (according to the conceptual model of Birkmeyer et al[33]).

Abbreviations: ICU, intensive care unit; MDT, multidisciplinary team.

Reprinted with permission from: Gouma DJ, Laméris HJ, Rauws EA, Busch OR. The centralisation of highly complex operations. *Ned Tijdschr Geneeskd* 2012;156:A4887.

was referred to as 'failure to rescue' in the high-mortality hospitals.[39]

To analyse this aspect, a small study was performed at the AMC, Amsterdam, the Netherlands. During a 15-week period, a consecutive group of patients with complex GI pathology was prospectively registered at the weekly preoperative outpatient MDT meeting. Preoperative changes in treatment strategy set by the referring hospital, additional findings by the MDT and alterations regarding postoperative management after the MDT meeting were scored. Of 128 patients, 41 were referred for a specific treatment strategy set by the referring hospital. A multidisciplinary team approach during preoperative meetings for patients with complex HPB pathology led to alterations of the initial treatment strategy in 14 of the 41 patients (34%). A separate cohort of patients presented at the postoperative MDT meeting on the surgical GI ward was also included. During these MDT meetings, additions and suggestions for change of the ongoing treatment strategies were made in 42 of the 149 patients (28%) in order to improve the recovery of those patients.[40] These findings underscore the substantial effects of the MDT concept on selection of the treatment strategy of such complex patients as well as early recognition of potential problems.

TRANSPARENCY IN MONITORING COMPLICATIONS AND OUTCOME

Transparency in monitoring the adverse effects of surgery, such as complications and surgery-related mortality, is crucial in order to improve care. By analysing the outcomes of different aspects of care, the quality can be assessed, monitored and, most importantly, warranted. National improvement programs set up by physicians often conduct this registration. These registrations should start with clear definitions of outcomes, as reported during the past decade. A generally accepted common definition of complications is, for example, the Clavien–Dindo classification[41] (see also Chapter 11). The challenge is to specify the definition to enable comparison. Another example is the LHCR (National Surgical Adverse Event Registration). This registry enables uniformity and comparison of outcomes at all surgical departments in the Netherlands and, indirectly, of the quality of care.[42,43] The next problem of any monitoring system is the source and registration manner; if one is incomplete, it will result in an incomplete registration, as we have shown in the past.[44] To avoid registration faults due to differences in the interpretation of the definition of a complication, the following definition was presented by the LHCR:

A complication is an unintended and undesirable event or condition following medical treatment, that is harmful for the patient and necessitates adjustment of medical treatment, or that leads to permanent harm.[43] Then, the complications should be graded depending on their severity, as also shown by the Clavien–Dindo classification. A sufficient complication registry that can be used for analysing outcomes in surgical care and improving that care. All patient and operative, epidemiological and disease characteristics can be linked. This enables risk adjustment and comparison.

To ensure validity for comparison between different hospitals, the National Surgical Quality Improvement Program (NSQIP) in the United States incorporated the following five elements[45] (see also Chapter 10):

- Standardisation of endpoints
- Standardisation of definitions and terms
- System for data collection and prospective collection
- Data collectors themselves grading and training
- Validated system for risk adjustment

The monitoring systems of complications and mortality and the structure and process of care in the different hospitals should be taken into account when reviewing data and publications on complications in surgery. An optimal quality of these data is a prerequisite for the start of the discussion on open access to all outcome data after surgery for the public, as currently is happening in the Netherlands.

New Assessment of Quality: From Mortality to Patient-Reported Outcome Measures and Patient-Reported Experience Measures

As mentioned above, evaluation of mortality is the early start of comparison of outcome data after surgery and medical treatment. This was an enormous, but relatively easy, step forward to compare outcome measurements in different hospitals. Currently, there is a trend to move from the 'simple' clinical data to more PROMs and PREMs. The use of PROMs in clinical practice is fast growing, but the lack of standardisation in PROMs used in cancer research makes it still difficult to use these data for quality monitoring, as stated recently by Howell et al.[46] They reviewed the literature, and the European Organization for Research and Treatment of Cancer (EORTC) Quality of Life questionnaire (QLQ)-30 was the most commonly used PROM, which is promising for further comparison. This was confirmed in two other studies describing patients with gastric and colorectal cancers; the most frequently used PROM was the EORTC QLQ.[47,48] Recently, a Delphi survey amongst 150 patients and 78 healthcare professionals in the Netherlands was performed to develop a core set of patient-reported outcomes in pancreatic cancer.[49] General quality of life, general health, physical ability, satisfaction with caregivers, satisfaction with services and care organisation, coping and defaecation, appetite, ability to work/do usual activities, medication use, weight changes, fatigue, negative feelings, positive feelings, fear of recurrence, relationship with partner/family, and pancreatic enzyme replacement therapy use were the outcomes that were reported as most important PROMs. One of these outcomes, satisfaction with services and care organisation, might be directly related to centralisation. Another study on PROMs in patients undergoing chemoradiotherapy for oesophageal cancer reported that the general questionnaires were an adequate tool to measure health-related quality of life.[50]

The International Consortium for Health Outcomes Measurement (ICHOM) is an important nonprofit consortium that was set up to define and recommend these relatively new patient outcomes in a standardised way (available at: www.ichom.org.) The ICHOM was developed in 2012 by the Harvard Business School, the Boston Consulting Group and the Karolinska Institute in Sweden and has developed several standard sets of outcomes meaningful to patients, and physicians can use those health outcomes data to evaluate their outcomes. McNair et al also published a core outcome set retracted from studies on patients with colorectal cancer, in order to develop a basic minimum of PROMs, which could be used in further studies; however, high grade of heterogeneity amongst the reported PROMs was seen.[48]

Although the objective measures such as morbidity, mortality and survival are easy to analyse and, therefore, the positive associations between volume and those measures are frequently being used in the past, PROMs such as quality of life, general health, physical ability and satisfaction should also be considered important for the future. The impact of cancer and treatments on patients' quality of life should be more recognised and researched. The eventual choice of treatment may be very well altered if we approach it in more detail from a patient-reported outcome point of view instead of an objective 'radical resection decreased mortality' physicians' perspective. However, if we look at the impact of PROMs on patient selection for surgery, its effect on physicians' behaviour has so far been minimal.[51] In order to incorporate PROMs as a decision tool, its implementation and lowering the degree of heterogeneity need more attention.

CONCLUSIONS

Hospital volume and surgeon volume are the most recognised and used variables to be correlated with mortality. Other hospital structures, facilities and availability such as fully equipped operating rooms, intensive care unit, interventional radiology and endoscopy, specialised surgeons, anaesthesiologists, microbiologists and nursing staff, and the high quality of every discipline are a prerequisite for quality of care, but correlations with mortality rates are difficult to quantify, resulting in limited data demonstrating any effect of these other factors on patient outcomes.

Through centralisation, better outcomes have been reported. High-volume hospitals ensure high-quality care throughout the hospital, by having invested in hospital structures and processes of care. The knowledge of experienced physicians is bundled, and through multidisciplinary teamwork, all aspects of care are addressed, pre-, per- and postoperatively. This can have an overall positive effect on the care given by physicians, as published previously by Khuri et al.[52] Furthermore, owing to centralisation, physicians might introduce a better patient selection. Overall, all these factors benefit the eventual outcome, which should, in the future, incorporate, in particular, the patient-related outcome criteria such as PROMs and PREMs.

REFERENCES

1. Luft HS, Bunker JP, Enthoven AC. Should operations be regionalized? The empirical relation between volume and mortality. *N Engl J Med* 1979;301:1364–9.
2. Gordon TA, Burleyson GP. The effectiveness of Whipple resection in patients with pancreatic cancer at Veterans Affairs (VA) hospitals. *Ann Surg* 1996;223:446.
3. Lieberman MD, Kilburn H, Lindsey M, Brennan MF. Relation of perioperative deaths to hospital volume among patients undergoing pancreatic resection for malignancy. *Ann Surg* 1995;222:638–45.
4. Birkmeyer JD, Siewers AE, Finlayson EV, et al. Hospital volume and surgical mortality in the United States. *N Engl J Med* 2002;346:1128–37.
5. Birkmeyer JD, Stukel TA, Siewers AE, Goodney PP, Wennberg DE, Lucas FL. Surgeon volume and operative mortality in the United States. *N Engl J Med* 2003;349:2117–27.
6. Brinkmeyer JD. Should we regionalize major surgery? Potential benefits and policy considerations. *J Am Coll Surg* 2000;190:341–9.
7. Merrill AL, Jha AK, and Dimick JB. Clinical Effect of Surgical Volume. *N Engl J Med* 2016;374:1380–2.

8. Gouma DJ, De Wit LT, Van Berge Henegouwen MI, Van Gulik TH, Obertop H. Hospital experience and hospital mortality following partial pancreaticoduodenectomy in The Netherlands. *Ned Tijdschr Geneeskd* 1997;141:1738–41.

9. Gouma DJ, van Geenen RC, van Gulik TM, et al. Rates of complications and death after pancreaticoduodenectomy: risk factors and the impact of hospital volume. *Ann Surg* 2000;232:786–95.

10. Van Heek NT, Kuhlmann KFD, Scholten RJ, et al. Hospital Volume and Mortality After Pancreatic Resection. *Ann Surg* 2005;242:781–90.

11. de Wilde RF, Besselink MG, van der Tweel I, et al. Impact of nationwide centralization of pancreaticoduodenectomy on hospital mortality. *Br J Surg* 2012;99:404–10.

12. Van Leersum NJ, Snijders HS, Henneman D, et al. The Dutch surgical colorectal audit. *Eur J Surg Oncol* 2013;39:1063–70.

13. Parry J, Jolly K, Rouse A, Wilson R. Re-organizing services for the management of upper gastrointestinal cancers: patterns of care and problems with change. *Public Health* 2004;118:360–9.

14. Groene O, Chadwick G, Riley S, Hardwick RH. Re-organisation of oesophago-gastric cancer services in England and Wales: a follow-up assessment of progress and remaining challenges. *BMC Res Notes* 2014;7:24.

15. Beenen E, Jao W, Coulter G, Roberts R. The high volume debate in a low volume country: centralisation of oesophageal resection in New Zealand. *NZ Med J* 2013;126:34–45.

16. Tol JA, van Gullik TM, Busch OR, Gouma DJ. Centralization of highly complex low-volume procedures in upper gastrointestinal surgery. A summary of systematic reviews and meta-analyses. *Dig Surg* 2012;29:374–83.

17. Brusselaers N, Mattsson F, Lagergren J. Hospital and surgeon volume in relation to long-term survival after oesophagectomy: systematic review and meta-analysis. *Gut* 2014;63:1393–400.

18. Lu CC, Chiu CC, Wang JJ, Chiu YH, Shi HY. Volume-outcome associations after major hepatectomy for hepatocellular carcinoma: a nationwide Taiwan study. *J Gastrointest Surg* 2014;18:1138–45.

19. Mamidanna R, Ni Z, Anderson O, Spiegelhalter SD, et al. Surgeon volume and cancer esophagectomy, gastrectomy, and pancreatectomy: a population-based study in England. *Ann Surg* 2016;263:727–32.

20. Hata T, Motoi F, Ishida M, et al. Effect of hospital volume on surgical outcomes after pancreaticoduodenectomy: a systematic review and meta-analysis. *Ann Surg* 2016; 263:664–72.

21. Gooiker GA, Lemmens VE, Besselink MG, et al. Impact of centralization of pancreatic cancer surgery on resection rates and survival. *Br J Surg* 2014;101:1000–5.

22. Onete VG, Besselink MG, Salsbach CM, et al. Impact of centralization of pancreatoduodenectomy on reported radical resections rates in a nationwide pathology database. *HPB (Oxford)* 2015;17:736–42.

23. Bakens MJ, van Gestel YR, Bongers M, et al. Hospital of diagnosis and likelihood of surgical treatment for pancreatic cancer. *Br J Surg* 2015;102:1670–5.

24. Hai Mohammad N, Bernards N, Besselink MG, et al. Volume matters in the systemic treatment of metastatic pancreatic cancer: a population-based study in the Netherlands. *J Cancer Res Clin Oncol* 2016;142:1353–60.

25. Varagunam M, Hutchings A, Black N. Relationship between patient-reported outcomes of elective surgery and hospital and consultant volume. *Med Care* 2015;53:310–6.

26. Khuri SF. Invited commentary: surgeons, not general motors, should set standards for surgical care. *Surgery* 2001;130:429–31.

27. van der Geest LG, van Rijssen LB, Molenaar IQ, et al. Volume-outcome relationships in pancreatoduodenectomy for cancer. *HPB* 2016;18:317–24.

28. Dikken JL, van Sandick JW, Allum WH, et al. Differences in outcomes of oesophageal and gastric cancer surgery across Europe. *Br J Surg* 2013;100:83–94.

29. Sullivan R, Alatise OI, Anderson BO, et al. Global cancer surgery: delivering safe, affordable, and timely cancer surgery. *Lancet Oncol* 2015;16:1193–224.

30. Meara JG, Leather AJ, Hagander L, et al. Global Surgery 2030: evidence and solutions for achieving health, welfare, and economic development. *Lancet* 386:569–624.

31. Ravaioli M, Pinna AD, Francioni G, et al. A partnership model between high- and low-volume hospitals to improve results in hepatobiliary pancreatic surgery. *Ann Surg* 2014;260:871–5; discussion 875–7.

32. Gooiker GA, van Gijn W, Wouters MWJM, et al. Systematic review and meta-analysis of the volume-outcome relationship in pancreatic surgery. *Br J Surg* 2011; 98:485–94.

33. Birkmeyer JD, Dimick JB. Understanding and reducing variation in surgical mortality. *Annu Rev Med* 2009;60: 405–15.

34. Gouma DJ, Lameris HJS, Rauws EAJ, Busch ORC. Centralisatie van hoogcomplexe chirurgie. *Ned Tijdschr Geneeskd* 2012;156:1–5.

35. Langer B. Role of volume outcome data in assuring quality in HPB surgery. *HPB* 2007;9:330–4.

36. Ghaferi A, Birkmeyer JD, Dimick JB. Complications, failure to rescue, and mortality with major inpatient surgery in medicare patients. *Ann Surg* 2009;250:1029–34.

37. Pawlik T, Laheru D, Hruban R, et al. Evaluating the impact of a single-day multidisciplinary clinic on the management of pancreatic cancer. *Ann Surg Oncol* 2008;15:2081–8.

38. Ghaferi A, Birkmeyer JD, Dimick JB. Variation in hospital mortality associated with inpatient surgery. *N Engl J Med* 2009;361:1368–75.

39. Silber JH, Williams S V, Krakauer H, Schwartz JS. Hospital and patient characteristics associated with death

after surgery. A study of adverse occurrence and failure to rescue. *Med Care* 1992;30:615–29.

40. Tol JA, Nieveen van Dijkum EJM, Klinkenbijl JHG, van Gulik TM, Busch ORC, Gouma DJ. Special issue: abstracts of the 11th World Congress of the International Hepato-Pancreato-Biliary Association, 22–27 March 2014, Seoul Korea. *HPB* 2014;16:146–7.

41. Clavien PA, Barkun J, de Oliveira ML, et al. The Clavien-Dindo classification of surgical complications: five-year experience. *Ann Surg* 2009;250:187–96.

42. Sokol DK, Wilson J, What is a surgical complication? *World J Surg* 2008;32,942–4.

43. Goslings JC, Gouma DJ. What is a surgical complication? *World J Surg* 2008;32:952.

44. Ubbink DT, Visser A, Gouma DJ, Goslings JC. Registration of surgical adverse outcomes: a reliability study in a university hospital. *BMJ Open* 2012;2:pii:e000891.

45. Khuri S, Daley J, Henderson W, et al. The Department of Veterans Affairs' NSQIP: the first national validated, outcome–based, risk-adjusted and peer-controlled program for the measurement and enhancement of the quality of surgical care. National VA Surgical Quality Improvement Program. *Ann of Surg* 1998;228:491–507.

46. Howell D, Molloy S, Wilkinson K, et al. Patient-reported outcomes in routine cancer clinical practice: a scoping review of use, impact on health outcomes, and implementation factors. *Ann Oncol* 2015;26:1846–58.

47. Straatman J, van der Wielen N, Joosten PJ, et al. Assessment of patient-reported outcome measures in the surgical treatment of patients with gastric cancer. *Surg Endosc* 2016;30:1920–9.

48. McNair AG, Whistance RN, Forsythe RO, et al. Synthesis and summary of patient-reported outcome measures to inform the development of a core outcome set in colorectal cancer surgery. *Colorectal Dis* 2015;17: O217–29.

49. Gerritsen A, Jacobs M, Henselmans I, et al. Developing a core set of patient-reported outcomes in pancreatic cancer: A Delphi survey. *Eur J Cancer* 2016;57:68–77.

50. Rees J, Hurt CN, Gollins S, et al. Patient-reported outcomes during and after definitive chemoradiotherapy for oesophageal cancer. *Br J Cancer* 2015;113:603–10.

51. Varagunam M, Hutchings A, Neuburger J, Black N. Impact on hospital performance of introducing routine patient reported outcome measures in surgery. *J Health Serv Res Policy* 2014;19:77–84.

52. Khuri SF, Daley J, Henderson WG. The comparative assessment and improvement of quality of surgical care in the Department of Veterans Affairs. *Arch Surg* 2002;137:20–7.

10

The American College of Surgeons National Surgical Quality Improvement Program: Standardised Data and Improved Outcomes

H.A. Pitt and E.P. Ceppa

ABSTRACT

Surgical quality is the modern form of assessment, for which surgeons gauge the results of surgical care in the 21st century. Reporting observed outcomes from surgical series has been replaced by process and procedure improvement to enhance surgical quality by maximising the benefits and diminishing postoperative morbidity. The American College of Surgeons National Surgical Quality Improvement Program (ACS–NSQIP) was at the forefront of the surgical quality evolution. This chapter describes the origin, the mechanisms and the improvements made in gastrointestinal surgery directly by ACS–NSQIP.

KEYWORDS

ACS–NSQIP, gastrointestinal surgery, ERAS, hepatopancreatobiliary surgery collaborative, procedure targeting, risk calculator, surgical quality

INTRODUCTION

The American College of Surgeons National Surgical Quality Improvement Program (ACS–NSQIP) is one of the most notable contributions to surgery in the 21st century. The ACS–NSQIP is the leading internationally validated, risk-adjusted, outcomes-based program to measure and improve the quality of surgical care in the United States within the private sector. The altered focus by surgeons on the quality of the outcomes, and not solely on the predictors of poor outcomes, was a fundamental change in course. The principle of trying to predict when a postoperative event would occur was no longer sufficient; instead, the idea of implementing a change to patient care before the occurrence of the sequence of events leading to a surgical complication was both novel and inspiring to a generation of surgeons. Thus, the aims of this chapter will be to describe the (1) inception of the ACS–NSQIP, (2) the construct of how it works and was validated, and (3) the noteworthy contributions by surgeons in improving the care of patients undergoing gastrointestinal surgery.

HISTORY

The nascent origins of the ACS–NSQIP began with the US federal government. The Veterans Health Administration (VHA), which provides medical services primarily to the veterans of the armed services, is the largest healthcare system in the United States in terms of number of patients, physicians, clinics and hospitals. During the 1980s, a widespread belief existed that the surgical care provided to the veterans was substandard relative to that provided to the private sector. In 1985, the US Congress passed Public Law 99–166, which mandated the VHA to report the following regarding veteran patients: (1) annual reports on surgical outcomes, (2) risk-adjusted expected outcomes, and (3) direct comparison of veteran patients' outcomes with national averages in the private sector.

The immediate result of this law was the realisation that no norms or national averages existed regarding surgical care anywhere. In order to address this gap in knowledge relative to the quality of surgical care delivered, the National Veterans Administration Surgical Risk Study Group (NVASRS) was created to fill this void with data. This study group existed between 1991 and 1993 and consisted of 44 veterans administration medical centres throughout the United States. This group benefitted from the strong computer informatics provided by the US Department of Defence to collect data in an automated fashion (something exceedingly novel and unique at that time). The study design included having a nurse at each medical centre to collect identical pre-, intra- and postoperative variables on every patient included in the study from the day of surgery until 30 days postoperatively. After 2 years of collecting data on 117,000 surgical patients undergoing various common surgical procedures across the surgical disciplines, risk models for 30-day morbidity and mortality were developed, which allowed for direct comparison of outcomes across the 44 participating hospitals.[1] An initial improvement was found via an 'observation' bias; however, further improvement in morbidity and mortality was found in the subsequent years. The validity of this method of collecting variables in a complete and prospective fashion was validated externally by a collective of three hospitals in the private sector (Emory University, University of Michigan, and University of Kentucky) in 1999. After 1 year of applying the identical methodology, improved surgical outcomes were seen in general and vascular surgical procedures.[2] Subsequently, 14 academic medical centres and four affiliated community hospitals confirmed that NSQIP was feasible in the private sector. As a result, the American College of Surgeons opened enrolment to all US hospitals in 2004. Currently, more than 700 hospitals in 11 countries participate in the ACS–NSQIP.

VALIDATION OF IMPACT ON MORBIDITY AND MORTALITY BY THE AMERICAN COLLEGE OF SURGEONS NATIONAL SURGICAL QUALITY IMPROVEMENT PROGRAM

The global effect of the ACS–NSQIP on hospitals has been assessed and reported previously to be beneficial on multiple levels. The most pertinent qualitative demonstration of the value of the ACS–NSQIP can be seen in the publication by Cohen et al, which assessed each participating ACS–NSQIP hospital's surgical outcomes over a period of time from 2006 to 2013.[3] The observed rate to expected rate (O/E) ratios were presented of individual participating hospitals, compared with oneself by year over the study time period. The trend consisted of a progressive, downward slope by year, demonstrating a gradual and sustained improvement in overall morbidity, mortality and surgical site infections (SSIs) over time.

Multiple varied quantitative reports exist that highlight the strength of quality improvement achieved through tracking outcomes with the ACS–NSQIP and changes in practice initiated by either individual hospitals or consortium of hospitals.[4] In fact, the reduction of postoperative morbidity, reported as O/E ratios over time, is a universally reported effect, as all types of NSQIP-participating hospitals (urban vs. rural, large vs. small and academic vs. private) have witnessed improvements, even after just a 3-year period of participation.[5] These reports established that the methodology was associated with improvement in surgical outcomes, even in heterogeneous practice environments. Multiple studies have described methods for reduction of SSIs, as reported through the ACS–NSQIP, with profound hospital cost savings as a result of fewer SSIs observed over study time periods.[6,7]

VARIABLES

The ACS–NSQIP collects 136 pre- and postoperative variables up to 30 days from the date of surgery. These variables fall into the following categories: (1) patient demographics, (2) comorbid conditions, (3) preoperative, (4) intraoperative, and (5) postoperative. A surgical clinical reviewer (SCR) abstracts all variables from the patient medical record; this role will be further described later in the chapter. The definition of each complication is strictly defined for each specific postoperative event (i.e., complication and morbidity); thus, no interpretation is made by the reviewer, highlighting the value of consistent data entry, irrespective of who is collecting the data from the medical record. Minimal year-to-year adjustments in the definitions have been made when the definitions were not precise, but these adjustments occurred only after a consensus to alter a definition was recorded by the leadership of the ACS–NSQIP. If an alteration ensues, a series of explanations of the changes is communicated via email, teleconference and/or oral presentations as part of the Annual National Conference. Once the variables are collected on all reported patients over a 6-month period (semiannual), a logistic regression analysis is performed to predict the risk of each recorded type of postoperative event after each surgical procedure. Then, risk adjustment is calculated, which is defined as the expected rate of postoperative events by weighing preoperative variables as a function of either a higher or lower rate of developing a postoperative event. Essentially, this process allows for calculating an expected rate for each postoperative event for all cases performed by a single hospital. An O/E ratio is determined for each variable by the hospital. The O/E ratios are then compared among all participating hospitals in the ACS–NSQIP that provide a ranking by deciles, with 1st decile being the best and 10th being the worst. This form of data reporting provides considerable motivation to each hospital to improve areas of poor performance by way of peer pressure.

OUTCOMES

Eight primary categories for postoperative events are (1) mortality, (2) morbidity, (3) wound occurrences, (4) respiratory occurrences, (5) urinary tract occurrences, (6) central nervous occurrences, (7) cardiac occurrences, and (8) other surgical occurrences (Table 10.1). The principal outcome is mortality, which is reported as either dead or alive at 30 days after the date of surgery. The rest of the primary outcomes tracked by the ACS–NSQIP are referred to as postoperative occurrences. Each patient

group is divided into categories as having zero, one, two, three, four or five or more total postoperative occurrences and is reported as a percentage of the total; the mean number of occurrences for the comparison groups is also provided. For the ACS–NSQIP, wound occurrences are divided into superficial SSIs, deep SSIs, organ/space SSIs and wound dehiscence (Table 10.2). These definitions are based on those developed by the Centers for Disease Control and Prevention. The ACS–NSQIP description for each has become the accepted definition, which other databases, retrospective studies and prospective trials use verbatim.

Pulmonary occurrences include pneumonia, prolonged intubation beyond 48 hours, pulmonary embolism and unplanned intubation. Urinary tract occurrences include acute renal failure, renal dysfunction and urinary tract infection (UTI). Central nervous system occurrences include cerebrovascular accident, coma for more than 24 hours and peripheral nerve injury. Cardiac occurrences include cardiac arrest with cardiopulmonary resuscitation and myocardial infarction. Other surgical occurrences that are not 'procedure-specific' include intra-/postoperative (up to 72 hours) transfusion, graft/flap/prosthesis failure,

Table 10.1 Routine postoperative occurrences

Category	Variable
Mortality	Death
Morbidity	Any complication Mean number of complications
Wound occurrences	Superficial SSI Deep SSI Organ/space SSI Wound dehiscence
Respiratory occurrences	Pneumonia Prolonged ventilation >48 hours postoperative Pulmonary embolism Unplanned intubation
Urinary tract occurrences	Acute renal failure Renal dysfunction Urinary tract infection
Central nervous occurrences	Cerebrovascular accident Coma >24 hours Peripheral nerve injury
Cardiac occurrences	Cardiac arrest with cardiopulmonary resuscitation Myocardial infarction
Other surgical occurrences	Transfusion (intraoperative or up to 72 hours postoperative) Graft/flap/prosthesis failure Deep vein thrombosis requiring treatment Sepsis Septic shock

Abbreviation: SSI, surgical site infection.

Table 10.2 The American College of Surgeons National Surgical Quality Improvement Program's definitions of surgical site infections

Wound occurrences

1. Superficial incisional surgical site infectionn (SSI): Superficial incisional SSI is an infection that occurs within 30 days after the operation, *and* infection involves only skin or subcutaneous tissue of the incision *and* at least *one* of the following:
- Purulent drainage, with or without laboratory confirmation, from the superficial incision.
- Organisms isolated from an aseptically obtained culture of fluid or tissue from the superficial incision.
- At least one of the following signs or symptoms of infection: pain or tenderness, localised swelling, redness or heat AND superficial incision is deliberately opened by the surgeon, unless incision is culture-negative.
- *Diagnosis of superficial incisional SSI by the surgeon or attending physician.*
- *Do not report the following conditions as SSI:*
  - Stitch abscess (minimal inflammation and discharge confined to the points of suture penetration).
  - Infected burn wound.
  - Incisional SSI that extends into the fascial and muscle layers (see **deep incisional SSI**).

2. Superficial incisional SSI—present at time of surgery (PATOS): If a 'Superficial incisional SSI' is noted as a postoperative outcome and an open wound, cellulitis (erythema, tenderness AND swelling) or wound infection was noted preoperatively or intraoperatively at the surgical site at the time of surgery, select 'YES'.
Guidance: If a superficial incisional SSI is assigned as a postoperative occurrence, only superficial incisional SSI PATOS can be assigned if the patient meets the criteria for superficial incisional PATOS (cannot assign deep or organ/space PATOS).

3. Deep incisional SSI: Deep incision SSI is an infection that occurs within 30 days after the operation and the infection appears to be related to the operation *and* infection involved deep soft tissues (e.g., fascial and muscle layers) of the incision *and* at least *one* of the following:
- Purulent drainage from the deep incision but not from the organ/space component of the surgical site.
- A deep incision spontaneously dehisces or is deliberately opened by a surgeon when the patient has at least one of the following signs or symptoms: fever (>38°C), localised pain or tenderness, unless site is culture-negative.
- An abscess or other evidence of infection involving the deep incision is found on direct examination, during reoperation or by histopathological or radiological examination.
- *Diagnosis of a deep incisional SSI by a surgeon or attending physician.*
Note:
- Report infection that involves both superficial and deep incision sites as deep incisional SSI.
- Report an organ/space SSI that drains through the incision as a deep incisional SSI.

4. Deep incisional SSI—PATOS: If a 'deep incisional SSI' is noted as a postoperative outcome, and an open wound, cellulitis (erythema, tenderness AND swelling) or infection was noted preoperatively or intraoperatively at the surgical site at the time of surgery, select 'YES'.
Guidance: If a deep incisional SSI is assigned as a postoperative occurrence, only deep incisional SSI PATOS can be assigned if the patient meets the criteria for deep incisional SSI PATOS (cannot assign superficial or organ/space PATOS).

5. Organ/space SSI: Organ/space SSI is an infection that occurs within 30 days after the operation and the infection appears to be related to the operation *and* the infection involves any part of the anatomy (e.g., organs and spaces), other than the incision, which was opened or manipulated during an operation *and* at least *one* of the following:
- Purulent drainage from a drain that is placed through a stab wound into the organ/space.
- Organisms isolated from an aseptically obtained culture of fluid or tissue in the organ/space.
- An abscess or other evidence of infection involving the organ/space that is found on direct examination, during reoperation or by histopathological or radiological examination.
- *Diagnosis of an organ/space SSI by a surgeon or attending physician.*
Note: Report an organ/space SSI that drains through the incision as a deep incisional SSI.

6. Organ/space SSI—PATOS: If an 'organ/space SSI' is noted as a postoperative outcome and an abscess or other evidence of infection involving the organ/space was noted preoperatively or intraoperatively at the surgical area at the time of surgery, select 'YES' for this variable (refer to the above **organ/space SSI** definition).
Guidance: if an organ/space SSI is assigned as a postoperative occurrence, only organ/space SSI PATOS can be assigned if the patient meets the criteria for organ/space SSI PATOS (cannot assign superficial or deep PATOS).

7. Wound disruption:
- **Abdominal site:** It refers primarily to loss of the integrity of fascial closure (or whatever closure was performed in the absence of fascial closure).
- **Other surgical sites:** There must be a total breakdown of the surgical closure, compromising the integrity of the procedure. Example: Tissue flap coverage where the surgical incisions, which were closed, have lost the integrity of closure. An ostomy with a small separation around it would NOT qualify.

deep vein thrombosis requiring therapy, sepsis and septic shock. Pertinent hospital discharge information, including death, discharge date and destination, index length of stay for more than 30 days, unplanned reoperation within 30 days and readmission events (<30 days, unplanned readmission, readmission related to principal procedure and primary cause of readmission), is also collected.

MECHANICS

The ACS–NSQIP variables are collected by a trained and certified SCR via a standardised process to maximise the accuracy of data collection. Various methods are used by the SCR to capture variables with abstracting data in real time from the medical record. Variables collected may be entered via a web-based software via the ACS–NSQIP encrypted website. Software exists for automatic populated data entry of some of the variables directly from the hospitals' electronic medical record. Internal controls inserted by the ACS for ascertaining and maintaining the quality of data collection performed by the SCR are present in various forms. These include web-based initial training, with subsequent completion of a certification examination annually, completion of training modules annually and Inter-Rater Reliability (IRR) audits.

The IRR audit is the most valued tool for assessment of data collection quality. Cases reviewed by an individual SCR are selected both at random and by intention. Cases selected by random are reviewed to assess if there was strict adherence to the sampling strategy for cases via review of the operative log and by intention are cases either with five or more higher-risk preoperative variables that were reported to not have suffered a complication or with two or less high-risk preoperative variables with a reported complication. A disagreement rate of less than 5% on the IRR audit is considered acceptable. If the disagreement rate is greater than 5%, IRR data are not provided in the next semiannual report and the SCR only resumes work after completing further education and training, followed by an additional IRR audit. For participating hospitals, the mean IRR is 1 to 2%.

Surgical procedures are sampled at a rate of 40 cases every 8 days. Thus, an ideal minimum number of cases collected annually for each program option is 1,680 cases. An ACS-validated sampling system called the '8-day cycle' is used to minimise bias in choosing cases for assessment. This sampling system divides the work year into 46 8-day cycles; 42 cycles are the minimum for participation in the ACS–NSQIP. The first 15 consecutive cases that meet the program's inclusion criteria within each 8-day cycle are selected, based on the program option's requirements. Each 8-day cycle begins on a different day of the week for each cycle to ensure that cases have an equal chance of being selected from each day of the week. Case selection and case mix are monitored by the program on a weekly basis to ensure that the sampling is appropriate. Exclusion criteria exist for cases and hospitals (Table 10.3).

Table 10.3 Exclusions

Case exclusion	
	Minor cases
	Patient age <18 years
	ASA score = 6 (brain-death organ donors)
	Any case involving hyperthermic intraperitoneal chemotherapy
	Any trauma patient
	Any transplant patient
	Case beyond three per 8-day cycle: 1. Inguinal herniorrhaphy 2. Breast lumpectomy 3. Laparoscopic cholecystectomy 4. Transurethral prostate/bladder resection
	Return to operating room of a prior NSQIP-captured case
	New case with a previously NSQIP-captured case within 30 days
Hospital exclusion	
	30-day follow-up rate <80%
	Interrater reliability audit disagreement rate >5%

Abbreviations: ASA, American Society of Anesthesiologists; NSQIP, National Surgical Quality Improvement Program.

PROCEDURE-TARGETED MODULE

An early criticism of the ACS–NSQIP was the collection of outcome variables on a large group of operations with very low morbidity and mortality. In response, the ACS–NSQIP decided to 'target' procedures with greater risk. In addition, risk adjustment focussing on the broad events leads to increased potential error because of the possible heterogeneity of reviewed cases. The ACS–NSQIP sought to augment the accuracy of risk adjustment by adding additional procedure-specific variables, in addition to the original 136 variables for a select number of high-risk procedures.[8] The original targeted procedures included colectomy, pancreatectomy, bariatric surgery, cholecystectomy and ventral hernia repair. Currently, 30 high-risk procedures are targeted across nine surgical specialties. We will highlight the procedures most pertinent to the gastrointestinal tract (Table 10.4).

Colectomy

Procedure-targeted variables for colectomy are numerous and detailed (Table 10.5). The additional preoperative variables include steroids/immunosuppression preoperatively, the use of an antibiotic and/or mechanical bowel preparation and preoperative chemotherapy. Indications for surgery (emergency vs. elective) and operative approach are new intraoperative variables. Surgical pathology variables are described as tumour size (T stage), nodal statuses (N stage), presence of metastasis and number of lymph nodes evaluations. Additional postoperative occurrences include anastomotic leak and prolonged 'nothing per os' or nasogastric tube use. Finally, the Enhanced Recovery After Surgery (ERAS) has a long list of pertinent additional variables included in Table 10.5.

Pancreatectomy

Pancreatectomy, generally considered a procedure with the most inherent risk, was ideally suited for a distinct procedure-targeted module. Thus, the module was created to provide great insight in some of the most pertinent variables that affect postoperative outcomes after pancreatectomy. Data are collected on pancreatoduodenectomy, distal pancreatectomy, total pancreatectomy, enucleation and ampullectomy. Twenty-four variables include (a) preoperative, (b) intraoperative, and (c) postoperative information (Table 10.5). Drain amylase data recorded include postoperative day 1, highest drain amylase between postoperative days 2 and 30, date of highest drain amylase and date of last pancreatic drain removal. Both pancreatic fistula and delayed gastric emptying are recorded as the most procedure-specific complications for pancreatectomy; percutaneous drainage within 30 days of surgery is recorded as the treatment of undrained symptomatic pancreatic fistula. Surgical pathology captured includes malignant versus benign tumour, TNM staging for malignant tumours and benign tumour size.

Hepatectomy

Similarly, hepatectomy is well suited for an independent procedure-targeted module because of the inherent grave risks of mortality and liver failure. Data are collected on major and partial hepatectomies. The novel postoperative variables (Table 10.5) include peak postoperative creatinine, total bilirubin and international normalised ratio (INR) (on or after postoperative day 5); postoperative drain bilirubin (on or after postoperative day 3) and date of last drain removal. Unique postoperative occurrences recorded include drain management, posthepatectomy liver failure, biliary fistula and the subsequent treatment with interventional radiology drainage and benign tumours. Surgical pathology is also captured for malignant tumours via TNM staging.

RISK CALCULATOR

As one of the most meaningful contributions made by the ACS–NSQIP, a web-based risk calculator, was to predict postoperative mortality and morbidity for individual patients being evaluated preoperatively. Only history and physical, not laboratory, data are entered into the risk calculator. The aim of a risk calculator is to provide precise, patient-specific risk to assist in shared surgical decision making and informed consent. The calculator combines 20 preoperative variables that are predictive of morbidity, with the planned surgical procedure listed by the Current Procedural Terminology code, to predict the risk of developing 15 distinct postoperative occurrences within 30 days of surgery. The 15 occurrences include serious complication, any complication, pneumonia, cardiac

Table 10.4 Gastrointestinal procedure targeted

Query 'NSQIP' + '...'	No. of citations	Time period
Oesophagectomy	17	2008–2016
Gastrectomy/bariatric surgery	31	2008–2016
Cholecystectomy	38	2008–2016
Pancreatectomy	36	2008–2016
Hepatectomy	33	2008–2016
Colectomy	108	2007–2016
Proctectomy	14	2008–2016

Table 10.5 Procedure-targeted variables

Colectomy	Pancreatectomy	Hepatectomy
Steroids/immunosuppression	Preoperative jaundice	Preoperative biliary stent
Mechanical bowel prep	Preoperative biliary stent	Preoperative chemotherapy
Oral antibiotic prep	Preoperative chemotherapy	Preoperative ablation
Chemotherapy within 90 days	Preoperative radiation therapy	Preoperative embolisation
Indication for surgery	Prophylactic antibiotics	History of hepatitis
Emergency surgery	Operative approach	Operative approach
Operative approach	Incision type	Liver texture
Pathology (TNM staging)	Pancreatic duct size	Concomitant resection
No. of lymph nodes harvested	Pancreatic gland texture	Intraoperative ablation
Anastomotic leak	Pancreatic anastomosis type	Drain placement
Prolonged NPO or NGT	Vascular resection	POD 3+ drain bilirubin
ERAS variables	Gastrointestinal reconstruction	Date of last drain removed
Preoperative counselling	Drains: number and location	Percutaneous drain placement
Clear liquids 3 hours preoperative	POD 1 drain amylase	Peak POD 5+ postoperative bilirubin
Epidural for open surgery	POD 2–30 highest drain amylase	Peak postoperative INR
Multimodal pain control	Date highest drain amylase	Postoperative creatinine
Normothermia in recovery	Date last drain removed	Biliary fistula
Goal-directed therapy	Pancreatic fistula	Posthepatectomy liver failure
Multimodal antiemetic prophylaxis	Delayed gastric emptying	Pathology (TNM staging)
Mobilisation, POD 0	Percutaneous drain placement	Benign tumour pathology
Clear liquids, POD 0	Drain type	Benign tumour size
Saline lock, POD 0	Pathology (TNM staging)	
Mobilisation, POD 1	Benign tumour pathology	
Solid diet, POD 1	Benign tumour size	
Foley removed by POD 1		
Mobilisation, POD 2		
Date return bowel function		
Date tolerating diet		
Date oral pain medication		

Abbreviations: INR, international normalised ratio; NGT, nasogastric tube; NPO, nil per os; POD, postoperative day.

complication, SSIs, UTIs, venous thromboembolism, renal failure, colonic ileus, colon anastomotic fistula, readmission, return to operating room, mortality, discharge to nursing/rehabilitation facility and predicted length of stay. In order to create the existing calculator, over 2.7 million ACS–NSQIP cases from 586 participating hospitals were reviewed between 2010 and 2014 to validate through linear regression models.[9]

The web link http://riskcalculator.facs.org/RiskCalculator/ provides access to the risk calculator free of charge. To navigate this site with ease, a disclaimer has to be acknowledged before use. The second page of the website consists of entry of the 20 preoperative variables plus the planned procedure (Figure 10.1). The third page of the website provides the summary report of the percentage chance of suffering each of the 15 postoperative occurrences included, based on the preoperative variables (Figure 10.2). The final page of the website allows for printing or emailing a copy of the results for documentation or record keeping (Figure 10.3).

PROCESS IMPROVEMENT IN GASTROINTESTINAL SURGERY

Many of the contributions within the ACS–NSQIP have occurred in surgery of the gastrointestinal tract. When performing literature searches using certain keywords such as 'NSQIP', in addition to any specific gastrointestinal surgery, the number of citations is impressive (Table 10.4). The cumulative effort has resulted in over 200 original

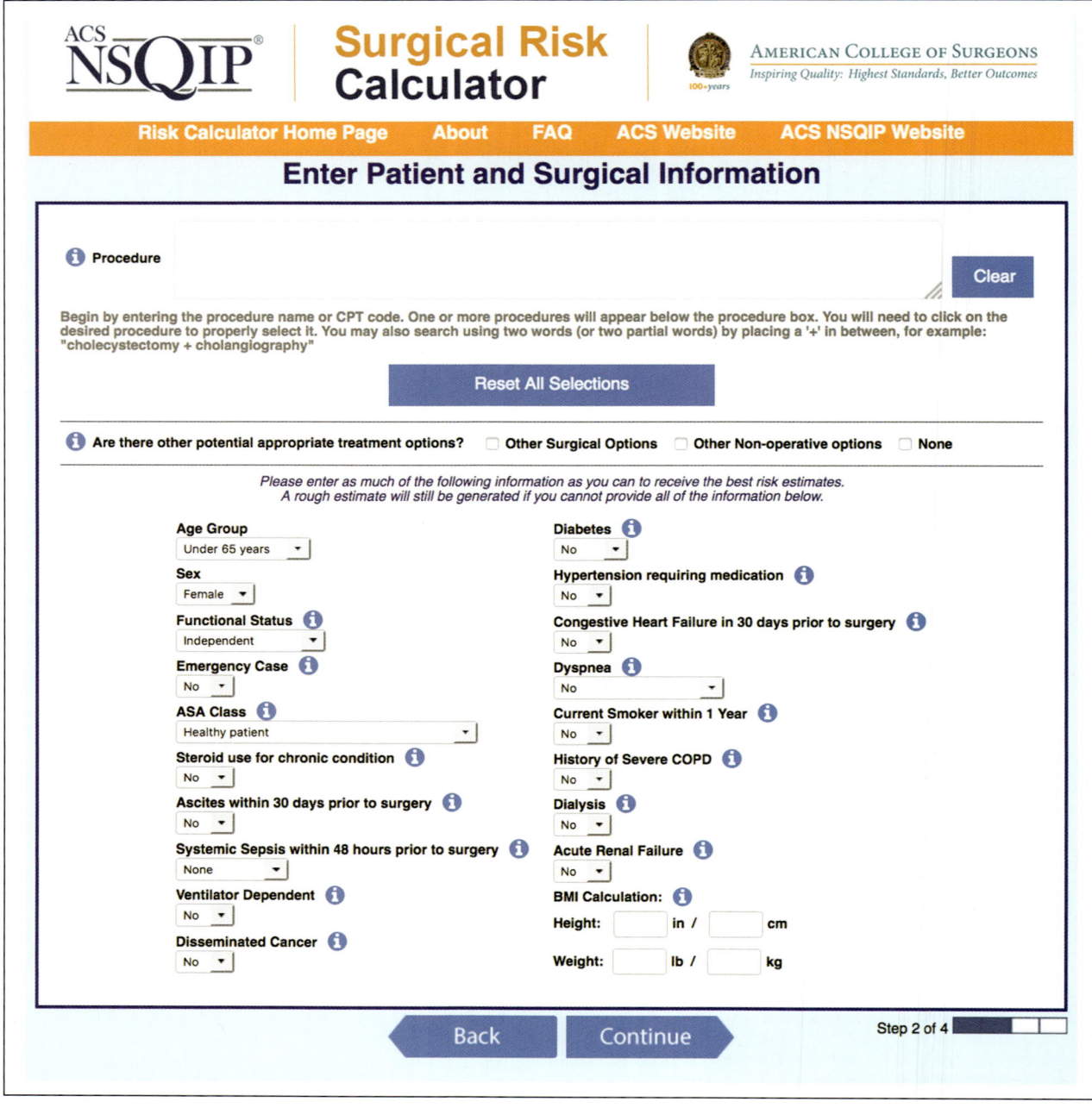

Figure 10.1 The American College of Surgeons National Surgical Quality Improvement Program's risk calculator 1.
Courtesy: Henry A. Pitt and Eugene P. Ceppa.

scientific publications focussed on the entire gastrointestinal track, ranging from oesophagectomy to proctectomy over a 10-year period. One of the purported assets of the ACS–NSQIP is the ability to compare trends in outcomes over time. An analysis of outcomes after major gastrointestinal surgical oncological procedures (oesophagectomy, gastrectomy, pancreatectomy, hepatectomy, colectomy and proctectomy) from 2005 to 2011 found that the overall complication rate decreased from 28 to 24% over this time period;

however, no change in mortality was witnessed.[10] This analysis suggests that improvements are possible with the structured format of the ACS–NSQIP data collection, strict definitions of postoperative events, the ability to monitor change over time and reporting that change occurred, with reporting of outcomes to directly surgeons.

The semiannual report consists of data demonstrating an institution's specific outcomes by each ACS–NSQIP postoperative event with the raw data as well as the

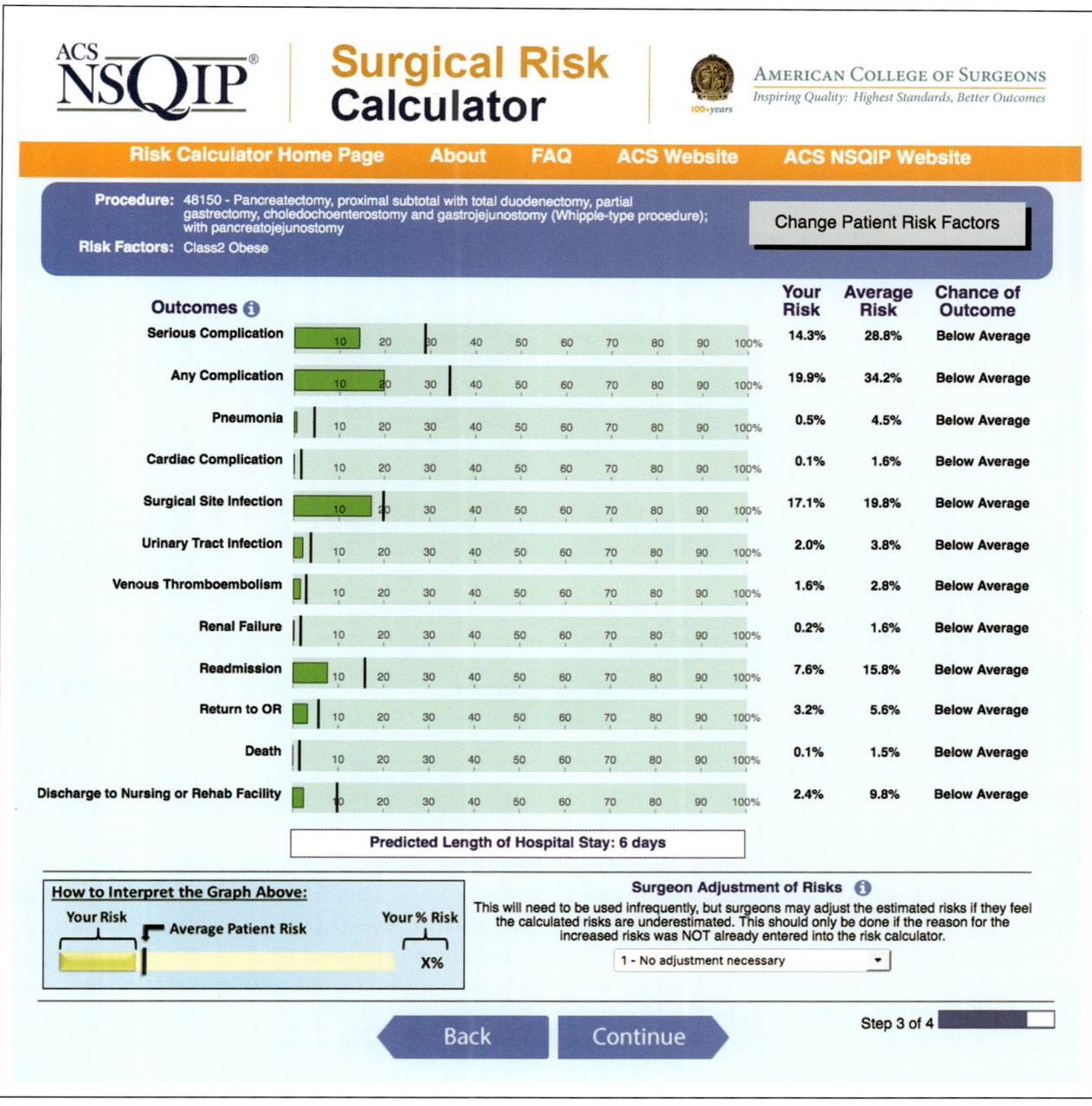

Figure 10.2 The American College of Surgeons National Surgical Quality Improvement Program's risk calculator 2.
Courtesy: Henry A. Pitt and Eugene P. Ceppa.

O/E and odds ratios, which account for preoperative risk adjustment to level the playing field for expected outcomes. Furthermore, decile scores (1st to 10th decile) are reported for the same categories; these perform a direct comparison by O/E and odds ratios, which indicate the institution's ranking among other participating hospitals as high performers (1st decile) or low performers (10th decile). The decile score provides an anonymous form of peer pressure for low-performing institutions to help guide

surgical leadership and hospital administration strategic planning for specific process improvement.

Oesophagectomy

The ACS–NSQIP has been critical in the analysis of predicting inpatient morbidity, prolonged length of stay and postdischarge morbidity after oesophagectomy. The reported rates of morbidity after oesophagectomy

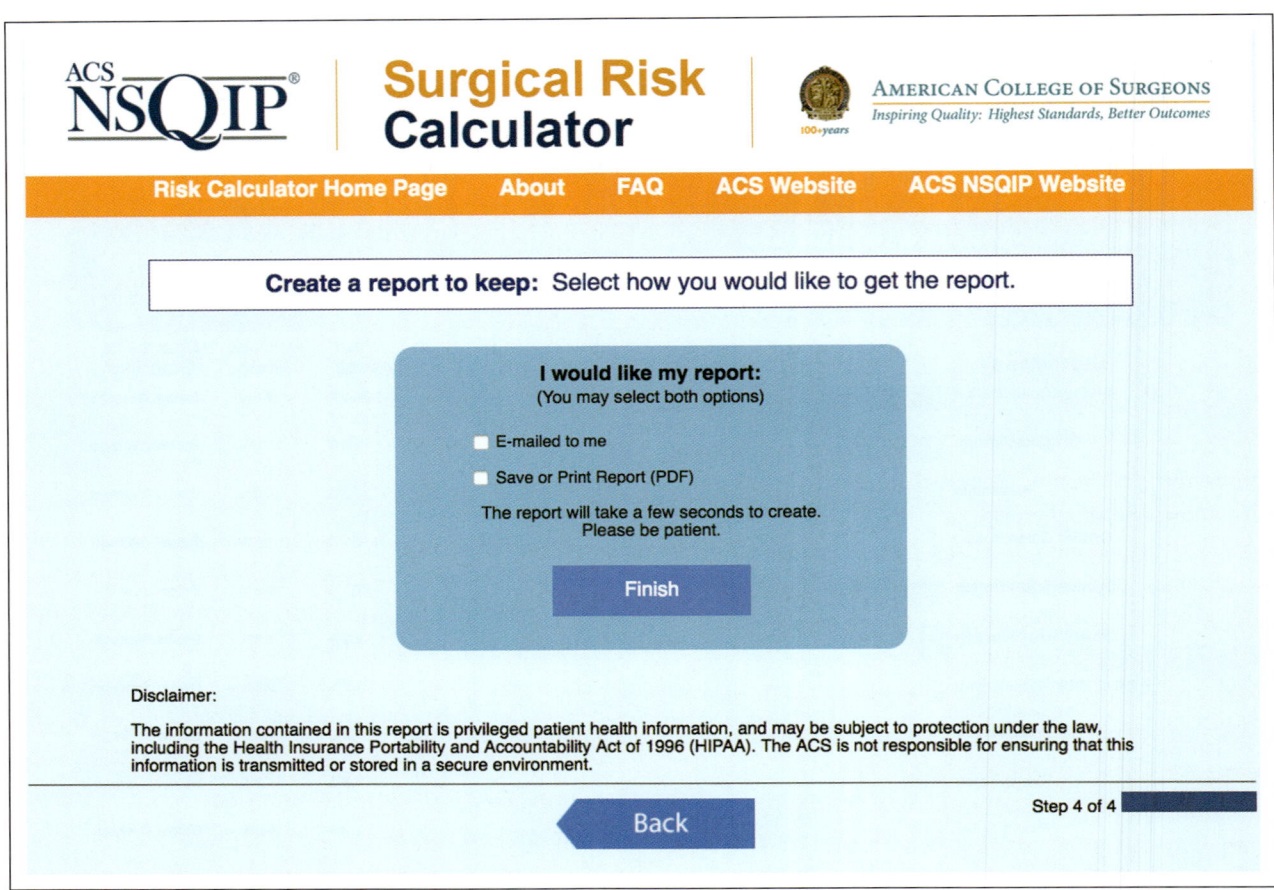

Figure 10.3   The American College of Surgeons National Surgical Quality Improvement Program's risk calculator 3.
Courtesy: Henry A. Pitt and Eugene P. Ceppa.

are 40 to 44%, depending on surgical approach.[11] The predictors for prolonged length of stay have been elucidated via the ACS–NSQIP with preoperative factors, such as emergency surgery and preoperative frailty, as well as postoperative events, such as prolonged mechanical ventilation, renal insufficiency and infectious events (pneumonia, organ site infection [OSI] and UTI).[12] The incidence of respiratory complications after oesophagectomy is 23%; a NSQIP multivariate analysis found that advanced age, alcohol consumption and tobacco consumption were predictive of respiratory morbidity, which ultimately leads to an increased mortality, increased morbidity, return to operating room and increased length of stay.[13] Although there are only 20% of patients with postoperative events after discharge, an analysis performed by Chen et al found that 50% of the severe morbidity and the majority of readmissions and returns to the operative theatre occurred in this small subset of patients.[14] This study highlighted that the patients without morbidity after discharge had a 4-day shorter length of stay (11 days)

from the index admission than those with an inpatient postoperative event (15 days). Potential room for improvement would be to delay discharge in higher-risk individuals to avoid the majority of the severe complications and return to operating theatre in such a small subgroup of patients.

Finally, oesophageal surgery is a multispecialty procedure crossing the diaphragmatic boundary between general surgeons and thoracic surgeons. Currently, the ACS–NSQIP for assessment of oesophagectomy has no procedure-specific variables, and as such, a recent study by Allen et al compared the sampling strategy of the ACS–NSQIP with the complete reporting through the Society of Thoracic Surgery database.[15] The authors compared institution-specific data to match postoperative outcomes and found that the ACS–NSQIP underreported postoperative events and overestimated mortality. This report highlights the lack of oesophagectomy-specific variables that contributes to this disparity and relative importance of evolving procedure-specific variables.

Gastrectomy/Bariatric Procedures

The impact of the ACS–NSQIP is evident when reviewing the literature regarding bariatric surgery. Many series in print use the large number of primary bariatric procedures reviewed at participating hospitals, which were not obtainable previously. The most pertinent and meaningful manuscript includes the modern comparison of the 'gold standard' laparoscopic Roux-en-Y gastric bypass, with the 'newcomer' laparoscopic sleeve gastrectomy. Young et al reported in their analysis that sleeve gastrectomy has a lower risk of morbidity, with equivalent mortality as gastric bypass.[16] Furthermore, complex questions have been addressed such as the risk profile of a band to sleeve gastrectomy conversion.[17] A metabolic and bariatric surgery collaborative of more than 700 hospitals has been developed in recent years. A unique aspect of this collaborative is that program accreditation is also involved.[18] Formal gastrectomy outcomes for malignancies such as gastrointestinal stromal tumours (GISTs) and gastric adenocarcinoma have also been reported in descriptive fashion via the ACS–NSQIP, identifying predictors of increased morbidity.[11,19]

Colectomy

Enhanced recovery after surgery has gained great notoriety and application based on an evidence-based approach. Thiele et al in 2015 published that, with the application of ERAS, all the modifiable factors, including length of stay, were improved.[20] Keenan et al took ERAS one step further and implemented an SSI bundle after introduction of ERAS and found a decrease in SSI from 16 to 6%; length of stay was also shortened and resulted in a savings of $8,000 per patient.[21] Moreover, Yuen et al reported that ERAS, when looked at from the quality aspect, found that both adverse events and readmission rates after colectomy were as safe in patients discharged early (postoperative day 2) as were seen for standard discharge with ERAS.[22]

Anastomotic leak is the principal source of major morbidity after colectomy. A recent study by Tevis et al demonstrated that failure to rescue was six times (6% vs. 1%) more likely in patients with an anastomotic leak after colectomy than those without a leak.[23] This study using NSQIP data and colectomy-specific variables confirmed what many had presumed to be true but did not have supporting data. Another study compared outcomes after laparoscopic and open colectomy and found anastomotic leak rates to be 2.8% and 4.5%, respectively. The associated mortality with a leak was 5.7% in those with a leak versus 0.6% in those without a leak.[24] Recent

studies have also demonstrated that the combination of mechanical and oral antibiotic bowel preparations results in fewer SSIs and anastomotic leaks.

Frailty has become an important variable preoperatively to predict postoperative events. Amrock et al performed an analysis of lower gastrointestinal procedures via NSQIP and applied multiple preoperative frailty indices.[25] The authors found that multiple models were predictive of morbidity in preoperative frail patients. The value of the ACS–NSQIP was the ability to provide complete data on each patient in order to validate the usefulness of these suggested indices of frailty, leading to morbidity.

Pancreatectomy

Pancreatectomy remains the area of gastrointestinal surgery that still carries the greatest associated morbidity. In turn, the heavy focus on attempting to predict causes of morbidity and to curtail negative outcomes is evident in the scientific literature. The ACS–NSQIP has been used to better understand the nature of clinical variables associated with outcomes primarily because of its ability to review a large number of patients across multiple institutions.

Pancreatic fistula remains the principal source of morbidity for patients undergoing pancreatectomy, and very little information has been identified to reduce fistula rates. Much has been published in defining predisposing factors, but little information is available to help prevent pancreatic fistulae. Pancreatic duct size and gland texture have historically been the principal factors to affect the rate of pancreatic fistula occurrence. Recent descriptions using the ACS–NSQIP have been reported to attempt to document methods towards decreasing fistula rates after either distal pancreatectomy or pancreatoduodenectomy. Stump closure method has been described to affect the fistula rate after distal pancreatectomy, with various conflicting reports. A contemporary comparison of sutured, stapled and saline-linked radiofrequency ablation of the pancreatic stump by using ACS–NSQIP data found that each method carried a 25% pancreatic fistula rate.[26] Recently, ACS–NSQIP data have been used to develop and validate risk-prediction models for pancreatic fistula. Procedure-specific data from pancreatoduodenectomy was used to augment the previously validated ACS–NSQIP risk calculator to enhance the predictive value of pancreatic fistula.[27] The authors found that their model accurately outperformed the ACS–NSQIP risk calculator alone; an improved prediction of 90-day mortality, major morbidity and reoperation was seen as a result.

Further evidence of ACS–NSQIP data serving as the platform to affect change in surgical quality was seen in a

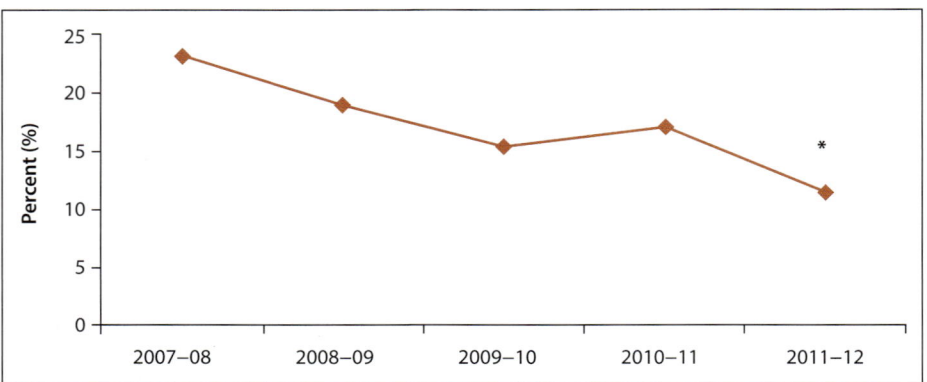

Figure 10.4   Readmissions over time. *p < 0.05 compared with that in 2007–08.

Reprinted with permission from: Ceppa EP, Pitt HA, Nakeeb A, et al. Reducing readmissions after pancreatectomy: limiting complications and coordinating the care continuum. *J Am Coll Surg* 2015;221:708–16.

recent publication focussed on reducing readmissions after pancreatectomy. Readmission rates after pancreatectomy remain the highest among all general surgical procedures, typically at 19% for the largest published series.[28] The ACS–NSQIP was used to track changes after a stepwise implementation of change year to year over a 5-year period (Figure 10.4). In this report, a multimodal approach was utilised to improving multiple processes, including lowering morbidity, establishing preferred sites for disposition, improving provider communication and relying on a 'discharge coach' to coordinate all details before discharge. The readmission rate steadily decreased year by year, starting at 23% and ending at 11.5%, without any change in case mix, complexity, length of stay or surgical volume.

Two studies, in particular, highlighted the limitations that ACS–NSQIP traditional variables were not sufficient in patients undergoing pancreatectomy because of the lack of tracking of delayed gastric emptying and underreporting of pancreatic fistula.[29,30] The glaring deficiency of tracking delayed gastric emptying was particularly notable, but, more importantly, organ space infection was not an adequate surrogate for pancreatic fistula. Evolution of the ACS–NSQIP has augmented the data available in two major ways over the last 5 years, including procedure-targeting and pancreatectomy-specific variables for the ACS–NSQIP. Procedure targeting allowed individual hospitals to track up to 100% of patients undergoing a specific procedure and not rely solely on the sampling strategy per cycle. Furthermore, pancreatectomy-specific variables are now present as an option following the ACS–NSQIP National Pancreatectomy Demonstration Project. A hepatopancreatobiliary (HPB)-specific NSQIP was first suggested in 2009[31] and gained momentum after the American College of Surgeons and the Americas Hepato-

Pancreato-Biliary Association supported the importance of conducting this pilot program. The Pancreatectomy Demonstration Project was conceived at 43 institutions to monitor these deficiencies, and pancreatectomy-specific variables were added to the traditional NSQIP variables. During 2011 to 2012, 43 high-volume pancreatectomy centres in North America using NSQIP collected additional variables (such as pancreatic fistula, delayed gastric emptying, surgical pathology and others; Table 10.5) as a pilot program to determine feasibility and completeness of the novel data. Multiple manuscripts have been published as a result of this pilot program.[32–34] The success of this program led to the incorporation of HPB-specific ACS–NSQIP, available to all participating hospitals in 2014.

Hepatectomy

Another area for which morbidity and mortality are significant preoperative considerations when choosing an operation and providing a recommendation for a patient is hepatectomy. A large number of factors are considered in planning a hepatectomy, with the goal to successfully remove the malignant tumour or symptomatic benign tumour while avoiding both biliary fistula and posthepatectomy liver failure. For many years, single-institution retrospective series provided data to guide care practices. However, recently, with the advent of hepatectomy-specific variables as a part of the ACS–NSQIP, a large, descriptive series presented data elucidating current trends of nearly 2500 hepatectomies in North America over a 12-month period.[35] Pertinent data included that 11% of patients had chronic viral hepatitis and 9% were cirrhotic at the time of resection. Perioperative therapies included neoadjuvant chemotherapy (25%), portal vein embolisation (2%) and intra-arterial chemotherapy (0.9%). Procedure approach found that 22.5% of cases were performed laparoscopically. Furthermore, data were present to distinguish minor versus major hepatectomy in specific postoperative events such as biliary fistula (4.9% vs. 10.9%) and liver insufficiency (1.9% vs. 6.9%). These types of data were not available previously and thus, have shed new light on current practices and possibilities for future improvements.

SURGICAL SITE INFECTION IN THE GASTROINTESTINAL TRACT

Process improvement in decreasing SSI has been accelerated throughout procedures of the gastrointestinal tract, as a result of the ACS–NSQIP. After documentation of SSIs after common procedures with the ACS–NSQIP, multiple strategies have been applied, and changes over time have been tracked with the ACS–NSQIP. Previously reported at a single institution, the ACS–NSQIP was used to determine what the baseline SSI rates were for hepatic, pancreatic and complex biliary surgical procedures. An SSI bundle that streamlined best practices across multiple surgeons, accounting for pre-, intra- and postoperative factors was created. The initial SSI rate observed was 24%, which decreased significantly to 16% after a 2-year period of application of the SSI bundle and observation using the ACS–NSQIP.[7] A similar study applied best practices in the form of both an SSI bundle and ERAS and decreased the SSI rate associated with colectomies from 18 to 5% and concomitantly reduced the length of stay.[36] Of note, the HPB Collaborative is planning a randomised controlled trial across the optimal prophylactic antibiotic for patients undergoing pancreatoduodenectomy.

HEPATO-PANCREATO-BILIARY COLLABORATIVE

In 2016, the ACS–NSQIP HPB Collaborative included 82 institutions in four countries. Both pancreatectomy and hepatectomy can be targeted, and almost all participating institutions target both. The HPB Collaborative was formed in October 2014, and the initial focus has been to reduce SSIs, which account for two-thirds of the morbidity after pancreatectomy and hepatectomy. Strategies have included a series of webinars to recommended best practices as well as symposia at the ACS–NSQIP National Conference. Next steps include initiation of the randomised controlled trial and more education regarding best practices to prevent pancreatic fistulas and bile leaks.

CONCLUSIONS

The contribution of the ACS–NSQIP to improvement of surgical care is an impactful innovation in surgery. Not only are the standardisation of care and clear evidence of improved outcomes observed as a result of the ACS–NSQIP novel, but also the ability to affect change of many patients, and not just one patient at a time, across multiple surgical disciplines leaves the most resounding impression. The full potential and global impact of the ACS–NSQIP have not been fully achieved and will continue to evolve at the direction of surgeons attempting to improve outcomes for patient benefit.

REFERENCES

1. Daley J, Khuri SF, Henderson W, et al. Risk adjustment of the postoperative morbidity rate for the comparative assessment of the quality of surgical care: results of the National Veterans Affairs Surgical Risk Study. *J Am Coll Surg* 1997;185:328–40.
2. Fink AS, Campbell DA Jr, Mentzer RM Jr, et al. The National Surgical Quality Improvement Program in non-veterans administration hospitals: initial demonstration of feasibility. *Ann Surg* 2002;236:344–53; discussion 353–4.
3. Cohen ME, Liu Y, Ko CY, et al. Improved surgical outcomes for ACS NSQIP hospitals over time: evaluation of hospital cohorts with up to 8 years of participation. *Ann Surg* 2016;263:267–73.
4. Guillamondegui OD, Gunter OL, Hines L, et al. Using the National Surgical Quality Improvement Program and the Tennessee Surgical Quality Collaborative to improve surgical outcomes. *J Am Coll Surg* 2012;214:709–14; discussion 714–6.
5. Hall BL, Hamilton BH, Richards K, Bilimoria KY, Cohen ME, Ko CY. Does surgical quality improve in the American College of Surgeons National Surgical Quality Improvement Program. *Ann Surg* 2009;250:363–76.
6. Ingraham AM, Richards KE, Hall BL, Ko CY. Quality improvement in surgery: the American College of Surgeons National Surgical Quality Improvement Program approach. *Adv Surg* 2010;44:251–67.
7. Ceppa EP, Pitt HA, House MG, et al. Reducing surgical site infections in hepatopancreatobiliary surgery. *HPB (Oxford)* 2013;15:384–91.
8. Dimick JB, Osborne NH, Hall BL, Ko CY, Birkmeyer JD. Risk adjustment for comparing hospital quality with surgery: how many variables are needed? *J Am Coll Surg* 2010;210:503–8.
9. Bilimoria KY, Liu Y, Paruch JL, Zhou L, Kmiecik TE, Ko CY, Cohen ME. Development and evaluation of the universal ACS NSQIP surgical risk calculator: a decision aid and informed consent tool for patients and surgeons. *J Am Coll Surg* 2013;217:833–42.
10. Lucas DJ, Pawlik TM. Quality improvement in gastrointestinal surgical oncology with American College

of Surgeons National Surgical Quality Improvement Program. *Surgery* 2014;155:593–601.

11. Papenfuss WA, Kukar M, Attwood K, et al. Transhiatal versus transthoracic esophagectomy for esophageal cancer: a 2005–2011 NSQIP comparison of modern multicenter results. *J Surg Oncol* 2014;110:298–301.

12. Park KU, Rubinfeld I, Hodari A, Hammoud Z. Prolonged Length of stay after esophageal resection: identifying drivers of increased length of stay using the NSQIP database. *J Am Coll Surg* 2016;223:286–90.

13. Molena D, Mungo B, Stem M, Lidor AO. Incidence and risk factors for respiratory complications in patients undergoing esophagectomy for malignancy: a NSQIP analysis. *Semin Thorac Cardiovasc Surg* 2014;26:287–94.

14. Chen SY, Molena D, Stem M, Mungo B, Lidor AO. Post-discharge complications after esophagectomy account for high readmission rates. *World J Gastroenterol* 2016;22:5246–53.

15. Allen MS, Blackmon S, Nichols FC, Cassivi SD, Shen KR, Wigle DA. Comparison of two national databases for general thoracic surgery. *Ann Thorac Surg* 2015;100:1155–61; discussion 1161–2.

16. Young MT, Gebhart A, Phelan MJ, Nguyen NT. Use and outcomes of laparoscopic sleeve gastrectomy vs laparoscopic gastric bypass: analysis of the American College of Surgeons NSQIP. *J Am Coll Surg* 2015;220:880–5.

17. Aminian A, Shoar S, Khorgami Z, Augustin T, Schauer PR, Brethauer SA. Safety of one-step conversion of gastric band to sleeve: a comparative analysis of ACS–NSQIP data. *Surg Obes Relat Dis* 2015;11:386–91.

18. Berger ER, Clements RH, Morton JM, et al. The impact of different surgical techniques on outcomes in laparoscopic sleeve gastrectomies: the first report from the Metabolic and Bariatric Surgery Accreditation and Quality Improvement Program (MBSAQIP). *Ann Surg* 2016;264:464–73.

19. Bellorin O, Kundel A, Ni M, Litong D. Surgical management of gastrointestinal stromal tumors of the stomach. *JSLS* 2014;18:46–9.

20. Thiele RH, Rea KM, Turrentine FE, et al. Standardization of care: impact of an enhanced recovery protocol on length of stay, complications, and direct costs after colorectal surgery. *J Am Coll Surg* 2015;220:430–43.

21. Keenan JE, Speicher PJ, Nussbaum DP, et al. Improving outcomes in colorectal surgery by sequential implementation of multiple standardized care programs. *J Am Coll Surg* 2015;221:404–14.

22. Yuen A, Elnahas A, Azin A, Okrainec A, Jackson TD, Quereshy FA. Is expedited early discharge following elective surgery for colorectal cancer safe? An analysis of short-term outcomes. *Surg Endosc* 2016;30:3904–9.

23. Tevis SE, Carchman EH, Foley EF, Heise CP, Harms BA, Kennedy GD. does anastomotic leak contribute to high failure-to-rescue rates? *Ann Surg* 2016;263:1148–51.

24. Murray AC, Chiuzan C, Kiran RP. Risk of anastomotic leak after laparoscopic versus open colectomy. *Surg Endosc* 2016;30:5275–82.

25. Amrock LG, Neuman MD, Lin HM, Deiner S. Can routine preoperative data predict adverse outcomes in the elderly? Development and validation of a simple risk model incorporating a chart-derived frailty score. *J Am Coll Surg* 2014;219:684–94.

26. Ceppa EP, McCurdy RM, Becerra DC, et al. Does pancreatic stump closure method influence distal pancreatectomy outcomes? *J Gastrointest Surg* 2015;19:1449–56.

27. McMillan MT, Allegrini V, Asbun HJ, et al. Incorporation of procedure-specific risk into the ACS–NSQIP surgical risk calculator improves the prediction of morbidity and mortality after pancreatoduodenectomy. *Ann Surg* 2016 [Epub ahead of print].

28. Ceppa EP, Pitt HA, Nakeeb A, et al. Reducing readmissions after pancreatectomy: limiting complications and coordinating the care continuum. *J Am Coll Surg* 2015;221:708–16.

29. Epelboym I, Gawlas I, Lee JA, Schrope B, Chabot JA, Allendorf JD. Limitations of ACS–NSQIP in reporting complications for patients undergoing pancreatectomy: underscoring the need for a pancreas-specific module. *World J Surg* 2014;38:1461–7.

30. Parikh JA, Beane JD, Kilbane EM, Milgrom DP, Pitt HA. Is American College of Surgeons NSQIP organ space infection a surrogate for pancreatic fistula? *Am Coll Surg* 2014;219:1111–6.

31. Pitt HA, Kilbane M, Strasberg SM, et al. ACS–NSQIP has the potential to create an HPB-NSQIP option. *HPB (Oxford)* 2009;11:405–13.

32. Beane JD, House MG, Pitt SC, et al. Distal pancreatectomy with celiac axis resection: what are the added risks? *HPB (Oxford)* 2015;17:777–84.

33. Cooper AB, Parmar AD, Riall TS, et al. Does the use of neoadjuvant therapy for pancreatic adenocarcinoma increase postoperative morbidity and mortality rates? *J Gastrointest Surg* 2015;19:80–6; discussion 86–7.

34. Tamirisa NP, Parmar AD, Vargas GMet al. Relative contributions of complications and failure to rescue on mortality in older patients undergoing pancreatectomy. *Ann Surg* 2016;263:385–91.

35. Spolverato G, Ejaz A, Kim Y, et al. Patterns of care among patients undergoing hepatic resection: a query of the National Surgical Quality Improvement Program-targeted hepatectomy database. *J Surg Res* 2015;196:221–8.

36. DeHaas D, Aufderheide S, Gano J, Weigandt J, Ries J, Faust B. Colorectal surgical site infection reduction strategies. *Am J Surg* 2016;212:175–7.

11

The Definition and Grading of Complications by Severity

K. Slankamenac, R.D. Staiger and P.-A. Clavien

ABSTRACT

Standardised methodologies are the keystone for reliable assessment and reporting of postoperative complications. Several intra- and postoperative complication grading systems were developed over time. This chapter summarises and compares the most influential complication classifications and indexes throughout the past 25 years, with an additional small outlook into the future of outcome research.

KEYWORDS

Clavien-Dindo classification, Comprehensive Complication Index, Accordion classification, Postoperative Morbidity Index, CLASSIC

INTRODUCTION

In the past, mortality was the most important measure to assess poor outcomes after surgical procedures, as it occurred frequently after many interventions.[1–3] Based on improvements in indications, surgical skills and technical advances, these mortality rates after surgeries have decreased continuously within the last 30 years. Therefore, the focus has shifted towards other endpoints, such as nonlethal complications, overall morbidity and quality of life.[4,5] The focus on morbidity and surgical complications led to various nonstandardised definitions.[6–11] Terms such as major, moderate, and minor complications were used in an inconsistent and subjective manner.[12,13] As a consequence, morbidity was reported in wide ranges, for example, after Whipple's procedure, it ranges between 18 and 72%.[14–16] This inconsistency has hampered conclusive comparisons among most studies. Therefore, reliable outcome reporting is essential to assess and compare the quality of surgical procedures.[17] Next to the problem of various definitions, most studies failed to report on the severity of complications.[18] Less than 20% of published articles reporting on postoperative complications provide some information about their severity.[18] In addition, many studies focussed only on surgery-specific complications, which were considered relevant to the surgeon. Events of lesser severity have been ignored and were therefore massively underreported.[9] The absence of a standardised methodology to assess, report and grade postoperative complications has hampered quality outcome research.[19] Being aware of these shortcomings, several research groups have developed different classification systems to grade the severity of postoperative complications in a standardised matter.[1,7,20–23]

VARIOUS DEFINITIONS OF ONE SPECIFIC COMPLICATION

In surgical research, short-term postoperative outcomes are the most frequently analysed endpoints. Mostly postoperative complications and mortality but also operating time and length of hospital stay are used to compare different surgical approaches. However, the quality of reporting complications has remained poor; there was no consistency or clarity in this documentation. In addition, the concern of disclosure of complications was also hindering an honest presentation.[24]

In 2001, Martin et al analysed prospective and large retrospective studies targeting three surgical procedures: hepatectomy, pancreatectomy and oesophagectomy.[18] The articles were assessed on the basis of 10 criteria, including, amongst others, the definition of complications, application of severity grading and identification of risk factors. They found that only one-third of the studies met at least 7 out of the 10 criteria.[18] They traced this great variability back to the lack of definitions for specific complications.[18]

Around the same time, Bruce et al analysed the quality of definitions, measurements and reporting of postoperative complications in the literature.[25] They selected four commonly reported complications or 'surgical adverse events' (surgical wound infection, anastomotic leak, deep vein thrombosis and surgical mortality) with different frequencies of occurrence.[25] The authors found significant inconsistencies in the quality of the reporting of those complications.[25] For example, in most studies, the definition of wound infection was missing. The description ranged from 'presence of pus' to criteria that distinguished levels of surgical would infections.[25] These authors concluded that this divergence prevented conclusive comparisons of complications over time as well as between institutions.[25] These analyses illustrated the need for a standardised complications grading system, preferably applicable to all surgical fields.

The Clavien-Dindo Classification

In 1992, Clavien et al proposed a new definition for what constitutes a negative outcome.[26] They designed a novel system to grade complications by severity based on the resources and invasiveness of treatments needed to correct the complications.[26] They differentiated three types of negative outcome after a surgical procedure[26]: complication, failure to cure and sequel.

Twelve years later, in 2004, Dindo et al published a revised version of this system based on the experience gained in several international surgical centres.[8] The revised classification was based on the same principle, while increasing the weight of life-threatening complications involving organ failure and eliminating subjective criteria such as length of hospital stay.[8] This revision, called the 'Clavien-Dindo classification', grades postoperative complications from grade I to V according to the need for treatment (such as additional medical, interventional, surgical or intensive care treatment)[8] (Table 11.1). Furthermore, Clavien and his coauthors emphasised patients' perspectives by adding postoperative persistent disability in the classification system, indicating the

Table 11.1 The Clavien-Dindo classification system adjusted and simplified from the original classification from 2004

Grade	Definition
Grade I	Any deviation from the normal postoperative course
Grade II	Pharmacological treatment
Grade III • IIIa • IIIb	Surgical treatment • Under local anaesthesia • Under general anaesthesia
Grade IV • IVa • IVb	Life-threatening complication, therapy on the intensive care unit • Single organ failure • Multiorgan failure
Grade V	Death

Adapted from: Dindo D, Demartines N, Clavien PA. Classification of surgical complications: a new proposal with evaluation in a cohort of 6336 patients and results of a survey. *Ann Surg* 2004;240:205–13.

need for further follow-up. The applicability, simplicity and interobserver variability of this classification system were tested and validated successfully on a large cohort concomitantly in the same study.[8]

In 2009, Clavien et al published the 5-year experience with the Clavien-Dindo classification by performing a systematic review of the literature and a survey in seven international centres that were routinely using the system.[11] In the survey, scenarios of so-far controversially graded severity of complications were discussed and ranked among an international panel of experts. It resulted in a high degree of agreement (89%) in complications' ranking.[11] In addition, the experts recommended avoiding terms such as 'minor' and 'major' to grade the severity of postoperative complications to prevent further subjectivity and imprecision in complication reporting.[11] This critical 5-year evaluation of the Clavien-Dindo classification showed that the system was well and widely established and did not need any further substantial adjustments.[11] Today, it is a valid measure for surgical quality assessment in databases, clinical practice and in morbidity and mortality (M&M) conferences. The Clavien-Dindo classification has been cited in more than 7000 studies from various surgical fields since 2004,[11,27–31] and the 5-year evaluation counts about 2000 citations to this day.[32–37]

Some Applications of the Clavien-Dindo Classification

The Clavien-Dindo classification has been used in various specialisations of medicine: general surgery,[16] gastroenterology/hepatology,[27,29,38] urology,[30,32,33] nephrology,[31] orthopaedic surgery[39] and transplant surgery.[40] To mention all subspecialisations and studies using this classification would go beyond the scope of this chapter; therefore, we will only present a small selection of studies and grade the postoperative complications according to this classification.

In 2006, surgeons from the Johns Hopkins Hospital applied the Clavien-Dindo classification system to their cohort of patients undergoing Whipple's procedures as one of the first research groups. They successfully showed that the use of the classification system facilitated analyses of incidence and severity of specific complications.

In 2010, Dindo et al investigated the reliability of residents in tracking complications after surgery according to the standardised Clavien-Dindo classification system.[17] They showed that residents failed to assess 80% of the complications.[17] However, regarding assessment of the complications, residents correctly graded 97% of the cases.[17] In addition, a survey in 108 European surgical centres released that in 80% of the participating centres, residents assessed the postoperative complications and were responsible for a correct reporting.[17] Despite the simplicity of the Clavien-Dindo classification, the assessment and reporting of postoperative complications are unreliable if performed by residents.[17] Therefore, it is of importance that a negative outcome is completely assessed and correctly graded by a trained data manager, so that reliable results can be used for interpretation and comparison.

A research group from Sydney reviewed the relevant urological literature from 2010 to 2012 for the incidence of reporting of postoperative complications according to the Clavien Dindo classification.[41] Almost 90% of published urological articles used the Clavien-Dindo classification for grading of negative outcomes.[41] They also presented an increased use of the classification from 21.4% in 2010 to 50.2% in 2012.[41] The European Association of Urology recommended in their guidelines from 2012 to assess and report postoperative complications after urological procedures according to the Clavien-Dindo classification.[32,33]

The lack of consensus on how to evaluate surgical complications was also an important point of discussion in the specialisation of transplant surgery.[40] The American Transplant Society applied the classification in their database for living-related liver transplantation in 2006.[42]

Mentula and Leppäniemi showed that the classification may also be applied for patients undergoing emergency surgery, both for acute and for life-threatening situations.[43]

This produces a new area of application, since the system was developed based on patients after an elective abdominal surgery. Nevertheless, the preoperative organ dysfunction status must be known; for example, a colon ischaemia may cause single- or multiorgan failure, and therefore, postoperative organ failures may not be classified as surgical complications but rather as sequela. If the organ failure was present before surgery, the authors recommended not to classify this as a complication, since the patient's condition remains unchanged.[43] A worsening of the organ dysfunction was considered a grade IV complication, and if the organ failure resulted in death, it was considered grade V.[43] For those reasons, the authors recommended risk stratification for patients' comorbidities, preoperative organ dysfunctions and the type of surgery.[43]

Modifications of the Clavien-Dindo Classification System

Although the 5-year evaluation stated that 'changes, unless clearly justified, are unwarranted, since they may only lead to confusion and inconsistencies in reporting outcome',[11] several modifications and adjustments of the classification system exist in the surgical literature.[18,44]

A group of orthopaedic surgeons from New York, United States, modified the Clavien-Dindo classification by eliminating the difference between grades IIIa and IIIb and between grades IVa and IVb.[39] According to the authors, the adapted classification system showed high interrater and intrarater reliabilities and facilitated the standardisation of complication reporting in orthopaedic surgery.[39]

The Comprehensive Complication Index

Nowadays, many surgical studies are reporting only the most severe postoperative complications, whereas complications of lower severities are usually ignored.[45] Despite the fact that the Clavien-Dindo classification system is widely used, it does not assess the 'overall' burden of postoperative complications of a surgical procedure[8,11,22] It is still not possible to simply add up complications to provide a value for the 'overall' morbidity after surgical or interventional procedures. To bridge this shortcoming, our group initiated a series of studies to develop an index that reflects all postoperative complications and their severities in a continuous scale from 0 (no complication) to 100 (death). This new metric was called the Comprehensive Complication Index (CCI).[23,46,47]

The development of the CCI was based on the Clavien-Dindo classification, adopting methods from operation-risk-index analysis in marketing research.[48–50] They designed a formula that considers any combination of complications, including the ones of lower severity. The CCI was calculated as the sum of all complications, which were weighted for their severity.[23]

This new index was internally and externally validated from several perspectives, that is, from the perspective of patients, nurses and doctors.[23,47] The validity of the CCI is supported by the negative correlation with the postoperative health status, assessed by the EQ-5D™.[23,51] The external validation demonstrated the superiority of the CCI over traditionally reported morbidity endpoints.[47] By the CCI, a cumulative overall morbidity may be presented at various times after surgery, typically at discharge, 3 months after surgery and 12 months after surgery. Another important finding was that the required sample size in trials using the CCI as a primary endpoint was significantly lower than that for other traditional endpoints.[47]

The CCI is currently being increasingly used in international databases as an outcome measure for overall morbidity. In the Oslo-CoMet trial, this index was used as an endpoint to investigate the outcome after laparoscopic versus open liver resection for colorectal liver metastases.[52]

The Accordion Severity Grading System

In 2009, Strasberg et al introduced the Accordion Severity Grading System.[22] The authors wished for a more flexible complication classification system, which could be adapted for the grading of postoperative complications of small versus major procedures. They evaluated published studies that have used the classification system reported in 1992.[26] The concept of the Accordion Classification is to adjust the grading system by expanding to the spectrum of complications of a complex procedure, for example, oesophageal or pancreatic resection and, alternatively, by tightening for studies with a small range of severe complications.[26]

The Accordion Classification includes four levels, using self-explanatory terms rather than grades.[22] The levels range from mild, moderate and severe complications to the fourth level,[22] death (Table 11.2). In the expanded version, the third level 'severe complications' is divided into three subcategories: 'invasive procedures without general anaesthesia', 'operation under general anaesthesia' and 'organ system failure' (Table 11.3). The applicability of the Accordion System was tested on an international board of experts that led to a revision of the classification by its authors.[53] Those changes affected only the expanded version of the Accordion Classification; single organ failure was added to severe complications subcategory

Table 11.2 The Accordion severity classification of postoperative complications: contracted classification

	Grade	Definition
1	Mild complication	Requires minor invasive procedures that can be done at bedside. Examples: Urinary catheter, drainage of wound infections and physiotherapy. Allowed drugs: Antipyretics, analgesics, antiemetics, diuretics and electrolytes.
2	Moderate complication	Requires pharmacological treatment Examples: Antibiotics, blood transfusion and parenteral nutrition
3	Severe complication	Complications requiring endoscopic, interventional radiological procedures, reoperations or those with organ failure
4	Death	Postoperative death

Adapted from: Strasberg SM, Linehan DC, Hawkins WG. The accordion severity grading system of surgical complications. *Ann Surg* 2009;250:177–86.

'operations under general anaesthesia' and 'operations under general anaesthesia' were joined to 'organ system failure'.[53]

Regarding the use of the Accordion Classification, gynaecologists used it on debulking surgeries in patients with ovarian cancer,[54] abdominal surgeons predicted the short-term outcome after right colectomy[55] or used it to classify complications after gastrectomy[56] and orthopaedic surgeons used it to assess carpal tunnel surgery.[57] On the other hand, assessment of complications of living-donor operations and of the transplanted organ could not be well captured by this classification.[22,58]

Modifications of the Accordion Severity Grading System

Some authors found that the Accordion System needed adjustments to be clinically relevant.[59] It was criticised for the absence of a definition regarding the length of the postoperative period and for the formal division into mild, moderate and severe, which seems to differ from the subjective perception of practicing surgeons.[59] In addition, the categorisation of grades 1 to 3 into 'minor complications' and grades 4 to 6 into 'major complications'

Table 11.3 The Accordion severity classification of postoperative complications: expanded classification

	Grade	Definition
1	Mild complication	Requires minor invasive procedures that can be done at bedside. Examples: Urinary catheter, drainage of wound infections, physiotherapy. Allowed drugs: Antipyretics, analgesics, antiemetics, diuretics and electrolytes.
2	Moderate complication	Requires pharmacological treatment Examples: Antibiotics, blood transfusion and parenteral nutrition
3	Severe: Invasive procedure without general anaesthesia	Requires management by an endoscopic, interventional procedure or reoperation, without general anaesthesia
4	Severe: Operation under general anaesthesia	Requires intervention/ operation under general anaesthesia
5	Severe: Organ system failure	Any type of organ system failure
6	Death	Postoperative death

Adapted from: Strasberg SM, Linehan DC, Hawkins WG. The accordion severity grading system of surgical complications. *Ann Surg* 2009;250:177–86.

was considered necessary because of the frequent use of this grading system by researchers and surgeons.

The Accordion Classification, however, has not gained wide acceptance. It is mostly used in Northern America,[60,61] in combination with the American College of Surgeons National Surgical Quality Improvement Program (ACS–NSQIP), a nationwide program in the United States that collects preoperative through 30-day postoperative data on randomly assigned patients. The goal of the NSQIP is to mirror the postoperative complications of each clinic to improve the quality of their surgery.[62,63]

The Postoperative Morbidity Index

Building on the Accordion Grading System, Strasberg and Hall developed the Postoperative Morbidity Index (PMI) to quantify complications.[64] To achieve this, they used the ACS–NSQIP complication data collection to investigate laparoscopic colectomy, appendectomy, hepatectomy, pancreatoduodenectomy and inguinal hernia repair.[64] The complications were rated with the extended Accordion System, but only the highest-graded event was used for this study.[64] The calculation of the PMI was done by grading each complication and then weighting each of them by a numerical weight previously calculated for each of the six Accordion grades.[64] Internal validation was performed, and they concluded that the PMI was a practical tool to demonstrate trends in decline or improvement of outcomes over time.[64] Beilan et al showed in an external validation of urological procedures that the PMI lacks of an individual risk adjustment by considering only the most severe complication.[65] In addition, the PMI failed to provide accurate information for patients with more than one complication.[65]

GRADING OF INTRAOPERATIVE COMPLICATIONS BY SEVERITY

Oslo Classification of Intraoperative Unfavourable Incidents

In 2005, Satava published a simple grading system to assess intraoperative complications (referred to as 'error') during surgery.[66] Grade I was defined as an error without consequence for the patient or a 'near miss'. Grade II was an error with immediate identification and correction, also referred to as 'recovery'. Grade III was defined as an error that stays unrecognised during the surgery and leads to significant consequences postoperatively for the patient. This system was initially developed to grade complications occurring during a surgical simulator training of laparoscopic interventions, with the goal of evaluating the development of surgical skills of trainees.[66] The Oslo classification system has been used in a few studies to grade intraoperative unexpected or negative incidents.[67,68]

Definition and Classification of Intraoperative Complications (CLASSIC)

Rosenthal et al, in 2015, published a new approach to define and classify intraoperative complications.[69] Those authors performed a pilot study evaluating the practicability and interrater agreement of this new Definition and Classification of Intraoperative Complications (CLASSIC) system.[69] The CLASSIC relates to any event occurring between skin incision and closure and should be rated directly after surgery.[69] Any event during the index surgery must be assessed, regardless of whether it is surgery- or anaesthesia-related.[69]

Complications that occurred after skin closure are recommended to be captured by the Clavien-Dindo classification system for postoperative complications.[69]

The CLASSIC was defined in four grades, ranging from I to IV[69]: grade 0 means that there is no deviation from the ideal intraoperative course. Grade I is defined as any deviation from the ideal intraoperative course, without the need for additional treatment or intervention. Grade II is identical to grade I, with demand of additional treatment or intervention to correct the incident. A grade II complication is not life-threatening and does not lead to permanent disability, in contrast to a grade III complication, which is considered life-threatening and/or leads to permanent disability. Grade IV represents any deviation from the ideal intraoperative course, with death of the patient as a consequence. The CLASSIC is developed and defined very alike the Clavien-Dindo classification and has demonstrated practicability as well as a good interrater agreement.[69] This simple classification still needs to be externally validated to show its advantages, practicability and establishment.

DISCUSSION

Many authors have called for the need of a standardised grading system for postoperative complications.[18,25] In today's connected world, where data and knowledge exchange is nearly limitless, uniform standards are essential for interpreting and comparing published data. Recognising these shortcomings, Clavien and Strasberg were pioneers of the outcome research by presenting their postoperative complication grading system in 1992.[26] Since then, significant progress has been made in improving this system. This initial study opened the door for a structural standardisation in postoperative complication grading by keeping individually advanced scores simple and practicable. Postoperative complications of every intervention in any surgical field could be captured by this principle of grading complications.

Despite several attempts of suggesting modifications to the initial proposal,[8,22] only the Clavien-Dindo classification system and, to a lesser degree, the Accordion Severity Grading System have established themselves as reliable and practical tools in outcome research.[8,22]

Differences Between the Clavien-Dindo Classification and the Accordion Severity Grading System

Dindo et al defined the complication grade IV as life-threatening complications requiring intensive care unit (ICU) management.[8] This grade is divided into single organ failure (grade IVa) and multiorgan failure (grade IVb).[8] Strasberg et al desisted from attributing the ICU admission and used organ system failure as the criterion for severe complications level 5.[22] Single or multiorgan failure was primarily not distinguished, but was implemented in a revised version.[22]

For complications with permanent disabilities, the Clavien-Dindo classification uses the suffix 'd'.[8] The authors of the Accordion System consider the division into 'complication leading to permanent disability', which is somewhat subjective.[22] An acute renal failure would be listed as a complication level 5. The authors believe that, for example, patients progressing to chronic renal failure are not given enough weight with this grading. They also introduced the term 'sequel of complications' separately,[22] which has not been adopted so far by others.

These grading systems served as a basis for the development of further complication grading systems. The CLASSIC, for example, was established analogous to the Clavien-Dindo classification and thus logically recommend using the Clavien-Dindo classification for postoperative complications.[70]

Advantages and Disadvantages of the Two Grading Systems

Clavien-Dindo Classification

Some clinicians criticise the clear underweight of permanent disabilities in this classification, arguing that the significance of such a complication is vast for each patient due to durability of impairment.[22] For example, a postoperative stroke is classified as grade IVa. However, unlike a transient renal failure (also grade IVa), the remaining decrease of life quality can be severe. To enable the classifications' use in operative medical fields with naturally more frequent permanent disabilities (e.g., neurosurgery and head and neck surgery), the Clavien-Dindo classification would need to level out this shortcoming.

Accordion Severity Grading System

The external validation of the grading system showed an inconsistency in the expanded version on the level of severe complications; this led to the revised Accordion System.[22] Owing to its new combination of organ failure and interventions needed, the grading system left its original path of simplicity. The attempt to improve the grading system led to confusion by the added specifications.

Differences Between the Comparison Comprehensive Complication Index and the Postoperative Morbidity Index

The CCI and the PMI share the same basic idea behind their development. The authors wanted to develop a metric system to accurately quantify the postoperative complications and give more credit to the weight of their severity. The main difference between those indexes is that the PMI integrates solely the most severe complication, meaning that multiple complications in one patient were ignored. The CCI, in contrast, takes all complications of a patient into account.

The authors of the PMI pointed out the lack of risk adjustment of their index.[64] They express the need for a comprehensive risk-adjusted modelling when assessing the impact of procedure-specific complications.[64] The PMI was developed on complication weighting of surgeons, whereas patients' opinions and estimates were ignored.

The CCI not only included all postoperative complications and their respective severities, but also estimates were gathered from both patients' and doctors' perspectives. The CCI may longitudinally measure the morbidity over time and may therefore become the needed standardised outcome parameter for longitudinal measurement of morbidity. It fulfils its primary goal of assessing the quality of surgery as a standardised outcome measure in surgical trials and other interventional fields of medicine. The authors also intended to facilitate decision making for patients regarding hospital choice and surgical alternatives. It may also serve as a tool for benchmarking and public health decisions.[71]

Although the CCI was developed on a broad spectrum of patients undergoing a variety of major and minor general surgical procedures, it is necessary to calibrate the weights used for the CCI and to test it in other specialised fields such as cardiac surgery, gynaecology and neurosurgery.

CONCLUSIONS

Standardised complication reporting systems were an important development for outcome research in the past decade. The Clavien-Dindo and the Accordion systems were enhanced by the CCI and the PMI. They led to a better and more comprehensive reporting of postoperative complications, so that data are correctly and consistently assessed and comparability between studies is possible, accurate and valid. With the CCI, trends of postoperative morbidity can be traced today.

In the future, this index may also serve as a tool for benchmarking surgical outcomes. Public health decisions, such as the issuing of surgical licensure, health insurance's financial coverage, and maybe even a patient's hospital choice, could be strongly influenced by such benchmarks.

The resolving of the insufficiently regulated grading of permanent disabilities should also be approached by the scientific field of outcome research.

FINANCIAL SUPPORT

PROSPER fellowship by the Swiss National Foundation (SNF 32333B_131633 and SNF 3233B_151049) to KS, Research Grant from the Olga Mayenfish Foundation to RDS and a grant from the Liver and Gastrointestinal Disease (LGID) Foundation to PAC.

REFERENCES

1. Clavien PA, Sanabria JR, Mentha G, et al. Recent results of elective open cholecystectomy in a North American and a European center. Comparison of complications and risk factors. *Ann Surg* 1992;216:618–26.
2. Pearse R, Moreno RP, Bauer P, et al. Mortality after surgery in Europe - authors' reply. *Lancet* 2013;381:370–1.
3. Vonlanthen R, Clavien PA. What factors affect mortality after surgery? *Lancet* 2012;380:1034–6.
4. Brennan MF, Radzyner M, Rubin DM. Outcome-more than just operative mortality. *J Surg Oncol* 2009;99: 470–7.
5. Finks JF, Osborne NH, Birkmeyer JD. Trends in hospital volume and operative mortality for high-risk surgery. *N Engl J Med* 2011;364:2128–37.
6. Feldman L, Barkun J, Barkun A, Sampalis J, Rosenberg L. Measuring postoperative complications in general surgery patients using an outcomes-based-strategy: comparison with complications presented at morbidity and mortality rounds. *Surgery* 1997;122:711–9.
7. Pomposelli JJ, Gupta SK, Zacharoulis DC, Landa R, Miller A, Nanda R. Surgical complication outcome (SCOUT) score: a new method to evaluate quality of care in vascular surgery. *J Vasc Surg* 1997;25:1007–14; discussion 1014–5.
8. Dindo D, Demartines N, Clavien PA. Classification of surgical complications: a new proposal with evaluation in a cohort of 6336 patients and results of a survey. *Ann Surg* 2004;240:205–13.
9. Strasberg SM, Linehan DC, Clavien PA, Barkun JS. Proposal for definition and severity, grading of pancreatic anastomosis failure and pancreatic occlusion failure. *Surgery* 2007;141:420–6.
10. Sugawara Y, Tamura S, Makuuchi M. Systematic grading of surgical complications in live liver donors. *Liver Transplant* 2007;13:781–2.

11. Clavien PA1, Barkun J, de Oliveira ML, et al. The Clavien-Dindo classification of surgical complications: five-year experience. *Ann Surg* 2009;250:187–96.

12. Gumbs AA, Grès P, Madureira FA, Gayet B. Laparoscopic vs. open resection of noninvasive intraductal pancreatic mucinous neoplasms. *J Gastrointest Surg* 2008;12:707–12.

13. Beck-Schimmer B, Breitenstein S, Urech S, et al. A randomized controlled trial on pharmacological preconditioning in liver surgery using a volatile anesthetic. *Ann Surg* 2008;248:909–18.

14. Trede M, Schwall G, Saeger HD. Survival after pancreatoduodenectomy. 118 consecutive resections without an operative mortality. *Ann Surg* 1990;211:447–58.

15. Seiler CA, Wagner M, Sadowski C, Kulli C, Büchler MW. Randomized prospective trial of pylorus-preserving vs. classic duodenopancreatectomy (Whipple procedure): initial clinical results. *J Gastrointest Surg* 2000;4:443–52.

16. DeOliveira ML, Winter JM, Schafer M, et al. Assessment of complications after pancreatic surgery: a novel grading system applied to 633 patients undergoing pancreaticoduodenectomy. *Ann Surg* 2006;244:931–9.

17. Dindo D1, Hahnloser D, Clavien PA. Quality assessment in surgery riding a lame horse. *Ann Surg* 2010;251:766–71.

18. Martin RC 2nd, Brennan MF, Jaques DP. Quality of complication reporting in the surgical literature. *Ann Surg* 2002;235:803–13.

19. Horton R. Surgical research or comic opera: questions, but few answers. *Lancet* 1996;347:984–5.

20. Pillai SB, van Rij AM, Williams S, Thomson IA, Putterill MJ, Greig S. Complexity- and risk-adjusted model for measuring surgical outcome. *Br J Surg* 1999;86:1567–72.

21. Veen MR, Lardenoye JW, Kastelein GW, Breslau PJ. Recording and classification of complications in a surgical practice. *Eur J Surg* 1999;165:421–4; discussion 425.

22. Strasberg SM, Linehan DC, Hawkins WG. The accordion severity grading system of surgical complications. *Ann Surg* 2009;250:177–86.

23. Slankamenac K, Graf R, Barkun J, Puhan MA, Clavien PA. The comprehensive complication index: a novel continuous scale to measure surgical morbidity. *Ann Surg* 2013;258:1–7.

24. Johnston L. *Healthcare Administration: Concept, Methodologies, Tools and Applications, Medical Information Science Reference*. Hershey, PA: IGI Global; 2015. ISBN: 978-1-4666-6339-8).

25. Bruce J, Russell EM, Mollison J, Krukowski ZH. The measurement and monitoring of surgical adverse events. *Health Technol Assess* 2001;5:1–194.

26. Clavien PA, Sanabria JR, Strasberg SM. Proposed classification of complications of surgery with examples of utility in cholecystectomy. *Surgery* 1992;111:518–26.

27. Chun YS, Vauthey JN, Ribero D, et al. Systemic chemotherapy and two-stage hepatectomy for extensive bilateral colorectal liver metastases: perioperative safety and survival. *J Gastrointest Surg* 2007;11:1498–504; discussion 1504–5.

28. Haynes AB, Weiser TG, Berry WR, et al. A surgical safety checklist to reduce morbidity and mortality in a global population. *N Engl J Med* 2009;360:491–9.

29. McKay A, Sutherland FR, Bathe OF, Dixon E. Morbidity and mortality following multivisceral resections in complex hepatic and pancreatic surgery. *J Gastrointest Surg* 2008;12:86–90.

30. Permpongkosol S, Link RE, Su LM, et al. Complications of 2,775 urological laparoscopic procedures: 1993 to 2005. *J Urol* 2007;177:580–5.

31. Sundaram CP, Martin GL, Guise A, et al. Complications after a 5-year experience with laparoscopic donor nephrectomy: the Indiana University experience. *Surg Endosc* 2007;21:724–8.

32. Mitropoulos D, Artibani W, Graefen M, et al. Reporting and Grading of Complications After Urologic Surgical Procedures: An ad hoc EAU Guidelines Panel Assessment and Recommendations. *Eur Urol* 2012;61:341–9.

33. Mitropoulos D, Artibani W, Graefen M, et al. Reporting and grading of complications after urologic surgical procedures: an ad hoc EAU Guidelines Panel assessment and recommendations. *Actas Urologicas Espanolas* 2013;37:1–11.

34. Oberkofler CE, Rickenbacher A, Raptis DA, et al. A multicenter randomized clinical trial of primary anastomosis or Hartmann's procedure for perforated left colonic diverticulitis with purulent or fecal peritonitis. *Ann Surg* 2012;256:819–27.

35. Seely AJ1, Ivanovic J, Threader J, et al. Systematic classification of morbidity and mortality after thoracic surgery. *Ann Thorac Surg* 2010;90:936–42.

36. Vonlanthen R, Slankamenac K, Breitenstein S, et al. The impact of complications on costs of major surgical procedures a cost analysis of 1200 patients. *Ann Surg* 2011;54:907–13.

37. Petrowsky H, Breitenstein S, Slankamenac K, et al. Effects of pentoxifylline on liver regeneration a double-blinded, randomized, controlled trial in 101 patients undergoing major liver resection. *Ann Surg* 2010;252:813–21.

38. de Santibañes E, Ardiles V, Gadano A, Palavecino M, Pekolj J, Ciardullo M. Liver transplantation: the last measure in the treatment of bile duct injuries. *World J Surg* 2008;32:1714–21.

39. Sink EL, Leunig M, Zaltz I, et al. Reliability of a complication classification system for orthopaedic surgery. *Clin Orthop Relat Res* 2012;470:2220–6.

40. Tamura S, Sugawara Y, Kaneko J, et al. Systematic grading of surgical complications in live liver donors according to Clavien's system. *Transplant Int* 2006;19:982–7.

41. Yoon PD, Chalasani V, Woo HH. Use of Clavien-Dindo classification in reporting and grading complications after

urological surgical procedures: analysis of 2010 to 2012. *J Urol* 2013;190:1271–4.

42. Barr ML, Belghiti J, Villamil FG, et al. A report of the Vancouver forum on the care of the live organ donor: lung, liver, pancreas, and intestine data and medical guidelines. *Transplantation* 2006;81:1373–85.

43. Mentula PJ, Leppäniemi AK. Applicability of the Clavien-Dindo classification to emergency surgical procedures: a retrospective cohort study on 444 consecutive patients. *Patient Saf Surg* 2014;8:31.

44. Kooby DA, Fong Y, Suriawinata A, et al. Impact of steatosis on perioperative outcome following hepatic resection. *J Gastrointest Surg* 2003;7:1034–43.

45. Strasberg SM, Linehan DC, Clavien PA, Barkun JS. Proposal for definition and severity grading of pancreatic anastomosis failure and pancreatic occlusion failure. *Surgery* 2007;141:420–6.

46. Slankamenac K, Graf R, Puhan MA, Clavein PA. Perception of surgical complications among patients, nurses and physicians: a prospective cross-sectional survey. *Patient Saf Surg* 2011;5:30.

47. Slankamenac K, Nederlof N, Pessaux P, et al. The comprehensive complication index a novel and more sensitive endpoint for assessing outcome and reducing sample size in randomized controlled trials. *Ann Surg* 2014;260:757–63.

48. Meffert H, Bolz J. Internationales Marketing-Management. 1998; S. 76 ff.

49. Welge MK, Holtbrügge D. Internationales Management: Theorien, Funktionen, Fallstudien. 2006; S. 100 ff.

50. Zentes J, Swoboda B, Schramm-Klein H. Internationales Marketing. 2006; S. 180.

51. EuroQol Group. EuroQol—a new facility for the measurement of health-related quality of life. *Health Policy* 1990;16:199–208.

52. Fretland AA, Kazaryan AM, Bjornbeth BA, et al. Open versus laparoscopic liver resection for colorectal liver metastases (the Oslo-CoMet study): study protocol for a randomized controlled trial. *Trials* 2015;16:73.

53. Porembka MR, Hall BL, Hirbe M, Strasberg SM. Quantitative weighting of postoperative complications based on the accordion severity grading system: demonstration of potential impact using the American College of Surgeons National Surgical Quality Improvement Program. *J Am Coll Surg* 2010;210:286–98.

54. Kumar A, Janco JM, Mariani A, et al. Risk-prediction model of severe postoperative complications after primary debulking surgery for advanced ovarian cancer. *Gynecol Oncol* 2016;140:15–21.

55. Klos CL, Safar B, Hunt SR, et al. Accordion complication grading predicts short-term outcome after right colectomy. *J Surg Res* 2014;190:510–6.

56. Jung MR, Park YK, Seon JW, Kim KY, Cheong O, Ryu SY. Definition and classification of complications of gastrectomy for gastric cancer based on the accordion severity grading system. *World J Surg* 2012;36:2400–11.

57. Noszczyk BH, Nowak M, Krześniak N. Use of the Accordion Severity Grading System for negative outcomes of carpal tunnel syndrome. *J Plast Reconstr Aesthet Surg* 2013;66:1123–30.

58. Chan EG, Bianco V 3rd, Richards T, et al. The ripple effect of a complication in lung transplantation: Evidence for increased long-term survival risk. *J Thorac Cardiovasc Surg* 2016;151:1171–9.

59. Kazaryan AM, Rosok BI, Edwin B. Morbidity assessment in surgery: refinement proposal based on a concept of perioperative adverse events. *ISRN Surg* 2013;2013:625093.

60. Kim YW, Yoon HM, Yun YH, et al. Long-term outcomes of laparoscopy-assisted distal gastrectomy for early gastric cancer: result of a randomized controlled trial (COACT 0301). *Surg Endosc* 2013;27:4267–76.

61. Agadzhanov VG, Shulutko AM, Kazaryan AM. Minilaparotomy for treatment of choledocholithiasis. *J Visc Surg* 2013;150:129–35.

62. Vollmer CM Jr, Lewis RS, Hall BL, et al. Establishing a quantitative benchmark for morbidity in pancreatoduodenectomy using ACS–NSQIP, the Accordion Severity Grading System, and the Postoperative Morbidity Index. *Ann Surg* 2015;261:527–36.

63. Reddy S, Contreras CM, Singletary B, et al. Timed stair climbing is the single strongest predictor of perioperative complications in patients undergoing abdominal surgery. *J Am Coll Surg* 2016;222:559–66.

64. Strasberg SM, Hall BL. Postoperative morbidity index: a quantitative measure of severity of postoperative complications. *J Am Coll Surg* 2011;213:616–26.

65. Beilan J, Strakosha R, Palacios DA, Rosser CJ. The postoperative morbidity index: a quantitative weighing of postoperative complications applied to urological procedures. *BMC Urology* 2014;14:1.

66. Satava RM. Identification and reduction of surgical error using simulation. *Minim Invasive Ther Allied Technol* 2005;14:257–61.

67. McClusky DA 3rd, Smith CD. Design and development of a surgical skills simulation curriculum. *World J Surg* 2008;32:171–81.

68. Rassweiler JJ, Teber D, Frede T. Complications of laparoscopic pyeloplasty. *World J Urol.* 2008;26:539–47.

69. Rosenthal R, Hoffmann H, Clavien PA, Bucher HC, Dell-Kuster S. Definition and Classification of Intraoperative Complications (CLASSIC): Delphi Study and pilot evaluation. *World J Surg.* 2015;39:1663–71.

70. Kazaryan AM, Marangos IP, Røsok B, et al. Laparoscopic resection of colorectal liver metastases surgical and long-term oncologic outcome. *Ann Surg* 2010;252:1005–12.

71. Rössler F, Sapisochin G, Song G, et al. Defining benchmarks for major liver surgery—a multicenter analysis of 5202 living liver donors. *Ann Surg* 2016;264:492–500.

12

The Impact of a Checklist on Complications after Surgery

J.F. Lange

ABSTRACT

Incidents during and after surgery can be reduced significantly by the use of surgical checklists as an important aspect of teamwork. The main advantages are represented by compensation of memory defects of the team members and collective situational awareness. Only if a blame-free climate with horizontal communication can be guaranteed in the surgical department, patient safety can be significantly improved by surgical checklists.

KEYWORDS

Protocols, surgical checklist, plan-do-check-act, PDCA, checklist fatigue, rush/time pressure

INTRODUCTION

The mortality rate after major surgery is estimated to be between 0.5 and 5%, and the morbidity rate is estimated to be up to 25%. Half of all hospital-adverse events occur in surgical care, and half of these occur during operation. Half of these incidents are considered preventable, most of these being caused by human error and not by technical failure. For the first time in healthcare, a preoperative checklist ('time out procedure' [Figure 12.1]) was introduced by American ophtalmologists to avoid wrong eye surgery.[1] This checklist was inspired by safety management in aviation, including checklists, especially to avoid human error, over a decade ago. In 2009, in the *New England Journal of Medicine*, the first results with regard to the WHO Safe Surgery Checklist (2008) were published by Gawande et al, with a reduction of mortality of over 30% in noncardiac surgery.[2] This checklist consists of three parts: a sign-in part, just before the induction of anaesthesia; a time-out part, just before the incision; and a sign-out part, just after closure of the incision. As the Safe Surgery Checklist does not cover the remaining half of incidents pre- and postoperatively, 1 year later,

in the same journal, Boermeester et al published a more complete, six-step checklist for all transfer moments during hospitalisation, with amelioration of outcomes by almost 50%.[3] Since then, several systemic reviews on the effect of checklists in surgery have been published, with favourable results as a rule.[4–6] From 2010, a surgical checklist for all operative disciplines is obligatory in Dutch hospitals.

SITUATIONAL AWARENESS

Apart from compensation for memory defects of team members, the main incentive of a surgical checklist is represented by the stimulation of situational awareness of the surgical team with regard to all risks of a certain surgical procedure in a certain patient. In the traditional model, each participant in the care process, from medical specialists and nurses to students, had their specific and relatively limited roles to play, often without the formal obligation and even intention to oversee and control all important aspects and risks of a specific treatment. Situational awareness can be regarded as a mutual mindset of all team members, in which the anticipation of the possibility of human error amidst ever-changing

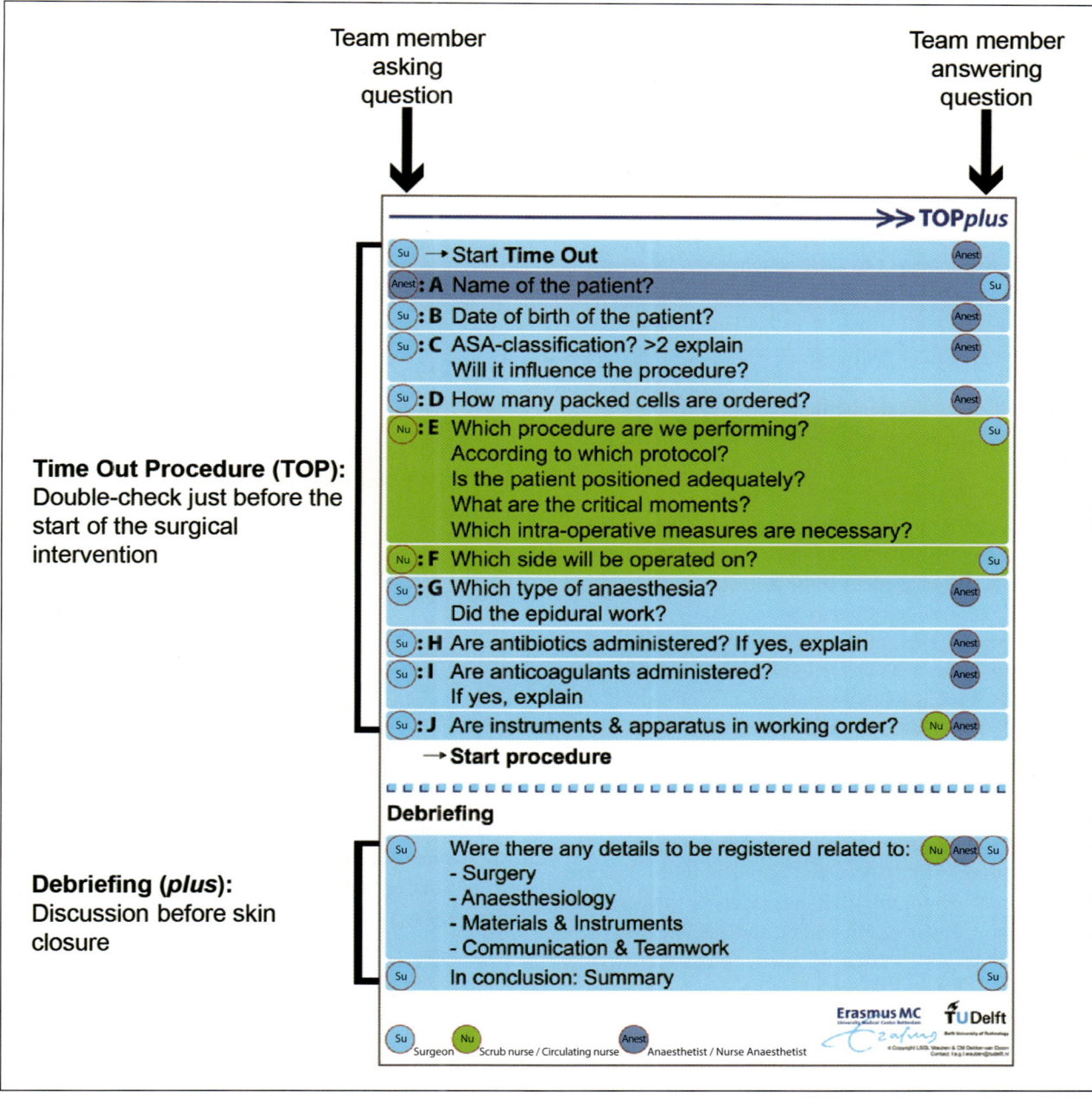

Figure 12.1 Time Out Procedure, Erasmus University Medical Center.

Courtesy: Johan F. Lange.

circumstances is considered paramount. Not only should the aspects of the specific patient and his type of surgery but also individual characteristics of all team members, including human factors such as fatigue, emotions, personality, and level of training, must be taken into account during the process of continuous risk estimation. Consequently, any member of the surgical team can not only anticipate specific measures to take, according to his or her role, but also must implement continuous cross-checking of all team members in a tension-free manner.

PROTOCOLS

It may be considered an additional advantage of the surgical checklists that they stimulate adherence to protocols, as these are standard subject of the checklist. In this respect, it is essential during the sign out (of the operation) to recapitulate the protocol and any deviation from it. As such, not only surgeons and residents but also all other team members will be acquainted with the protocols.

CULTURE

The favourable effects of surgical checklists will be optimal only if the culture within the surgical setting, such as the department and the hospital, is transparent and sound. Unfortunately, fear and dependence are, even in the 21st century, factors not to be neglected, especially in invasive disciplines such as surgery, sometimes even overtly mimicking a military hierarchy. Under these circumstances, it is to be expected that at least some team members, such as residents, nurses and students, will be reluctant to speak up when necessary. Other members such as medical specialists will probably interpret cross-checking by traditionally 'lower' colleagues as improper criticism. Wrong organs have, indeed, been removed, as team members have withheld from commenting. To avoid this, checklist management must not only be considered to be an isolated component of care but should also be an essential part of structured team training, just like crew resource management. In such a training, care workers of all levels learn to communicate effectively and horizontally, with both respect and confidence. Anyhow, a safety management instrument such as a safety climate questionnaire can be considered very useful and even conditional to estimate the effectiveness of checklists in certain settings of surgical care. In this sense, checklists can also be considered an additional opportunity to get used to horizontal communication, prerequisite for a blame-free climate, consistent teamwork and patient safety.[7,8] Teamwork in all its aspects, such as shared decision making, interchanging leader and follower roles, horizontal communication and cross-checking, makes the checklist flourish but by all means must not exclude hierarchy. On the contrary, functional hierarchy with horizontal and respectful communication, instead of traditional hierarchy with a conventional top-down approach, is obligatory in all types of complex-task performance, such as surgery, not implicating the type of surgeon manifesting himself as the 'captain of the ship' in all circumstances of the intervention. Moreover, he must often be a follower when the specific expertise of another team member, for example, the scrub nurse, will be involved.

CONTENT OF THE SURGICAL CHECKLIST

There is no universal format for a surgical checklist. Its efficacy and support by care workers are optimal only if the checklist is customised with regard to the category of patients and the specific surgical team within its own 'habitat'. In this regard, it certainly works best if the team has also participated proactively in the development of the checklist's format. However, in all surgical checklists, some common elements can be discerned: apart from the identity of the patient and the side of the surgery in case of a unilateral procedure, the principal elements of the preoperative checklist must not outnumber about 10 different components; these principal elements are generally considered as follows: medication and allergies; haemostasis; specifications of the type of anaesthesia/analgesia and operation, including any deviation of the protocol; complications and blood loss; antibiotic prophylaxis; position of the patient; bladder catheterisation; imaging; and equipment, including instruments and apparatus (Figure 12.2). Aspects of the checklist as to the sign-out procedure at the termination of the procedure must be as follows: number of gauzes and instruments, any incidents or complications, deviation of the protocol, quality of communication between team members and instructions for postoperative management. In case of gastrointestinal surgery, specific elements might be added to the checklist, such as checks with regard to the laparoscopy apparatus.[9]

ERRORS USING A SURGICAL CHECKLIST

Checklists are complex instruments to manage; in fact, many hazards have already proved to exist in industries such as aviation and care, including surgery. The most common errors are as follows:

- Incomplete participating team, resulting in insufficient situational awareness; lack of team members is still a common phenomenon and can evenly occur at the beginning and ending of the surgery.
- Traditional hierarchy and reluctance to speak up, if necessary.
- Lack of standardisation of the checklist procedure and/or specific roles of team members during the checklist procedure.
- Lack of protocols for operative procedures.
- Checklist fatigue, especially if items are too many.
- Absence of a plan-do-check-act (PDCA) quality system, making debriefing during the sign-out phase irrelevant and demotivating team members; it is a well-known fact that especially the sign out is a weak element of the checklist procedure, as until now, many surgical wards do not feature structured debriefings with feedback to the team members.
- Rush/time pressure.

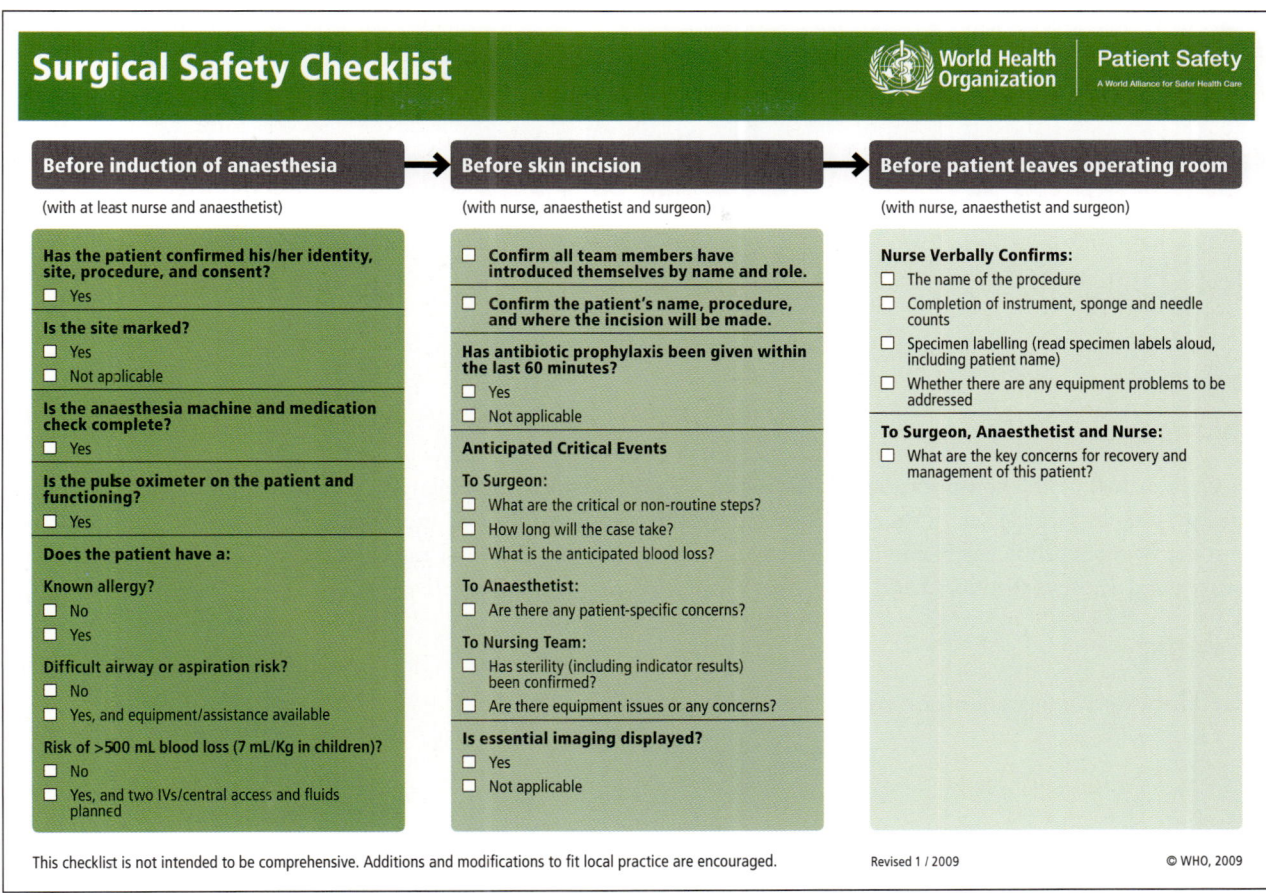

Figure 12.2 Surgical safety checklist.

Reprinted from: Patient Safety, World Health Organization, Surgical Safety Checklist, 2009.

CONCLUSIONS

In conclusion, surgical checklists have become an essential part of the patient safety and quality system of the surgical department. However, the development and implementation of checklists are complex and time consuming. It is of the utmost importance that the team itself participate in the entire process of implementation, including development. At least yearly, the surgical checklist should be evaluated and updated, if necessary. In addition, compliance should also be checked on a regular basis. Finally, condition sine qua non is an appropriate safety culture, without traditional hierarchy and dependence of team members.

REFERENCES

1. Simon JW. Preventing surgical confusions in ophthalmology (an American Ophthalmological Society thesis). *Trans Am Ophthalmol Soc* 2007;105:513–29.

2. Haynes AB, Weiser TG, Berry WR, et al. A surgical safety checklist to reduce morbidity and mortality in a global population. *N Engl J Med* 2009;360:491–9.

3. de Vries EN, Prins HA, Crolla RM, et al; SURPASS Collaborative Group. Effect of a comprehensive surgical safety system on patient outcomes. *N Engl J Med* 2010;363:1928–37.

4. Treadwell JR, Lucas S, Tsou AY. Surgical checklists: a systematic review of impacts and implementation. *BMJ Qual Saf* 2014;23:299–318.

5. Pucher PH, Johnston MJ, Aggarwal R, Arora S, Darzi A. Effectiveness of interventions to improve patient handover in surgery: a systematic review. *Surgery* 2015;158:85–95.

6. Molina G, Jiang W, Edmondson L, et al. Implementation of the surgical safety checklist in South Carolina hospitals is associated with improvement in perceived perioperative safety. *J Am Coll Surg* 2016;222:725–36.

7. Pugel AE, Simianu VV, Flum DR, Patchen Dellinger E. Use of the surgical safety checklist to improve communication and reduce complications. *J Infect Public Health* 2015;8:219–25.

8. Korkiakangas T. Mobilising a team for the WHO Surgical Safety Checklist: a qualitative video study. *BMJ Qual Saf* 2016 Feb 29 (Epub ahead of print).

9. Verdaasdonk EG, Stassen LP, Hoffmann WF, van der Elst M, Dankelman J. Can a structured checklist prevent problems with laparoscopic equipment? *Surg Endosc* 2008;22:2238–43.

13

Impact of Checklists in Developing Countries

N. Chaudhary

ABSTRACT

More than half of the complications after surgery are preventable. Implementation of a cost-effective and simple strategy such as surgical safety checklists can reduce the complications and mortality during surgical perioperative period. However, problems remain in complete implementation of checklists, and close coordination and monitoring are required at the institutional and government levels to bring about a positive outcome.

KEYWORDS

Checklists, developing countries, complications

INTRODUCTION

Adverse events after surgery are common and result in substantial financial burden on healthcare, more so in resource-poor settings. The surgical mortality in developing countries is 10-fold higher as compared with that in the developed world.[1] Nearly half of the complications after surgery are preventable.[2] Surgical safety checklists have evolved gradually as a powerful weapon for reducing complications and deaths attributed to surgery. The beneficial effect of checklists in the developing world has been proven beyond doubt, with more and more studies coming from low- and middle-income countries (LMICs).[3] However, with the emergence of quality evidence from this part of the world, difficulties in implementation of checklists have come to the forefront in terms of compliance and completeness. This chapter focusses on surgical disease burden in the developing countries, the urgent need for strict implementation of checklists and the challenges ahead.

SURGICAL DISEASE BURDEN AND BARRIERS IN ACHIEVING UNIVERSAL SURGICAL CARE IN DEVELOPING COUNTRIES

Quantification of surgical disease burden globally is difficult. The reasons are multifactorial: from underreporting of diseases to inadequate data collection.

Furthermore, patients travel across countries for surgical care. Initial estimates by Debas et al indicated that 11% of global disease burden needs surgery.[4] However, recent estimates suggest that 30% of diseases across the world need surgical treatment.[5] This estimate was similar in both low-income countries and middle-income countries. The increase is mainly due to the rise in chronic and noncommunicable diseases owing to epidemiologic shift. More than three-fourths of deaths due to these noncommunicable diseases occur in low-income countries.[6]

Huge disparity exists between high-, low- and middle-income countries in the performance of surgical procedures. The number of surgical procedures varies from 295 procedures per 100,000 population in Ethiopia to 23,369 procedures per 100,000 population in Hungary.[1] The number of surgical procedures per year correlates with per capita spending on health expenditure. The LMICs, which constitute 70% of the total world population, have disproportionately low number (28.5%) of surgical procedures per year.[7] This not only explains the limited accessibility of this population to healthcare but also underlies the fact that a large proportion of disease burden globally remains unaddressed. According to an estimate, approximately 321 million surgical procedures need to be performed globally per year.[8]

Barriers in delivery of surgical care could be due to accessibility, availability, affordability and acceptability at patient, physician or institutional level.[9] To overcome these hurdles, coordination between governmental agencies, nongovernment organisations (NGOs) and healthcare professionals is a must. A unique strategy of cross-subsidisation has been adopted by an Indian centre to overcome financial problems in delivering quality eye care treatment.[10]

Surgical Care: Global Public Health Concern

Initial research suggested that surgical care was neither cost-effective nor generated public attention because of the treatment of chronic and noncommunicable diseases. This resulted in reluctance in accepting surgical care as a public health concern. However, recent research states that the number of disability adjusted life years averted by a surgical procedure compares favourably with nonsurgical interventions.[4] Hence, at present, surgical care has gained priority and scaling up of surgical infrastructure has been suggested to improve healthcare.

WHY DO WE NEED SURGICAL SAFETY CHECKLISTS?

We need surgical safety checklists to achieve the following goals.

To Prevent Complications/Deaths

Surgery is an essential component of healthcare. Complications after major surgical procedures are common and occur in 3 to 16% of patients. Mortality varies from 0.4 to 0.8%; this means that around 1 million patients die after surgery and 7 million would have some complications. These figures are from the developed world. Nearly half of these complications are said to be preventable.[2,11] The data from the developing countries are scarce. The mortality rates are in the range of 5 to 10% after major surgeries.[12,13] In sub-Saharan Africa, the mortality after general anaesthesia is estimated to be 0.7%.[14] Extrapolation of data from the developed world would then mean a higher and significant number of complications, and deaths could be preventable. Implementation of the World Health Organization (WHO) surgical safety checklist has shown beneficial effect of checklist in both developed and developing countries.[3,15] A systematic review and meta-analysis concluded that checklists are effective and economic means to reduce complications.[16]

Checklists are the means to pre-empt mistakes and thereby decrease the risk of complications to infinitesimal levels. Operative room fatigue and stress are a common phenomenon; in such circumstances, cognitive decline may occur, leading to 'errors', which could have been avoided.[17] Such situations are more likely to happen in the developing countries, where a surgeon is forced to operate upon a large number of patients. Besides, inadequate infrastructure and manpower of other healthcare professionals involved in surgical care add to the risks.

To Enhance Teamwork and Communication

Surgical care is a complex process and involves close coordination between surgeons, anaesthetists, nurses and other operating room staff. The traditional operating room structure, with surgeon as the 'head' of the operating room, promotes autonomy, which may be counterproductive. A checklist completion requires individual inputs from surgeons, anaesthetists and nurses, and this enhances teamwork. Lingard et al performed a prepost interventional study and concluded that use of preoperative checklist resulted in better teamwork in the operating room.[18]

Improper interprofessional communication in an operating room has negative effects on outcomes. Gawande et al conducted confidential interviews of 38 surgeons at Massachusetts regarding surgical adverse events.[19] Of all the incidents reported, two-thirds occurred during the operation. Communication failure was cited as the main reason in 43% of incidents. Surgical checklists decreases communication gap. Preoperative briefings involving surgeons, anaesthetists and nurses reduce miscommunication errors.[20]

EVOLUTION OF CHECKLISTS

Checklists were initially incorporated in intensive care unit (ICU) protocols to reduce catheter-related bloodstream infections (CR-BSI). Five percent of all ICU patients with central lines would acquire a CR-BSI.[21] A study from John Hopkins used simple protocols and a checklist to prove that CR-BSIs are preventable. The CR-BSIs reduced from 11 per 1000 catheter days to 0 per 1000 catheter days in the study group over a period of 4 years. No change in infection rates were observed in the control group.[22] As a result of the significant benefit, the checklists were then included in surgical protocols.

The WHO Surgical Safety Checklist

Safe Surgery Saves Lives (SSSL) study group in 2007 to 2008 implemented a 19-item surgical safety checklist in patients undergoing noncardiac surgeries (both elective and urgent) at eight centres across the world.[15] Data were collected from 3733 consecutive patients and 3955 patients, before and after the implementation of checklists, respectively. The overall mortality reduced from 1.5 to 0.8%, and inpatient complications reduced from 11 to 7% (both statistically significant). Out of the eight centres, four were from high-income countries and the remaining four were from LMICs. Although the reduction in complication rates was similar in both high-income countries and LMICs, the reduction in mortality rates was more significant only in LMICs after the implementation of checklists. This multicentre study proved that checklists can be implemented in diverse economic environments. The Hawthorne effect (improvements in results when the performance is directly observed) was mentioned as a major limitation of the study because of its nonrandomised design. Following this landmark publication, several studies were conducted that showed beneficial outcomes.

The role of surgical safety checklists in urgent noncardiac surgeries was evaluated by SSSL study group.[23] The study included 842 patients and 908 patients, before and after the implementation of checklist, respectively. This pre–post intervention observation study found complications to reduce by almost one-third and deaths by 60% after checklists usage. Even adherence to six safety steps improved.

Modified Checklists in Surgery

One of the limitations pointed out in the WHO checklist was the low number of items in checklists and the absence of adequate handover of surgical patients to the postoperative room staff and, hence, not maintaining safety culture over the entire surgical pathway. Many modifications were then proposed and studied.

- Veterans Hospital Administration used preoperative briefings and postoperative debriefings checklists and found a significant increase in antibiotic and deep vein thrombosis (DVT) prophylaxis compliance rates after checklist implementation.[24]
- SURPASS checklist: A comprehensive checklist to cover the entire surgical pathway was studied across six centres in the Netherlands.[25] This prospective study included 3760 patients and 3820 patients, before and after the implementation of checklists, respectively. The total number of complications decreased from 27.3 to 16.7 per 100 patients and mortality decreased from 1.5 to 0.8% in the study period. No significant changes in complications or mortality were observed in the control hospitals.

Subgroup analysis revealed that complications rates were significantly lower in the group where the adherence to completion of checklists was higher. Although the SURPASS checklist represented an ideal scenario, where all aspects of surgical care pathway were looked into, it has its own limitations in requiring a considerable time and effort and more manpower in its implementation because of its comprehensive and multidisciplinary design.

- Several modified checklists have been compiled, suited according to the local environments. These modifications in checklists have been studied in different specialties, such as ophthalmology and neurosurgery.

CHECKLISTS IN DEVELOPING COUNTRIES

The need of strict implementation of surgical safety checklists is probably more in the developing countries. The higher disease burden, poor accessibility to healthcare and low healthcare expenditure in the developing countries put increased burden on existing professionals involved in surgical care. The number of physicians in Ethiopia is only 0.2 per 10,000 population.[26] The healthcare professionals in such an environment are more likely to commit errors. Moreover, less than one-fourth of the population in the developing countries have medical insurance and the rest of population is paying out of their pockets. Thus, the financial burden of healthcare on the patient and family is huge, and reducing complications by any means would be useful. Thus, a cost-effective intervention, such as surgical checklist, is likely to have more impact in LMICs. The data of checklist use and outcomes from the developing countries is scarce.

The beneficial effect of checklist in the developing countries has been shown in several studies. Chaudhary et al conducted a randomised controlled trial in India to observe the effects of implementation of the WHO surgical safety checklist on patient outcomes (Figure 13.1).[3] The study was done in a tertiary care academic centre and included patients requiring both elective and emergent operations. Only the patients were blinded to the intervention. The number of complications per patient reduced from 0.97 in the nonintervention group to 0.80 in the intervention group. The effect of checklist on mortality and higher-grade complications was even more significant; higher-grade complications (Clavien grade 3 or 4 complications) per patient reduced by 30% and mortality decreased by 43% in the checklist group as compared with the group in which the checklist was not implemented. On subgroup analysis, the study

WHO SURGICAL SAFETY CHECKLIST WITH MODIFICATIONS

Before induction of anaesthesia ▶▶▶▶▶▶▶▶ Before skin incision ▶▶▶▶▶▶▶▶▶▶▶▶ Before patient leaves operating room

SIGN IN

☐ PATIENT HAS CONFIRMED
  • IDBNTITY
  • SITE
  • PROCEDURE
  • CONSENT

☐ SITE MARKED/NOT APPLICABLE

☐ ANAESTHESIA SAFETY CHECK COMPLETED

☐ PULSE OXIMETER ON PATIENT AND FUNCTIONING

DOES PATIENT HAVE A:

KNOWN ALLERGY?
☐ NO
☐ YES

DIFFICULT AIRWAY/ASPIRATION RISK?
☐ NO
☐ YES, AND EQUIPMENT/ASSISTANCE AVAILABLE

RISK OF >500ML BLOOD LOSS
(7ML/KG IN CHILDREN)?
☐ NO
☐ YES, AND ADEQUATE INTRAVENOUS ACCESS AND FLUIDS PLANNED

Has the imaging been discussed with radiologist preoperatively—yes/no/not

TIME OUT

☐ CONFIRM ALL TEAM MEMBERS HAVE INTRODUCED THEMSELVES BY NAME AND ROLE

☐ SURGEON, ANAESTHESIA PROFESSIONAL AND NURSE VERBALLY CONFIRM
  • PATIENT
  • SITE
  • PROCEDURE

ANTICIPATED CRITICAL EVENTS

☐ SURGEON REVIEWS: WHAT ARE THE CRITICAL OR UNEXPECTED STEPS, OPERATIVE DURATION, ANTICIPATED BLOOD LOSS?

☐ ANAESTHESIA TEAM REVIEWS: ARE THERE ANY PATIENT-SPECIFIC CONCERNS?

☐ NURSING TEAM RIVIEWS: HAS STERILITY (INCLUDING INDICATOR RESULTS) BEEN CONFIRMED? ARE THERE EQUIPMENT ISSUES OR ANY CONCERNS?

HAS ANTIBIOTIC PROPHYLAXIS BEEN GIVEN WITHIN THE LAST 60 MINUTES?
☐ YES
☐ NOT APPLICABLE

IS ESSENTIAL IMAGING DISPLAYED?
☐ YES
☐ NOT APPLICABLE

Has DVT prophylaxis been administered—yes/no/not required

SIGN OUT

NURSE VERBALLY CONFIRMS WITH THE TEAM:

☐ THE NAME OF THE PROCEDURE RECORDED

☐ THAT INSTRUMENT, SPONGE AND NEEDLE COUNTS ARE CORRECT (OR NOT APPLICABLE)

☐ HOW THE SPECIMEN IS LABELLED (INCLUDING PATIENT NAME)

☐ WHETHER THERE ARE ANY EQUIPMENT PROBLEMS TO BE ADDRESSED

☐ SURGEON, ANAESTHESIA PROFESSIONAL AND NURSE REVIEW THE KEY CONCERNS FOR RECOVERY AND MANAGEMENT OF THIS PATIENT

Figure 13.1 World Health Organization's surgical safety checklist with some modifications, as was used in a study.
Based on the WHO Surgical Safety Checklist, http://www.who.int/patientsafety/safesurgery/checklist/en/index.html, © World Health Organization 2009. All rights reserved.

found better results in the group in which the checklist was fully completed as compared with the group with incomplete checklist. This is the first RCT from a developing country to show positive effects of checklists on outcomes.

A comparative study conducted in a referral academic centre in Iran before and after the implementation of surgical safety checklist showed a decrease of 57% in the number of complications.[27] Yuan et al studied the effect of the WHO surgical safety checklist in Liberia and concluded that the checklist was associated with improvements in outcome.[28] A South American study concluded that adherence to checklist's completion was associated with improved patient outcomes.[29]

The impact of checklists, along with usage of pulse oximetry in Moldova (an European LMIC), was studied by Kwok et al.[30] It was a pre–post intervention study, and data of more than 2000 patients in each group were collected. The adherence to safety protocols increased from 0 to 67%. The number of overall complications and hypoxaemic episodes reduced significantly.

Only a few centres from the African continent have evaluated the effect of checklists on outcomes. A Ugandan study showed significant decrease in complications with checklist use.[31] A study from Tunisia noted a significant decrease in surgical site infections and unplanned return to the operating room.[32] The authors concluded that surgical checklist greatly enhances surgical safety culture during the operation.

DRAWBACKS WITH CHECKLISTS

Although checklists have proved their utility in improving outcomes, certain problems do exist with checklists.

• Incompleteness: It may be impossible for checklists to include items to avoid all possible complications.

It has been suggested, therefore, to target a specific complication.

- Checklist fatigue: This problem specifically comes when checklists are used on a large scale, in broad situations and/or when they are extensive. With continued usage in such situations, the compliance decreases with time; this is termed checklist fatigue.
- Extra effort and time: This is more so a problem with exhaustive checklists containing large number of items to be completed, for example, the SURPASS checklist, which is a comprehensive checklist requiring multiple disciplines to complete. This particular issue is more important in the developing countries, where the healthcare professionals involved in surgical care are already stressed by heavy workload.

CHALLENGES IN IMPLEMENTING CHECKLISTS IN DEVELOPING COUNTRIES

The most important problem lies in compliance and completion of checklists. Only 4% of the checklists were completely filled in a Brazilian study.[29] Some centres have reported compliance rates of as low as 40 to 45%.[33,34] A descriptive study from Thailand included 4340 patients over a period of 6 months. In this study, the surgical site was marked in only 20% of patients; antibiotic prophylaxis was not given in 30% of patients; and the instrument, sponge and needle counts were missed in 3.2% of patients.[35] Strong correlations exist between adherence to surgical safety protocols and reduction in complications.[36] A comparative study found that noncompliance with checklists' implementation was more likely to occur in LMICs as compared with high-income countries.[37]

Most of the observational studies with pre- and postintervention study design have reported an increase in compliance rates after intervention in the form of checklists. This could possibly be due to Hawthorne effect, as described in the Safe Surgery Saves Lives study group.[15] However, an Ethiopian centre showed a decrease in compliance rates with time. The compliance rates fell from 89% at the start of the study to less than 20% after 6 months of checklist's implementation.[33] Bashford suggested several reasons for this reduction: loss or turnover of staff or local leadership; perception that continued efforts are not required; and inadequate infrastructure, for example, lack of a printer, paper or even a pen to fill the checklists. Lack of manpower and equipment was suggested as possible challenge to compliance and completing of checklists in another African study.[31]

Quite often, the checklist implementation in resource-poor settings is managed by overseas agency, which is not sustainable in the long term. Close coordination between hospital administration, local governments and nongovernmental organisations would result in better implementation on a long-term basis. An African study even proposed an external observer, who could be from a different department from the same hospital or from a different hospital, to oversee the implementation of checklists on a regular basis, so as to improve compliance.[33] Yearly audits should be done regarding compliance and completeness of checklists and should be published to observe the effects over a time. Lack of training was cited as an important reason for noncompliance, and therefore, proper training sessions should be conducted at the time of introducing the checklists.[34]

Cultural barriers have been elucidated as a reason for noncompliance and incomplete checklists.[36] Marking on another's body is against the norm of the society in Thailand; surgical sites were marked in less than 20%. Similarly, the introduction of the team members at time-out period was less often completed, since the people in Thailand introduce themselves only initially and are reluctant and shy of repeating it again. Cultural practices should be taken into account, and modifications in checklist should be done to suit the local needs.

CONCLUSIONS

Surgical complications are unavoidable but preventable. Postoperative complications pose a heavy financial burden on patients and healthcare providers. Surgical safety checklists are a simple and cost-effective measure to decrease the complications and mortality in the developing countries. Developing countries have specific barriers to the implementation of checklists, and checklists should be adapted to best suit the local environments. Noncompliance and incomplete checklists are major problems in the way of achieving sustainable positive outcomes. Strict checklist implementation should be mandatory in the developing countries. The challenge lies in overcoming cultural barriers and increasing the coordination between hospital administration and government and nongovernment agencies to have a significant and positive outcome in reducing complications and mortality.

REFERENCES

1. Weiser TG, Regenbogen SE, Thompson KD, et al. An estimation of the global volume of surgery: a modelling strategy based on available data. *Lancet* 2008;372:139–44.

2. Gawande AA, Thomas EJ, Zinner MJ, Brennan TA. The incidence and nature of surgical adverse events in Colorado and Utah in 1992. *Surgery* 1999;126:66–75.

3. Chaudhary N, Varma V, Kapoor S, Mehta N, Kumaran V, Nundy S. Implementation of a surgical safety checklist and postoperative outcomes: a prospective randomized controlled study. *J Gastrointest Surg* 2015;19:935–42.

4. Debas HT, Gosselin R, McCord C, et al. *Disease Control Priorities in Developing Countries*. 2nd ed. Disease Control Priorities Project. Washington, DC: International Bank for Reconstruction and Development/World Bank; 2006:1245–60.

5. Shrime MG, Bickler SW, Alkire BC, Mock C. Global burden of surgical disease: an estimation from the provider perspective. *Lancet Glob Health* 2015;3:S8–9.

6. Daar AS, Singer PA, Persad DL, et al. Grand challenges in chronic non-communicable diseases. *Nature* 2007; 450:494–6.

7. Weiser TG, Haynes AB, Molina G, et al. Size and distribution of the global volume of surgery in 2012. *Bull World Health Organ* 2016;94:201–9F.

8. Rose J, Weiser TG, Hider P, Wilson L, Gruen RL, Bickler SW. Estimated need for surgery worldwide based on prevalence of diseases: a modelling strategy for the WHO Global Health Esimate. *Lancet Glob Health* 2015;3: S13–20.

9. Grimes CE, Bowman KG, Dodgion CM, Lavy CB. Systematic review of barriers to surgical care in low-income and middle-income countries. *World J Surg* 2011;35:941–50.

10. Howitt P, Darzi A, Yang GZ, et al. Technologies for global health. *Lancet* 2012;380:507–35.

11. Kable AK, Gibberd RW, Spigelman AD. Adverse events in surgical patients in Australia. *Int J Qual Health Care* 2002;14:269–76.

12. Bickler SW, Sanno-Duanda B. Epidemiology of paediatric surgical admissions to a government referral hospital in the Gambia. *Bull World Health Organ* 2000;78:1330–6.

13. Yii MK, Ng KJ. Risk-adjusted surgical audit with the POSSUM scoring system in a developing country. *Br J Surg* 2002;89:110–3.

14. Ouro-Bang'na Maman AF, Tomta K, Ahouangbévi S, Chobli M. Deaths associated with anaesthesia in Togo, West Africa. *Trop Doct* 2005;35:220–2.

15. Haynes AB, Weiser TG, Berry WR, et al. Safe Surgery Saves Lives Study Group: a surgical safety checklist to reduce morbidity and mortality in a global population. *N Engl J Med* 2009;360:491–509.

16. Borchard A, Schwappach DLB, Barbir A, Bezzola P. A systematic review of the effectiveness, compliance, and critical factors for implementation of safety checklists in surgery. *Ann Surg* 2012;256:925–33.

17. Arora S, Sevdalis N, Nestel D, Woloshynowych M, Darzi A, Kneebone R. The impact of stress on surgical performance: a systematic review of the literature. *Surgery* 2010;147:318–30.

18. Lingard L, Regehr G, Orser B, Reznick R, Baker GR, Doran D, et al. Evaluation of a preoperative checklist and team briefing among surgeons, nurses, and anaesthesiologists to reduce failures in communication. *Arch Surg* 2008;143:12–7.

19. Gawande AA, Zinner MJ, Studdert DM, Brennan TA. Analysis of errors reported by surgeons at three teaching hospitals. *Surgery* 2003;133:614–21.

20. Lingard L, Whyte S, Espin S, Baker GR, Orser B, Doran D. Towards safer interprofessional communication: constructing a model of "utility" from preoperative team briefings. *J Interprof Care* 2006;20:471–83.

21. Saint S, Veenstra DL, Lipsky BA. The clinical and economic consequences of nosocomial central venous catheter-related infection: are antimicrobial catheters useful? *Infect Control Hosp Epidemiol* 2000;21:375–80.

22. Berenholtz SM, Pronovost PJ, Lipsett PA, et al. Eliminating catheter-related bloodstream infections in the intensive care unit. *Crit Care Med* 2004;32:2014–20.

23. Weiser TG, Haynes AB, Dziekan G, et al. Effect of a 19-item surgical safety checklist during urgent operations in a global patient population. *Ann Surg* 2010;251: 976–80.

24. Paull DE, Mazzia LM, Wood SD, et al. Briefing guide study: preoperative briefing and postoperative debriefing checklists in the Veterans Health Administration medical team training program. *Am J Surg* 2010;200:620–3.

25. de Vries EN, Prins HA, Crolla RM, et al. Effect of a comprehensive surgical safety system on patient outcomes. *N Engl J Med* 2010;363:1928–37.

26. World Health Organisation: Ethiopia: health profile. [Online]; 2011 [cited 2011 May 8]. Available from: http://www.who.int/gho/countries/eth.pdf.

27. Askarian M, Kouchak F, Palenik CJ. Effect of surgical safetychecklists on postoperative morbidity and mortality rates, Shiraz, Faghihy Hospital: a 1-year study. *Qual Manage Health Care* 2011;20:293–7.

28. Yuan CT, Walsh D, Tomarken JL, Alpern R, Shakpeh J, Bradley EH. Incorporating the World Health Organization Surgical Safety Checklist into practice at two hospitals in Liberia. *Jt Comm J Qual Patient Saf* 2012;38:254–60.

29. Freitas MR, Antunes AG, Lopes BN, Fernandes FdaC, MonteLdeC, Gama ZA. Assessment of adherence to the WHO surgical safety checklist in urological and gynecological surgeries at two teaching hospitals in Natal, *Rio Grande do Norte State, Brazil. Cad Saúde Pública* 2014;30:137–48.

30. Kwok AC, Funk LM, Baltaga R, et al. Implementation of the World Health Organization surgical safety checklist, including introduction of pulse oximetry in a resource-limited setting. *Ann Surg* 2013;257:633–9.

31. Lilaonitkul M, Kwikiriza A, Ttendo S, et al. Implementation of the WHO surgical safety checklist and surgical swab and instrument counts at a regional referral hospital in Uganda—a quality improvement project. *Anaesthesia* 2015;70:1345–55.

32. El Mhamdi S, Letaief M, Cherif Y, Bouanene I, Kallel W, Hamdi A. Implementation of the safe surgery checklist of the World Health Organization at the University Hospital of Monastir (Tunisia). *Tunis Med* 2014;92: 385–90.

33. Bashford T, Reshamwalla S, McAuley J, Allen NH, McNatt Z, Gebremedhen YD. Implementation of the WHO Surgical Safety Checklist in an Ethiopian Referral Hospital. *Patient Saf Surg* 2014;8:16.

34. Melekie TD, Getahun GM. Compliance with surgical safety checklist completion in the operating room of University of Gondar Hospital, Northwest Ethiopia. *BMC Res Notes* 2015;19:8.

35. Kasatpibal N, Senaratana W, Chitreecheur J, Chotirosniramit N, Pakvipas P, Junthasopeepun P. Implementation of the World Health Organization surgical safety checklist at a university hospital in Thailand. *Surg Infect* 2012;13:50–6.

36. Bergs J, Hellings J, Cleemput I, Zurel O, De Troyer V, Van Hiel M, et al. Systematic review and meta-analysis of the effect of the World Health Organization surgical safety checklist on postoperative complications. *Br J Surg* 2014;101:150–8.

37. Aveling EL, McCulloch P, Dixon-Woods M. A qualitative study comparing experiences of the surgical safety checklist in hospitals in high-income and low-income countries. *BMJ Open* 2013;3:e003039.

14

The Dutch Surgical Colorectal Audit: Reducing Complications by Nationwide Feedback on Process and Outcome

N.J. van Leersum, E.H. Eddes, M.W.J.M. Wouters and R.A.E.M. Tollenaar

ABSTRACT

In 2009, the Association of Surgeons of the Netherlands initiated the Dutch Surgical Colorectal Audit (DSCA) with the objective to implement a quality instrument that would improve outcomes in colorectal cancer surgery and provide stakeholders with reliable quality information on hospital performance. The intrinsic motivation of the healthcare professionals and their active management of the audit are among the key factors that led to the success of the nationwide audit: all Dutch hospitals participate and include more than 98% of eligible patients in the audit. After 7 years, over 60% reduction in 30-day mortality has been achieved in both colon and rectal cancer surgeries. In addition, complication rates have decreased substantially. In rectal cancer surgery, the incidence of circumferential resection margin involvement has decreased by 65%. These performance indicators were all made transparent to stakeholders (e.g., payers and patient organisations) on hospital level. In this chapter, the merits of the DSCA are described, along with the resulting insights and effects on quality of colorectal cancer care.

KEYWORDS

Quality of care, healthcare, colorectal cancer, surgery, clinical audit, performance indicator, quality improvement, colorectal surgery

INTRODUCTION

Since 2009, the Dutch Surgical Colorectal Audit (DSCA) has resulted in large improvements in the treatment and outcomes of colorectal cancer in the Netherlands. In this chapter, the rationale for using clinical auditing as a quality instrument is explained, and specifically, the merits of the DSCA and the resulting insights and effects on quality of colorectal cancer care are described.

CLINICAL AUDITING

The idea of a hospital register to help doctors improve the quality of care was first discussed by the British doctor Sir Thomas Percival (1803): 'By the adoption of the register, physicians and surgeons would obtain clearer insight into the comparative success of their hospital and private practice; and would be incited to a diligent investigation of the causes of such difference'.[1] In addition, Dr. Ernest Codman (1869–1940), an American surgeon, advocated clinical registries, as he stated that evaluating outcomes of care in every patient is an intrinsic need and responsibility of every healthcare professional: 'Every hospital should follow every patient it treats long enough to determine whether the treatment has been successful, and then to inquire 'if not, why not' with a view to preventing similar failures in the future'.[2] The systematic gathering of follow-up data provides the opportunity to identify errors and areas for improvement. Doctor Codman's so-called end-result idea is considered the foundation of modern clinical audits that have emerged internationally since the end of the 20th century.[3]

Clinical auditing is a quality improvement tool that is used to expose quality of care by continuous and meticulous evaluation of patients' outcomes. It compares these outcomes between hospitals (benchmarking) and provides feedback on their results to participants. A clinical audit is typically a continuous plan-do-check-act cycle: 'a process that seeks to improve patient care and outcomes through systematic review of care against explicit criteria and the implementation of change'.[4]

A literature review shows that clinical auditing has a positive effect on both the process and the outcomes of care.[5] Moreover, the effect on quality improvement is further amplified when improvement interventions are actively implemented next to clinical auditing. As underlying mechanisms for the effect of clinical auditing on quality improvement, the following are considered: (1) feedback information enabling performance monitoring, benchmarking with peers and the identification of best practices, and (2) the 'Hawthorne effect'.[6,7] Feedback information raises doctors' awareness and provides the opportunity to identify areas for improvement. The 'Hawthorne effect' is the psychological phenomenon in which individuals improve in response to their awareness of being observed.

In addition to improving clinical outcomes, clinical auditing has also been associated with significant cost reduction, especially in high-risk procedures, such as colorectal cancer surgery.[8] As undesired outcomes, such as complications and unplanned reinterventions, are very costly, it is credible that improved outcome will go hand in hand with cost reduction.

Internationally, many clinical audits have been initiated since the past three decades, especially in the surgical and oncological domains. Examples of national clinical audits are the National Surgical Quality Improvement Program (NSQIP) in the United States, the National Bowel Cancer Project (NBOCAP) in the United Kingdom, the Swedish Rectal Cancer Audit and the Norwegian Colorectal Cancer Project.[9–12]

THE INITIATION OF THE DUTCH SURGICAL COLORECTAL AUDIT

In 2010, a report of the signalling committee of the Dutch Cancer Society revealed that large variation in colorectal cancer care existed between hospitals, resulting in an almost 2-fold higher risk of dying in one hospital compared with another.[13] In addition, under- and overtreatment were identified in some hospitals regarding (neo-) adjuvant therapies. The committee considered differences in the care process, local preferences and delayed implementation of new therapeutic options underlying the variation between hospitals. To reduce variation and improve quality of care, the authors recommended (1) the development of minimal quality standards, (2) the implementation of clinical auditing on a national level, and (3) centralisation of cancer care in those hospitals meeting the quality standards and showing high-quality care processes and outcomes for their patients.

Prompted by this call for improvement, the Association of Surgeons in the Netherlands (ASN) developed a set of minimal procedural volume standards and requirements regarding institutional infrastructure and medical specialties available.[14] Furthermore, they initiated the Dutch Surgical Colorectal Audit (DSCA).[15] This nationwide clinical audit was initiated with the purpose to evaluate and improve quality of care for primary colorectal cancer surgery in the Netherlands. Hereby, the audit should meet the professional need both to evaluate and benchmark their quality of colorectal cancer care and, simultaneously, to provide reliable data for the public demand for transparency on quality of care.

Hereafter, the main features of the DSCA are described and the results of 7 years of auditing are shown. Subsequent to this success, the Dutch Institute of Clinical Auditing (DICA) was founded in 2011, with the objective to facilitate and organise the start-up of new nationwide audits, currently covering 23 major diagnoses.

Main Features of the Dutch Surgical Colorectal Audit

Bottom-up Initiative

Contrary to some international audits that are government-driven, the DSCA was set up by a professional association of surgeons, the ASN. This association serves as a central protector of common interests of surgeons and wants to ensure that every surgical patient in the Netherlands receives high-quality colorectal cancer care. Membership is compulsory for all surgeons in the Netherlands. The ASN has integrated the evaluation of audit results in their quality assurance program and provided counselling to negative outliers to improve their outcomes. The lead and intensive engagement of surgeons in audit is considered one of the largest merits of the DSCA.

Governance of the Audit

A scientific committee of mandated clinical experts in colorectal cancer care (surgeons, oncologists, pathologists and epidemiologists) was formed to oversee the audit. It defined performance indicators to highlight trends and identify potential quality concerns, areas for improvement and best practices. The data set consists of case-mix, process and outcome variables and is evaluated yearly. Besides the development of the database, the committee designed the registration process and evaluates the audit results on a quarterly basis. The findings are reported on in medical conferences and in an annual report and are published in peer-reviewed journals.

Data Collection

The DSCA uses a web-based program to enable manual data entry in a secured web environment. In addition, automated processes for data registration from the hospital administration in the form of electronic patient files to the national database are possible. A front office is available for participants regarding technical issues and medical content. Depending on the complexity of the patient and perioperative course, 56 to 179 variables have to be completed per patient. Unifying definitions and helping texts are attached to each variable to improve data quality. Data quality is highly important, as doctors will use the results to implement change in practice only if they believe that the data accumulation is accurate.

Performance Feedback to Participants

All participating hospitals have access to a secured personalised website called 'my DICA'. Performance feedback is given by presenting reports on quality and completeness of the registered data, procedural volume, basic characteristics, performance indicators and outcomes of care. The individual results are shown with the benchmark of all other hospitals and a national average and can be compared between different time periods. Case-mix adjusted hospital outcomes are presented in funnel plots, using 95% confidence limits. The reports are updated on a weekly basis.

Independent Data Verification

When working with self-reported data, the mantra among surgeons is 'high trust, high penalty'. On a cyclical basis, 'data verification teams' randomly check the registered data of the DSCA with the electronic patient files in the hospitals. In addition, they validate whether all patients that meet the inclusion criteria are registered in the national database. The results per hospital are judged by an independent committee and are publicly reported on. Hereby, the quality and reliability of the audit are ensured.

Transparent Quality Information for Stakeholders

The results of the DSCA are used not only for an internal quality improvement cycle but also for providing healthcare insurers and patients with transparent quality information on hospitals. Regularly, the different stakeholders gather on a national level to discuss which performance indicators are available from the audit and are suitable for this purpose. Then, master classes are provided to educate different stakeholders on the right interpretation of each indicator result. Not only have these consensus-based gatherings led to a higher quality of the indicators and a better mutual understanding on what quality of care entails, but also the registration burden of hospitals has decreased compared with the situation before, when hospitals had to manually collect and deliver instant data after noncoordinated individual data requests of different stakeholders.

A Platform for Quality of Care

An extensive annual report with the results of the audit is published and discussed on the DICA conference each year.[16] The conference is accessible to clinicians, patients, patient advocates, healthcare insurers and policy makers and politicians. Hereby, the audit functions as a platform for all stakeholders to address their (common) interests and to discuss diverse healthcare topics together.

Funding of the Audit

The onset of the DSCA was funded by quality improvement grants donated by a healthcare insurance company. Since 2013, each participating hospital pays a subscription fee for the audit. Thereby, the association of healthcare insurers funds the costs of DICA that functions as umbrella organisation. The subscription costs are returned to the hospitals, as they are enclosed in the payments of treating patients with colorectal cancer. Costs of the data registration itself are not compensated and are borne by the hospitals.

QUALITY IMPROVEMENT

From its introduction in 2009, the DSCA has shown to be a valuable quality improvement tool. Within 2 years, high-quality data have been collected, as all hospitals in the Netherlands participated and a near-complete case ascertainment was established.[17] Within 3 years, hospital variation diminished remarkably and both the quality of the care process and postoperative outcomes improved.[18]

The following outcomes regarding complications were defined: reinterventions, nonsurgical complications (e.g., lung infection), severe complications (any complication leading to a reinterventions, prolonged hospital stay, ICU stay or death), 30-day mortality, failure to rescue (a complication resulting in death, proxy for the quality of the management of complications) and a positive circumferential resection margin (CRM) in rectal cancer.

Mortality after colon cancer surgery was 5.8% in the first registration year. Today, after 7 years since the initiation of the DSCA, mortality rates are as low as 2.3%,[19,20] a risk reduction of 61% (Figure 14.1a). For rectal cancer, the difference was 2.7 to 1.2% (63% risk reduction) (Figure 14.1b). Severe complications decreased from 19 to 14% and from 23 to 20% after colon and rectal cancer surgeries, respectively. Research of the data resulted in the following insights that were used for quality improvement: (1) the risk of failure to rescue was two times higher after elective colon than that after rectal cancer surgery, especially due to nonsurgical complications.[21] (2) Failure to rescue was three times higher in high-mortality hospitals.[22] (3) Of total hospital costs in this study, 31% was spent on management of complications and the top 5% most expensive patients were accountable for 23% of hospitals budgets.[23] (4) Nonelective colon cancer surgery was associated with a 2-fold higher mortality risk, especially after right-sided resections and patients with tumour perforation at presentation.[24] (5) The Hartmann's procedure and low anterior resection (LAR) with diverting ileostomy

were associated with fewer infective complications and reoperations than LARs with primary anastomosis (6.5% and 10.1% vs. 16.2%; p<0.001) and reoperation (7.3% and 8.1% vs. 16.5%; p<0.001).[25] (6) The percentage of laparoscopic resection increased in 2009 to 2015 from 33 to 71% and 34 to 79% in colon and rectal cancers, respectively, and was associated with a decreased risk of postoperative mortality compared with open resection in elective setting in patients with nonlocally advanced, nonmetastasised colorectal cancer[20,26] (Figure 14.2).

At the start of the DSCA, the registration of the CRM status in the pathology report was only 48% and CRM involvement was seen in 14% of cases. After increased attention and feedback on this topic in the audit, registration improved from 48 to 98% and the incidence of CRM-positive margins after rectal cancer surgery decreased from 14 to 5% (65% risk reduction).[18,20] Although CRM involvement after abdominoperineal excision (APE) was higher than that after LAR, it was found that the risk of CRM involvement was not necessarily related to the selected therapy (APE or LAR) but was associated with differences in quality of care, as hospital variation in CRM involvement is considerable and hospital factors such as annual hospital volume and type of hospital are of influence.[27,28]

It is difficult to prove a direct causal effect of clinical auditing on quality improvement, because time, as a proxy for innovation, is a confounding factor. However, there

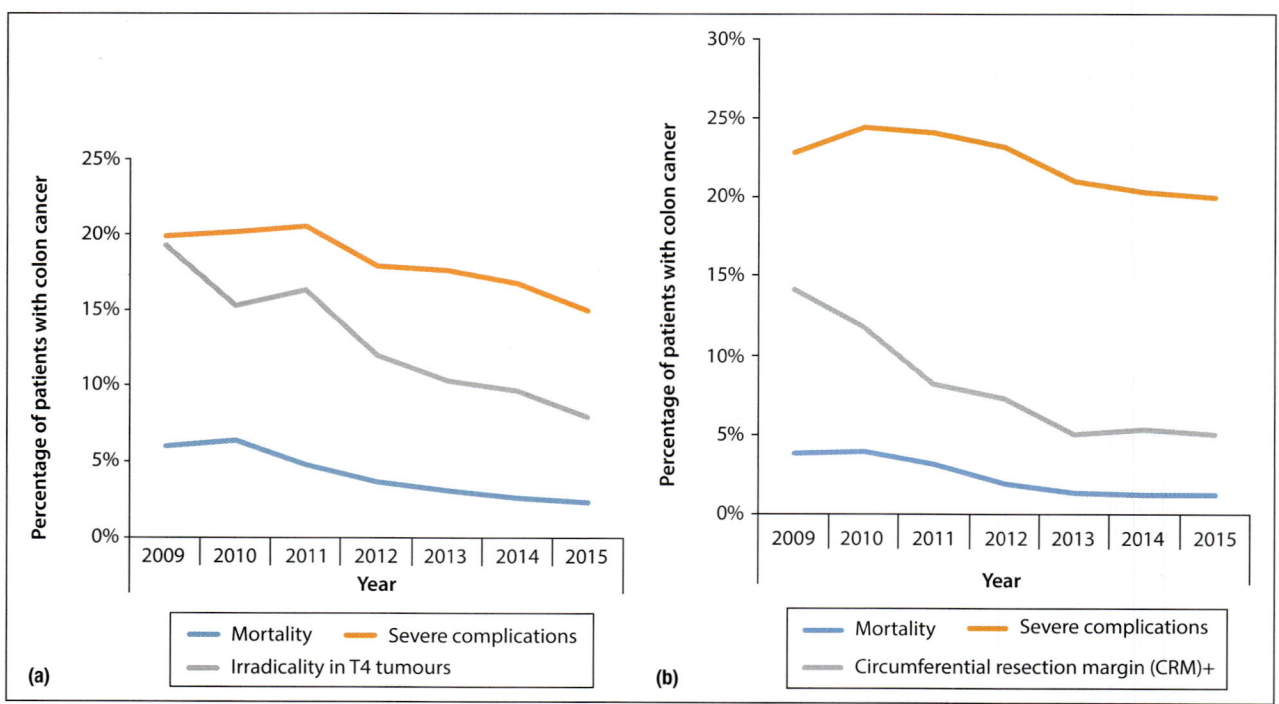

Figure 14.1 Line diagrams presenting trends in outcomes after (a) colon and (b) rectal cancer surgery from 2009 to 2015.

Courtesy: Nicoline J. van Leersum, Eric Hans Eddes, Michel W.J.M. Wouters and Rob A.E.M. Tollenaar.

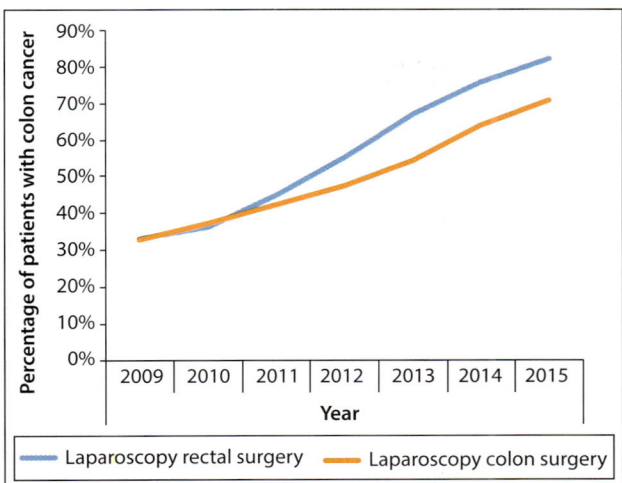

Figure 14.2 Line diagram presenting trends in the percentage of laparoscopic procedures in colorectal cancer from 2009 to 2015.

Courtesy: Nicoline J. van Leersum, Eric Hans Eddes, Michel W.J.M. Wouters and Rob A.E.M. Tollenaar.

is consensual view that the awareness and continuous evaluation of doctors of their outcomes, in relation to those of their peers, has led to a change in internal quality culture. Furthermore, during the same period, in the Netherlands, a similar improvement in outcome either did not occur in other gastrointestinal surgical procedures or started only after outcome registries were also introduced for these procedures.

In addition, we should take into account that although technical improvements in care are certainly important, it is the cultural component that is perhaps the most critical element in quality improvement.[29]

FUTURE

Patient Feedback

Notwithstanding its valuableness as a quality improvement tool, the data gathered for the DSCA provide only a limited view on quality of care: the clinical process and outcome measures that are important from a clinician's perspective with regard to safety and effectiveness of care. The perspective of patients may provide essential information to doctors to improve quality of care. In recent years, patient-reported outcome measures (PROMs) have been introduced.[30] The joint evaluation of clinical data and patient-reported outcomes on a patient level may be the key to better interpretation of PROMs, as demographic (such as socioeconomic status) and other confounding factors are available in the database to calculate risk-adjusted PROMs. Since 2013, PROMs data have been gathered on a voluntary basis.

International Benchmarking

New movements state that not only should patients take part in the registration process by registering PROMs, but also they should pronounce which outcomes really matter to them, when choosing a hospital, doctor or therapy, as these should be the similar outcomes that doctors should strive for when treating patients.[31] In 2012, a joint force of Michael Porter at the Harvard Business School, the Boston Consulting Group and the Karolinska Institute in Sweden initiated the International Consortium for Health Outcomes Measurement (ICHOM).[32] The purpose of this organisation is to define global standard sets of outcome measures that really matter to patients and drive adoption and reporting of these measures worldwide. The first sets are currently implemented in Dutch healthcare, enabling international benchmarking in the future.

Integrating Quality and Patient Feedback with Costs

As costs of healthcare are growing stronger than the gross domestic product in the Netherlands (in 2009, accounting for 15%),[33] our current healthcare system is not sustainable in the future. Where current payment models incentivise volume, there is a growing movement aiming to tie reimbursements to the quality and the value of healthcare (cost per gained health). Porter advocates that competition between hospitals on quality of care (outcomes) will reduce costs, owing to diminishing preventable complications and overtreatment and, thereby, will increase value of healthcare.[34] Recently, the Dutch Value-Based Health Care study showed that the addition of in-hospital costs to DSCA data may provide benchmark information on the value of care, and as variation exists between hospitals, there may be an opportunity to learn from each other's results.[35] An integral view on clinical outcomes, patient-reported outcomes and costs might be the holy grail to strive for in healthcare.

CONCLUSIONS

The joint effort of various stakeholders involved in the DSCA has led to large improvements in the outcomes of patients, more transparency of hospital performance information and significant cost reductions after colorectal cancer care. This makes the DSCA an international example of how to successfully improve healthcare on a national level. The leading role of the medical specialist association in the design and conduct of the audit has been essential for medical specialists to embrace the audit as a quality improvement instrument.

REFERENCES

1. Percival T. *Medical Ethics or a Code of Institutes and Precepts, Adapted to the Professional Interests of Physicians and Surgeons.* Manchester, UK: S. Russell; 1803.

2. Neuhauser D. Heroes and martyrs of quality and safety-Ernest Amory Codman MD. *Qual Saf Health Care* 2002;11:104–5.

3. Donabedian A. Ernest A. Codman, MD, the end result idea and the product of a hospital. A commentary. *Arch Pathol Lab Med* 1990;114:1105.

4. NICE. *Principles of Best Practice in Clinical Audit.* Oxon, UK: Radcliffe Medical Press Ltd; 2002.

5. van Leersum NJ, Kolfschoten NE, Klinkenbijl JH, Tollenaar RA, Wouters MW. 'Clinical auditing', a novel tool for quality assessment in surgical oncology. *Nederlands tijdschrift voor geneeskunde* 2011;155:A4136.

6. Mugford M, Banfield P, O'Hanlon M. Effects of feedback of information on clinical practice: a review. *BMJ* 1991;303:398–402.

7. Jamtvedt G, Young JM, Kristoffersen DT, O'Brien MA, Oxman AD. Does telling people what they have been doing change what they do? A systematic review of the effects of audit and feedback. *Qual Saf Health Care* 2006;15:433–6.

8. Govaert JA, van Bommel AC, van Dijk WA, van Leersum NJ, Tollenaar RA, Wouters MW. Reducing healthcare costs facilitated by surgical auditing: a systematic review. *World J Surg* 2015;39:1672–80.

9. Wibe A, Moller B, Norstein J, et al. A national strategic change in treatment policy for rectal cancer—implementation of total mesorectal excision as routine treatment in Norway. A national audit. *Dis Colon Rectum* 2002;45:857–66.

10. Pahlman L, Bohe M, Cedermark B, et al. The Swedish rectal cancer registry. *Br J Surg* 2007;94:1285–92.

11. NHS. National Bowel Cancer Audit. 2016. Available from: http://www.ic.nhs.uk/services/national-clinical-audit-support-programma-ncasp/cancer/bowel

12. American College of Surgeons. ACS National Surgical Quality Improvement Program® (ACS NSQIP®). Available from: http://www.acsnsqip.org

13. Kankerbestrijding SKVK. *Kwaliteit van kankerzorg in Nederland.* Oisterwijk: VandenBoogaard Print & Media Management; 2010.

14. NVvH. http://www.heelkunde.nl

15. The Dutch Surgical Colorectal Audit. 2009. Available from: http://www.dica.nl

16. Dutch Institute for Clinical Auditing. Annual Reports. 2011. Available from: http://www.dica.nl

17. Auditing DIfC. Annual Report 2010. 2010.

18. Van Leersum NJ, Snijders HS, Henneman D, et al. The Dutch surgical colorectal audit. *Eur J Surg Oncol.* 2013;39:1063–70.

19. Auditing DIfC. Annual Report 2014. 2015.

20. Dutch Institute for Clinical Auditing: Annual Report 2015.

21. Henneman D, Ten Berge MG, Snijders HS, et al. Safety of elective colorectal cancer surgery: non-surgical complications and colectomies are targets for quality improvement. *J Surg Oncol* 2014;109:567-73.

22. Henneman D, Snijders HS, Fiocco M, et al. Hospital variation in failure to rescue after colorectal cancer surgery: results of the Dutch Surgical Colorectal Audit. *Ann Surg Oncol* 2013;20:2117–23.

23. Govaert JA, Fiocco M, van Dijk WA, et al. Costs of complications after colorectal cancer surgery in the Netherlands: Building the business case for hospitals. *Eur J Surg Oncol* 2015;41:1059–67.

24. Bakker IS, Snijders HS, Grossmann I, Karsten TM, Havenga K, Wiggers T. High mortality rates after nonelective colon cancer resection: results of a national audit. *Colorectal Dis* 2016;18:612–21.

25. Jonker FH, Tanis PJ, Coene PP, Gietelink L, van der Harst E, Dutch Surgical Colorectal Audit G. Comparison of a low Hartmann's procedure with low colorectal anastomosis with and without defunctioning ileostomy after radiotherapy for rectal cancer: results from a national registry. Colorectal Dis. 2016;18:785–92.

26. Gietelink L, Wouters MW, Bemelman WA, et al. Reduced 30-Day Mortality After Laparoscopic Colorectal Cancer Surgery: A Population Based Study From the Dutch Surgical Colorectal Audit (DSCA). *Ann Surg* 2016;264:135–40.

27. van Leersum N, Martijnse I, den Dulk M, et al. Differences in circumferential resection margin involvement after abdominoperineal excision and low anterior resection no longer significant. *Ann Surg* 2014;259:1150–5.

28. Gietelink LH, D. van Leersum N.J., de Noo, M. Wouters, MWJM, Manusama E. Tollenaar, R.A.E.M. Tanis, P.J. The influence of hospital volume on circumferential resection margin involvement: results of the Dutch Surgical Colorectal Audit (DSCA). *Ann Surg* 2016;263:745–50.

29. The Commonwealth Fund. *Hospital Quality: Ingredients for Success—Overview and Lessons Learned.* 2004. Cambridge, MA: Institute for Healthcare Improvement.

30. Soreide K, Soreide AH. Using patient-reported outcome measures for improved decision-making in patients with gastrointestinal cancer – the last clinical frontier in surgical oncology? *Front Oncol* 2013;3:157.

31. Michael E, Thomas HL. *The Strategy That Will Fix Health Care.* Boston, MA: Harvard Business School Bublishing. 2013.

32. http://www.ichom.org

33. Kuenen JW Mohr R, Larsson S, Leeuwen van W *Zorg voor waarde.* Amsterdam, the Netherlands: The Boston Consulting Group; 2011.

34. Porter ME. A strategy for health care reform–toward a value-based system. *N Engl J Med* 2009;361:109–12.

35. Govaert JA, van Dijk WA, Fiocco M, et al. Nationwide Outcomes measurement in colorectal cancer surgery: improving quality and reducing costs. *J Am Coll Surg* 2016;222:19–29e2.

15

Impact of Chemotherapy on Postoperative Complications after Gastrointestinal Surgery

B. Sirohi, A. Mitra and S.V. Shrikhande

ABSTRACT

Neoadjuvant, perioperative and adjuvant chemotherapy/chemoradiotherapy form an integral part of treating gastrointestinal cancers to improve response rates, sphincter preservation surgery and survival. Multidisciplinary care has improved overall outcomes. The timing of surgery, chemotherapy and radiotherapy have an impact on the postsurgical morbidity and mortality. This chapter brings out the key issues highlighting these aspects.

KEYWORDS

Morbidity, mortality, chemotherapy, chemoradiotherapy, gastrointestinal cancers

INTRODUCTION

Neoadjuvant and adjuvant treatments are integral part of the multidisciplinary management of gastrointestinal malignancies. The use of neoadjuvant, perioperative and adjuvant strategies has affected the overall outcome and quality of life (QOL) of patients. However, these treatment strategies can potentially affect the postoperative outcomes and increase morbidity after surgery. The start of adjuvant treatment is dependent on the postoperative recovery. In this review, we aim to discuss the impact of neoadjuvant therapies on postoperative outcome and how the complications after surgical resections affect the use of adjuvant therapy.

CARCINOMA OF THE OESOPHAGUS

There has always been a debate about the best neoadjuvant strategy in oesophageal cancer: chemoradiotherapy (CRT) versus chemotherapy alone versus upfront surgery. Preoperative concurrent CRT using carboplatin and paclitaxel is the current standard of care for resectable oesophageal and oesophagogastric cancers, irrespective of histology. This regimen has shown to significantly improve overall survival (OS), when compared with surgery alone (49.4 vs. 24 months) within the ChemoRadiotherapy for Oesophageal cancer followed by Surgery Study (CROSS) trial. The recently published long-term follow-up of the CROSS study with a median follow up of 84 months confirms the survival benefit.[1] A meta-analysis of randomised controlled trials (RCT) has shown that both neoadjuvant chemotherapy and CRT provide significant survival benefit for carcinoma of the oesophagus, when compared with surgery alone, but a clear advantage of neoadjuvant CRT over chemotherapy could not be shown in the meta-analysis.[2]

The key issue with neoadjuvant therapy is its toxicity and impact on the postoperative outcome.[3] However, neoadjuvant CRT has been shown to increase the risk of respiratory, septic and cardiovascular complications but not mortality.[3] The risk of cardiovascular complications is increased, especially, in elderly patients.[3] A recent meta-analysis of 23 RCTs has shown that neoadjuvant chemotherapy does not contribute to increased postoperative morbidity and mortality, but neoadjuvant

CRT was associated with a significant increase in the risk of postoperative mortality for squamous cell carcinoma (SCC).[4] A recent multicentre European study also showed that neoadjuvant CRT leads to a significant increase in chylothorax, cardiovascular complications and thromboembolic events but does not influence anastomotic leak rates after oesophagectomy.[5] This increased risk after CRT may be attributed to increase in the cardiopulmonary insult due to underlying risk factors for SCC, such as tobacco and alcohol, and radiation-induced lung damage. A recent RCT compared neoadjuvant CRT and chemotherapy and found no difference in the overall morbidity and mortality.[6]

The mortality rates after oesophagectomy have reduced considerably over time; however, the procedure is still associated with considerable morbidity, ranging from 36 to 64%.[7] There is a differing opinion on the effect of postoperative complications on long-term outcome. These have been shown to negatively impact survival in some studies but not in others.[8,9]

CARCINOMA OF THE STOMACH

There is a distinct difference in approach to treating gastric cancers globally: Europeans and South-East Asians tend to favour perioperative chemotherapy regimens; East Asia tends to favour adjuvant chemotherapy and the Americans favour adjuvant CRT.[10–15] There is a debate about the extent of nodal dissection, D1 versus D2 versus D3 lymphadenectomies, but the general consensus is to perform a D2 lymphadenectomy.[16,17]

The two large RCTs that have shown a clear benefit in favour of adjuvant chemotherapy in gastric carcinoma are the ACTS-GC (adjuvant chemotherapy S-1) and CLASSIC (adjuvant chemotherapy with capecitabine-oxaliplatin [CAPOX]) trials in patients after gastrectomy and D2 lymphadenectomy.[10,11] Adjuvant CRT is currently the standard of care in the United States in view of the results of the INT 0116 trial, which showed a survival benefit for patients after surgery (the majority had undergone D1 lymphadenectomy).[12] The benefit of adjuvant CRT has also been shown within a subgroup analysis of the ARTIST trial for patients with node-positive disease, and this is now being studied in the ARTIST II trial.[18]

D2 gastrectomy is associated with morbidity and mortality rates of 35 to 45% and 4 to 16%, respectively. [16,17] The factors that have been shown to be significantly associated with morbidity include American Association of Anesthesiologists (ASA) grade, body mass index (BMI), combined organ resection and increased duration

of surgery.[19,20] Postoperative complications have been shown to be associated with a negative impact on survival.[21,22] In one of these studies, the grade of complication was an independent prognostic factor, with the survival being 43.0%, 42.5%, 25.5% and 9.6% for no complications, grade I, II and III complications, respectively.[21] The proposed mechanisms related to detrimental survival are immunosuppression and inflammation associated with postoperative complications. Immunosuppression allows proliferation and survival of residual cells in the host, whereas inflammation promotes the release of proinflammatory cytokines, which affect the function of natural killer (NK) cells, cytotoxic T cells and antigen-presenting cells (APCs), and also stimulates vascular endothelial growth factor (VEGF), which promotes metastases.[19] However, a recent study has found that Clavien-Dindo complication grade > II, sepsis and intra-abdominal sepsis do not contribute to a negative effect on the oncological outcome, but the predictors for OS were pTNM stage, male gender, age and adjuvant therapy.[23] In another recent study, the rates of completion of adjuvant therapy were compared to those of neoadjuvant therapy. Patients undergoing surgery first were less likely than patients treated with neoadjuvant therapy to complete at least one cycle of chemotherapy (56% vs. 100%; p = 0.001) and all recommended therapy (44% vs. 66%; p = 0.013).[24] One of the factors that might contribute to a detrimental survival in patients who develop postoperative complications is decreased use of adjuvant therapy, that is, the inability to initiate or complete adjuvant treatment. However, no study, till date, has investigated the impact of postoperative complications on the use of adjuvant therapy for gastric carcinoma.

Neoadjuvant chemotherapy comprising at least three cycles of perioperative chemotherapy is currently the standard of care for carcinoma of the gastroesophageal junction and stomach in European countries. This is based on the results of two landmark randomised trials: the Medical Research Council Adjuvant Gastric Infusional Chemotherapy (MAGIC) and the French Fédération nationale des centres de lutte contre le cancer/ Fédération française de cancérologie digestive (FNLCC/ FFCD).[13,14] In these trials, perioperative chemotherapy was compared with surgery alone and resulted in a better R0 resection (84% vs. 73%; p = 0.04), pathological downstaging and an improvement in 5-year progression-free survival (PFS) and OS (36% vs. 23%; p = 0.0009). Neoadjuvant chemotherapy, however, did not result in an increase in the rate of postoperative complications and 30-day mortality in the MAGIC trial (46% vs. 45% and 5.6% vs. 5.9%, respectively). Similar results have been shown in a recent meta-analysis of 12 RCTs, which showed that neoadjuvant chemotherapy resulted in a significantly better 3-year PFS, tumour downstaging and R0 resection rate when compared with surgery alone; but there was no difference in the postoperative complications and perioperative mortality.[25] However, the EORTC 40954 study showed that postoperative complications were more frequent in the neoadjuvant group.[26]

PANCREATIC ADENOCARCINOMA

Despite curative surgery in selected cases, the overall 5-year OS remains at 5% for pancreatic adenocarcinoma, as this is a systemic disease. Neoadjuvant strategies are increasingly being employed to improve the survival in resectable, borderline resectable and locally advanced pancreatic cancers.

Three randomised trials (ESPAC-1, ESPAC-3 and CONKO-001) have demonstrated that adjuvant chemotherapy is associated with improved survival and gemcitabine is the agent of choice in the adjuvant setting.[27–29] Adjuvant chemoradiation was found to be detrimental when compared with adjuvant chemotherapy or surgery alone in the ESPAC-1 trial.[27] However, it has been shown to provide a survival advantage in the GITSG and EORTC trials and recently in a John Hopkins–Mayo Clinic collaborative study.[30–32] Despite a decline in mortality after pancreatic resections, they are still associated with morbidity, which ranges from 30 to 40%, even at high-volume centres.[33,34]

The occurrence of postoperative complications and ability to commence and complete adjuvant chemotherapy have affected long-term outcomes. In a study from the MD Anderson Cancer Center, one-fourth of the patients were unable to receive adjuvant therapy, owing to delayed postoperative recovery.[35] A recent study looked at the association between postoperative complications and adjuvant chemotherapy use for all resected pancreatic cancers as per the American College of Surgeons National Surgical Quality Improvement Program (ACS–NSQIP) database.[36] Overall, 58% of the 2047 patients were treated with adjuvant chemotherapy and the chemotherapy usage was affected by the occurrence and nature of complications. Chemotherapy was given to 62% patients without complications compared with that given to 44% with at least one serious complication. Labori et al documented that early disease progression (34.7%), postoperative complications/poor performance status (32.2%) and age greater than 75 years (24.6%) were the reasons why patients (58%) were unable to initiate (p < 0.001) or complete adjuvant chemotherapy (p = 0.007).[37]

In a study by Kamphues et al, the occurrence of severe postoperative complications (grades III–IV) was an independent prognostic factor and associated with a significantly shortened survival (16.5 months vs. 12.4 months; p = 0.002).[38] In a study by Murakami et al, chemotherapy started within 20 days of surgery for pancreatic cancer was associated with a 5-year OS and PFS of 53% and 52%, respectively, versus 26% and 22%, respectively, when chemotherapy was started after 20 days.[39] However, a study from ESPAC-3 group has shown that completeness of all six cycles, rather than early initiation of chemotherapy, is an independent prognostic factor, and there is no impact on the long-term outcome in patients who are able to complete six cycles, even if chemotherapy is delayed up to 12 weeks.[40] The ability to identify a subgroup of patients who are at risk of developing postoperative complications and are unable to receive adjuvant therapy is important, as they can be treated with neoadjuvant therapy to maximise the survival benefit of a multimodal approach.

The use of neoadjuvant therapy is not supported by robust evidence, but many centres have adopted it owing to the advantages that it offers: decrease in local recurrence, delivery of radiation to well-oxygenated tissues, lower chances of bowel toxicity compared with postoperative radiation, earlier initiation of and increase in the chances of completion of treatment, in vivo assessment of response, decrease in the rate of futile laparotomies, no increase in postopertaive morbidity and improved cost-effectiveness.[41–43] In a large ACS–NSQIP database study, the factors affecting postoperative outcomes were age greater than 70 years, ASA class more than 2, preoperative sepsis, dyspnoea, weight loss, impaired functional status, peripheral vascular disease and operation time of longer than 8 hours.[42] In addition, it has been seen that preoperative CRT significantly decreases the occurrence of pancreatic fistulae, which may be attributed to an increase in pancreatic fibrosis after CRT.[44]

COLORECTAL CARCINOMA

En bloc resection of the primary and regional lymph nodes along with adjacent involved organs is the mainstay of curative treatment of carcinoma of the colon. Similarly, total mesorectal excision is the mainstay of treatment of middle and lower one-third rectal cancers.

Patients with high-risk stage II and stage III colorectal cancer (CRC) are candidates for adjuvant chemotherapy. The first randomised trial published in 1990 showed that fluorouracil (5-FU) and levamisole decreased the risk of recurrence by 41% in stage C colon cancer, and later,

5-FU and folinic acid were found to be more effective.[45,46] The MOSAIC trial has showed that addition of oxaliplatin to 5-FU and folinic acid significantly improves PFS, albeit with an increase in the adverse events.[47] Colorectal surgery is associated with a significant morbidity, ranging from 18 to 38%. In a recent study, approximately 15.8 of 2368 patients experienced at least one serious complication.[48] The common complications in this study were surgical site infections (SSIs) (10.9%), superficial SSIs (7.7%), return to the operating room (5.0%) and sepsis and septic shock (5.0%).[48]

The use of adjuvant chemotherapy for colon cancer is suboptimal. In a recent study, adjuvant chemotherapy was not used in 34% of stage III colon cancers, and this was influenced by patient comorbidities, demographic factors, hospital volume and individual hospital. The demographic factors include age, marital status, socioeconomic status and race.[49] In a recent large SEER database study, which included 17108 stage III CRC patients, 18% had at least one complication.[50] Adjuvant chemotherapy was not used in 46% of patients with complications versus 31% of patients without complications (p < 0.0001). The occurrence of complications was an independent factor responsible for omission of chemotherapy and contributed to delay in its use.[50]

The only retrospective study to study the impact of postoperative complications on delay in adjuvant chemotherapy and outcome for rectal cancer patients has shown that complications are associated with a delay in the commencement of chemotherapy of 8 weeks or more and are associated with a significantly lower OS in patients who received chemotherapy after 8 weeks or more in the presence of complications.[51,52] The occurrence of at least one complication increased the likelihood of treatment delay by 21 to 65%.[48,50] The types of complications that were associated with a significant delay in the initiation of adjuvant chemotherapy were overall SSIs, superficial SSIs, organ/space SSIs and sepsis or septic shock. The study also showed that the chemotherapy use decreased from 67 to 31% as the number of complications increased from zero to three.[48] The usage also differed according to the type of complication: 66% for superficial SSIs and 18% for renal failure.[48] A recent retrospective study focussed on the impact of anastomotic leaks after colorectal surgery on chemotherapy usage and outcomes. Patients with leaks had a higher local recurrence rate, as the usage of adjuvant chemotherapy was significantly lower (63% vs. 87%, p = 0.007), and the time to initiation was also longer but not significant.[53]

A delay in the timing of adjuvant chemotherapy for CRC has been shown to be linked to survival. However, it is still not clear as to what constitutes a delay. Two recent large retrospective studies have shown that there is no impact on OS and PFS in CRC if adjuvant chemotherapy is administered within 12 weeks of surgery.[54,55] However, a large meta-analysis of 14 studies, of which eight studies used an 8-week cut-off, showed that a delay in starting adjuvant chemotherapy of more than 8 weeks is associated with a significant decrease in OS but there is no impact on PFS.[56] Studies have shown that surgical resection increases the number of cells in the cycling phase and proliferation of the residual cancer cells and, therefore, leads to an activation of the dormant micrometastases.[57] A mathematical model has shown that the best window of opportunity to commence adjuvant chemotherapy is within 100 days.[58] A laparoscopic approach has been shown to negate the detrimental oncological impact of delay in the initiation of adjuvant chemotherapy.[59] A retrospective study has shown that laparoscopic surgery did not result in an earlier initiation of adjuvant chemotherapy, whereas in another study, the laparoscopic group received it 25 days earlier than the open group.[59,60]

The superiority of preoperative over postoperative CRT for patients with stage II and stage III rectal cancer was established by Sauer et al in the landmark German RCT. The preoperative continuous infusion of 5-FU–based concurrent CRT resulted in a significant decrease in the local recurrence (6% vs. 13%), without an improvement in OS. Since then, preoperative long-course CRT has been established as the standard of care for T3 and/or N+ rectal cancer. The recently published long-term results of the same trial also show a significant decrease in the local recurrence (7.1% vs. 10.1%).[61]

Sauer et al also showed that there was a reduction in acute (27% vs. 40%) and late toxicity (14% vs. 24%) with the use of preoperative chemoradiation.[61] However, various retrospective studies have tried to define the role of neoadjuvant treatment in the outcome after surgery for rectal cancer. Neoadjuvant CRT was found to impair the function of the rectal remnant in one of these studies.[62] An increased low anterior resection syndrome score was observed in 80% of irradiated patients versus 20% in nonirradiated patients. Similarly, in a large population-based observation study, neoadjuvant radiotherapy was also associated with a significant increase in the frequency of intra-abdominal abscesses requiring intervention after a Hartmann's procedure.[63] However, a recent phase II trial (EXPERT-C) has used an intensified preoperative combination of CAPOX and CRT and did not observe any significantly detrimental impact on the QOL and bowel function.[64] The prognostic factors for occurrence of postoperative complications after neoadjuvant treatment include a low serum albumin, intra- and postoperative transfusion, ypT0-1 stage, prolonged duration of surgery and ASA status III/IV.[65] The neoadjuvant strategies in rectal cancer are now focussing on whether it is possible to avoid CRT in view of long-term side effects—randomised trials are underway and comparison of neoadjuvant CRT with chemotherapy and initial data looks encouraging.

Patients presenting with features of obstruction require a stoma before initiation of neoadjuvant CRT. Whether or not a patient should have a stoma should be dictated by clinical rather than endoscopic findings.[66] According to two recently published studies, for patients who had a stoma, the initiation of neoadjuvant CRT was delayed but did not have an impact on complications or the percentage of patients treated and OS.[66,67]

COLORECTAL CANCER: LIVER METASTASES

Liver metastases develop in nearly 50% of patients at some stage of the natural history of CRC and approximately 20% patients present with metastases at the time of diagnosis. The survival time for untreated colorectal liver metastases (CRLM) is 4 months.[68] Curative resection is the best treatment strategy for CRLM and 5-year survival rates ranging from 36 to 58% have been achieved.[69,70] Colorectal liver metastases can be resectable, potentially resectable and unresectable at presentation. The goal of preoperative therapy in the first two settings is to prolong survival, as compared with resection alone (neoadjuvant), and improve respectability by downsizing (conversion). Three meta-analysis of RCTs showed no effect on OS of neoadjuvant therapy on resectable CRLM.[71–73] However, a subgroup analysis showed a significant improvement in PFS with the use of hepatic arterial infusion (HAI) and systemic chemotherapy and a trend towards an improved OS with systemic chemotherapy.[72,73] The real impact of neoadjuvant therapy on long-term outcome of CRLM needs to be explored further. The use of systemic agents for unresectable CRLMs has yielded an R0 resection rate of 13 to 38% in large series, with a 5-year OS ranging from 33 to 50%.[74,75]

However, the use of various systemic agents has been shown to impact the outcomes after liver resections. Chemotherapeutic agents such as oxaliplatin and irinotecan lead to morpholocal changes in the liver parenchyma, namely the sinusoidal obstructive syndrome (SOS) and chemotherapy-associated steatohepatitis (CASH), respectively.[76]

The SOS is histologically characterised by dilatation and congestion of the sinusoidal spaces, with discontinuity in the sinusoidal membrane and deposition of collagen in the perisinusoidal spaces. Macroscopically, it presents as a 'blue liver.' Rubbia-Brandt et al were the first to document the presence of the SOS in patients with CRLM treated with chemotherapy.[77] Histological changes were documented in 29% of patients who were treated with chemotherapy preoperatively versus none in those who underwent surgery alone. These changes were seen in 79% of patients who received oxaliplatin versus 23% of patients treated with other regimens, and their presence was not related to the dose of oxaliplatin.[77] Other studies have also shown that patients with CRLM treated with oxaliplatin-based chemotherapy had vascular abnormalities and sinusoidal injury.[78,79] These patients were more likely to require intraoperative blood transfusion, especially those with the severest vascular abnormalities.[78] Some studies have shown that there is no significant increase in mortality and morbidity in chemotherapy-treated CRLM patients, whereas others have shown a significantly increased morbidity, without an impact on mortality. In a study by Aloia et al, treatment with more than 12 courses of chemotherapy was associated with a significant increase in hospital stay and the percentage of patients requiring reoperations.[78] Other studies have also shown that a prolonged course of oxaliplatin-based chemotherapy (nine cycles or more) was significantly associated with liver insufficiency, without an improvement in the pathological response rates.[80] Patients with sinusoidal injury were more likely to have a prolonged preoperative ICG R-15 of more than 10%, raised postoperative bilirubin and prolonged hospital stay.[79] Factors predictive of sinusoidal injury included female gender, administration of six cycles or more of oxaliplatin-based chemotherapy, an abnormal value of the preoperative aspartate aminotransferase (>36 IU/L) and an abnormal preoperative ICG-R15 (>10%).[79]

Nonalcoholic fatty liver disease is a spectrum of disease ranging from steatosis to steatohepatitis.[81] Administration of chemotherapy is associated with similar changes and is thus termed CASH. The CASH can result from oxaliplatin and 5-FU, but the most common agent is irinotecan.[76] Behrns et al were the first to show that moderate to severe steatosis is associated with an increased likelihood of liver insufficiency and mortality after major liver resections.[82] Fernandez et al calculated the mean biopsy scores of patients treated with or without chemotherapy and concluded that administration of irinotecan-/oxaliplatin-based chemotherapy, especially in obese patients, was significantly associated with severe steatohepatitis.[83] In a study by Vauthey et al, administration of irinotecan was associated with steatohepatitis in 20.2% versus 4.4% (p < 0.001) in those without chemotherapy. Steatohepatitis was also associated with a 90-day mortality of 14.7% versus 1.6% (p = 0.001) and an increased risk of death from liver failure of 5.8% versus 0.8% (p = 0.01).[76] Another study showed that a greater degree of steatosis was significantly associated with admission to the intensive care unit, morbidity, infective complications and biochemical profile changes and that steatosis was an independent predictor of morbidity.[84] However, Parikh et al showed that irinotecan-based chemotherapy was associated with development of steatosis but not associated with an increase in the perioperative morbidity and mortality after liver resection.[85]

The best evidence for the use of targeted agents in combination with chemotherapy is in the setting of unresectable CRLM as conversion therapy. Addition of bevacuzimab to irinotecan has resulted in an improvement in OS and PFS; however, its addition to oxaliplatin has furnished no such results.[86,87] Cetuximab combined with both irinotecan and oxaliplatin has been shown to be the first-line neoadjuvant treatment strategy for CRLM.[88,89] The response rates with these combinations have ranged from 45 to 55%, with R0 resection rates as high as 25%.[88–90] Animal studies in mice have shown that anti-VEGF antibodies result in an impaired liver regeneration and hepatocyte proliferation, whereas anti-epidermal growth factor receptor (EGFR) antibodies are not associated with any impact on liver parenchyma.[91] Majority of studies have found bevacuzimab to be a safe agent, with no impact on morbidity and mortality if a gap of more than 6 to 8 weeks is kept between administration and surgery; however, a pooled data set of seven RCTs showed an increased incidence of wound complications.[92–96] A recent meta-analysis has shown that bevacuzimab has a protective effect on the liver parenchyma, without an increase in morbidity and mortality.[95] Two recent case–control studies have shown that the addition of cetuximab to the neoadjuvant chemotherapy regimens does not appear to increase the morbidity rate after hepatectomy for CRLM.[97,98]

HEPATOCELLULAR CARCINOMA

Resection or liver transplantation can be considered for hepatocellular carcinomas (HCC) within the Milan criteria with Child–Pugh A liver function. However, liver resection can also be performed for high-risk HCCs, including large-sized, multinodular HCCs, with acceptable outcomes.[99] Transarterial chemoembolisation (TACE) has been used in preoperative and adjuvant settings for HCC. Various strategies, including TACE, have been tried as bridge to liver transplantation, with the aim of decreasing progression and drop out rate, while on the waiting list.[100] Although there are no randomised trials recommending the use of this approach, a recent study has shown that drug-eluting bead (DEB) TACE is associated with a higher response rate (44.7% vs. 32.0%; p = 0.2834) and higher 3-year PFS (87.4% vs. 61.5%; p = 0.0493) when compared with conventional TACE.[101]

An additional use of TACE is for downsizing the tumour to be within the transplantation criteria. Prospective studies have shown that the survival of those with transplanted HCCs downsized with TACE to within Milan or UCSF criteria is similar to those who initially met these criteria.[102,103] However, preoperative TACE before liver transplantation has been found to be safe in retrospective comparative studies and did not result in an increase in the operative difficulty, perioperative morbidity or mortality.[104] Transarterial chemoembolisation is used preoperatively in the setting of resectable HCC, with the aim to improve response, PFS and OS. However, a systematic review of randomised and nonrandomised trials and another meta-analysis of four RCTs have shown a higher pathological response rate but no improvement in PFS and OS with the use of preoperative TACE.[105,106] Preoperative TACE has also been found to be associated with a higher cost but similar morbidity and mortality as compared with surgery alone.[106,107] In a recent retrospective comparative study, preoperative TACE therapy was found to be associated with significantly raised enzymes preoperatively and longer duration of surgery, though without an increase in complication rates.[108]

BILIARY TRACT CANCERS

The surgical treatment of cholangiocarcinomas and gallbladder cancers has been improving steadily, with broader indications, decreased morbidity and improved outcomes. However, the overall outcome for these cancers remains poor, mainly because of advanced disease stage presentation and refractoriness to most treatments. Randomised data on the use of adjuvant strategies, including chemotherapy, CRT and TACE, are lacking, and currently, there is no standard of care.

A retrospective study has shown that patients with major postoperative morbidity after resection for hilar cholangiocarcinoma had a worse OS and PFS.[109] Neoadjuvant strategies are also being used for gallbladder and biliary tract cancers safely and with acceptable morbidity; however, detailed analysis on postoperative mortality and morbidity is lacking.[110,111]

CONCLUSIONS

Overall, the judicious use of neoadjuvant strategies has had an impact on the overall outcome of many gastrointestinal cancers, without compromising surgical safety. The data are compelling in patients with rectal, oesophageal and gastric cancers as well as in those with CRLM; however, robust level 1 evidence has to be awaited in hepatopancreatobiliary cancers. Adjuvant treatment has an effect on cancer-specific survivals for most stage II and beyond cancers. The future for neoadjuvant strategy, hopefully, will be careful selection of chemotherapy and targeted drugs based on specific actionable mutations or targets. Whether or not a patient receives adjuvant treatment may be decided by the ct-DNA (circulating tumour DNA), the data for which looks promising in colon cancer.[112]

REFERENCES

1. Shapiro J, van Lanschot JJ, Hulshof MC, et al; CROSS study group. Neoadjuvant chemoradiotherapy plus surgery versus surgery alone for oesophageal or junctional cancer (CROSS): long-term results of a randomised controlled trial. *Lancet Oncol* 2015;16:1090–8.

2. Sjoquist KM, Burmeister BH, Smithers BM, et al. Survival after neoadjuvant chemotherapy or chemoradiotherapy for resectable oesophageal carcinoma: an updated meta-analysis. *Lancet Oncol* 2011;12:681–92.

3. Ruol A, Portale G, Castoro C, et al. Effects of neoadjuvant therapy on perioperative morbidity in elderly patients undergoing esophagectomy for esophageal cancer. *Ann Surg Oncol* 2007;14:3243–50.

4. Kumagai K, Rouvelas I, Tsai JA, et al. Meta-analysis of postoperative morbidity and perioperative mortality in patients receiving neoadjuvant chemotherapy or chemoradiotherapy for resectable oesophageal and gastro-oesophageal junctional cancers. *Br J Surg* 2014;101:321–38.

5. Gronnier C, Tréchot B, Duhamel A, et al. Impact of neoadjuvant chemoradiotherapy on postoperative outcomes after esophageal cancer resection: results of a European multicenter study. *Ann Surg* 2014;260:764–70.

6. Klevebro F, Johnsen G, Johnson E, et al. Morbidity and mortality after surgery for cancer of the oesophagus and gastro-oesophageal junction: a randomized clinical trial of neoadjuvant chemotherapy vs. neoadjuvant chemoradiation. *Eur J Surg Oncol* 2015;41:920–6.

7. Atkins BZ, Shah AS, Hutcheson KA, et al. Reducing hospital morbidity and mortality following esophagectomy. *Ann Thorac Surg* 2004;78:1170–6.

8. Rizk NP, Bach PB, Schrag D, et al. The impact of complications on outcomes after resection for esophageal and gastroesophageal junction carcinoma. *J Am Coll Surg* 2004;198:42–50.

9. Ancona E, Cagol M, Epifani M, et al. Surgical complications do not affect long term survival after esophagectomy for carcinoma of the thoracic esophagus and cardia. *J Am Coll Surg* 2006;203:661–9.

10. Sasako M, Sakuramoto S, Katai H, et al. Five-year outcomes of a randomized phase III trial comparing adjuvant chemotherapy with S-1 versus surgery alone in stage II or III gastric cancer. *J Clin Oncol* 2011;29:4387–93.

11. Bang YJ, Kim YW, Yang HK, Chung HC, Park YK, Lee KH, Adjuvant capecitabine and oxaliplatin for gastric cancer after D2 gastrectomy (CLASSIC): a phase 3 open-label, randomised controlled trial. *Lancet* 2012;379:315–21.

12. Macdonald JS, Smalley SR, Benedetti J, et al. Chemoradiotherapy after surgery compared with surgery alone for adenocarcinoma of the stomach or gastroesophageal junction. *N Engl J Med* 2001;345:725–30.

13. Cunningham D, Allum WH, Stenning SP, et al. MAGIC Trial Participants. Perioperative chemotherapy versus surgery alone for resectable gastroesophageal cancer. *N Engl J Med* 2006;355:11–20.

14. Ychou M, Boige V, Pignon JP, et al. Perioperative chemotherapy compared with surgery alone for resectable gastroesophageal adenocarcinoma: an FNCLCC and FFCD multicenter phase III trial. *J Clin Oncol* 2011;29:1715–21.

15. Sirohi B, Barreto SG, Singh A, et al. Epirubicin, oxaliplatin, and capectabine is just as "MAGIC" al as epirubicin, cisplatin, and fluorouracil perioperative chemotherapy for resectable locally advanced gastro-oesophageal cancer. *J Cancer Res Ther* 2014;10:866–70.

16. Bonenkamp JJ, Songun I, Hermans J, et al. Randomised comparison of morbidity after D1 and D2 dissection for gastric cancer in 996 Dutch patients. *Lancet* 1995;345:745–8.

17. Cuschieri A, Fayers P, Fielding J, et al. Postoperative morbidity and mortality after D1 and D2 resections for gastric cancer: preliminary results of the MRC randomised controlled surgical trial. The Surgical Cooperative Group. *Lancet* 1996;347:995–9.

18. Lee J, Lim do H, Kim S, et al. Phase III trial comparing capecitabine plus cisplatin versus capecitabine plus cisplatin with concurrent capecitabine radiotherapy in completely resected gastric cancer with D2 lymph node dissection: the ARTIST trial. *J Clin Oncol* 2012;30:268–73.

19. Li QG, Li P, Tang D, Chen J, Wang DR. Impact of postoperative complications on long-term survival after radical resection for gastric cancer. *World J Gastroenterol* 2013;19:4060–5. doi: 10.3748/wjg.v19.i25.4060.

20. Schumacher G, Schlechtweg N, Chopra SS, et al. Impact of the body mass index on the prognosis and complication rate after surgical resection of cancers at the oesophagogastric junction. *Zentralbl Chir* 2009;134:66–70.

21. Jiang N, Deng JY, Ding XW, et al. Effect of complication grade on survival following curative gastrectomy for carcinoma. *World J Gastroenterol* 2014;20:8244–52.

22. Tokunaga M, Tanizawa Y, Bando E, Kawamura T, Terashima M. Poor survival rate in patients with postoperative intra-abdominal infectious complications following curative gastrectomy for gastric cancer. *Ann Surg Oncol* 2013;20:1575–83.

23. Climent M, Hidalgo N, Vidal Ó, et al. Postoperative complications do not impact on recurrence and survival after curative resection of gastric cancer. *Eur J Surg Oncol* 2016;42:132–9.

24. Fuentes E, Ahmad R, Hong TS, et al. Adjuvant therapy completion rates in patients with gastric cancer undergoing perioperative chemotherapy versus a surgery-first approach. *J Gastrointest Surg* 2016;20:172–9.

25. Xiong BH, Cheng Y, Ma L, Zhang CQ. An updated meta-analysis of randomized controlled trial assessing the effect of neoadjuvant chemotherapy in advanced gastric cancer. *Cancer Invest* 2014;32:272–84.

26. Schuhmacher C, Gretschel S, Lordick F, et al. Neoadjuvant chemotherapy compared with surgery alone for locally advanced cancer of the stomach and cardia: European Organisation for Research and Treatment of Cancer randomized trial 40954. *J Clin Oncol* 2010;28:5210–8.

27. Neoptolemos JP, Stocken DD, Friess H, et al. A randomized trial of chemoradiotherapy and chemotherapy after resection of pancreatic cancer. *N Engl J Med* 2004;350:1200–1210.

28. Neoptolemos JP, Stocken DD, Bassi C, et al. Adjuvant chemotherapy with fluorouracil plus folinic acid vs gemcitabine following pancreatic cancer resection. *JAMA* 2010;304:1073–81.

29. Oettle H, Post S, Neuhaus P, et al. Adjuvant chemotherapy with gemcitabine vs observation in patients undergoing curative-intent resection of pancreatic cancer. *JAMA* 2007;297:267–77.

30. Kalser MH, Ellenberg SS. Pancreatic cancer. Adjuvant combined radiation and chemotherapy following curative resection. *Arch Surg* 1985;120:899–903.

31. Garofalo MC, Regine WF, Tan MT. On statistical reanalysis, the EORTC trial is a positive trial for adjuvant chemoradiation in pancreatic cancer. *Ann Surg* 2006;244:332–3.

32. Hsu CC, Herman JM, Corsini MM, et al. Adjuvant chemoradiation for pancreatic adenocarcinoma:the Johns Hopkins Hospital-Mayo Clinic collaborative study. *Ann Surg Oncol* 2010;17:981–90.

33. de Rooij T, Tol JA, van Eijck CH, et al; Dutch Pancreatic Cancer Group. outcomes of distal pancreatectomy for pancreatic ductal adenocarcinoma in the Netherlands: a nationwide retrospective analysis. *Ann Surg Oncol* 2016;23:585–91.

34. Shrikhande SV, Barreto SG, Somashekar BA, et al. Evolution of pancreatoduodenectomy in a tertiary cancer center in India: improved results from service reconfiguration. *Pancreatology* 2013;13:63–71.

35. Spitz FR, Abbruzzese JL, Lee JE, et al. Preoperative and postoperative chemoradiation strategies in patients treated with pancreaticoduodenectomy for adenocarcinoma of the pancreas. *J Clin Oncol* 1997;15:928–37.

36. Merkow RP, Bilimoria KY, Tomlinson JS, et al. Postoperative complications reduce adjuvant chemotherapy use in resectable pancreatic cancer. *Ann Surg* 2014;260:372–7.

37. Labori KJ, Katz MH, Tzeng CW, et al. Impact of early disease progression and surgical complications on adjuvant chemotherapy completion rates and survival in patients undergoing the surgery first approach for resectable pancreatic ductal adenocarcinoma: a population-based cohort study. *Acta Oncol* 2016;55:265–77.

38. Kamphues C, Bova R, Schricke D, et al. Postoperative complications deteriorate long-term outcome in pancreatic cancer patients. *Ann Surg Oncol* 2012;19:856–63.

39. Murakami Y, Uemura K, Sudo T, et al. Early initiation of adjuvant chemotherapy improves survival of patients with pancreatic carcinoma after surgical resection. *Cancer Chemother Pharmacol* 2013;71:419–29.

40. Valle JW, Palmer D, Jackson R, et al. Optimal duration and timing of adjuvant chemotherapy after definitive surgery for ductal adenocarcinoma of the pancreas: ongoing lessons from the ESPAC-3 study. *J Clin Oncol* 2014;32:504–12.

41. Abbott DE, Tzeng CW, Merkow RP, et al. The cost-effectiveness of neoadjuvant chemoradiation is superior to a surgery-first approach in the treatment of pancreatic head adenocarcinoma. *Ann Surg Oncol* 2013;20:S500–8.

42. Cho SW, Tzeng CW, Johnston WC, et al. Neoadjuvant radiation therapy and its impact on complications after pancreaticoduodenectomy for pancreatic cancer: analysis of the American College of Surgeons National Surgical Quality Improvement Program (ACS–NSQIP). *HPB (Oxford)* 2014;16:350–6.

43. Araujo RL, Gaujoux S, Huguet F, et al. Does pre-operative chemoradiation for initially unresectable or borderline resectable pancreatic adenocarcinoma increase post-operative morbidity? A case-matched analysis. *HPB (Oxford)* 2013;15:574–80.

44. Takahashi H, Ogawa H, Ohigashi H, et al. Preoperative chemoradiation reduces the risk of pancreatic fistula after distal pancreatectomy for pancreatic adenocarcinoma. *Surgery* 2011;150:547–56.

45. Moertel CG, Fleming TR, Macdonald JS, et al. Levamisole and fluorouracil for adjuvant therapy of resected colon carcinoma. *N Engl J Med* 1990;322:352–8.

46. Haller DG, Catalano PJ, MacDonald JS, et al. Phase III study of fluorouracil, leucovorin, and levamisole (LEV) in high-risk stage II and III colon cancer: final report of Intergroup 0089. *J Clin Oncol* 2005;23:8671.

47. André T, Boni C, Mounedji-Boudiaf L, et al. Oxaliplatin, fluorouracil, and leucovorin as adjuvant treatment for colon cancer. *N Engl J Med* 2004;350:2343–51.

48. Merkow RP, Bentrem DJ, Mulcahy MF, et al. Effect of postoperative complications on adjuvant chemotherapy use for stage III colon cancer. *Ann Surg* 2013;258:847–53.

49. Becerra AZ, Probst CP, Tejani MA, et al. Opportunity lost: adjuvant chemotherapy in patients with stage III colon cancer remains underused. *Surgery* 2015;158:692–9.

50. Hendren S, Birkmeyer JD, Yin H, Banerjee M, Sonnenday C, Morris AM. Surgical complications are associated with omission of chemotherapy for stage III colorectal cancer. *Dis Colon Rectum* 2010;53:1587–93.

51. Tevis SE, Kohlnhofer BM, Stringfield S, Foley EF, Harms BA, Heise CP, Kennedy GD. Postoperative complications in patients with rectal cancer are associated with delays in chemotherapy that lead to worse disease-free and overall survival. *Dis Colon Rectum* 2013;56:1339–48.

52. van der Geest LG, Portielje JE, Wouters MW, et al. Complicated postoperative recovery increases omission, delay and discontinuation of adjuvant chemotherapy in patients with Stage III colon cancer. *Colorectal Dis* 2013;15:e582–91.

53. Kim IY, Kim BR, Kim YW. The impact of anastomotic leakage on oncologic outcomes and the receipt and timing of adjuvant chemotherapy after colorectal cancer surgery. *Int J Surg* 2015;22:3–9.

54. Lima IS, Yasui Y, Scarfe A, Winget M. Association between receipt and timing of adjuvant chemotherapy and survival for patients with stage III colon cancer in Alberta, Canada. *Cancer* 2011;117:3833–40.

55. Cheung WY, Neville BA, Earle CC. Etiology of delays in the initiation of adjuvant chemotherapy and their impact on outcomes for Stage II and III rectal cancer. *Dis Colon Rectum* 2009;52:1054–63.

56. Des Guetz G, Nicolas P, Perret GY, Morere JF, Uzzan B. Does delaying adjuvant chemotherapy after curative surgery for colorectal cancer impair survival? A meta-analysis. *Eur J Cancer* 2010;46:1049–55.

57. Fisher B, Gunduz N, Coyle J, et al. Presence of a growth-stimulating factor in serum following primary tumor removal in mice. *Cancer Res* 1989;49:1996–2001.

58. Harless W, Qiu Y. Cancer: a medical emergency. *Med Hypotheses* 2006;67:1054–9.

59. Gantt GA Jr, Ashburn J, Kiran RP, Khorana AA, Kalady MF. Laparoscopy mitigates adverse oncological effects of delayed adjuvant chemotherapy for colon cancer. *Surg Endosc* 2015;29:493–9.

60. Strouch MJ, Zhou G, Fleshman JW, Birnbaum EH, Hunt SR, Mutch MG. Time to initiation of postoperative chemotherapy: an outcome measure for patients undergoing laparoscopic resection for rectal cancer. *Dis Colon Rectum* 2013;56:945–51.

61. Sauer R, Liersch T, Merkel S, Fietkau R, Hohenberger W, Hess C, et al. Preoperative versus postoperative chemoradiotherapy for locally advanced rectal cancer: results of the German CAO/ARO/AIO-94 randomized phase III trial after a median follow-up of 11 years. *J Clin Oncol* 2012;30:1926–33.

62. Bondeven P, Emmertsen KJ, Laurberg S, Pedersen BG. Neoadjuvant therapy abolishes the functional benefits of a larger rectal remnant, as measured by magnetic resonance imaging after restorative rectal cancer surgery. *Eur J Surg Oncol* 2015;41:1493–9.

63. Jonker FH, Tanis PJ, Coene PP, van der Harst E; Dutch Surgical Colorectal Audit Group. Impact of neoadjuvant radiotherapy on complications after Hartmann procedure for rectal cancer. *Dis Colon Rectum* 2015;58:931–7.

64. Sclafani F, Peckitt C, Cunningham D, et al. Short-and long-term quality of life and bowel function in patients with MRI-defined, high-risk, locally advanced rectal cancer treated with an intensified neoadjuvant strategy in the randomized phase 2 EXPERT-C trial. *Int J Radiat Oncol Biol Phys* 2015;93:303–12.

65. Valenti V, Hernandez-Lizoain JL, Baixauli J, et al. Analysis of early postoperative morbidity among patients with rectal cancer treated with and without neoadjuvant chemoradiotherapy. *Ann Surg Oncol* 2007;14:1744–51.

66. Patel JA, Fleshman JW, Hunt SR, et al. Is an elective diverting colostomy warranted in patients with an endoscopically obstructing rectal cancer before neoadjuvant chemotherapy? *Dis Colon Rectum* 2012;55:249–55.

67. Anderson BJ, Hill EG, Sweeney RE, et al. The impact of surgical diversion before neoadjuvant therapy for rectal cancer. *Am Surg* 2015;81:444–9.

68. Wood CB, Gillis CR, Blumgart LH. A retrospective study of the natural history of patients with liver metastases from colorectal cancer. *Clin Oncol* 1976;2:285–8.

69. Rees M, Tekkis PP, Welsh FK, O'Rourke T, John TG. Evaluation of long-term survival after hepatic resection for metastatic colorectal cancer: a multifactorial model of 929 patients. *Ann Surg* 2008;247:125–35.

70. Choti MA, Sitzmann JV, Tiburi MF, et al. Trends in long-term survival following liver resection for hepatic colorectal metastases. *Ann Surg* 2002;235:759–66.

71. Nelson R, Freels S. Hepatic artery adjuvant chemotherapy for patients having resection or ablation of colorectal cancer metastatic to the liver. *Cochrane Database Syst Rev* 2006;4:CD003770.

72. Wieser M, Sauerland S, Arnold D, Schmiegel W, Reinacher-Schick A. Peri-operative chemotherapy for the treatment of resectable liver metastases from colorectal cancer: a systematic review and meta-analysis of randomized trials. *BMC Cancer* 2010;10:309. doi: 10.1186/1471-2407-10-309.

73. Wang ZM, Chen YY, Chen FF, Wang SY, Xiong B. Peri-operative chemotherapy for patients with resectable colorectal hepatic metastasis: a meta-analysis. *Eur J Surg Oncol* 2015;41:1197–203.

74. Adam R, Delvart V, Pascal G, et al. Rescue surgery for unresectable colorectal liver metastases downstaged by chemotherapy: a model to predict long-term survival. *Ann Surg* 2004;240:644–57.

75. Giacchetti S, Itzhaki M, Gruia G, et al. Long-term survival of patients with unresectable colorectal cancer liver metastases following infusional chemotherapy with

5-fluorouracil, leucovorin, oxaliplatin and surgery. *Ann Oncol* 1999;10:663–9.

76. Vauthey JN, Pawlik TM, Ribero D, et al. Chemotherapy regimen predicts steatohepatitis and an increase in 90-day mortality after surgery for hepatic colorectal metastases. *J Clin Oncol* 2006;24:2065–72.

77. Rubbia-Brandt L, Audard V, Sartoretti P, et al. Severe hepatic sinusoidal obstruction associated with oxaliplatin-based chemotherapy in patients with metastatic colorectal cancer. *Ann Oncol* 2004;15:460–6.

78. Aloia T, Sebagh M, Plasse M, et al. Liver histology and surgical outcomes after preoperative chemotherapy with fluorouracil plus oxaliplatin in colorectal cancer liver metastases. *J Clin Oncol* 2006;24:4983–90.

79. Nakano H, Oussoultzoglou E, Rosso E, et al. Sinusoidal injury increases morbidity after major hepatectomy in patients with colorectal liver metastases receiving preoperative chemotherapy. *Ann Surg* 2008;247:118–24.

80. Kishi Y, Zorzi D, Contreras CM, et al. Extended preoperative chemotherapy does not improve pathologic response and increases postoperative liver insufficiency after hepatic resection for colorectal liver metastases. *Ann Surg Oncol* 2010;17:2870–6.

81. Saito T, Misawa K, Kawata S. Fatty liver and non-alcoholic steatohepatitis. *Intern Med* 2007;46:101–3.

82. Behrns KE, Tsiotos GG, DeSouza NF, Krishna MK, Ludwig J, Nagorney DM. Hepatic steatosis as a potential risk factor for major hepatic resection. *J Gastrointest Surg* 1998;2:292–8.

83. Fernandez FG, Ritter J, Goodwin JW, Linehan DC, Hawkins WG, Strasberg SM. Effect of steatohepatitis associated with irinotecan or oxaliplatin pretreatment on resectability of hepatic colorectal metastases. *J Am Coll Surg* 2005;200:845–53.

84. Gomez D, Malik HZ, Bonney GK, et al. Steatosis predicts postoperative morbidity following hepatic resection for colorectal metastasis. *Br J Surg* 2007;94:1395–402.

85. Parikh AA, Gentner B, Wu TT, Curley SA, Ellis LM, Vauthey JN. Perioperative complications in patients undergoing major liver resection with or without neoadjuvant chemotherapy. *J Gastrointest Surg* 2003;7:1082–8.

86. Hurwitz H, Fehrenbacher L, Novotny W, et al. Bevacizumab plus irinotecan, fluorouracil, and leucovorin for metastatic colorectal cancer. *N Engl J Med* 2004;350:2335–42.

87. Saltz LB, Clarke S, Díaz-Rubio E, et al. Bevacizumab in combination with oxaliplatin-based chemotherapy as first-line therapy in metastatic colorectal cancer: a randomized phase III study. *J Clin Oncol* 2008;26:2013–9.

88. Van Cutsem E, Köhne CH, Hitre E, et al. Cetuximab and chemotherapy as initial treatment for metastatic colorectal cancer. *N Engl J Med* 2009;360:1408–17.

89. Bokemeyer C, Bondarenko I, Makhson A, et al. Fluorouracil, leucovorin, and oxaliplatin with and without cetuximab in the first-line treatment of metastatic colorectal cancer. *J Clin Oncol* 2009;27:663–71.

90. Ye LC, Liu TS, Ren L, et al. Randomized controlled trial of cetuximab plus chemotherapy for patients with KRAS wildtype unresectable colorectal liver-limited metastases. *J Clin Oncol* 2013;31:1931–8.

91. Van Buren G 2nd, Yang AD, Dallas NA, et al. Effect of molecular therapeutics on liver regeneration in a murine model. *J Clin Oncol* 2008;26:1836–42.

92. Kesmodel SB, Ellis LM, Lin E, et al. Preoperative bevacizumab does not significantly increase postoperative complication rates in patients undergoing hepatic surgery for colorectal cancer liver metastases. *J Clin Oncol* 2008;26:5254–60.

93. Utsumi H, Honma Y, Nagashima K, et al. Bevacizumab and postoperative wound complications in patients with liver metastases of colorectal cancer. *Anticancer Res* 2015;35:2255–61.

94. Hurwitz HI, Tebbutt NC, Kabbinavar F, et al. Efficacy and safety of bevacizumab in metastatic colorectal cancer: pooled analysis from seven randomized controlled trials. *Oncologist* 2013;18:1004–12.

95. Volk AM, Fritzmann J, Reissfelder C, Weber GF, Weitz J, Rahbari NN. Impact of Bevacizumab on parenchymal damage and functional recovery of the liver in patients with colorectal liver metastases. *BMC Cancer* 2016; 16:84.

96. Reddy SK, Morse MA, Hurwitz HI, et al. Addition of bevacizumab to irinotecan- and oxaliplatin-based preoperative chemotherapy regimens does not increase morbidity after resection of colorectal liver metastases. *J Am Coll Surg* 2008;206:96–106.

97. Pessaux P, Panaro F, Casnedi S, et al. Targeted molecular therapies (cetuximab and bevacizumab) do not induce additional hepatotoxicity: preliminary results of a case-control study. *Eur J Surg Oncol* 2010;36:575–82.

98. Pessaux P, Marzano E, Casnedi S, Bachellier P, Jaeck D, Chenard MP. Histological and immediate postoperative outcome after preoperative cetuximab: case-matched control study. *World J Surg* 2010;34:2765–72.

99. Truty MJ, Vauthey JN. Surgical resection of high-risk hepatocellular carcinoma: patient selection, preoperative considerations, and operative technique. *Ann Surg Oncol* 2010;17:1219–25.

100. Fujiki M, Aucejo F, Kim R. General overview of neo-adjuvant therapy for hepatocellular carcinoma before liver transplantation: necessity or option? *Liver Int* 2011;31:1081–9.

101. Nicolini D, Svegliati-Baroni G, Candelari R, et al. Doxorubicin-eluting bead vs conventional transcatheter arterial chemoembolization for hepatocellular carcinoma before liver transplantation. *World J Gastroenterol* 2013;19:5622–32.

102. Yao FY, Kerlan RK, Hirose R, et al. Excellent outcome following down-staging of hepatocellular carcinoma prior to liver transplantation: an intention-to-treat analysis. *Hepatology* 2008;48:819–827.

103. Ravaioli M, Grazi GL, Piscaglia F, et al. Liver transplantation for hepatocellular carcinoma: results of down-staging in patients initially outside the Milan selection criteria. *Am J Transplant* 2008;8: 2547–57.

104. Richard HM 3rd, Silberzweig JE, Mitty HA, Lou WY, Ahn J, Cooper JM. Hepatic arterial complications in liver transplant recipients treated with pretransplantation chemoembolization for hepatocellular carcinoma. *Radiology* 2000;214:775–9.

105. Chua TC, Liauw W, Saxena A, et al. Systematic review of neoadjuvant transarterial chemoembolization for resectable hepatocellular carcinoma. *Liver Int* 2010; 30:166–74.

106. Cheng X, Sun P, Hu QG, Song ZF, Xiong J, Zheng QC. Transarterial (chemo)embolization for curative resection of hepatocellular carcinoma: a systematic review and meta-analyses. *J Cancer Res Clin Oncol* 2014;140:1159–70.

107. Jianyong L, Jinjing Z, Wentao W, et al. Preoperative transcatheter arterial chemoembolization for resectable hepatocellular carcinoma: a single center analysis. *Ann Hepatol* 2014;13:394–402.

108. Rong W, Yu W, Wu F, et al. Effect of preoperative transcatheter arterial chemoembolization on the perioperative outcome of patients with hepatocellular carcinoma. *Zhonghua Zhong Liu Za Zhi* 2015;37:671–5. PMID: 26813431.

109. Chauhan A, House MG, Pitt HA, et al. Post-operative morbidity results in decreased long-term survival after resection for hilar cholangiocarcinoma. *HPB (Oxford)* 2011;13:139–47.

110. Sirohi B, Mitra A, Jagannath P, et al. Neoadjuvant chemotherapy in patients with locally advanced gallbladder cancer. *Future Oncol* 2015;11:1501–9.

111. Kobayashi S, Tomokuni A, Gotoh K, et al. Evaluation of the safety and pathological effects of neoadjuvant full-dose gemcitabine combination radiationtherapy in patients with biliary tract cancer. *Cancer Chemother Pharmacol* 2015; 76:1191–8.

112. Gingras I, Salgado R, Ignatiadis M. Liquid biopsy: will it be the 'magic tool' for monitoring response of solid tumors to anticancer therapies? *Curr Opin Oncol* 2015;27: 560–7.

Part III

Organ-Specific Problems

Oesophagus and Stomach

16

Complications after Oesophageal Surgery

M. Reeh, Y.K. Vashist and J.R. Izbicki

ABSTRACT

Prevention, early detection and sufficient management of intra- and postoperative complications during and after oesophagectomy are the key steps of safety improvement and reduction of still-high morbidity and mortality rates after this complex surgical intervention. Preoperative detection of specific and individual risk factors with consequent treatment of these risk factors can sufficiently decrease morbidity and mortality related to oesophagectomy. The implementation of preoperative risk scores into the clinical routine is a promising tool for outcome improvement of this highly invasive and complex technique. Pneumonia is one of the most common postoperative complications and one of the main factors of mortality after oesophagectomy. Intensive preoperative lung training can reduce the risk of pneumonia. Restrictive fluid administration and early extubation within 24 hours after oesophagectomy are the main factors for prevention of pneumonia. Anastomotic insufficiency and necrosis of the interposition graft are the main surgical risk factors of mortality after oesophagectomy with reconstruction by gastric tube or colonic interposition. A precise suturing technique, the avoidance of tension and the providence of an optimal perfusion of the conduit (stomach and/or colon) reduce the rate of anastomotic insufficiencies. Sufficient treatment of complications after oesophagectomy demands conservative therapy by intensive care specialists, interventional experts (e.g., endoscopic and radiologic interventions such as stent or drainage placement) and, of course, operative procedures such as reoperation in cases of uncovered anastomotic leakages, fistulas or empyema. Optimal patient outcome after oesophagectomy can be achieved only by interdisciplinary treatment approach, which enables low morbidity and mortality rates in high-volume centres.

KEYWORDS

Oesophagectomy, complications, prevention, diagnostics, treatment

INTRODUCTION

Oesophagectomies are most commonly performed for malignancies, and patients with oesophageal cancer usually have multiple comorbidities, which influence their intra- and postoperative outcome. In patients with adenocarcinomas, the main risk factors are obesity and cardiovascular diseases, whereas patients with squamous cell carcinomas suffer from lung and hepatic diseases, for example, chronic obstructive lung disease (COPD) and liver cirrhosis after alcohol or nicotine abuse. A further risk factor with a major impact on the perioperative course is cachexia due to the disease. Thus, oesophageal resections represent surgical procedures with high morbidity and mortality rates. This chapter will systematically describe the most relevant complications after oesophageal surgery, and we will present different strategies to prevent severe intra- and postoperative complications after the procedures.

PREVENTION OF COMPLICATIONS

The most important factor for prevention of complications in oesophageal surgery is the selection of the patient for operation. Objective diagnostic and several risk scores help to detect high-risk patients. This begins with a precise and detailed medical history. Further diagnostic tests are needed to define the patient's health status. Especially, objective cardiovascular, liver and lung function tests enable sufficient preoperative risk stratification before oesophagectomy. A low vital capacity (VC) of less than 80% and a low forced expiratory volume (FEV_1) (of less than 70%) are associated with a high risk of perioperative complications. The biological age is also a significant risk factor.

Several risk scores have been published for sufficient risk stratification in oesophageal surgery.[1] Most of them enable no adequate risk predication and others (such as the Physiological and Operative Severity Score for the enumeration of Mortality and morbidity [POSSUM] score) are too complex for daily clinical use. The preoperative oesophagectomy risk (PER) score published in 2016 includes objective diagnostics of the cardiovascular, lung and liver function systems.[2] The score has not been validated until today, but it may be a promising tool for sufficient risk prediction.

Especially high-risk patients need preoperative special recommendations for improvement of their health status. Some of these recommendations are as follows:

- Stopping alcohol and nicotine abuse
- Intensive lung training
- Avoidance of cachexia or malnutrition by adding preoperative enteral or parenteral nutrition
- Treatment of coronary heart disease
- Improvement of the liver function (e.g., transjugular intrahepatic portosystemic shunt [TIPS] installation in patients with severe liver cirrhosis)

NONSURGICAL COMPLICATIONS

Pneumonia

Pneumonia is one of the most common postoperative complications and one of the main factors of mortality after oesophagectomy (Figure 16.1). The main risk factors for the development of pneumonia are nicotine abuse and diseases of the lung parenchyma such as COPD.

Prevention

Intensive preoperative lung training can reduce the risk of pneumonia. Restrictive fluid administration and early extubation within 24 hours after oesophagectomy are the main factors for the prevention of pneumonia. Anaesthesia and mechanical ventilation lead to hospital-acquired infections. Thus, early tracheotomy should be performed in patients in which extubation is not possible.[3]

Sufficient analgesia is another crucial factor in the prevention of pneumonia. Continuous pain control by a peridural catheter enables sufficient breathing, and a strong cough also prevents the development of pneumonia.[4] Postoperative antibiotic prophylaxis treatment is not indicated and leads to bacterial resistance.

During surgery, careful handling of the lung during the preparation and dissection of the oesophagus and mediastinal lymph nodes is important for the prevention of pneumonia. Not only can the intraoperative mechanical irritation of the lung lead to lung injury and infection, but also the surgical procedure itself carries the risk of postoperative intermittent aspiration owing to the removal of the lower oesophageal sphincter and denervation of the

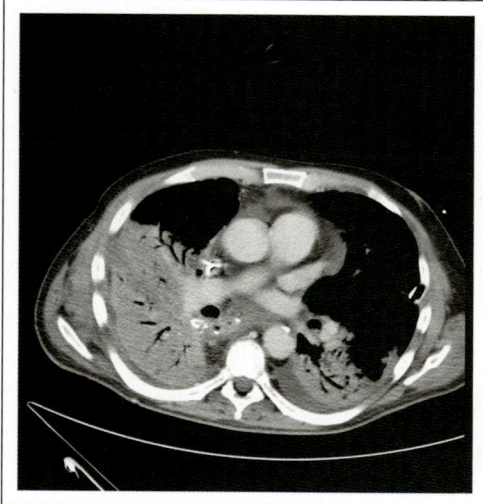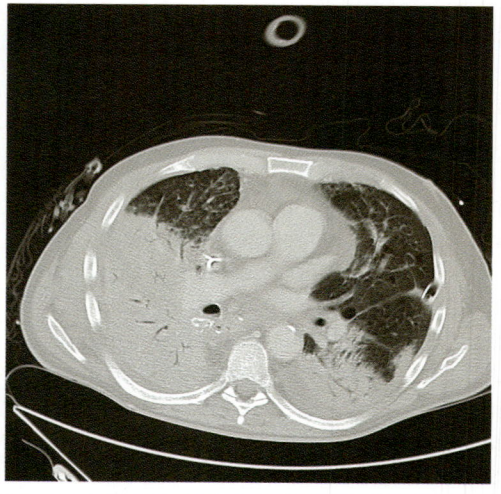

Figure 16.1   Computed tomography: Pneumonia after oesophagectomy.
Courtesy: Matthias Reeh, Yogesh K. Vashist and Jakob R. Izbicki.

gastric tube. Paresis of the recurrent laryngeal nerve can also cause severe pneumonia. Intermittent bronchoscopy with removal of obstructing mucous is the treatment of choice for the prevention and treatment of atelectasis and leads to an improvement of lung function when there is respiratory insufficiency or inadequate coughing.

Cardiac Arrhythmias

A cardiac arrhythmia can be the first sign of an anastomotic insufficiency, sepsis or mediastinitis.[5] Especially, tachyarrhythmia should be treated according to the cardiac guidelines by adjustment of the electrolyte balance, digitalis therapy or the use of a beta-blocker. Another option is the use of an electric cardioversion or a medicinal cardioversion with amiodarone. However, secondary to the cardiac treatment, surgical complications such as anastomotic insufficiency have to be excluded by further diagnostic tests, for example, endoscopy and computed tomography.

SURGICAL COMPLICATIONS

Anastomotic Insufficiency and Necrosis of the Interposition Graft

Prevention and Surgical Technique

Anastomotic insufficiency and necrosis of the interposition graft are one of the main surgical risk factors of mortality following oesophagectomy with reconstruction by gastric tube or colonic interposition.[6] Incidences are between 4.5% and 13% in the literature.[7–9] The insufficiencies are subdivided into the insufficiencies that occur early due to a surgical problem and late anastomotic insufficiency, which is usually caused by ischaemia and disorders of wound healing.

To prevent anastomotic insufficiency, the surgeon has to make sure that there are:

- Sufficient arterial perfusion
- A sufficient venous down gradient
- A tension-free anastomosis

This can be achieved by meticulous preparation of the gastric tube or colonic conduit, with careful dissection and protection of the feeding vessels. Thus, during the preparation of the gastric tube, the arteria and vena gastroepiploicae dextra and the arteria gastroduodenalis have to be preserved carefully. An oesophagogastrostomy should not be performed if there is ischaemia of the cranial part of the gastric tube. In this case, a colonic interposition should be considered. The effects of

preoperative embolisation of the left gastric artery or a two-staged ligature of the artery to improve perfusion of the gastric tube have been proposed, but there is no general agreement on the benefit of this manoeuvre.[7]

To achieve a tension-free anastomosis, a Kocher manoeuvre should be performed routinely before a gastric tube interposition. Further, avoiding torsion of the gastric tube or colonic conduit is crucial. Concerning the technique of the anastomosis, studies have shown no significant differences between a stapled anastomosis compared with a hand-sewn one for gastric tube reconstruction as well as colonic interposition.[10] However, the cervical anastomosis should be performed using the hand-sewn technique.

Clinical Symptoms and Diagnostic Studies

A continuous monitoring of the patient after oesophagectomy is needed for early detection of surgical complications such as anastomotic insufficiency and ischaemia of the interposition graft. Clinical signs are patient's delirium, increase in laboratory infection parameters, hypotension, tachycardia, fever, cardiac arrhythmia and a change in colour of the drainage fluids, especially of the thoracic drains that are placed in the area of the anastomosis. The aim of the diagnostic tests, especially of endoscopy, is to detect an anastomotic leakage, measure its size and evaluate the perfusion of the interposition graft (Figures 16.2 and 16.3). Further, treatment procedures such as EndoVAC™ therapy or drainage application can be performed simultaneously, if indicated. Studies have shown that postoperative

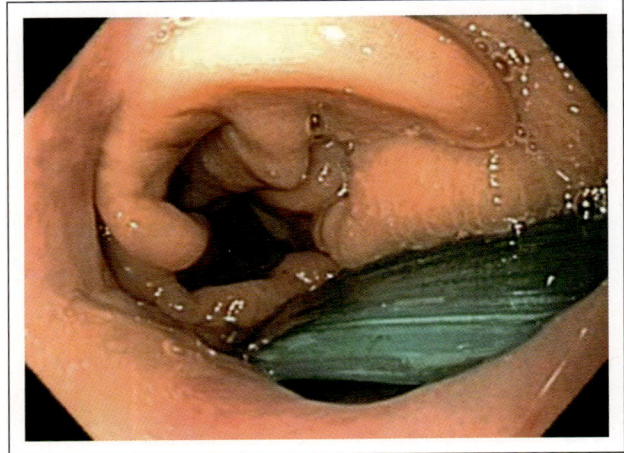

Figure 16.2 Endoscopy: Anastomotic insufficiency of an oesophagogastrostomy, with gastric tube reconstruction after oesophagectomy.

Courtesy: Matthias Reeh, Yogesh K. Vashist and Jakob R. Izbicki.

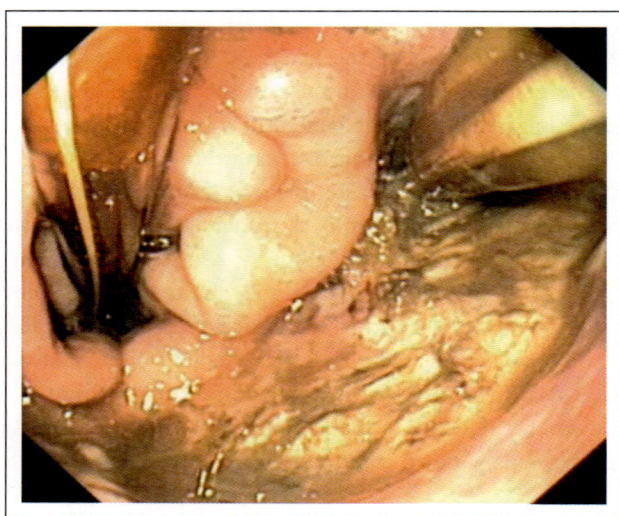

Figure 16.3 Endoscopy: Anastomotic insufficiency of an oesophagogastrostomy, with gastric tube reconstruction after oesophagectomy with thoracic abscess.

Courtesy: Matthias Reeh, Yogesh K. Vashist and Jakob R. Izbicki.

endoscopy is not correlated with higher morbidity rates. In contrast, smaller anastomotic leaks can be missed by endoscopy.

The second step in the diagnosis is computed tomography (CT).[11] The aim of this technique is to locate the thoracic, abdominal or mediastinal fluid collection (Figure 16.4), which should be drained simultaneously by CT-navigated drainage placements. Furthermore, CT can detect small anastomotic leaks by using oral contrast agents.

Treatment Options for Anastomotic Insufficiencies

The main goals of the treatment of an anastomotic insufficiency are the avoidance of sepsis and, in a septic patient, the removal of the septic focus.[12,13]

Thus, the treatment of anastomotic insufficiency depends on several parameters:

- Location of the insufficiency (thoracic vs. cervical)
- Perfusion quality of the interposition graft (ischaemia and necrosis)
- Patients' health constitution (noncompromised vs. septic shock)
- Time interval between operation and diagnosis of insufficiency (early [<48 hours] vs. late [>48 hours])
- Presence of a thoracic abscess or mediastinitis

Early insufficiencies often show no coverage by the mediastinal structures and show a free leakage of contrast agents. Thus, these insufficiencies, in general, require timely, operative revision. In contrast, late insufficiencies are often covered by mediastinal parenchyma or pleura without mediastinal abscesses or mediastinitis. In these cases, a conservative treatment regime can be followed.[7] In summary, the evidence for the treatment of oesophagoenteric anastomotic leakages is limited and the optimal treatment remains under discussion. Thus, we initiated a randomised trial (Esoleak trial) in 2015 that analyses the conservative treatment in comparison with the endoscopic treatment in case of anastomotic insufficiency after oesophagectomy. The first results are expected in 2017.

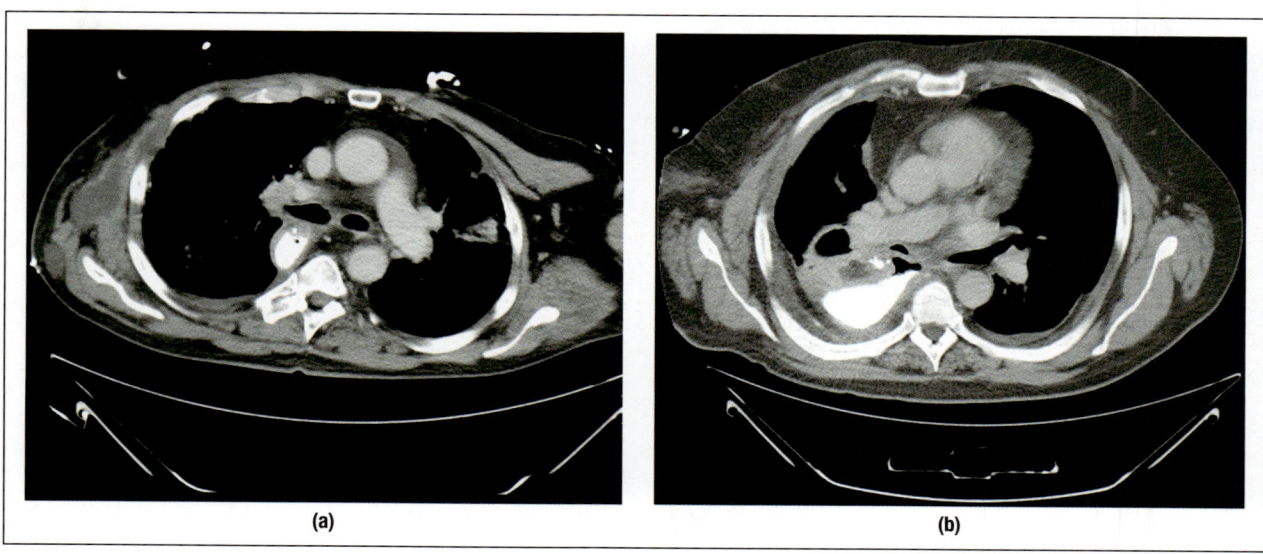

(a)   (b)

Figure 16.4 Computed tomography: Anastomotic insufficiency of an oesophagogastrostomy, with gastric tube reconstruction after oesophagectomy. (a) Intraluminal contrast agent, (b) extraluminal contrast agent.

Courtesy: Matthias Reeh, Yogesh K. Vashist and Jakob R. Izbicki.

Thoracic Versus Cervical Anastomotic Insufficiency

Thoracic anastomotic insufficiency can be subclassified into three stages[11]:

Stage 1 insufficiency
- Small insufficiency (see below under Stage 3 also, anastomotic insufficiency)
- Drained sufficiently (no fluid collections)
- Absence of septic signs
- Adequate perfusion of the interposition graft

Stage 1 insufficiencies are conservatively treated by sufficient drainage of the insufficiency, antibiotics and enteral nutrition by a feeding catheter placed in the jejunum. Continuous monitoring of these patients is inalienable. In case of an imminent sepsis, the conservative treatment regime should be re-evaluated. Small insufficiencies can be well treated by EndoVAC™ therapy. This treatment procedure is only possible in those parts of the gastrointestinal tract where endoscopic evaluation of anastomotic insufficiencies is applicable (oesophagus, stomach or rectum). EndoVAC™ therapy contains a sponge, which is placed into the insufficiency. Subsequently, a drain in the sponge that is nasal-channelled performs a continuous suction. The sponge is left in place for 3 to 4 days.

Stage 2 insufficiency
- Large insufficiency (see below also, anastomotic insufficiency)
- Drained adequately
- Adequate perfusion of the interposition graft
- Early septic signs

The adequate treatment regime of stage 2 insufficiencies is controversial. A consensus meeting in 2011 recommended the endoscopic placement of a self-expanding stent, which is positioned into the area of the insufficiency.[14,15] The stent should be removed after 3 to 4 weeks. Furthermore, thoracic or mediastinal abscesses have to be sufficiently drained, for example, by CT-navigated drain placement. At the beginning of septic signs, the patient has to be monitored in an intensive care unit.

Stage 3 insufficiency
- Large anastomotic insufficiency with wound healing disorder
- Ischaemic interposition graft/necrosis
- Sepsis or septic shock

Stage 3 anastomotic insufficiency demands emergency operative revision. In these severe cases, a resection of the interposition graft with installation of a cervical esophagostomy is often the only treatment option. The reconstruction can be performed after 3 months. Sometimes, the interposition graft can be shortened and a new anastomosis can be fashioned.

Cervical anastomotic insufficiencies can mostly be treated by reopening the wound and sufficient wound lavage. This conservative treatment regime often heals the insufficiency in 4 to 6 weeks. Inadequate reopening of the cervical wound can lead to mediastinitis and sepsis. The wound should be cleaned daily; furthermore, drinking of water and tea also cleans the wound.

In case of sepsis, mediastinitis or necrosis of the interposition graft, the interposition graft should be resected. A surgical revision with shortening of the interposition graft and reinstallation of a cervical anastomosis is often impossible. Stenosis of the anastomoses often occurs after healing of a cervical anastomotic insufficiency. In these cases, early endoscopic dilatation is the treatment of choice, sometimes followed by a surgical procedure in case of fixed anastomotic strictures.

ANASTOMOTIC STRICTURES

Anastomotic strictures often occur after healing of an anastomotic leak or are the consequence of a poorly perfused interposition graft (Figure 16.5). The clinical symptoms are dysphagia, nausea and persistent weight loss. The treatment of choice is early endoscopic dilatation. This can be challenging in stapled anastomoses. Thus, at the minimum, a 25-mm stapler should be used for anastomosis to prevent an anastomotic stenosis.[7]

POSTOPERATIVE DELAYED GASTRIC EMPTYING

Delayed gastric emptying and stenosis of the pylorus are often the consequence of the vagotomy of the gastric tube. A prophylactic pyloroplasty is obsolete and can lead to

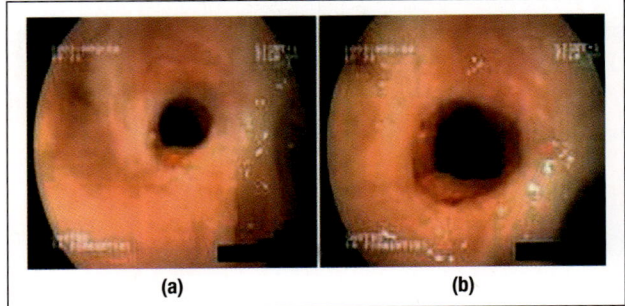

(a)   (b)

Figure 16.5 Endoscopy: Scarred stenosis of a cervical anastomosis after oesophagectomy, with gastric tube reconstruction. (a) Before endoscopic dilatation, (b) after endoscopic dilatation.

Courtesy: Matthias Reeh, Yogesh K. Vashist and Jakob R. Izbicki.

strictures. The first choice of treatment is the placement of a nasogastric tube with slowly increasing feeding volumes. Further, prokinetic drugs such as metoclopramide and erythromycin can be used. If the conservative treatment regime does not lead to a decrease of the clinical symptoms, endoscopic dilatation or the injection of botulinum toxin into the pylorus should be performed. Only in very rare cases is an operative pyloroplasty necessary.

DYSPHAGIA

Dysphagia can be the consequence of an injury or paresis of the recurrent nerve.[16] Thus, the radical lymphadenectomy demands a detailed anatomic knowledge of the mediastinum and the route of the recurrent laryngeal nerve. The right recurrent nerve can be easily injured in the area of the subclavian artery. In contrast, the left recurrent nerve is compromised in the area of the dorsal trachea. Paresis of both recurrent nerves is extremely rare and demands the performance of a tracheostomy. One-sided injury of the recurrent nerve leads to hoarseness and dysphagia. Both symptoms have to be treated by intensive logopaedic training and interdisciplinary therapy. Sometimes, a lateralisation of the vocal chords can be necessary.

CHYLE FISTULA

A chyle fistula can be easily diagnosed by the colour shift of the drain fluid. The drain fluid looks like milk. The incidence is between 2% and 5% in the literature.[17,18] For further diagnosis, chylomicrons can be analysed in the drain fluid. In most cases, conservative treatment is done by using parenteral or middle-chain-triglyceride (MCT) enteral nutrition. A high-output chyle fistula with a fluid volume of more than 1 L per 24 hours should be surgical treated by operative revision, with closure of the thoracic duct.

The duct should be dissected and closed by ligature directly cranial to the diaphragm to prevent a chyle fistula. Studies have shown that this technique reduces the incidence of chyle fistula from 2.1 to 0.3%[19] Thus, this procedure should be a routine step of an oesophagectomy.

INJURY OF THE TRACHEOBRONCHIAL SYSTEM

Owing to its close, anatomic location, the pars membranacea of the trachea and, especially, the left main bronchus can easily be injured during the dissection part of an oesophagectomy. In particular, neoadjuvant radiochemotherapy can cause severe adhesions between the oesophagus and trachea, which may complicate the dissection of the oesophagus.

During preoperative staging of T4 tumours, bronchoscopy should be performed. Definitive radiotherapy is the treatment of choice in patients with tumour infiltration of the trachea. In case of an intraoperative diagnosis of tumour infiltration of the trachea, an R2 resection should be performed, avoiding injuries to the trachea and the main bronchus.[7] In case of injury to the trachea or the main bronchus, primary closure by suture and additional coverage of the lesion by using well-perfused parenchyma, for example, pericardial flap, vena azygos and latissimus muscle, should be performed. In endoscopic treatment, double stenting of the oesophagus and the tracheobronchial system should be done to avoid the development of a bronchoenteric fistula.

CONCLUSIONS

Prevention, early detection and sufficient management of intra- and postoperative complications during and after oesophagectomy are the keys steps of safety improvement and reduction of still high morbidity as well as mortality rates after this complex surgical intervention. Best patients' outcome after oesophagectomy can be achieved only by interdisciplinary treatment approach, which enables low morbidity and mortality rates in high-volume centres.

REFERENCES

1. Abunasra H, Lewis S, Beggs L, Duffy J, Beggs D, Morgan E. Predictors of operative death after oesophagectomy for carcinoma. *Br J Surg* 2005;92:1029–33.

2. Reeh M, Metze J, Uzunoglu FG, et al. The PER (Preoperative Esophagectomy Risk) score: a simple risk score to predict short-term and long-term outcome in patients with surgically treated esophageal cancer. *Medicine (Baltimore)* 2016;95:e2724.

3. Tandon S, Batchelor A, Bullock R, et al. Peri-operative risk factors for acute lung injury after elective oesophagectomy. *Br J Anaesth* 2001;86:633–8.

4. Cense HA, Lagarde SM, De Jong K, et al. Association of no epidural analgesia with postoperative morbidity and mortality after transthoracic esophageal cancer resection. *J Am Coll Surg* 2006;202:395–400.

5. Stippel DL, Taylan C, Schroder W, Beckurts KT, Holscher AH. Supraventricular tachyarrhythmia as early indicator of a complicated course after esophagectomy. *Dis Esophagus* 2005;18:267–73.

6. Meyer T, Merkel S, Gohl J, Stumpf P, Hohenberger W. Changes and complication rate in surgery for thoracic esophageal carcinoma. *Zentralbl Chir* 2003;128:631–9.

7. Holscher AH, Schroder W, Bollschweiler E, Beckurts KT, Schneider PM. How safe is high intrathoracic esophagogastrostomy?. *Chirurg* 2003;74:726–33.

8. Mariette C, Taillier G, Van Seuningen I, Triboulet JP. Factors affecting postoperative course and survival after en bloc resection for esophageal carcinoma. *Ann Thorac Surg* 2004;78:1177–83.

9. Orringer MB, Marshall B, Iannettoni MD. Transhiatal esophagectomy for treatment of benign and malignant esophageal disease. *World J Surg* 2001;25:196–203.

10. Korolija D. The current evidence on stapled versus hand-sewn anastomoses in the digestive tract. *Minim Invasive Ther Allied Technol* 2008;17:151–4.

11. Palmes D, Bruwer M, Bader FG, et al; German Advanced Surgical Treatment Study. Diagnostic evaluation surgical technique and perioperative management after esophagectomy: consensus statement of the German Advanced Surgical Treatment Study Group. *Langenbecks Arch Surg* 2011;396:857–66.

12. Crestanello JA, Deschamps C, Cassivi SD, et al. Selective management of intrathoracic anastomotic leak after esophagectomy. *J Thorac Cardiovasc Surg* 2005;129:254–60.

13. Schubert D, Pross M, Nestler G, et al. Endoscopic treatment of mediastinal anastomotic leaks. *Zentralbl Chir* 2006;131:369–75.

14. Leers JM, Vivaldi C, Schafer H, et al. Endoscopic therapy for esophageal perforation or anastomotic leak with a self-expandable metallic stent. *Surg Endosc* 2009;23:2258–62.

15. Schubert D, Scheidbach H, Kuhn R, et al. Endoscopic treatment of thoracic esophageal anastomotic leaks by using silicone-covered self-expanding polyester stents. *Gastrointest Endosc* 2005;61:891–6.

16. Liebermann-Meffert DM, Walbrun B, Hiebert CA, Siewert JR. Recurrent and superior laryngeal nerves: a new look with implications for the esophageal surgeon. *Ann Thorac Surg* 1999;67:217–23.

17. Svanes K, Stangeland L, Viste A, Varhaug JE, Gronbech JE, Soreide O. Morbidity ability to swallow and survival after oesophagectomy for cancer of the oesophagus and cardia. *Eur J Surg* 1995;161:669–75.

18. Rao DV, Chava SP, Sahni P, Chattopadhyay TK. Thoracic duct injury during esophagectomy: 20 years experience at a tertiary care center in a developing country. *Dis Esophagus* 2004;17:141–5.

19. Lai FC, Chen L, Tu YR, Lin M, Li X. Prevention of chylothorax complicating extensive esophageal resection by mass ligation of thoracic duct: a random control study. *Ann Thorac Surg* 2011;91:1770–4.

17

Management of Pancreatic Fistula after Gastrectomy for Gastric Cancer

S. Morita, A. Okaro, T. Wada, T. Fukagawa and H. Katai

ABSTRACT

Pancreatic fistula (PF) is one of the major complications after D2 gastrectomy. The management of PF has a significant impact on the outcome. Two thousand three hundred and ninety two patients had surgical resections for gastric cancer at the National Cancer Center between 2005 and 2009. Patients with PF were managed by tube drainage and saline irrigation. Fistulograms via the drains were used to assess the cavity size and guide treatment. One hundred fifty two (6.4%) patients developed PF. This pancreas-related complication occurred more commonly after total gastrectomy with either pancreas-preserving splenectomy or pancreatosplenectomy. Eleven (7%) patients developed secondary haemorrhage, necessitating angiography and embolisation. There were 12 (8%) reoperations for drainage. There were two (1%) deaths refractory to the treatment. The meticulous and careful management in this group of patients by using tube drainage and irrigation methods is an effective means of treatment, which can prevent fatalities.

KEYWORDS

Gastric cancer, pancreatic fistula, drain amylase, lymphadenectomy, saline irrigation

INTRODUCTION

Gastric resection with D2 lymphadenectomy is the standard treatment for locally advanced gastric cancer in Eastern Asia.[1–3] Completing D2 lymphadenectomy requires extensive tissue dissection along major vascular structures in the retroperitoneum and around the pancreas, which increases the likelihood of pancreatic juice leakage.[4–9] Suprapancreatic lymph node dissection using surgical energy devices, such as the electric scalpel, ultrasonic coagulation scissors and vessel-sealing instruments, occasionally causes mechanical and chemical pancreatic parenchyma damage, as well as compression of the pancreatic parenchyma, resulting in pancreatic juice leakage from the damaged area into the surrounding tissues. Poor drainage has the potential of causing serious secondary complications such as intra-abdominal abscesses, anastomotic leakage and massive bleeding from the pseudoaneurysm formed by the leaking pancreatic fluid. The appropriate management of such serious complications has a direct and significant impact on overall outcomes. Therefore, it is critical to predict the occurrence of a pancreatic fistula (PF) and initiate appropriate treatment promptly, in order to minimise morbidities and fatalities. However, there are only few published studies in the world's literature that aim at offering guidance in the management of patients who develop a PF after gastric surgery.[10,11] This chapter outlines an approach to diagnosing and managing patients who develop this potentially fatal complication after gastric cancer surgery, based on retrospective data accumulated in our unit and a review of the relevant literature.

PATIENTS' DATA

Two thousand three hundred ninety two patients underwent surgical resections for gastric cancer at the National Cancer Center Hospital between January

2005 and December 2009. Information collected retrospectively and stored in our databases, relating to each patient, was accessed. All patients underwent gastrectomy with either curative or palliative intent. Patients who underwent wedge resection were excluded. In addition, those patients in whom surgery involved excision of synchronous other malignancies were excluded from this study. Gastric resections were classified as either total or partial, for the purpose of conducting this analysis. The former group included completion gastrectomy cases, whereas the latter group comprised patients undergoing proximal gastrectomy, distal gastrectomy and also those receiving pylorus-preserving procedures. As appropriate, we also performed a pancreas-preserving splenectomy, as described by Maruyama et al.[12] Patients were fully evaluated and staged after the diagnosis of gastric cancer within a multidisciplinary team structure. The extent of the lymphadenectomy performed depended on the type of resection and the stage of the gastric tumour, in accordance with Japanese classifications.[1,13]

DEFINITION

To date, no unified diagnostic criteria for PF after gastric cancer surgery have been established; however, an international consensus was reached for postoperative PF after pancreatic cancer surgery.[14] Specifically, the absence of a postoperative PF is defined as D-AMY, whereas a fistula on or after the third postoperative day (3POD) is indicated by a serum amylase level at least three times the normal upper limit. Grade A is defined as no specific treatment being required, despite a 3-fold or more elevation of D-AMY on 3POD. Grade B is defined as requiring a change in the management or adjustment of the clinical management. Grade C is defined as requiring a major change in the clinical management. Clinical intervention is aggressive and often carried out in the intensive care unit setting. However, the situation surrounding gastrectomy differs from that of pancreatectomy, because there can be pancreatic capsule damage during suprapancreatic lymph node dissection. Gastrectomy with lymphadenectomy by using electrical surgical devices has been a focal point in the development of PF. In clinical practice, at the physician's discretion or on radiological images, PF is diagnosed if there is prolonged purulent discharge containing pancreatic juice from the drainage tube. In particular, PF has reportedly been defined as a condition in which fluid with an amylase concentration more than three times the normal serum concentration is

drained from the peripancreatic area for more than 7 days postoperatively or purulent fluid containing turbid necrotic debris is drained from the peri-pancreatic area for more than 7 days.[15,16] Recently, Clavien-Dindo classification has come into use in some randomised control trials.[17]

It is certain that the D-AMY levels reflect the probability of occurrence for PF. However, high concentration of D-AMY does not necessarily follow PF if we could ensure delivery of the suitable drainage tube to the right place. It is crucial to be alert to the signs of infection for about 1 week.

INCIDENCE RATE AND RISK FACTORS

The published incidences in retrospective analyses range from 1 to 22%.[10,15,16,18–24] In our unit, the overall incidence was 6.4% (152 of 2392 patients). When focussing on PF defined as grade 3 or higher, according to the Clavien-Dindo Classification,[25] the incidence was 5.3% (126 of 2392 patients). There are some studies that look prospectively at the incidence rates that are quoting figures from 0.5 to 12%.[5,7,26–31] Two well-known European randomised studies, the Dutch and British trials, demonstrated operative mortality rates of 10% and 13%, respectively.[5,29] These high ratios were strongly related to distal pancreatectomy or splenectomy, which carried a significant risk of PF development; however, the reported incidence of PF was considerably lower. On the other hand, an Italian group reported that an acceptable operative mortality with an extremely low PF rate was achieved in phase 2 trials in selected institutions.[22,28] A single German facility also reported a low mortality rate, with 2.7% of cases developing a PF.[30] As a risk factor for PF development, total gastrectomy with either pancreas-preserving splenectomy or distal pancreatectomy and splenectomy was reported to be independent risk factor for this complication.[16] Furthermore, we found that 65 (24%) out of 276 patients who had undergone pancreas-preserving gastrectomy and 12 (60%) out of 20 patients who had received distal pancreatectomy with splenectomy developed a PF (Tables 17.1). We previously reported on risk factors associated with the development of PF and abscess in our experience.[15] The patients in that study underwent surgery between 1992 and 1999. In brief, the analysis showed age, body mass index (BMI), duration of surgery, tumour stage, splenectomy and pancreatosplenectomy to be the risk factors for PF development. In this more recent study, multivariate analysis of patients with PF revealed advanced age, male gender, high BMI, prolonged

Table 17.1 Patient and surgical information from both pancreatic fistula and nonpancreatic fistula patient groups

Background	Patients without pancreatic fistula (n=2240)	Patients with pancreatic fistula (n=152)	p value
Age (years)			
Median (range)	63 (21–90)	66 (30–85)	0.007
Sex ratio			
Male	1492 (66.6%)	130 (85.5%)	<0.001
Female	748 (33.4%)	22 (14.5%)	
Body mass index (Kg/m^2)			
Median (range)	22.3 (12.8–42.6)	23.6 (16.4–37.7)	<0.001
Surgical depth of invasion			
T1	1345 (60.0%)	37 (24.3%)	<0.001
T2/T3/T4	895 (40.0%)	115 (75.7%)	
Type of gastrectomy			
Total	524 (23.4%)	90 (59.2%)	<0.001
Partial	1716 (76.6%)	62 (40.8%)	
Operative time			
Median (range)	228 (80–575)	293 (145–555)	<0.001
Blood loss			
Median (range)	200 (2–5100)	453.5 (35–2820)	<0.001
Extent of lymph node dissection			
D0/D1	1205 (53.8%)	38 (25%)	<0.001
D2≤	1035 (46.2%)	114 (75%)	
Combined resection			
Splenectomy	211 (9.4%)	65 (42.8%)	<0.001
Pancreatosplenectomy	8 (0.4%)	12 (7.9%)	
Pancreatoduodenectomy	1 (0.04%)	0	
Neither	2020 (90.2%)	75(49.3%)	

Table 17.2 Multivariate Cox regression analysis for risk factors in patients with pancreatic fistula

Variables	p value	Hazard ratio	95% confidence interval
Gender (male/female)	0.004	2.094	1.275–3.439
Age	0.002	1.028	1.010–1.046
Body mass index	<0.001	1.124	1.064–1.187
Operative time	<0.001	1.006	1.004–1.008
Splenectomy or pancreatosplenectomy	<0.001	4.624	2.972–7.194
Surgical diagnosis of depth	0.001	2.189	1.385–3.460

operative time, splenectomy and surgical depth to be independent prognostic factors (Table 17.2). There is little to distinguish between these two analyses. This issue needs to be kept in mind when proactively managing postoperative care.

INTRAOPERATIVE DRAINAGE

For the purpose of obtaining information useful for judging the possibility of postoperative complications and ensuring efficient drainage, prophylactic placement of a

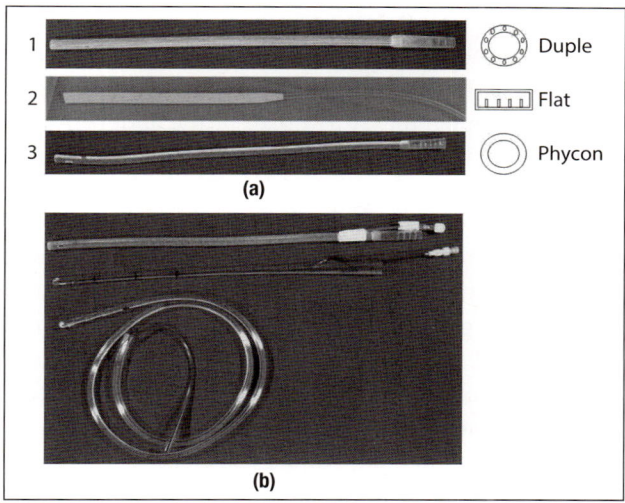

Figure 17.1 The type of drainage tube. (a) Single-lumen type: (1) with multiple intramural and side holes, (2) featuring tooth-like structure, and (3) without multiple intramural holes. (b) Double-lumen type.

Courtesy: Shinji Morita, Abuchi Okaro, Takeyuki Wada, Takeo Fukagawa and Hitoshi Katai.

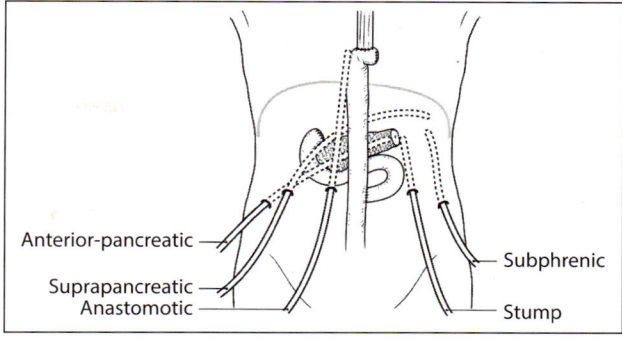

Figure 17.2 Schematic position of prophylactic drains is shown after total gastrectomy with pancreatosplenectomy and lower oesophagectomy.

Courtesy: Shinji Morita, Abuchi Okaro, Takeyuki Wada, Takeo Fukagawa and Hitoshi Katai.

drainage tube with multiple intramural and side holes is the standard strategy, with placement in a closed state, at our centre (Figure 17.1 a1). The positions and number of drains placed around the operative field depend on the type of gastrectomy and any additional organ(s) removed. We routinely place a single soft tube drain along the upper border of the pancreas (suprapancreatic region), after any type of gastrectomy. After a total gastrectomy with pancreas-preserving splenectomy, a second drain is required and it is placed in the left subphrenic space. In patients undergoing pancreatosplenectomy, an additional drain is placed in proximity to the tips of the drains in the suprapancreatic region. In patients undergoing bursectomy, an extra flat drain is placed on the pancreatic body over its entire length. After inferior mediastinal lymphadenectomy, one or two drains are usually placed around the oesophagojejunoanastomotic sites on either side (Figure 17.2). To prevent dislocation of the drainage tube, a soft drain with a flat shape is quite helpful (Figure 17.1 a2).

CLINICAL AND MANAGEMENT INFORMATION OF PATIENTS WITH PANCREATIC FISTULAS IN OUR UNIT

Five hundred sixty three (23.5%) of the 2392 patients who underwent gastric surgery developed at least one postoperative complication. Pancreatic fistula was the most common complication, occurring in 152 (6.4%)

patients. In this group, there were 11 (7.2% of pancreatic fistula group) patients with both a PF and an anastomotic leak. We had 10 (0.4%) patients with an intra-abdominal abscess unrelated to pancreatic leakage.

The majority of patients with PF (98; 64.5%) had a fluid amylase level in one or more of the drains, exceeding 4000 IU/L within the first 72 hours after surgery. A red wine–colored drain discharge in the first 72 hours was documented in 76 (50%) of these patients. Among the 152 patients who developed PF, intermittent irrigation was sufficient for treating 71 (47%) patients, whereas 43 (28%) patients required continuous irrigation. No irrigation was needed in 38 patients. The majority of patients were treated by employing one to two drains (105; 69%). Cultures from the drains were positive in 121 (80%) patients. Of these patients, 11 (9%) had coagulase-negative *Staphylococcus* and/or methicillin-resistant *S. aureus* (MRSA), which was thought to be due to a retrograde infection through the drainage tubes. Eleven patients developed secondary haemorrhage, necessitating angiography. The median length of hospital stay in patients with PF was 45 days, with 74% staying longer than 30 days. Two patients died of sepsis or sepsis-related multiple-organ failure during this period, due to a PF refractory to treatment (Table 17.3).

DIAGNOSIS AND MANAGEMENT

Early detection and effective management of PF are critical for preventing unnecessary morbidity and mortality. During the first 3POD, routine patient care is composed of daily blood collections, for measuring serum amylase, as well as determination of drain amylase levels, as previously reported.[15] In addition, the colour, volume and viscosity of the drainage fluid are monitored and recorded.

Table 17.3 Clinical and management information of patients with pancreatic fistula

Clinical/operative/management	Number of patients (n = 152)
Drain amylase (IU/L)	
Median over 72 hours (range)	5978 (282–397300)
More than 4000 IU/L over 72 hours	98 (64.5%)
Drain color over 72 hours	
Red wine (Bordeaux)	76 (50%)
Sero-bloody	39 (26%)
Serous	19 (13%)
White blood cell over 72 hours (median)	13,200 (5600–25,600)
C-reactive protein over 72 hours (median)	22.8 (8.1–41.33)
Method of irrigation	
Intermittent	71 (47%)
Continuous	43 (28%)
None	38 (25%)
Number of drains in situ	
One	47 (31%)
Two	58 (38%)
Three	32 (21%)
Four or more	15 (10%)
Angiography	11 (7%)
Positive drain microbiology	121 (80%)
Positive for CNS or MRSA	11 (9%)
Postoperative hospital stay	
Less than 30 days	40 (26%)
Greater than 30 days	112 (74%)
Reoperation	12 (8%)
Operation-related death	2 (1%)

Abbreviations: CNS, coagulase-negative *Staphylococcus*; MRSA, methicillin-resistant *Staphylococcus aureus*.

In the majority of cases, we are able to clinically identify within the first 3POD those patients with pancreatic juice leakage who are at risk of developing a PF by measuring the amylase level in the drain fluid and observing the colour (characteristically resembling that of Bordeaux wine due to haemolysis by pancreatic enzymes) and the consistency of the drainage material. In addition, we check whether C-reactive protein is elevated, accompanied by a high fever.

As previously indicated, a PF is said to exist when a patient is found to have a persistently cloudy or purulent discharge originating from the peripancreatic region for more than 1 week.[7] Patients diagnosed of having a PF are initially assessed by obtaining a computed tomography (CT) scan of the abdomen and pelvis to look for any intra-abdominal or retroperitoneal undrained fluid collections. This CT scan serves as a baseline. When the amount of daily discharge from the drains is deemed to be excessive or has a greenish-brown colour suggestive of an associated anastomotic or stump leakage, an urgent gastrointestinal contrast study should be performed.

The key to successfully managing PF patients is a 2-fold approach. The first principle is to guide the drainage tubes into any undrained spaces, in proper positions, under radiographic guidance. A guide-wired exchange technique under radiological control is our preference. Therapeutic replacement of a drainage tube, which has side holes without multiple intramural holes, is recommended to prevent fungi from propagating via the drainage tube itself (Figure 17.1 a3). This measure allows minor PF development to be prevented.

When a fistula persists despite this treatment, the second treatment approach involves decontaminating the cavity by aspirating or flushing out tissue debris. Both of these measures will minimise the exposure of surrounding vascular structures and other vital tissues to highly corrosive pancreatic juice and can thereby be anticipated to control infection. It is necessary to be mindful of drain blockages that can be caused by rather tenacious drainage fluid or debris, when identifying spillage from the side of the drainage tube or a sharp decline in drainage fluids. To prevent this, it is usually necessary to cut the drain short to allow for intermittent aspiration down the drain by using a sterile fine catheter and a 20 mL syringe (Figure 17.3). When PF exacerbation occurs, saline irrigation is carried out intermittently. The usual practice is to perform it once or twice a day with a 20 mL syringe, delivered through the drains. Intermittent irrigation tends to be used when the cavity is small, relatively clean and produces only small amounts of daily discharge. However, before irrigation can be safely commenced, the fistulous tract needs to be walled off from the general peritoneal cavity. This usually takes a minimum of 7 days. Alternatively, the drains can be placed on gentle suction. In this early stage, if the patient is found to be septic, broad-spectrum antibiotic administration is begun, pending any microbiology results. Patients are allowed to eat and drink about 3 days after the operation, provided there are no contraindications, and are encouraged to be ambulatory the day after surgery. A fistulogram is performed, usually by the 10th postoperative day, by

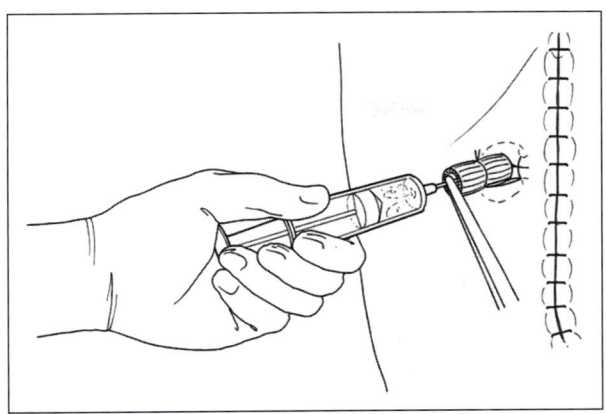

Figure 17.3 Intermittent aspiration down the drain by using a sterile catheter and a syringe.

Courtesy: Shinji Morita, Abuchi Okaro, Takeyuki Wada, Takeo Fukagawa and Hitoshi Katai.

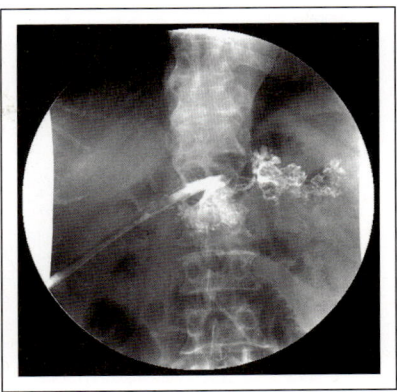

Figure 17.4 Fistulogram providing valuable information about the size and structure of the peripancreatic abscess cavity

Courtesy: Shinji Morita, Abuchi Okaro, Takeyuki Wada, Takeo Fukagawa and Hitoshi Katai.

injection of contrast down the drains. This very first fistulogram not only confirms the presence of a mature tract but also provides valuable information about the size and structure of the cavity (Figure 17.4). However, if an immature tract is identified, an additional fistulogram needs to be performed several days later. Fistulograms are repeated once or twice a week to check the position of the drain(s) within the cavity and to monitor changes in the size of the cavity, which is a good means of assessing the effectiveness of irrigation.

When managing intractable cases, the next step is to exchange the previously cut drains for double-lumen drains in preparation for continuous irrigation, once a mature tract has been demonstrated (Figure 17.1 b). Continuous irrigation is far more effective for any larger, contaminated and more productive cavities. Irrigation is usually started at an initial flow rate of 50 to 100 mL/h. An accurate hour-by-hour measurement of the fluid balance is important for early detection of any excessive fluid retention that may result from inadequate drainage of the irrigated cavity. The flow rate can always be adjusted later, according to the results of fluid balance measurements and subsequent fistulograms. Irrigation is continued until the fistulograms confirm complete obliteration of the cavity and the drainage fluid becomes clear and free of debris. In some instances, when the fistulogram shows an extremely small cavity and there are only small amounts of nonpurulent daily discharge, we elect to delay the drain exchange for some days while continuing to monitor the drain output. Finally, we begin to withdraw the drainage tube gradually over several days.

The drains can usually be removed shortly after the irrigation has been stopped. We prefer to observe the discharge from the drains for several days. If the amount is small and the fluid is clear, we deem the cavity to have been successfully drained. The drains are then shortened about an inch every other day until complete removal.

If the drainage effect is insufficient, it can be difficult to manage patients developing a second complication. Eleven (7.2%) patients in our series had both a PF and an anastomotic leak. We have found that there are two different types of anastomotic leaks in this group of patients. This conclusion is based on the time the anastomotic leak becomes evident and on patient's clinical behaviour. The early or primary leak usually becomes clinically evident very early in the postoperative period and generally leads to significant sepsis and large amounts of fluid drainage. These patients, though few in number, can be very difficult to manage. The primary leak was confirmed in 23 (1.0%) of the 2392 patients (14 in the oesophagogastric anastomosis, 7 in the duodenal stump and 2 in the gastro-gastro anastomosis) in our series. To evaluate postoperative patients in whom anastomotic leakage is suspected, passage was examined by contrast radiology. When the patients show little clinical symptoms and obscure imaging findings, intravenous therapy in the fasting state is provided in conjunction with drainage therapy. With progressive objective deterioration, the precautions for the next step should be the same as those for the management of PF. Therapeutic replacement of a drainage tube without multiple intramural holes is also recommended, as previously described. This is because the anastomotic leakage is bound to stir up intra-abdominal infection. In case the fistulous tract is still not walled off from the cavity, low-pressure continuous aspirator helps lower the risk for intra-abdominal infection from

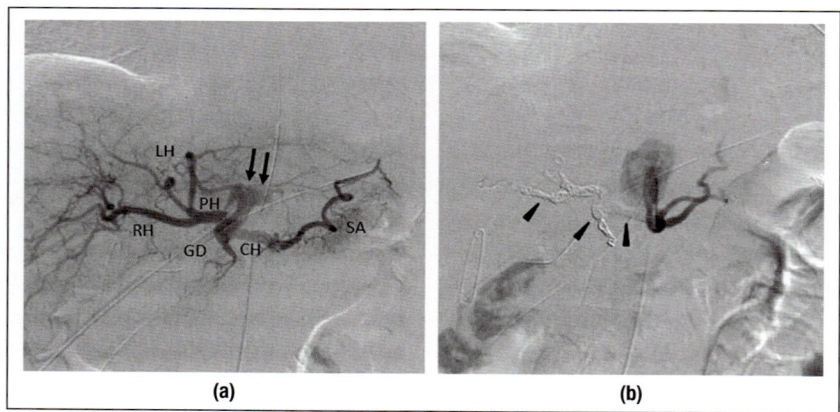

Figure 17.5 Control of secondary haemorrhage by means of transcatheter embolisation. (a) Celiac artery angiogram demonstrates massive contrast extravasation (arrowheads) from the bifurcation of proper hepatic artery and gastroduodenal artery. (b) Arterial embolisation (arrows) of CH, GD and PH.

Abbreviations: CH, common hepatic artery; GD, gastroduodenal artery; LH, left hepatic artery; PH, proper hepatic artery; RH, right hepatic artery; SA, splenic artery.

Courtesy: Shinji Morita, Abuchi Okaro, Takeyuki Wada, Takeo Fukagawa and Hitoshi Katai.

spreading. Reoperation was performed successfully in five patients for septic peritonitis caused by excessive leakage. It is necessary to provide quick and appropriate treatment in response to the severity. The second and more common of the two arises as a secondary event, usually later in the postoperative period, and occurs when the fistula cavity drains into the gastrointestinal tract via the anastomosis (internal drainage). Notably, such patients usually experience clinical improvement.

Secondary haemorrhage occurred in 11 of our patients, most of whom were successfully managed by selective angiography and embolisation (Figure 17.5). Since the early to the mid-90s, as standard practice, we have been performing angiography and embolisation when this potentially fatal complication of vascular erosion and rupture occurs. Previously, most patients underwent an emergency laparotomy to control the bleeding, but the procedure was technically demanding, as the tissues were difficult to handle and suture. This is now only rarely necessary in our unit, as interventional radiologists are much more skilled at locating and controlling the source of the haemorrhage. We have not needed to reoperate on any of our patients with PF for haemorrhage control in the last 5 years.

The mortality figure was 5.3% in the earlier period compared with 0.1% in our most recent study. We feel that a combination of refinement of the management protocol for patients with PF and changes in the way we approach patients with bleeding may have contributed to these differences.

Whenever the condition of a previously stable patient with PF is found to deteriorate, with signs of sepsis, a local cause such as an undrained/poorly drained primary cavity or a new secondary cavity is likely. Computed tomography and fistulography are clearly warranted in such cases, but a more general cause such as chest infection, urinary tract infection and line sepsis must also be considered.

Our unit's advancements in the field of interventional radiology have meant that reoperative procedures in this particular group of patients can now be avoided much more readily, and in our opinion, there are few reasons for a patient with PF to be subjected to reoperation. One valid reason for subjecting the patient to reoperation is when pancreatic juice leakage produces excessive amounts of fluid drainage, with accompanying sepsis. This scenario, although rare, usually results from a coexisting anastomotic leak. Surgery is performed to thoroughly clean out the peritoneal cavity, and multiple drains (in some cases up to seven) are placed throughout the abdomen and pelvis. Another reason is drains having accidentally become dislodged before the tract matures and hence need replacement. Finally, when haemorrhage cannot be stanched, direct surgical ligation is usually the last and only option. Twelve of our patients required reoperation: combined PF and a primary anastomosis in four, uncontrolled PF in three, delayed intestinal perforation in two and other indications in three. Drainage, as demonstrated radiologically, was not feasible in these cases.

We, sometimes, see one or two patients in a year whose drains have been removed early, after a normal amylase level and normal-coloured drainage fluid, who later develop an intra-abdominal abscess, usually in the left subphrenic region. We previously reported that a certain proportion of such cases are likely to result from an undetected/undiagnosed pancreatic juice leakage, and this possibility should always be kept in mind.[16,22] However, the treatment is the same with radiological drain placement for irrigation.

EVIDENCE-BASED VALUE OF PROPHYLACTIC DRAINAGE IN GASTRIC CANCER SURGERY

Few prospective studies on prophylactic drainage versus no drainage after gastric surgery have been reported. A 2004 systematic review and meta-analysis concluded that prophylactic drainage remains indicated after total gastrectomy. For fear of mediastinitis caused by disruption of the oesophagojejunostomy, which occurs in 3 to 11% cases, drains are normally placed prophylactically, without any adequate evidence of efficacy.[32] Recently, several randomised trials have compared drainage against no drainage in this type of procedure to clarify the clinical usefulness of this strategy.

Kim et al conducted a randomised prospective trial involving 170 patients with gastric cancer assigned to either a drainage group or a no-drainage group. In their study, there was no significant difference in the incidence of postoperative complications between these two groups. They concluded that prophylactic drain placement does not offer additional benefit for patients undergoing gastric cancer surgery with extended lymph node dissection.[33] Alvarez et al conducted a trial, enrolling 60 patients with gastric cancer assigned to two groups. They do not recommend the use of drains in patients with total gastrectomies for gastric cancer, as the group with drains experienced a higher rate of complications and longer hospital stays.[34] Kumar et al reported that prophylactic drainage placement is not necessary after subtotal gastrectomy for gastric cancer, since it does not offer additional benefits to patients.[35] In their trial, 108 patients were divided into a drainage group and a no-drainage group. These studies involved limited numbers of patients, and good evidence to support the usefulness of prophylactic drainage tubes could not be obtained.

SUMMARY

Reoperation within a short time after surgery usually poses a high risk, especially in patients with septic complications. Reoperation should be avoided in patients who have diabetes, vascular disease and respiratory disorders, since visceral tissue is fragile and the diseases tend to be intractable. For this reason, the prophylactic use of drainage tubes is strongly recommended to reduce the incidence of pancreas-related complications, which are fatal in a significant proportion of patients.

On the other hand, drainage tube removal is normally recommended in the immediate postoperative period in patients undergoing D0/D1 lymphadenectomy, without splenectomy and partial gastrectomy, which carry a low risk of PF development.

The key feature of the widely held scepticism about the value of routinely using drainage tubes[36] is the negative impact of retrograde infection. Claims that it does not reduce postoperative complications, despite drainage placement being carried out appropriately, have been made. The idea is that interventional drainage or embolisation under radiographic or ultrasonic guidance is much more effective in solving clinical problems, even if serious complications such as leakage, abdominal abscess and bleeding occur. However, these treatments need a back-up system, including image processing methods, computer programs and related radiation equipment, as well as the skills of interventional radiologists. It must be strictly acknowledged that insertion of a drainage tube into a proper position involves a high degree of difficulty as compared with intraoperative placement, and percutaneous puncture carries potential risk of intra-abdominal organ injury, with patients experiencing pain, anxiety and discomfort.

CONCLUSIONS

Meticulous and careful management with the tubal drainage and irrigation systems monitored and guided both clinically and radiologically using regular fistulograms is effective for managing patients with PF and can thereby prevent morbidities and fatalities. A drainage tube in proper position provides a wealth of information about the inside of the abdominal cavity. To quickly and accurately detect an abnormality, it is clearly important to accurately observe and ensure proper timing of drainage tube removal in clinical practice.

REFERENCES

1. Nakajima T. Gastric cancer treatment guidelines in Japan. *Gastric Cancer* 2002;5:1–5.
2. Sano T, Katai H, Sasako M, Maruyama K. One thousand consecutive gastrectomies without operative mortality. *Br J Surg* 2002;89:123.

3. Sasako M. Principles of surgical treatment for curable gastric cancer. *J Clin Oncol* 2003;21:274s–5s.

4. Bonenkamp JJ, van de Velde CJ, Sasako M, Hermans J. R2 compared with R1 resection for gastric cancer: morbidity and mortality in a prospective, randomised trial. *Eur J Surg* 1992;158:413–8.

5. Cuschieri A, Fayers P, Fielding J, et al. Postoperative morbidity and mortality after D1 and D2 resections for gastric cancer: preliminary results of the MRC randomised controlled surgical trial. The Surgical Cooperative Group. *Lancet* 1996;347:995–9.

6. Ichikawa D, Kurioka H, Yamaguchi T, et al. Postoperative complications following gastrectomy for gastric cancer during the last decade. *Hepatogastroenterology* 2004;51: 613–7.

7. Sano T, Sasako M, Yamamoto S, et al. Gastric cancer surgery: morbidity and mortality results from a prospective randomized controlled trial comparing D2 and extended para-aortic lymphadenectomy—Japan Clinical Oncology Group study 9501. *J Clin Oncol* 2004;22:2767–73.

8. Kodera Y, Sasako M, Yamamoto S, et al. Identification of risk factors for the development of complications following extended and superextended lymphadenectomies for gastric cancer. *Br J Surg* 2005;92:1103–9.

9. Kostic Z, Cuk V, Ignjatovic M, Usaj-Knezevic S. Early complications following radical surgical treatment of patients with gastric adenocarcinoma. *Vojnosanit Pregl* 2006;63:249–56.

10. Sasako M, Katai H, Sano T, Maruyama K. Management of complications after gastrectomy with extended lymphadenectomy. *Surg Oncol* 2000;9:31–4.

11. Okabayashi T, Kobayashi M, Sugimoto T, Okamoto K, Matsuura K, Araki K. Postoperative pancreatic fistula following surgery for gastric and pancreatic neoplasm; is distal pancreaticosplenectomy truly safe? *Hepatogastroenterology* 2005;52:233–6.

12. Maruyama K, Sasako M, Kinoshita T, Sano T, Katai H, Okajima K. Pancreas-preserving total gastrectomy for proximal gastric cancer. *World J Surg* 1995;19:532–6.

13. Japanese Gastric Cancer A. Japanese classification of gastric carcinoma – 2nd English Edition. *Gastric Cancer* 1998;1:10–24.

14. Bassi C, Dervenis C, Butturini G, et al. Postoperative pancreatic fistula: an international study group (ISGPF) definition. *Surgery* 2005;138:8–13.

15. Sano T, Sasako M, Katai H, Maruyama K. Amylase concentration of drainage fluid after total gastrectomy. *Br J Surg* 1997;84:1310–2.

16. Katai H, Yoshimura K, Fukagawa T, Sano T, Sasako M. Risk factors for pancreas-related abscess after total gastrectomy. *Gastric Cancer* 2005;8:137–41.

17. Katayama H, Kurokawa Y, Nakamura K, et al. Extended Clavien-Dindo classification of surgical complications: Japan Clinical Oncology Group postoperative complications criteria. *Surg Today* 2016;46:668–85.

18. Kobayashi D, Iwata N, Tanaka C, et al. Factors related to occurrence and aggravation of pancreatic fistula after radical gastrectomy for gastric cancer. *J Surg Oncol* 2015;112:381–6.

19. Miki Y, Tokunaga M, Bando E, Tanizawa Y, Kawamura T, Terashima M. Evaluation of postoperative pancreatic fistula after total gastrectomy with D2 lymphadenectomy by ISGPF classification. *J Gastrointest Surg* 2011;15: 1969–76.

20. Nobuoka D, Gotohda N, Konishi M, Nakagohri T, Takahashi S, Kinoshita T. Prevention of postoperative pancreatic fistula after total gastrectomy. *World J Surg* 2008;32:2261–6.

21. Pacelli F, Doglietto GB, Bellantone R, Alfieri S, Sgadari A, Crucitti F. Extensive versus limited lymph node dissection for gastric cancer: a comparative study of 320 patients. *Br J Surg* 1993;80:1153–6.

22. Schmid A, Thybusch A, Kremer B, Henne-Bruns D. Differential effects of radical D2-lymphadenectomy and splenectomy in surgically treated gastric cancer patients. *Hepatogastroenterology* 2000;47:579–85.

23. Tomimaru Y, Miyashiro I, Kishi K, et al. Is routine measurement of amylase concentration in drainage fluid necessary after total gastrectomy for gastric cancer? *J Surg Oncol* 2011;104:274–7.

24. Yu HW, Jung do H, Son SY, et al. Risk factors of postoperative pancreatic fistula in curative gastric cancer surgery. *J Gastric Cancer* 2013;13:179–84.

25. Clavien PA, Barkun J, de Oliveira ML, et al. The Clavien-Dindo classification of surgical complications: five-year experience. *Ann Surg* 2009;250:187–96.

26. Furukawa H, Hiratsuka M, Ishikawa O, et al. Total gastrectomy with dissection of lymph nodes along the splenic artery: a pancreas-preserving method. *Ann Surg Oncol* 2000;7:669–73.

27. Wu CW, Hsiung CA, Lo SS, Hsieh MC, Shia LT, Whang-Peng J. Randomized clinical trial of morbidity after D1 and D3 surgery for gastric cancer. *Br J Surg* 2004;91:2832–7.

28. Degiuli M, Sasako M, Ponti A, Soldati T, Danese F, Calvo F. Morbidity and mortality after D2 gastrectomy for gastric cancer: results of the Italian Gastric Cancer Study Group prospective multicenter surgical study. *J Clin Oncol* 1998;16:1490–3.

29. Bonenkamp JJ, Songun I, Hermans J, et al. Randomised comparison of morbidity after D1 and D2 dissection for gastric cancer in 996 Dutch patients. *Lancet* 1995;345: 745–8.

30. Roukos DH, Lorenz M, Encke A. Evidence of survival benefit of extended (D2) lymphadenectomy in western patients with gastric cancer based on a new concept: a prospective long-term follow-up study. *Surgery* 1998;123: 573–8.

31. De Sol A, Cirocchi R, Di Patrizi MS, et al. The measurement of amylase in drain fluid for the detection of pancreatic

fistula after gastric cancer surgery: an interim analysis. *World J Surg Oncol* 2015;13:65.

32. Petrowsky H, Demartines N, Rousson V, Clavien PA. Evidence-based value of prophylactic drainage in gastrointestinal surgery: a systematic review and meta-analyses. *Ann Surg* 2004;240:1074–84; discussion 84–5.

33. Kim J, Lee J, Hyung WJ, et al. Gastric cancer surgery without drains: a prospective randomized trial. *J Gastrointest Surg* 2004;8:727–32.

34. Alvarez Uslar R, Molina H, Torres O, Cancino A. Total gastrectomy with or without abdominal drains. A prospective randomized trial. *Rev Esp Enferm Dig* 2005;97:562–9.

35. Kumar M, Yang SB, Jaiswal VK, Shah JN, Shreshtha M, Gongal R. Is prophylactic placement of drains necessary after subtotal gastrectomy? *World J Gastroenterol* 2007;13:3738–41.

36. Dougherty SH, Simmons RL. The biology and practice of surgical drains. Part 1. *Curr Probl Surg* 1992;29:559–623.

18

Immediate and Long-term Complications after Antireflux Surgery

I. Rouvelas, T. Irino and L. Lundell

ABSTRACT

Despite multiple prospective randomised trials documenting the efficacy of antireflux surgery in the management of gastroesophageal reflux disease and hiatal hernia complication, surgical treatment is currently probably underused. Minor complications are expected to develop in between 10% and 15% after laparoscopic antireflux surgery, with about double the numbers after redo interventions. Most of these will all resolve with noninvasive treatment. Major complications in laparoscopic antireflux surgery are rare, where the indications for treatment are straightforward and prompt actions resolve the problem in most cases, without permanent disability. Nevertheless, because complications occur twice as often during reoperations, surgery for failed previous antireflux operations is difficult and should be undertaken by an experienced team with profound knowledge and skills in laparoscopic as well as open surgical procedures. Commonly, symptoms of paraoesophageal hernia are abdominal fullness, nausea, swallowing disorders and heartburn. A generally valid recommendation is immediate surgery after diagnosis of an intrathoracic stomach with severe complaints and well-described clinical symptoms. The most frequent postfundoplication problems are dysphagia, gas bloat complaints and recurrent reflux. A summary can be given, based on consensus document, over the technical details to master the most common antireflux surgical procedures, including the following steps. Preserve the hepatic branch of the anterior vague nerve. Complete a generous transhiatal mobilisation of the oesophagus to allow approximately 3 cm of the distal oesophagus to be positioned within the abdominal cavity. All short gastric vessels shall be left intact, if possible. A posterior crural repair is always added by nonabsorbable sutures. In case of a very large hiatus defect, the addition of a few anterior crural sutures can be done. A total wrap shall be created by bringing the right and left portions of the mobile fundus around the distal oesophagus and suturing together in front of the anterior part of the abdominal portion of the oesophagus. The length of the wrap should be 1.5 to 2 cm, and the most distal suture (nonabsorbable) shall incorporate the anterior musculature wall of the oesophagus. At the time of the construction of the wrap, the introduction of a large boogie through the oesophagus can be recommended but cannot be defined as essential.

KEYWORDS

GERD, antireflux surgery, perioperative complications, postoperative complications, dysphagia, bloating, oesophageal perforation, paraoesophageal hernia

INTRODUCTION

Data are accumulating to show an increasing point prevalence of gastroesophageal reflux disease (GERD) throughout the western world, with a delayed but evident change emerging also in Asia.[1–6] It is most likely that these findings truly reflect a real increase in the incidence of the disease. During the last decades, we have experienced a dramatic change in the efficacy by which medical therapy for GERD is offered. Proton-pump inhibitor (PPI) therapeutic trials have not only delineated the efficacy in the short- and long-term perspectives but also clarified the impact of uncontrolled GERD on the patient's health-related quality of life.[7,8] Tentatively, as a consequence of the awareness of similar therapeutic achievements, surgical therapy in chronic GERD has been met by an enhanced interest. In fact, the prescription rates of PPI drugs have had very little, if any, negative impact on the operative activities, but the reverse seems more likely to be true. No doubt, the introduction of the laparoscopic approach to antireflux surgery meant a more liberal attitude to and frequent use of the procedure in many institutions throughout the world.[9,10] Having said this, it is also relevant to point out that substantial regional differences are prevailing between and within the individual countries, suggesting the impact of individual surgeons' interest and attitudes. Despite multiple prospective randomised trials documenting equivalent or superior outcomes of antireflux surgery, when compared with long-term PPI treatment, surgical treatment has probably been underused, and this seems to be the case currently as well.[11–14] Multiple factors account for this fact, importantly including the side effects of fundoplication. Side effects, including dysphagia, bloating, and flatulence, can be minimised with careful surgical technique and patient selection; however, they remain an important barrier to surgical referral. Postoperative morbidity has been diminished considerably by the introduction of laparoscopic fundoplication; however, the degree to which this is true will remain uncertain.[9,15–18]

Because laparoscopic antireflux operations are performed widely and the number of surgeons who perform this technically demanding operation is increasing, it is important to evaluate the spectrum of intraoperative and immediate postoperative complications, as reported from centres with a large volume of laparoscopic antireflux operations. For unclear reasons, there seems to be an increasing age of patients undergoing inpatient antireflux surgery; this suggests that referring gastroenterologists might be reserving surgical therapy for older patients with longstanding reflux disease. There are now increasing concerns about the side effects of long-term PPI use, including increased risks of community-acquired pneumonia, *Clostridium difficile* colitis and hip fracture, and the interaction with clopidogrel therapy for patients with coronary heart disease.[19–26] Accordingly, it can be hypothesised that a decrease in long-term PPI use may renew some interests in antireflux surgery.

DEFINITION OF COMPLICATIONS

For the purposes of this chapter, a complication has been defined as a deviation from the normal postoperative course, as delineated by long clinical experience. The

routine postoperative use of a nasogastric tube (NGT) is not justified; that is why someone who needed it for distention, bloating or vomiting can be considered to have had a minor complication. Moreover, all patients shall receive full-liquid diet on the night after surgery or the next morning and should be discharged home on the second or third postoperative day (if not offered day-care surgery). Patients who could not progress on their diet as expected can again be considered to have a mechanical bowel obstruction. Minor complications are those that require no treatment other than, for example, intravenous fluids, NGT, bladder catheterisation and antibiotics, and might be considered simple deviations of the expected recovery course. Major complications were defined as those that had the potential for death, a reoperation or permanent disability and that required repeated or more invasive treatment.

MINOR COMPLICATIONS

Minor complications are expected to develop in between 10% and 15% of people after laparoscopic antireflux surgery (LARS), with about double the numbers after redo surgery.

Liver Haematoma

Small lacerations or contusions of the left lobe of the liver are usually uneventful and self-limited and thus were not considered as complications. However, a few patients may require treatment or hospitalisation for a liver laceration, which, in these situations, seldom can convert into a major complication due to rupture. These latter patients need blood transfusion, angiography and embolisation of a bleeding vessel.

Bowel Obstruction

Symptoms suggestive of small bowel obstruction are reported in about 5% and occur significantly more frequently after reoperations (15%) than after primary operations. Most of these patients required insertion of an NGT in the immediate postoperative course to treat the problem. Their mean length of hospital stay is usually doubled because of distention, nausea and abdominal pain. An ileus was diagnosed by means of abdominal X-ray and treated with NGT suction. The vast majority of these patients recover, without further operative intervention.

Urinary Retention

Urinary retention necessitating reinsertion of a bladder catheter occurs in a few percentages. However, some males have to be discharged with a catheter and evaluated by a urologist.

Others

Other minor complications were pneumonia, atelectasis, temporary atrial fibrillation and wound infection, all of which resolve with noninvasive treatment.

ACUTE MAJOR PERIOPERATIVE COMPLICATIONS

Major complications are expected to develop in between % after laparoscopic antireflux surgery. No doubt, the impact of the experience of the operating surgeon is apparent and just illustrates the importance of controlling factors relevant for the safety and quality of the operative procedure.[27,28] With the introduction of laparoscopy, a significant reduction in the need for splenectomy has been recorded. The most common complications are listed as follows:

- The importance of the operator
- Bleeding
- Tension pneumothorax
- Perforation
- Acute herniation of the wrap

Tension Pneumothorax

A common complication during the laparoscopic procedure is intraoperative pneumothorax, which is diagnosed by means of observation of the paradoxical motion of the diaphragm or an obvious dissection-induced defect in the pleura. This complication occurred in about 5% of patients undergoing reoperation and in 2% of patients undergoing an index operation. Clinical manifestations of pneumothorax do not develop in most of these patients but can exceptionally develop where the patient becomes haemodynamically unstable for a short time. As soon as the pneumoperitoneum is released and the patient is resuscitated with intravenous fluids, the operation can be finished uneventfully at a lower insufflation pressure (10 mmHg). Postoperative chest X-ray shall be performed, mainly for documentation.

Iatrogenic Intraoperative Oesophageal or Gastric Perforation

Regardless of which approach is used, one of the most serious complications is *iatrogenic intraoperative oesophageal or gastric perforation*. The consequences of perforation may be especially troublesome if the perforation is unrecognised intraoperatively, leading to significant postoperative complications and even fatal outcome. Data from the 1990s suggest that open surgery has a 1 to 3% risk of iatrogenic perforation, with a resultant 25% mortality rate.[29–32] The risk of intraoperative perforation in the beginning of the laparoscopic era suggests that the intraoperative perforation rate remained unchanged and that most of these occurred during the retroesophageal dissection and bougie insertion. Subsequently, many advances in laparoscopic surgery have occurred, including improved equipment and energy devices but, perhaps, the most important is the increased surgeon experience with these operations. A review of more recent data seems to indicate fewer perforations that occurred during the retroesophageal portion of the dissection.[33] Instead, perhaps, more common mechanisms during LARS and laparoscopic paraoesophageal hernia (PEH) repair seem to be traction injuries and suture placement. This shift in mechanism could be due to surgeons' heightened awareness of the potential danger during retroesophageal dissection, improved visualisation and greater experience. The issue of prevention of bougies-related damages is either to avoid the use of such devices or to use softer, more flexible bougies. Other strategies that may help minimise the risk of an adverse event related to bougie insertion include avoiding oesophagus tenting during passage and fostering clear communication between the surgeon and the anaesthetist. The most common mechanism of injury during PEH repair seems to be traction. The possible means for mitigating this risk are sac mobilisation before attempting to reduce the stomach and avoidance of undue tension as the PEH is reduced.

If a perforation does occur, it is important to close the lesion by sutures or with an endoscopic liner stapler. Often, the site can also be incorporated into the fundoplication, which may further decrease the risk of a subsequent leak. Redo hiatal hernia repairs are considerably more technically challenging and are associated with a greater risk of intraoperative complications and postoperative morbidity. In a meta-analysis of 17 papers,[33] a 14% intraoperative perforation rate was reported during redo Nissen fundoplication, as for redo hiatal hernia repair, which is 10 times greater than that during primary LARS and PEH repairs. Notably, most of these perforations were recognised intraoperatively, possibly due to the heightened awareness of the risk and vigilance in identifying and repairing perforations in these difficult cases. Postoperative radiographic swallow studies are often obtained in many patients with known intraoperative perforations, which shall be expected to show leaks in about 5% of the patients. A wise strategy is to take these few patients back to the theatre for complementary surgical repair. Although iatrogenic perforations can be a major adverse event during LARS and PEH surgery, it has been clearly shown that this is of no consequence as long as these tears/lesions are repaired intraoperatively. In contrast, when they are not accordingly identified, significant postoperative complications and reinterventions ensue, which often require an intensive care unit (ICU) stay, a prolonged hospitalisation and even impaired quality of life.

Acute Herniation

Acute herniation of the wrap seems to be frequently overlooked due to the sometimes-diffuse symptomatology. The persistence of epigastric and/or retrosternal pain in the postoperative situation is typical for this potentially lethal complication. A plain X-ray of the chest always gives the diagnosis if there is suspicion from the very beginning, which nowadays is often replaced by CT scan (Figure 18.1). These patients have to be re-explored immediately in order to prevent a fatal outcome. The less common types II, III and IV are all varieties of PEHs. The type IV hernia is associated with a large defect in the phrenoesophageal membrane, allowing various parts of the stomach or other organs to enter the hernia sac.[34,35] Potential complications include gastric volvulus with gastric outlet obstruction or strangulation, gastric wall necrosis and perforation, haemorrhage and respiratory distress secondary to compression of the left main stem bronchus.[36–44]

Commonly, symptoms of PEH are abdominal fullness, nausea, swallowing disorders and heartburn. A generally valid recommendation is immediate surgery after diagnosis of an intrathoracic stomach with severe complaints. The following guidelines are recommended to be followed to manage these patients successfully:

- Exact interpretation of the clinical history, inclusive onset and duration of complaints, as well as of previous diagnostic steps and medical treatments
- Clinical examination in view of acute cardiac and pulmonary diseases
- Chest X-ray (intrathoracic bubble)
- Standardised blood analysis: serum lactate, C-reactive protein (CRP), kidney, electrolytes and coagulation, including heart enzymes and d-dimer
- Cautious approach of gastroscopy, if necessary, with children gastroscope
- Video Gastrografin® swallow (optional)
- Multislice contrast CT of the trunk

Dysphagia

Persistent dysphagia more than 2 months postoperatively may occur in around 2% of the patients. No diagnostic test or intervention is usually required during the first 8 weeks postoperatively. Endoscopy and contrast oesophagography and endoscopy are then indicated in all patients with similar remaining complaints. The treatment in these few remaining patients consists of endoscopic dilation (sometimes pneumatic up to a diameter of 30 mm). The vast majority of these patients will become asymptomatic after a few dilations.

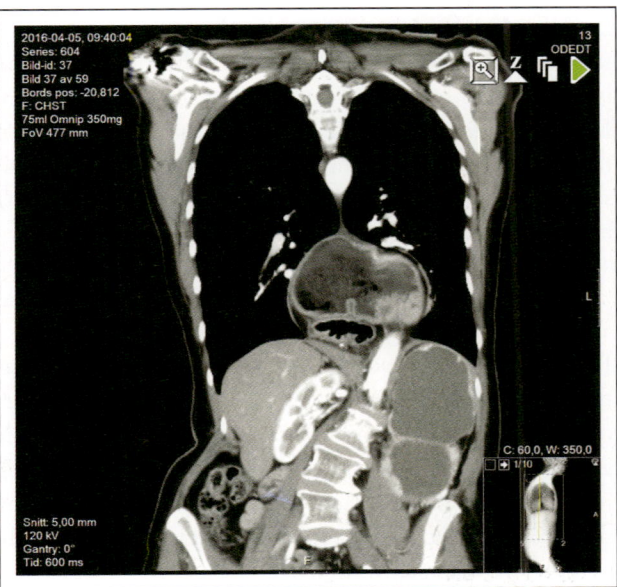 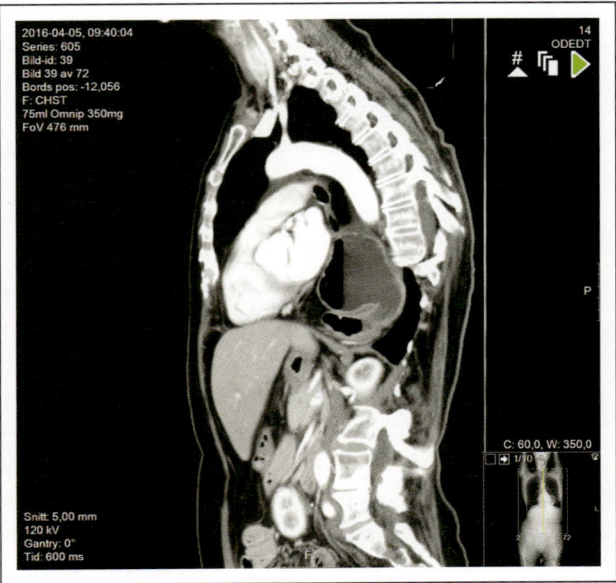

Figure 18.1   Computed tomography scan of the upper abdomen and lower chest demonstrating a type IV paraoesophageal hernia.
Courtesy: Ioannis Rouvelas, Tomoyuki Irino and Lars Lundell.

It can be concluded that major complications in LARS are rare and the treatment is straightforward and resolves the problem in most cases, without permanent disability. Nevertheless, because complications occur twice as often during reoperations, surgery for failed previous antireflux operations is difficult and should be undertaken by an experienced team with advanced laparoscopic skills.

CHRONIC POSTFUNDOPLICATION PROBLEMS

The mode of action of a fundoplication is to restore the reflux barrier in the gastroesophageal junction (GEJ). The fundoplication reinforces the lower oesophageal sphincter pressure by increasing the resting pressure and the relaxation (nadir) pressure.[45–47] Thereafter follows the reduction of the sliding (or alternatively the PEH) hernia, followed by mobilisation of the distal oesophagus and repair of the crus, establishing a positive intra-abdominal pressure; this offers an important component of the reflux barrier and a better synchronisation and overlap of the intrinsic and extrinsic sphincters. Moreover, fundoplication reduces the number of transient lower esophageal sphincter relaxations and also those being associated with reflux. However, as a consequence, the procedure results in a supracompetent valve, which tends to impair the other two functions of the gastroesophageal junction. Accordingly, the main side effects of fundoplication are impaired swallowing of solids and liquids and gas-related symptoms caused by inability to vent air from the stomach.[48–51]

The most frequent postfundoplication problems are as follows:

- Dysphagia
- Gas bloat complaints
- Recurrent reflux

Dysphagia

Early dysphagia in the postoperative period is a frequent problem, particularly after a total fundoplication (Nissen type). Usually, these complaints subside with the passage of time.[52,53] Instructions have to be given to each patient about these expected postoperative symptoms. If similar complaints remain after 6 months, repeated dilatation (30-mm diameter) could be performed, but if incomplete or no response is seen, reoperation should be considered. In those instances, the suggested strategy should be to redo the wrap to a partial posterior type of fundoplication, but most importantly, it should be carried out by an experienced surgeon (see below).

Gas Bloat Complaints

The natural history of severe gas bloat complaints is not very well researched, but recent data suggest that these symptoms seem to remain fairly stable throughout the years.[54] These symptoms are difficult to treat effectively and require careful investigations before specific treatments are instituted. Owing to the difficulties in venting air from the stomach after a fundoplication, in general, and a total wrap, in particular, it remains a delicate matter how to deal with these patients from a surgical perspective. The best data suggest that a reoperation converting a total into a partial fundoplication can offer some relief to the patient from similar complaints, but the surgical literature is not very helpful to give guidance, in this particular situation, as to which preventive strategy should be preferred.[55–57]

Recurrent Reflux

Recurrent reflux occurs in around 10 to 15% patients, depending on a variety of factors, of which the level of expertise of the operating or assisting surgeon seem to be the best documented.[33] Many of these symptoms can be controlled by modern medical therapies, but some patients maintain the opinion that they want to have another operation to avoid drug dependency. Furthermore, we have the problem with recurrent reflux combined with obstructive complaints and those who suffer from severe regurgitation.

Redo operations have to be concentrated to specialised tertiary referral centres, both for the actual operative procedure and, definitely, for the final (preoperative) investigations and evaluations. Redo operations carry a significant risk of postoperative morbidity, and mortality is about 10 times higher than that after an index operation. During this reoperation, the surgeon has to be prepared to take the final decision on the type of reconstruction that should be carried out during this procedure after anatomy has been clarified entirely.

PREVENTION IS THE BEST STRATEGY

Rudolf Nissen discovered in 1956 serendipitously that fundoplication prevented reflux on a patient 16 years of age, after partial esophagectomy. He described it as 'a simple operation to influence reflux esophagitis' and called it 'fundoplication'.[58] The original publication describes the wrap utilising the posterior wall of the stomach. Over time, the total fundoplication according to Nissen has become the most widely performed operation for gastroesophageal reflux disease. Nissen fundoplication has then been modified several times, especially by the work of

Donahue et al[59] and DeMeester et al,[60] who introduced the concept of reducing the length of the fundic wrap and the tightness of the encircled fundus. The procedure includes mobilisation of the distal oesophagus; division of the short gastric vessels; posterior repair of the crural diaphragm; and wrapping of the fundus of the stomach around the oesophagus, covering its entire circumference. The Nissen-Rossetti variation has also been introduced and includes mobilisation of the distal oesophagus and posterior crural repair.[61–63] The only difference between the two operations is that the short gastric vessels are not divided and that the fundoplication is created by using the anterior wall of the stomach only. Further modifications of the total Nissen wrap have been the incorporation of a component as the fixation to the anterior wall of the stomach with three sutures and to the right crus with one suture. Subsequent analyses have demonstrated that there are no differences, neither in the short- nor in the long-term perspective between the original Nissen and the Nissan-Rossetti modified fundoplication.[62,63] Other parts of the total fundoplication technique have been launched, for example, dividing the short gastric vessels, to ensure the construction of a 'floppy Nissen', but studies have shown diverging results when comparing dividing the vessels with leaving them intact. The conclusion emerging is that vessel should mostly be left intact and divided only if the wrap otherwise would be too tight.

A summary can be given based on the consensus document over the technical details to master the most common antireflux surgical procedure.[64]

- Open the phrenicoesophageal ligament to approach the hiatus and the distal oesophagus from the left to the right.
- Attempts should be made to preserve the hepatic branch of the anterior vague nerve.
- Both crura should be carefully and completely dissected, all the way distally to where the right and left crura connect.
- A generous transhiatal mobilisation of the oesophagus should be completed to allow approximately 3 cm of the distal oesophagus to be positioned within the abdominal cavity.
- All short gastric vessels should be left intact, if possible. They may be divided, if necessary, to create a tension-free wrap.
- A posterior crural repair is always added by nonabsorbable sutures. In case of a very large hiatus defect, the addition of a few anterior crural sutures can be allowed.
- The total wrap should be created by bringing the right and left portions of the mobile funds around the distal oesophagus and sutured together in front

of the anterior part of the abdominal portion of the oesophagus.
- The length of the wrap should be 1.5 to 2 cm, and the most distal suture (nonabsorbable) should incorporate the anterior musculature wall of the oesophagus.
- The number of sutures used should be recorded, and two to four sutures are recommended in order to prevent a telescoping of the wrap into the thoracic aperture; this is called 'slipped fundoplication'.
- At the time of the construction of the wrap, the introduction of a large boogie through the oesophagus may recommended but cannot be defined as essential.

CONCLUSIONS

The chronic postfundoplication problems can have a major negative impact on patients' quality of life, and a reoperation should be then considered. However, the evaluation of these type of problems as well as the 'redo' procedures should be concentrated to specialised tertiary referral centres.

REFERENCES

1. Vakil N. Disease definition, clinical manifestations, epidemiology and natural history of GERD. *Best Pract Res Clin Gastroenterol* 2010;24:759–64.
2. Locke GR, Talley NJ, Fett SL, et al. Prevalence and clinical spectrum of gastroesophageal reflux: a population-based study in Olmsted County, Minnesota. *Gastroenterology* 1997;112:1448–56.
3. Jones RH, Hungin AP, Phillips J, et al. Gastro-oesophageal reflux disease in primary care in Europe: clinical presentation and endoscopic findings. *Eur J Gen Pract* 1995;1:149–54.
4. El-Serag HB, Sweet S, Winchester CC, Dent J. Update on the epidemiology of gastro-oesophageal reflux disease: a systematic review. *Gut* 2014;63:871–80. doi: 10.1136/gutjnl-2012-304269.
5. Ho KY. From GERD to Barrett's esophagus: is the pattern in Asia mirroring that in the West? *J Gastroenterol Hepatol* 2011;26:816–24.
6. Bai Y, Du Y, Zou D, et al. Gastroesophageal Reflux Disease Questionnaire (GerdQ) in real-world practice: a national multicenter survey on 8065 patients. *J Gastroenterol Hepatol* 2013;28:626–31.
7. Vakil N, Veldhuyzen van Zanten S, Kahrilas P, et al. The Montreal definition and classification of gastro-esophageal reflux disease (GERD)—a global evidence-based consensus. *Am J Gastroenterol* 2006;101:1900–20.
8. McDougall NI, Johnston BT, Kee F, Collins JS, McFarland RJ, Love AH. Natural history of reflux oesophagitis: a 10 year follow up of its effect on patient symptomatology and quality of life. *Gut* 1996;38:481–6.

9. Watson DI, Jamieson GG. Antireflux surgery in the laparoscopic era. *Br J Surg* 1998;85:173–84.

10. Wang YR, Dempsey DT, Richter JE. Trends and perioperative outcomes of inpatient antireflux surgery in the United States, 1993–2006. *Dis Esophagus* 2011; 24:215–23.

11. Anvari M, Allen C, Borm A. Laparoscopic Nissen fundoplication is a satisfactory alternative to long term omeprazole therapy. *Br J Surg* 1995;82:938–42.

12. Mehta S, Bennett J, Mahon D, Rhodes M. Prospective trial of laparoscopic Nissen fundoplication versus proton pump inhibitor therapy for gastroesophgeal reflux disease: seven-year follow-up. *J Gastrointest Surg* 2006;10:1312–7.

13. Grant AM, Wileman SM, Ramsay CR, et al. Minimal access surgery compared with medical management for chronic gastro-oesophageal reflux disease: UK collaborative randomised trial. *BMJ* 2008;337:a2664.

14. Galmiche JP, Hatlebakk J, Attwood S, et al. Laparoscopic antireflux surgery vs esomeprazole treatment for chronic GERD: the LOTUS randomized clinical trial. *JAMA* 2011;305:1969–77.

15. Hinder RA, Filipi CJ, Wetscher G, et al. Laparoscopic Nissen fundoplication is an effective treatment for gastroesophageal reflux disease. *Ann Surg* 1994; 220:472–83.

16. Salminen P, Hurme S, Ovaska J Fifteen-year outcome of laparoscopic and open Nissen fundoplication: a randomized clinical trial. *Ann Thorac Surg* 2012;93:228–33.

17. Grotenhuis BA, Wijnhoven BP, Bessell JR, Watson DI. Laparoscopic antireflux surgery in the elderly. *Surg Endosc* 2008;22:1807–12.

18. Gill J, Booth MI, Stratford J, Dehn TC. The extended learning curve for laparoscopic fundoplication: a cohort analysis of 400 consecutive cases. *J Gastrointest Surg* 2007;11:487–92.

19. Yang YX, Lewis JD, Epstein S, Metz DC. Long-term proton pump inhibitor therapy and risk of hip fracture. *JAMA* 2006;296:2947–53.

20. Yu EW, Blackwell T, Ensrud KE, et al. Acid-suppressive medications and risk of bone loss and fracture in older adults. *Calcif Tissue Int* 2008;83:251–9.

21. Corley DA, Kubo A, Zhao W, Quesenberry C. Proton pump inhibitors and histamine-2 receptor antagonists are associated with hip fractures among at-risk patients. *Gastroenterology* 2010;139:93–101.

22. Burkard T, Kaiser CA, Brunner-La Rocca H, et al. Combined clopidogrel and proton pump inhibitor therapy is associated with higher cardio-vascular event rates after percutaneous coronary intervention: a report from the BASKET trial. *J Intern Med* 2012;271:257–63.

23. Fohl AL, Regal RE. Proton pump inhibitor-associated pneumonia: not a breath of fresh air after all? *World J Gastrointest Pharmacol Ther* 2011;2:17–26.

24. Howell MD, Novack V, Grgurich P, et al. Iatrogenic gastric acid suppression and the risk of nosocomial Clostridium difficile infection. *Arch Intern Med* 2010;170:784–90.

25. Cundy T, Mackay J. Proton pump inhibitors and severe hypomagnesaemia. *Curr Opin Gastroenterol* 2011;27:180–5.

26. Attwood SE, Ell C, Galmiche JP, et al. Long-term safety of proton pump inhibitor therapy assessed under controlled, randomised clinical trial conditions: data from the SOPRAN and LOTUS studies. *Aliment Pharmacol Ther* 2015;41:1162–74.

27. Broeders JA, DraaismaWA, Rijnhart-de Jong HG, et al. Impact of surgeon experience on 5-year outcome of laparoscopic Nissen fundoplication. *Arch Surg* 2011;146: 340–6.

28. Tsuboi K,Gazallo J, Yano F, et al. Good training allows excellent results for laparoscopic Nissen fundoplication even early in the surgeon's experience. *Surg Endosc* 2010;24:2723–9.

29. Zhang LP, Chang R, Matthews BD, et al. Incidence, mechanisms, and outcomes of esophageal and gastric perforation during laparoscopic foregut surgery: a retrospective review of 1,223 foregut cases. *Surg Endosc* 2014;28:85–90.

30. Niebisch S, Fleming FJ, Galey KM, et al. Perioperative risk of laparoscopic fundoplication: safer than previously reported—analysis of the American College of Surgeons National Surgical Quality Improvement Program 2005 to 2009. *J Am Coll Surg* 2012;215:61–9.

31. Schauer PR, Meyers WC, Eubanks S, et al. Mechanisms of gastric and esophageal perforation during laparoscopic Nissen fundoplication. *Ann Surg* 1996;223:43–52.

32. Lowham AS, Filipi CJ, Hinder RA, et al. Mechanisms and avoidance of esophageal perforation by anesthesia personnel during laparoscopic foregut surgery. *Surg Endosc* 1996;10:979–82.

33. van Beek DB, Auyang ED, Soper NJ. A comprehensive review of laparoscopic redo fundoplication. *Surg Endosc* 2011;25:706–12.

34. Lidor AO, Chang DC, Feinberg RL, et al. Morbidity and mortality associated with antireflux surgery with or without paraesophogeal hernia: a large ACS–NSQIP analysis. *Surg Endosc* 2011;25:3101–8.

35. Dean C, Etienne D, Carpentier B, Gielecki J, Tubbs RS, Loukas M. Hiatal hernias. *Surg Radiol Anat* 2012;34:291–9.

36. Rashid F, Thangarajah T, Mulvey D. A review article on gastric volvulus: a challenge to diagnosis and management. *Int J Surg* 2010;8:18.

37. Davis SS Jr. Current controversies in paraesophageal hernia repair. *Surg Clin North Am* 2008;88:959.

38. Vas W, Malpani AR, Singer J. Computed tomographic evaluation of paraesophageal hernia. *Gastrointest Radiol* 1989;14:91–4.

39. Krähenbuehl L, Schäfer M, Farhadi J. Laparoscopic treatment of large paraesophageal hernia with totally intrathoracic stomach. *J Am Coll Surg* 1998;187:231.

40. Ponsky J, Rosen M, Fanning A, Malm J Anterior gastropexy may reduce the recurrence rate after laparoscopic paraesophageal hernia repair. *Surg Endosc* 2003;17:1036.

41. Casabella F, Sinanan M, Horgan S, Pellegrini CA. Systematic use of gastric fundoplication in laparoscopic repair of paraesophageal hernias. *Am J Surg* 1996;171:485.

42. Wu MH, Chang YC, Wu CH. Acute gastric volvulus: a rare but real surgical emergency. *Am J Emerg Med* 2010;28:e5.

43. Chau B, Dufel S. Gastric volvulus. *Emerg Med J* 2007; 24:446.

44. Köhler G, Koch OO, Antoniou SA, Emmanuel K, Pointner R. "Acute intrathoracic stomach!" How should we deal with complicated type IV paraesophageal hernias? *Hernia* 2015;19:627–33.

45. Rydberg L, Ruth M, Lundell L. Mechanism of action of the antireflux procedure. *Br J Surg* 1999;86:405–10.

46. Engström C, Blomqvist A, Dalenbäck J, Lönroth H, Ruth M, Lundell L. Mechanical consequences of short gastric vessel division at the time of laparoscopic total fundoplication. *J Gastroenterol Surg* 2004;8:442–7.

47. Johnsson F, Holloway RH, Irelande AC, Jamieson GG, Dent D. Effect of fundoplication on transient lower esophageal relaxations and gas reflux. *Br J Surg* 1997;84:686–9.

48. Wescher GJ, Glaser K, Wieschmeyer T, et al. Tailored antireflux surgery for gastrooeophageal reflux disease: effectiveness and risk of postoperative dysphagia. *World J Surg* 1997;21:605–10.

49. Alexiou C, Beggs D, Myers JC, et al. A tailored approach for gastro oesophageal reflux disease: the Nottingham experience. *Eur J Cardiothorac Surg* 2000;17:389–95.

50. Baigre RJ, Watson DI, Myers JC, et al. Outcome of laparoscopic Nissen fundoplication in patients with disordered preoperative peristalsis. *Gut* 1997;40:381–5.

51. Rydberg L, Ruth M, Abrahamson H, et al. Tailoring antireflux surgery: a randomized clinical trial. *Worl J Surg* 1999;23:612–8.

52. Funch-Jensen P, Jacobsen B. Dysphagia after laparoscopic Nissen fundoplication. *Scand J Gastroenterol* 2007;42: 428–31.

53. Swanstrom L, Wayne R (1994) Spectrum of gastrointestinal symptoms after laparoscopic fundoplication. *Am J Surg* 167:538–41.

54. Lundell L, Miettinen P, Myrvold HE, et al. Seven-year follow-up of a randomized clinical trial comparing proton-pump inhibition with surgical therapy for reflux oesophagitis. *Br J Surg* 2007;94:198–203.

55. Lundell L, Abrahamsson H, Ruth M, Rydberg L, Lönroth H, Olbe L. Long-term results of a prospective radnomised comparison of total fundic wrap (Nissen-Rossetti) or semifundoplication (Toupet) for gastro-esophageal reflux. *Br J Surg* 1996;83:830–83.

56. Hagedorn C, Lönroth H, Rydberg L, et al. Long-term efficacy of total (Nissen-Rossetti) and posterior partial (Toupet) fundoplication: result of a randomized clinical trial. *J Gastrointest Surg* 2002;6:540–5.

57. Ludemann R, Watson DI, Jamieson GG, et al. Five-year follow-up of a randomized clinical trial of laparoscopic total versus anterior 180 degrees fundoplication. *Br J Surg* 2005;92:240–3.

58. Nissen R. Eine eifache Opertion zür Beeinflussung der reflux Oesophagitis. *Schweiz Med Wochenschr* 1956;86:590.

59. Donahue PE, Samelson S, Nyhus LM, et al. The floppy Nissen fundoplication. *Arch Surg* 1985;120:663–8.

60. DeMeester TR, Bonnavina L, Albertucci M. Nissen fundoplication for gastroesophageal reflux disease. An evaluation of primary repair in 100 consecutive patients. *Ann Surg* 1986;204:9–20.

61. Rosetti M, Hell K. Fundoplication in the treatment of gastroesophageal reflux in hiatal hernia. *World J Surg* 1977;1:439–44.

62. Mardani J, Lundell L, Engström C. Total and posterior fundoplication in the treatment of GERD. Results of a randomised trial after two decades of follow up. *Ann Surg* 2011;253:875–8.

63. Engström C, Jamieson GG, Devitt PG, Watson DI. Meta-analysis of two randomised clinical trials to identify long-term symptoms after division of the short gastric vessels during Nissen fundoplication. *Br J Surg* 2011;98:1063–7.

64. Attwood SE, Lundell L, Ell C, et al; LOTUS Trial Group. Standardization of surgical technique in antireflux surgery: the LOTUS Trial experience. *World J Surg* 2008;32:995–8.

19

Prevention and Management of Complications after Bariatric Surgery

M. Lakdawala, A.G. Bhasker and J.W.M. Greve

ABSTRACT

Morbidly obese patients have limited physiological reserves and high abdominal fat content, which adds to the difficulty of the complex bariatric procedures being performed on them. Early recognition of complications may be challenging, owing to very subtle signs and symptoms. Mild-grade fever, tachycardia and tachypnoea may be the early signs that must alert surgeons and raise an alarm. High degree of clinical suspicion is critical for early detection of complications and proves to be life-saving. Early intervention is the key to decreasing the morbidity and mortality due to complications. As bariatric surgery rises in the popularity charts among the surgeons and patients, it is high time that our efforts be strongly directed towards minimising the surgical morbidity and mortality. This chapter describes the common complications after bariatric surgery and evaluates the current evidence that is available for their management.

KEYWORDS

Complications, morbidly obese, leaks, obstruction, stricture, cholelithiasis, wound infection, bariatric surgery

INTRODUCTION

The worldwide epidemic of obesity and, parallel to that, the obesity-related comorbidities is a tremendous concern in the modern healthcare. Prevention is, of course, the best option, but for the huge number of patients that suffer from obesity and, in particular, morbid obesity [body mass index (BMI) >40 Kg/m^2 or BMI >35 Kg/m^2 with type 2 diabetes mellitus, hypertension and/or obstructive sleep apnoea syndrome), treatment options are limited. Lifestyle intervention, diet and medical treatment have failed to show substantial long-term weight loss.[1] In the past 50 years, surgical treatment has evolved as a reliable and effective treatment, in which the laparoscopic approach has significantly reduced the complication rates and improved postoperative outcomes. The number of procedures performed annually (>465,000 in the world in 2013)[2] is still increasing, so despite the reduced complication rates, hospitals and surgeons are confronted with bariatric surgery-related complications.[3]

Morbidly obese patients have limited physiological reserves and high abdominal fat content, which add to the difficulty of the complex bariatric procedures being performed on them. The importance of training and crossing the learning curve before practicing bariatric surgery cannot be undermined. Good patient selection policies and team work go a long way in decreasing the complication rates further.

Early recognition of complications may be challenging, owing to very subtle signs and symptoms. Mild-grade fever, tachycardia and tachypnoea may be the early signs that must alert surgeons and raise an alarm. High degree of clinical suspicion is critical for early detection of complications and proves to be life saving.

LAPAROSCOPIC VERSUS OPEN BARIATRIC SURGERY

Laparoscopic bariatric surgery has a lower complication rate compared with open bariatric surgery and should be the preferred option (level of evidence-1, grade of recommendation-A).

The first report of a laparoscopic Roux-en-Y gastric bypass (RYGB) was published by Wittgrove et al in 1994.[4] Since then, there have been multiple retrospective reports and a few randomised controlled trials that have established the superiority of laparoscopic technique over open surgery.[5,6] Patients undergoing laparoscopic surgery recover faster; return to work earlier; and have less postoperative pain, less wound complications, lesser incidence of venous thromboembolism (VTE) and better postoperative pulmonary function. Patients undergoing open surgery have been reported to have a higher rate of iatrogenic splenectomy and abdominal wall hernias. The earlier laparoscopic series reported a higher rate of gastrointestinal bleeding, anastomotic strictures and internal hernias, but these are seen to decline with increasing experience with the laparoscopic technique.[7]

COMPLICATIONS COMMON TO ALL PROCEDURES

Venous Thromboembolism

Venous thromboembolism prophylaxis must be mandatory for all patients undergoing bariatric surgery (level of evidence-1, grade of recommendation-A).

Obesity is regarded as a prothrombotic state, and morbidly obese people are 2.5 times as likely to develop VTE as compared with their nonobese counterparts.[8] Morbidly obese patients undergoing bariatric surgery have an unexpectedly high rate of clinically silent pulmonary emboli (PE), and PE remains one of the biggest causes of perioperative mortality in patients undergoing bariatric surgery.[9]

Venous thromboembolism can be catastrophic, and prophylaxis is a must in morbidly obese population undergoing bariatric surgery. A combination of unfractionated heparin and low-molecular-weight heparin (LMWH), compression devices, elastic stockings and early mobilisation have been recommended. Although weight-adjusted dosing is being practiced in most centres, it may lead to overdosing and haemorrhage, as total body weight does not have a linear relationship with intravascular volume. On the other hand, inadequate dosing may have its own perils. The American College of Chest Physicians (ACCP) in 2004 adopted a pragmatic view in this regard and stated that 'in the absence of clear data, it seems prudent to consider a 25% increase in the thrombo-prophylactic dose of LMWH in very obese patients(10)'.

There is no consensus yet on the optimum dose and duration for VTE prophylaxis or on the preoperative use of inferior vena cava filters.

Cholelithiasis

There is a significantly higher incidence of cholelithiasis after bariatric surgery. Postoperative ursodiol administration reduces the incidence of gall stone formation and must be recommended (level of evidence-1, grade of recommendation-A).

Rapid weight loss after bariatric surgery is associated with increased incidence of gall stone formation. A total of 7.8 to 52% patients tend to develop cholelithiasis after 10 months to 1 year after bariatric surgery.[11,12] Patients may be asymptomatic or present with cholecystitis, cholangitis or acute gall stone pancreatitis. Although definitive cholecystectomy is the treatment of choice, an endoscopic retrograde cholangiopancreatography (ERCP), when indicated, may be difficult or impossible to perform after RYGB, single anastomosis gastric bypass (SAGB) and duodenal switch (DS), owing to altered gastrointestinal anatomy. Prophylactic ursodiol administration is said to decrease postoperative gall stone formation. Sugerman et al reported that a daily dose of 600 mg of ursodiol for the first 6 months significantly reduced gall stone formation to 2% versus 32% with placebo.[13] In general, there is no evidence that cholecystectomy in patients that have underwent bypass type of surgery is more complicated than in patients without previous surgery; this is an important argument against routine cholecystectomy during the bariatric procedure.[14] Prophylactic cholecystectomy does add the risk of biliary complications in a large number of patients that otherwise never would require cholecystectomy.

Role of prophylactic cholecystectomy for all patients remains to be controversial.

Trocar Site Hernia and Trocar Injuries

Trocar site hernias can lead to significant postoperative morbidity, and proper fascial closure is recommended for all trocar sizes of 10 mm and above (level of evidence-3, grade of recommendation-C).

Trocar site hernias (Figure 19.1) are known to occur after laparoscopic bariatric surgery.[15] Failure to close fascial defects at the time of surgery can lead to these hernias. If bowel is involved, these can lead to intestinal obstruction and early strangulation due to the small size of defects. Intestinal obstruction may, in turn, lead to a leak from the proximal staple lines, as in the case of a sleeve gastrectomy, RYGB or DS. A high degree of suspicion for diagnosis and an early surgery to reduce the hernia contents and close

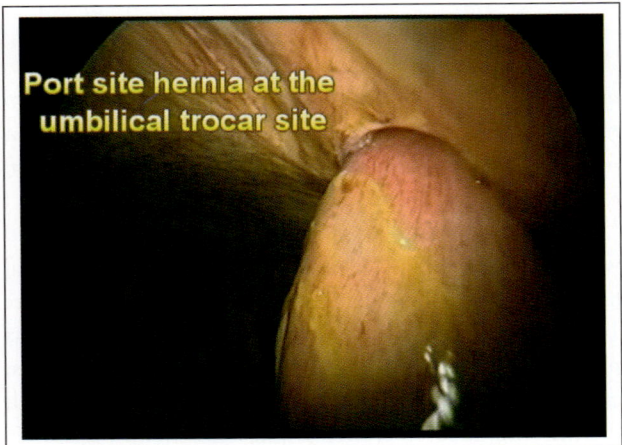

Figure 19.1 Trocar site hernia.

Courtesy: Muffazal Lakdawala, Aparna Govil Bhasker and Jan Willem M. Greve.

hernia defects is warranted. Another trocar-related issue is trocar injuries. A large nationwide survey derived from the Scandinavian Obesity Surgery Registry revealed that the reported incidence is low, 0.07% (12/17,446 laparoscopic gastric bypass procedures), and consisted of bleeding (n = 8 omentum, small bowel mesentery and liver) and perforation (n = 4 stomach or small bowel).[16] Interestingly, most procedures were done with the Veress needle technique (59%), followed by direct introduction of an optical trocar (30%) and other techniques, including the Hasson technique (11%). The complications were evenly distributed over Veress versus optical trocar, whereas there were no complications reported with the Hasson technique.

Gastrointestinal Haemorrhage

Gastrointestinal haemorrhage is a significant cause for morbidity and mortality in postoperative patients. Staple line re-enforcement may help in preventing bleeding (level of evidence-2, grade of recommendation-B).

The incidence of postoperative haemorrhage is seen in less than 4% patients undergoing bariatric surgery.[17] Bleeding commonly occurs from the omental or mesenteric vessels but can also occur from the staple lines, anastomotic sites or the remnant stomach and usually presents with tachycardia, haematemesis and/or melaena. A long staple line in sleeve gastrectomy has an increased risk of postoperative haemorrhage. Use of appropriate staple length for the right tissue thickness, especially in presence of scar tissue, plays a role in postoperative haemorrhage. Techniques such as oversewing and buttressing may

prevent hemorrhage from the staple line; however, evidence for the use of re-enforcement of any kind is still lacking.[18,19] Even the use of biosurgical material such as glue lacks evidence. Other causes of bleeding can be lesions of the liver or spleen; these injuries are usually encountered during the procedure. If the patient is being administered hypotensive anaesthesia during surgery, it is a good practice to increase the patient's blood pressure to normal levels before extubation. It is also important to check all port sites on removal of the trocars for bleeding to prevent intra-abdominal haemorrhage. Although haemorrhage is self-limiting in majority of cases, an emergency laparoscopy may be warranted in patients who are haemodynamically unstable.

For intraluminal bleeding from either the pouch or gastrojejunal anastomosis, resuscitation and blood replacement along with proton-pump inhibitors is the first line of management. If bleeding persists or the patient is haemodynamically unstable, then it would be advisable to do a gastroscopy with saline adrenaline injection, glue application, clipping or argon plasma cauterisation of the bleeder. If bleeding site is from jejunojejunostomy, a long mother–daughter scope, if available, or a long scope that can reach the jejunojejunostomy may be used. Other obscure sites of the bleed can be detected and tackled by angiography and selective embolisation.

Wound Infection

The incidence of wound infections has decreased significantly after the advent of laparoscopic surgery. In case of other bariatric procedures, the incidence of wound infection can be minimised by reducing the contact of the contents of the gut with the wound. It may be prudent to remove the cut ends of the intestine or the specimens of resected stomach in an endobag. Laparoscopic port site infections can be managed easily by a short course of antibiotics and local wound care. Care should be taken when using foreign material such as a mesh, a band or a ring, as infection of the foreign material can lead to a sinus tract (Figure 19.2).

Leaks

Leaks after bariatric surgery are one of the biggest causes of morbidity and mortality. Early recognition and management are mandatory (level of evidence-2A, grade of recommendation-B).

Detection of leak (Figures 19.3–19.5) may be difficult in morbidly obese patients, and subtle signs such as tachycardia, tachypnoea and mild-grade fever must prompt further investigations.

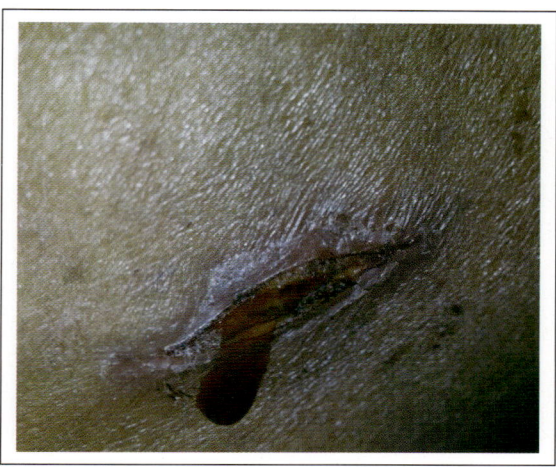

Figure 19.2 Wound infection.

Courtesy: Muffazal Lakdawala, Aparna Govil Bhasker and Jan Willem M. Greve.

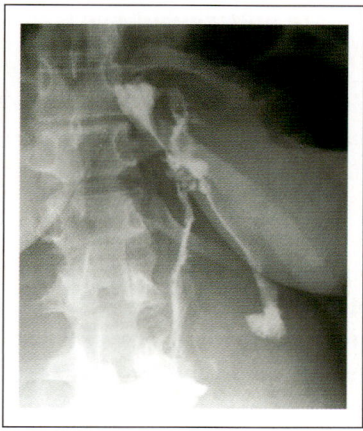

Figure 19.3 Oral contrast study depicting a gastroesophageal junction leak in sleeve gastrectomy.

Courtesy: Muffazal Lakdawala, Aparna Govil Bhasker and Jan Willem M. Greve.

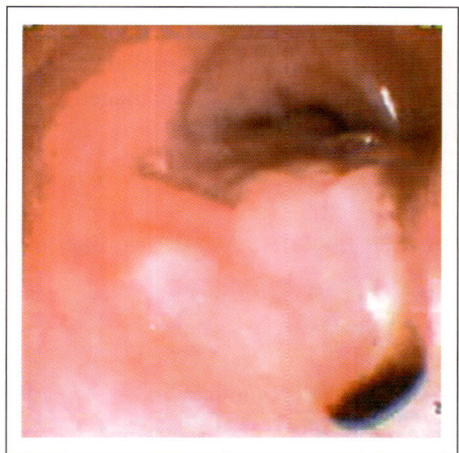

Figure 19.4 Endoscopic image of a gastroesophageal junction leak in sleeve gastrectomy.

Courtesy: Muffazal Lakdawala, Aparna Govil Bhasker and Jan Willem M. Greve.

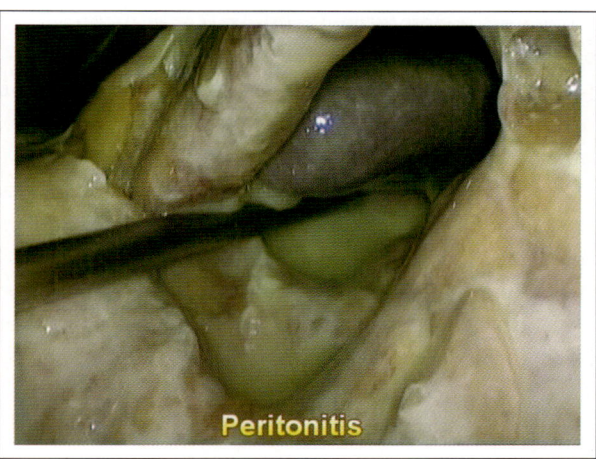

Figure 19.5 Diagnostic laparoscopy for peritonitis secondary to a leak.

Courtesy: Muffazal Lakdawala, Aparna Govil Bhasker and Jan Willem M. Greve.

Interpretations of radiology findings also vary, making it even more difficult to diagnose leaks. Early intervention is the key to successful management in this patient population, and there must be a low threshold for relaparoscopy. In particular, a pulse rate of over 115 per minute is considered an absolute indication for relaparoscopy. Early relaparoscopy is preferred over a computed tomography (CT) scan, because sometimes, these patients may not even fit on to the CT scan tables and there may be unnecessary waste of time. Time is crucial here, and an early relaparoscopy, even if negative, is justified.

The incidence of anastomotic leak after RYGB is 0.4 to 5.2% and may carry a mortality rate of 30 to 50%.[20–22]

Most leaks occur at the gastrojejunostomy. Intraoperative methylene blue or air leak tests may help reduce the occurrence of leaks. Leaks may occur due to technical failure, excessive traction or ischaemia at the anastomotic site.

In case of mini-gastric bypass (MGB) or the omega loop gastric bypass, leak rates range from 0.8 to 1.6%. These are more dangerous and need immediate attention because of biliary peritonitis. Same is the case of a leak from a jejunojejunostomy in a Roux-en-Y gastric bypass or a duodenojejunostomy in a sleeve with duodenojejunal bypass (DJB) or a duodenoileostomy in a single anastomosis duodenoileostomy (SADI) or a DS.[23]

Staple Line Leaks After Laparoscopic Sleeve Gastrectomy

Staple line leaks after laparoscopic sleeve gastrectomy are the biggest cause for short- and long-term morbidities after laparoscopic sleeve gastrectomy (LSG) (level of evidence-2A, grade of recommendation-B).

Reported in 1 to 7% of patients, a leak is the most dreaded complication after LSG.[24] Staple line leaks after LSG are notoriously difficult to treat. They have been classified into acute (within 7 days), early (within 1–6 weeks), late (after 6 weeks) and chronic (after 12 weeks).[25] A total of 85.7% of the leaks happen from the proximal third of the staple line and about 14.3% happen from the distal third of the staple line.[26] The three main causes of leaks are increased intraluminal pressure, ischaemia and technical failure.

The first sleeve consensus meeting showed wide technical variations between surgeons, and usefulness of staple line re-enforcement/suturing in leak prevention remains controversial.[27]

Unresolved leaks can lead to chronic complications such as gastrocutaneous, oesophagopleural and gastrocolic fistulas in the long term.

Relaparoscopy with or without concomitant endoscopic stenting remains the mainstay of treatment for acute and early leaks after LSG. Chronic leak management is challenging, and surgery remains the best option. Management options for leaks after bariatric surgery are shown in Algorithm 19.1.

Strictures

Most strictures at the gastrojejunostomy site can be managed by endoscopic balloon dilatation (level of evidence-2A, grade of recommendation-B).

Reported incidence of gastrojejunal strictures ranges from 2.9 to 23%.[28,29] Gastrojejunal anastomosis can be done using a circular stapler or a linear stapler or it may be hand-sewn. The highest incidence of strictures has been observed with the use of a 21-mm circular stapler. Other causes for stricture are tension and ischaemia at the site of anastomosis. Patients present with dysphagia and vomiting, usually within the first 3 months after surgery. Two to three sittings of endoscopic balloon dilatation are sufficient in most cases. Rarely, surgical revision involving excision of the gastrojejunostomy and redoing the anastomosis may be needed in a patient with multiple failed dilatations. Strictures at jejunojejunostomy site are

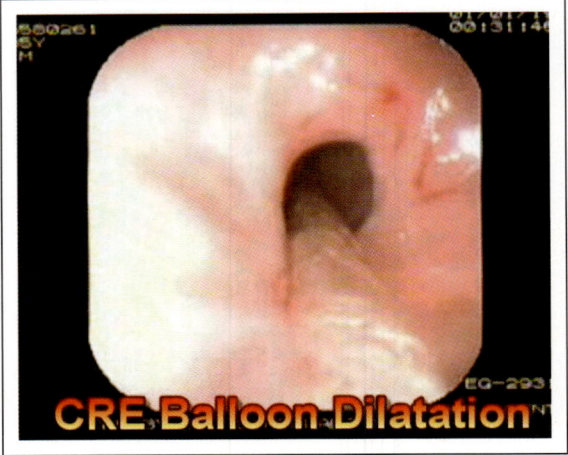

Figure 19.6 CRE™ balloon dilatation of a stricture post gastrojejunostomy.

Courtesy: Muffazal Lakdawala, Aparna Govil Bhasker and Jan Willem M. Greve.

mainly iatrogenic/technique-related and are rarely seen in the long term. These can be managed by an omega anastomosis (Figure 19.6).

Strictures after Laparoscopic Sleeve Gastrectomy

Special care must be taken not to cause narrowing at the incisura angularis (level of evidence-2A, grade of recommendation-B).

Strictures are a late complication of LSG and are seen in 07 to 3.5% of patients.[30–32]

The most common site for stricture formation is at the incisura angularis.[33] Patients usually present with dysphagia, vomiting and excessive weight loss. Diagnosis is made on an upper gastrointestinal (UGI) endoscopy and a contrast series. Management depends on the site and length of the stricture. Management entails either endoscopic dilatation with an achalasia balloon or seromyotomy or conversion to an RYGB.[32]

Internal Herniation

Closure of mesenteric defects decreases the incidence of internal hernias after RYGB, and proper closure of all mesenteric defects is recommended (level of evidence-2A, grade of recommendation-B).

Internal hernias are the most common cause of small bowel obstruction after RYGB. The reported incidence of

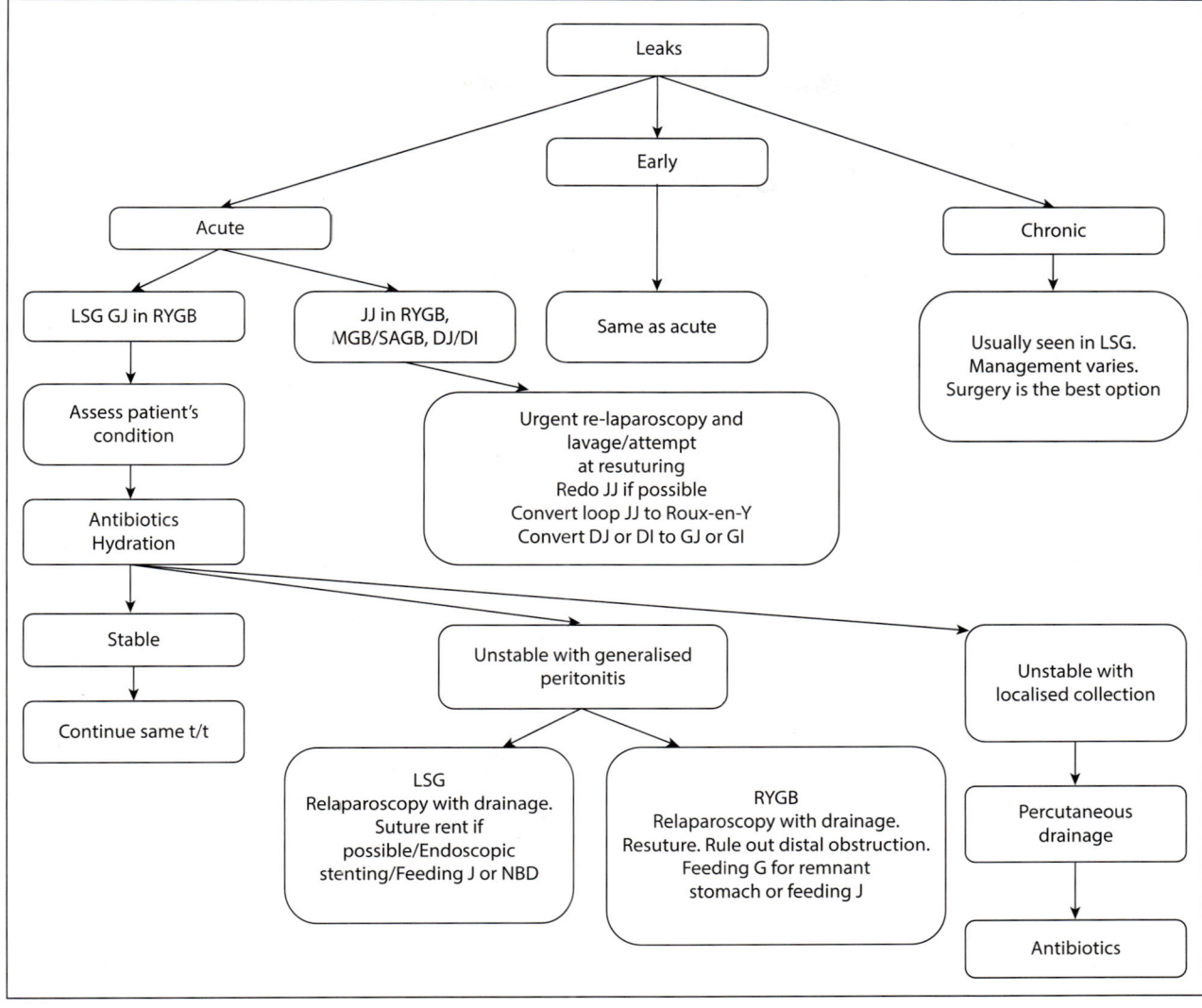

Algorithm 19.1   Algorithm for management of leaks after bariatric surgery.
Abbreviations: DI, duodenoileostomy; DJ, duodenojejunostomy; LSG, laparoscopic sleeve gastrectomy; MGB, mini-gastric bypass; RYGB, Roux-en-Y gastric bypass; SAGB, single anastomosis gastric bypass; GI, gastroileostomy; GJ, gastrojejunostomy; JJ, jejunojejunostomy.
Courtesy: Muffazal Lakdawala, Aparna Govil Bhasker and Jan Willem M. Greve.

internal hernias ranges from 1 to 9%.[34–37] Most surgeons use the antecolic approach in RYGB. This approach has reduced the rate of Peterson's hernia as compared with the retrocolic approach. The antecolic approach creates two defects: one at the jejunojejunostomy mesenteric site and the other is the Peterson defect between the alimentary loop and transverse mesocolon. Closure of these defects with a nonabsorbable continuous suture has been recommended for prevention of internal herniation. This was confirmed in a large randomised Scandinavian study (closure vs. nonclosure), despite the fact that closure of

the mesenteric defect resulted in significantly more early complication, owing to kinking of the small bowel.[38] The overall conclusion from this study is that closure of both defects is adviced.

Diagnosis is difficult as the hernia may reduce spontaneously and the imaging modalities may not be able to detect any abnormality. A low threshold for surgical intervention is advised when there is a suspicion of an internal hernia. Delay in diagnosis and management can lead to disastrous consequences such as bowel gangrene.

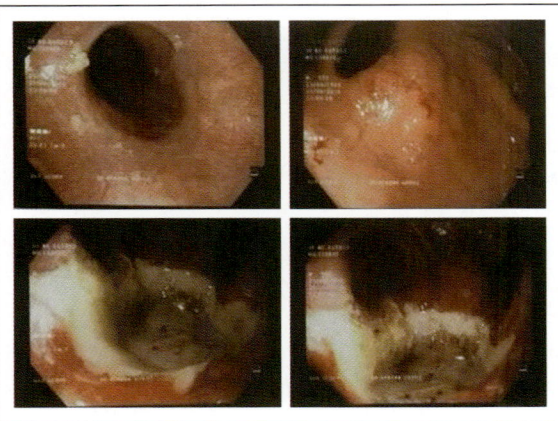

Figure 19.7 Marginal ulcer at gastrojejunostomy post Roux-en-Y gastric bypass.

Courtesy: Muffazal Lakdawala, Aparna Govil Bhasker and Jan Willem M. Greve.

Marginal Ulcers

Most marginal ulcers after RYGB can be managed by conservative treatment (level of evidence-2A, grade of recommendation-B).

Marginal ulcers (Figure 19.7) are reported in 1 to 16% of patients undergoing RYGB and up to 14.3% of patients after SAGB/MGB.[39,40] Ischaemia at the anastomotic site, presence of a foreign body, regular use of nonsteroidal anti-inflammatory drugs (NSAIDs), *Helicobacter pylori* infection and smoking have been implicated in the development of marginal ulcers. Patients present with epigastric pain, nausea and vomiting. Haematemesis or melaena may occur due to haemorrhage from the ulcer. Marginal ulcer perforation is a rare but possible complication and is associated with high morbidity and mortality rates.

A UGI endoscopy usually nails the diagnosis. Surgical intervention is rarely required, and most ulcers heal with the administration of proton-pump inhibitors and sucralfate.

Gastrogastric Fistula

Gastrogastric fistula is a rare complication after RYGB. It may be iatrogenic or may present as a sequel of a marginal ulcer perforation or a delayed presentation of a contained leak. The incidence is between 1% and 6%.[41,42] Most patients present with inadequate weight loss or weight regain. Other symptoms may be epigastric pain, intractable marginal ulceration and haemorrhage. Diagnosis is done by a UGI endoscopy and a contrast series. Surgical management may be indicated in symptomatic patients or those with weight regain (Figure 19.8).

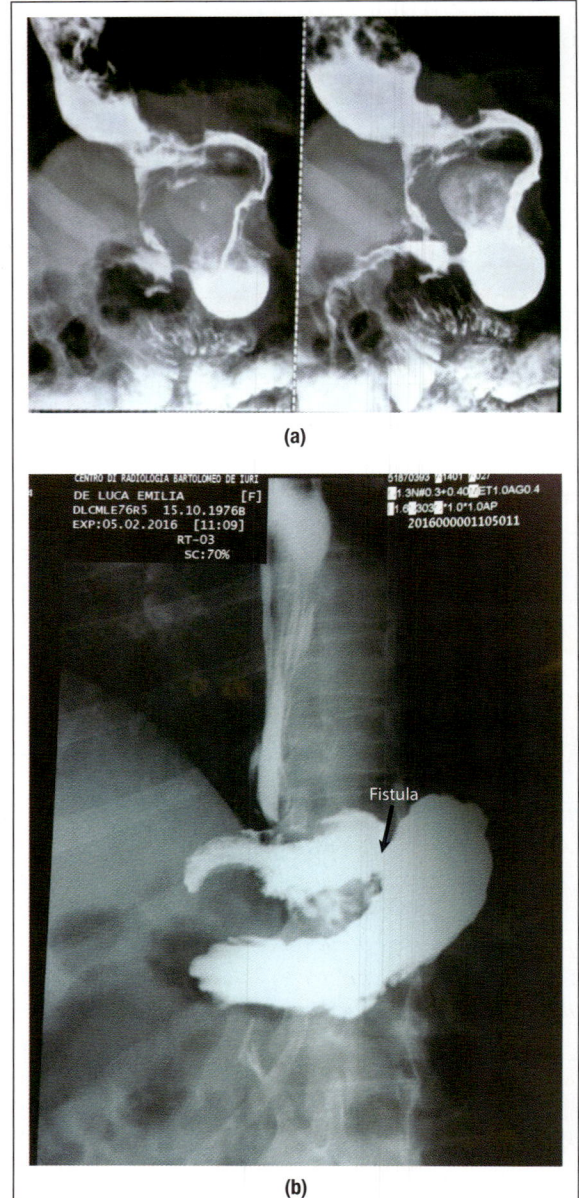

Figure 19.8 Gastrogastric fistula.

Courtesy: Muffazal Lakdawala, Aparna Govil Bhasker and Jan Willem M. Greve.

Small Bowel Obstruction after RYGB/MGB/DJB/DS

Small bowel obstruction after RYGB can be due to an inadvertent Roux-en-O reconstruction, a bezoar, internal herniation, port site herniation or adhesive bands. Kinking of the bowel at the site of the jejunojenunal or jejunoileal anastomosis, in particular, after closure of the mesenteric defect is another cause for small bowel obstruction (Figure 19.9).

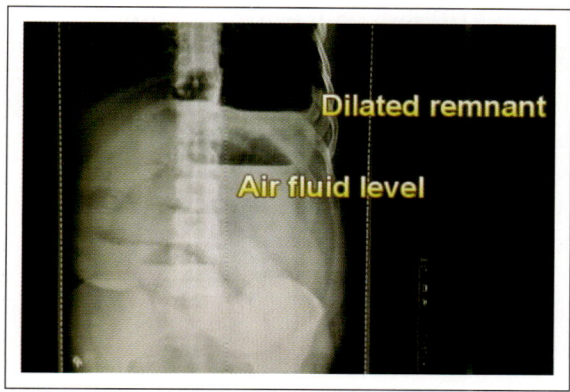

Figure 19.9 Small bowel obstruction post Roux-en-Y gastric bypass.

Courtesy: Muffazal Lakdawala, Aparna Govil Bhasker and Jan Willem M. Greve.

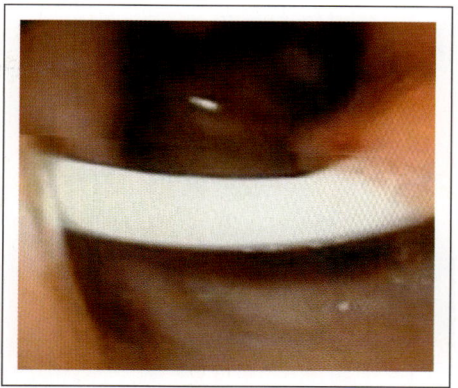

Figure 19.10 Eroded GaBp ring in the stomach pouch.

Courtesy: Dr. Perveen Bhatia and Dr. Vivek Bindal.

Band-Related Complications in Banded Gastric Bypass

Band-specific complications are seen in 4.1% of patients; erosion and slippage in 2.3% and 1.5%, respectively.[43] (Figure 19.10).

COMPLICATIONS SPECIFIC TO LAPAROSCOPIC GASTRIC BANDING

Laparoscopic gastric banding (LGB) may be the safest bariatric procedure in terms of short-term morbidity and mortality but has a high rate of long-term morbidity associated with the silicon prosthesis (level of evidence-2A, grade of recommendation-B).

Laparoscopic gastric banding is considered the safest bariatric procedure. The mean short-term mortality rate after LGB is 0.05% as compared with 0.5% after RYGB.[44] In a review, Chapman et al reported an 11.3% overall median morbidity after LGB.[44] Although the rate of short-term complications after LGB is lower as compared with other bariatric procedures, the silicon prosthesis has up to 24% rate of long-term complications.[45]

Band Prolapse/Slippage

The reported incidence of band slippage ranges from 1 to 25% and is said to decrease with the increasing surgical experience and the pars flaccida approach.[46] In case of slippage or pouch dilation, surgical repositioning of the band can be effective.[47,48] However, most patients with a failing band are switched to a gastric bypass, which, in general, is successful.[48] Acute slippage may lead to gastric outlet obstruction and intractable vomiting.

Diagnosis is mainly done by a plain radiograph of the abdomen, which reveals the position of the band (angle of phi). Management entails immediate band deflation. Surgical treatment includes band removal or repositioning of the band, based on the experience of the operating surgeon. Most important is to recognise acute herniation of the stomach through the band. This presents with severe epigastric pain and acute obstruction. Immediate action, deflation of the band and, in most cases, laparoscopic opening of the band are required to prevent severe necrosis of the stomach (Figure 19.11).

Band Erosion

Band erosion has been reported in up to 11% of cases.[49] It can happen months or years after band placement. Overall erosion rate, in particular, after introduction of the pars flaccida technique is about 1%.[50] Erosion is usually asymptomatic but can also be a cause for pain, bleeding, perforation and infection. Port site infection is a cardinal sign of band erosion. Loss of restriction and weight regain must also alert the surgeon. Eroded band can be diagnosed on UGI endoscopy and contrast studies. Management is endoscopic or surgical removal of the band, depending on the severity of erosion. A concomitant revisional bariatric procedure is avoided at the same sitting (Figure 19.12).

Mega Oesophagus

A very high placement of band or a very tight band may lead to oesophageal dilatation and stasis. This can, in turn, lead to symptoms of severe reflux. Management involves deflation of the band. If symptoms do not improve, removal of band may be considered; however, the best option (in particular when the patient has insufficient weight loss) is conversion to a gastric bypass.

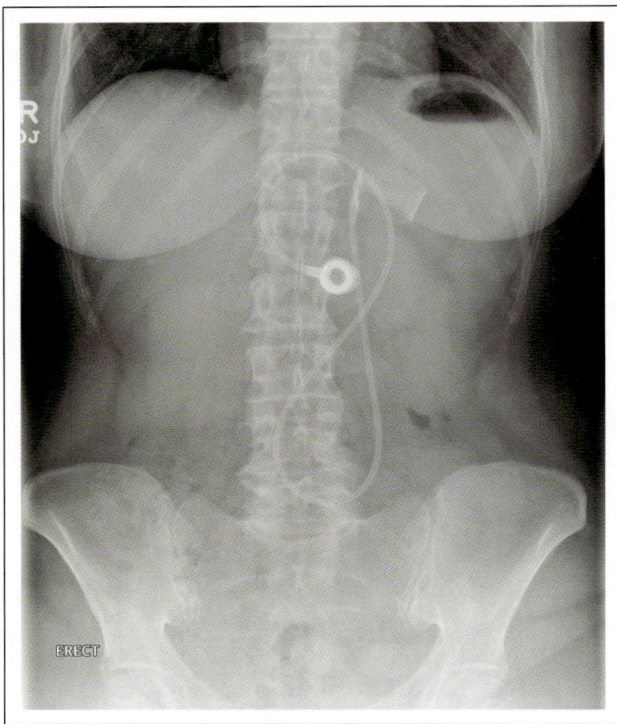

Figure 19.11   Slipped gastric band.

Courtesy: Muffazal Lakdawala, Aparna Govil Bhasker and Jan Willem M. Greve.

COMPLICATIONS SPECIFIC TO LAPAROSCOPIC SLEEVE GASTRECTOMY

Laparoscopic sleeve gastrectomy is a technically simpler operation, but its complications are more difficult to manage.

Complications include strictures, corkscrew rotation of the sleeve and gastroesophageal reflux disease (GERD).

Gastroesophageal Reflux Disease after Laparoscopic Sleeve Gastrectomy

An LSG must not be performed on a patient with grade B or above oesophagitis (the Los Angeles classification), a large sliding hiatus hernia or a grade III or above flap valve (Hill's classification). Aggressive identification of a crural defect and a concomitant crural repair with LSG may prevent postoperative GERD (level of evidence-2A, grade of recommendation-B).

Along with the rise in the popularity of LSG, there are concerns about the increasing incidence of postoperative GERD and future occurrence of Barrett's oesophagus after LSG (Figure 19.13). Himpens et al reported a decrease in the GERD symptoms after LSG at 3 years and attributed it to the restoration of the angle of His. However, at 6-year follow-up, de novo GERD was observed in 21.9%

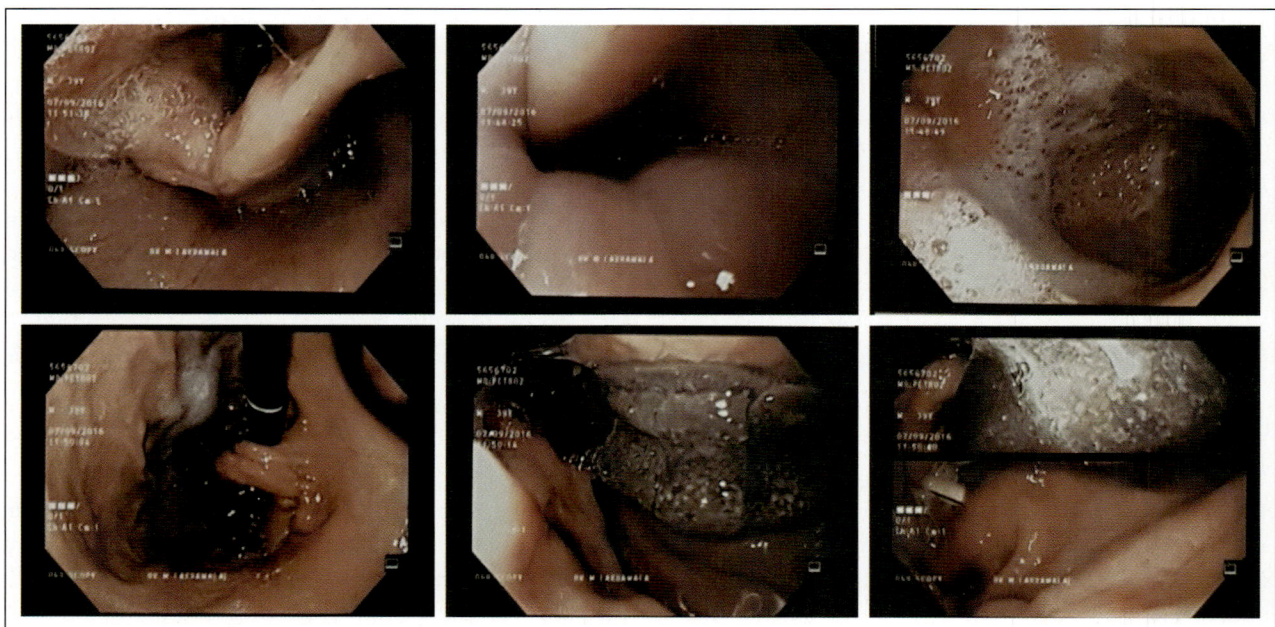

Figure 19.12   Eroded gastric band.

Courtesy: Muffazal Lakdawala, Aparna Govil Bhasker and Jan Willem M. Greve.

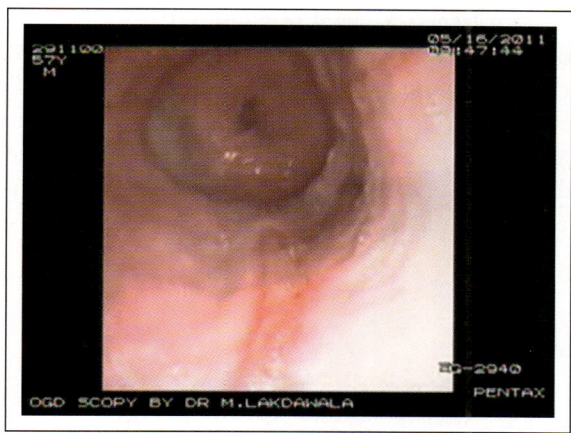

Figure 19.13 Gastroesophageal reflux disease post sleeve gastrectomy.

Courtesy: Muffazal Lakdawala, Aparna Govil Bhasker and Jan Willem M. Greve.

of their patients.[51] In a systematic review by Chiu et al, the data regarding GERD after LSG was found to be inconclusive. Four studies reported an increase in the rate of GERD and seven studies reported a decrease in its rate.[52] Some units prescribe proton-pump inhibitors for the first 6 months to all postoperative patients; however, the evidence for the same is lacking. In a recent study, Soricelli et al reported that LSG with crural repair may be a safe technique for the prevention of postoperative GERD.[53]

An UGI endoscopy and contrast studies are useful for the diagnosis of GERD in post-LSG patients. Although most patients may settle down with antireflux therapy, severe cases may require conversion to an RYGB.

A preoperative UGI endoscopy is recommended in all patients undergoing bariatric surgery. Patients with grade B and above reflux oesophagitis and large hiatal hernias must not be selected for an LSG in the first place.

COMPLICATIONS AFTER LAPAROSCOPIC DUODENAL SWITCH

In a systematic review on trends in mortality after bariatric surgery, Buchwald et al reported that biliopancreatic diversion (BPD)/DS had the highest early mortality, with a rate of 0.29 to 1.23% for open and 0.0 to 2.7% for laparoscopic procedures.[54] Major complication rate after DS has been reported to be between 5 and 7%.[55,56]) An LSG and a duodenoileostomy are the two components of a DS. Complications such as staple line and anastomotic leaks, intestinal obstruction, internal hernias, deep vein thrombosis (DVT) and pulmonary

complications are seen as commonly after a DS as in any other bariatric surgery. The bigger concern after DS is protein energy malnutrition and the metabolic complications. Iron-deficiency anaemia; vitamins B_1 and B_{12} deficiency; deficiencies of fat-soluble vitamins A, D, E and K; secondary hyperparathyroidism, etc. are seen more commonly after DS than with any other bariatric procedure.[57–59] There are concerns regarding hepatic failure after DS, but the available data are inconclusive.[60,61]

OTHER PROCEDURES

Recently, there has been a surge in newer bariatric procedures such as the ileal transposition, omega loop gastric bypass, gastric imbrication, banded gastric imbrication, SADI, sleeve with DJB and endoscopic techniques. Every new surgical procedure comes with a set of complications. The literature on these procedures is scarce, and it is beyond the scope of this review to discuss these at the moment. However, surgeons are advised to bear caution while practicing these procedures and to follow similar principles of complication management.

Metabolic Complications after Bariatric Surgery

Metabolic and nutritional complications are known after bariatric surgery, and hence, there is a significance of life-long follow-up. Electrolyte abnormalities such as low potassium and sodium along with deficiencies of trace elements (e.g., magnesium) can lead to cardiac arrhythmias and myopathies. Iron deficiencies are often found, in particular, after gastric bypass type of procedures; these cause anaemia and are also associated with fatigue, weakness and sometimes pica (craving for ice, chalk, dirt, etc.). Vitamin D deficiency and calcium deficiency can lead to secondary hyperparathyroidism, causing renal calculi. More importantly, these can also lead to osteoporosis and osteomalacia in the long term. Increased bacterial overgrowth after bariatric surgery may lead to diarrhoea and abdominal distension. An important and early complication can be severe vitamin B_1 (thiamin) deficiency due to the initial low values and low intake (no vitamin supplementation) and frequent vomiting directly after surgery. When not recognised and treated immediately, this can lead to irreversible neurological defects (Wernicke's encephalopathy) and even death.

Hypoglycaemia has been recognised as a complication after almost all kinds of bariatric procedures. Pathophysiology of hypoglycaemia after bariatric surgery is still unclear, but dumping syndrome, alteration in beta cell function and increase in beta cell mass have all been implicated. Hypoglycaemia is probably the result of increased hepatic insulin sensitivity and decreased peripheral insulin resistance. Increased islet cell hypertrophy or nesidioblastosis is a late complication that can give rise to neuroglycopaenic symptoms a few years after gastric bypass surgery. An often underdiagnosed cause of the hyperinsulinaemic hypoglycaemia is chronic abuse of refined sugars. Early and strict correction of the diet can prevent this condition in a compliant patient.

Mortality after Bariatric Surgery

Mortality after bariatric surgery is lower than many other surgical procedures, thus making it an equally safe procedure. Early recognition and management of complications must be done at more experienced centres dedicated to bariatric surgery to decrease mortality rates (level of evidence-1, grade of recommendation-A).

In a systematic review published in 2007, Buchwald et al studied all papers published between 1990 and 2006 and reported an overall 30-day mortality of 0.28%. Mortality rate between 30 days and 2 years was found to be 0.35%.[54] The mortality rates after bariatric surgery are lower than other gastrointestinal surgeries such as oesophagectomy and gastrectomy.

CONCLUSIONS

With the current obesity epidemic and the huge increase in obesity-related type 2 diabetes mellitus, along with the lack of valid alternative treatment options for the treatment of morbid obesity, the numbers of bariatric surgery will significantly increase in the years to come. Bariatric or metabolic surgery has become a very important part of gastrointestinal surgery.

This, coupled with the fact that some of these surgeries may need to last a lifetime in one of the most difficult group of patients, has led to an increase in the short- and long-term complications associated with this type of surgery, though the minimal invasive approach and the currently available surgical tools have significantly reduced complication and mortality rates.

The severely obese patients present a unique challenge to the surgeon, as the patients usually do not present with the typical signs and symptoms seen in patients with normal gastrointestinal surgery. High degree of suspicion is necessary for early diagnosis of complications

in these patients. A raised respiratory rate or mild fever may be the only telltale signs of septicaemia at times. Early intervention is the key to decreasing the morbidity and mortality due to complications. As bariatric surgery rises in the popularity charts among surgeons and patients, it is high time that our efforts be strongly directed towards minimising the surgical morbidity and mortality.

REFERENCES

1. Sjostrom L. Review of the key results from the Swedish Obese Subjects (SOS) trial—a prospective controlled intervention study of bariatric surgery. *J Intern Med* 2013;273:219–34.
2. Angrisani L, Santonicola A, Iovino P, Formisano G, Buchwald H, Scopinaro N. Bariatric Surgery Worldwide 2013. *Obes Surg* 2015;25:1822–32.
3. Buchwald H, Avidor Y, Braunwald E, et al. Bariatric surgery: a systematic review and meta-analysis. *JAMA* 2004;292:1724–37.
4. Wittgrove AC, Clark GW, Tremblay LJ. Laparoscopic gastric bypass, Roux-en-Y: preliminary report of five cases. *Obes Surg* 1994;4:353–7.
5. Nguyen NT, Goldman C, Rosenquist CJ, et al. Laparoscopic versus open gastric bypass: a randomized study of outcomes, quality of life, and costs. *Ann Surg* 2001;234:279–89; discussion 89–91.
6. Westling A, Gustavsson S. Laparoscopic vs open Roux-en-Y gastric bypass: a prospective, randomized trial. *Obes Surg* 2001;11:284–92.
7. Schauer P, Ikramuddin S, Hamad G, Gourash W. The learning curve for laparoscopic Roux-en-Y gastric bypass is 100 cases. *Surg Endosc* 2003;17:212–5.
8. Stein PD, Beemath A, Olson RE. Obesity as a risk factor in venous thromboembolism. *Am J Med* 2005;118:978–80.
9. Melinek J, Livingston E, Cortina G, Fishbein MC. Autopsy findings following gastric bypass surgery for morbid obesity. *Arch Pathol Lab Med* 2002;126:1091–5.
10. Geerts WH, Pineo GF, Heit JA, et al. Prevention of venous thromboembolism: the Seventh ACCP Conference on Antithrombotic and Thrombolytic Therapy. *Chest* 2004;126:338S–400S.
11. Iglezias Brandao de Oliveira C, Adami Chaim E, da Silva BB. Impact of rapid weight reduction on risk of cholelithiasis after bariatric surgery. *Obes Surg* 2003;13:625–8.
12. Li VK, Pulido N, Fajnwaks P, Szomstein S, Rosenthal R, Martinez-Duartez P. Predictors of gallstone formation after bariatric surgery: a multivariate analysis of risk factors comparing gastric bypass, gastric banding, and sleeve gastrectomy. *Surg Endosc* 2009;23:1640–4.
13. Sugerman HJ, Brewer WH, Shiffman ML, et al. A multicenter, placebo-controlled, randomized, double-

blind, prospective trial of prophylactic ursodiol for the prevention of gallstone formation following gastric-bypass-induced rapid weight loss. *Am J Surg* 1995;169:91–6; discussion 6–7.

14. Tsirline VB, Keilani ZM, El Djouzi S, et al. How frequently and when do patients undergo cholecystectomy after bariatric surgery? *Surg Obes Relat Dis* 2014;10:313–21.

15. Pilone V, Di Micco R, Hasani A, et al. Trocar site hernia after bariatric surgery: our experience without fascial closure. *Int J Surg* 2014;12:S83–6.

16. Sundbom M, Ottosson J. Trocar injuries in 17,446 laparoscopic gastric bypass—a nationwide survey from the Scandinavian Obesity Surgery Registry. *Obes Surg* 2016;26:2127–30.

17. Dick A, Byrne TK, Baker M, Budak A, Morgan K. Gastrointestinal bleeding after gastric bypass surgery: nuisance or catastrophe? *Surg Obes Relat Dis* 2010;6: 643–7.

18. Angrisani L, Lorenzo M, Borrelli V, Ciannella M, Bassi UA, Scarano P. The use of bovine pericardial strips on linear stapler to reduce extraluminal bleeding during laparoscopic gastric bypass: prospective randomized clinical trial. *Obes Surg* 2004;14:1198–202.

19. Nguyen NT, Longoria M, Welbourne S, Sabio A, Wilson SE. Glycolide copolymer staple-line reinforcement reduces staple site bleeding during laparoscopic gastric bypass: a prospective randomized trial. *Arch Surg* 2005;140: 773–8.

20. Fernandez AZ, Jr., DeMaria EJ, Tichansky DS, et al. Experience with over 3,000 open and laparoscopic bariatric procedures: multivariate analysis of factors related to leak and resultant mortality. *Surg Endosc* 2004;18:193–7.

21. Marshall JS, Srivastava A, Gupta SK, Rossi TR, DeBord JR. Roux-en-Y gastric bypass leak complications. *Arch Surg* 2003;138:520–3; discussion 3–4.

22. Fullum TM, Aluka KJ, Turner PL. Decreasing anastomotic and staple line leaks after laparoscopic Roux-en-Y gastric bypass. *Surg Endosc* 2009;23:1403–8.

23. Georgiadou D, Sergentanis TN, Nixon A, Diamantis T, Tsigris C, Psaltopoulou T. Efficacy and safety of laparoscopic mini gastric bypass. A systematic review. *Surg Obes Relat Dis* 2014;10:984–91.

24. Deitel M, Gagner M, Erickson AL, Crosby RD. Third International Summit: current status of sleeve gastrectomy. *Surg Obes Relat Dis* 2011;7:749–59.

25. Rosenthal RJ, International Sleeve Gastrectomy Expert P, Diaz AA, et al. International Sleeve Gastrectomy Expert Panel Consensus Statement: best practice guidelines based on experience of >12,000 cases. *Surg Obes Relat Dis* 2012;8:8–19.

26. Burgos AM, Braghetto I, Csendes A, et al. Gastric leak after laparoscopic-sleeve gastrectomy for obesity. *Obes Surg* 2009;19:1672–7.

27. Deitel M, Crosby RD, Gagner M. The First International Consensus Summit for Sleeve Gastrectomy (SG), New York City, October 25–27, 2007. *Obes Surg* 2008;18: 487–96.

28. Alasfar F, Sabnis AA, Liu RC, Chand B. Stricture rate after laparoscopic Roux-en-Y Gastric bypass with a 21-mm circular stapler: the Cleveland Clinic experience. *Med Princ Pract* 2009;18:364–7.

29. Mathew A, Veliuona MA, DePalma FJ, Cooney RN. Gastrojejunal stricture after gastric bypass and efficacy of endoscopic intervention. *Dig Dis Sci* 2009;54: 1971–8.

30. Frezza EE, Reddy S, Gee LL, Wachtel MS. Complications after sleeve gastrectomy for morbid obesity. *Obes Surg* 2009;19:684–7.

31. Sarkhosh K, Birch DW, Sharma A, Karmali S. Complications associated with laparoscopic sleeve gastrectomy for morbid obesity: a surgeon's guide. *Can J Surg* 2013; 56:347–52.

32. Parikh A, Alley JB, Peterson RM, et al. Management options for symptomatic stenosis after laparoscopic vertical sleeve gastrectomy in the morbidly obese. *Surg Endosc* 2012;26:738–46.

33. Cottam D, Qureshi FG, Mattar SG, et al. Laparoscopic sleeve gastrectomy as an initial weight-loss procedure for high-risk patients with morbid obesity. *Surg Endosc* 2006;20:859–63.

34. Higa KD, Ho T, Boone KB. Internal hernias after laparoscopic Roux-en-Y gastric bypass: incidence, treatment and prevention. *Obes Surg* 2003;13:350–4.

35. Schneider C, Cobb W, Scott J, Carbonell A, Myers K, Bour E. Rapid excess weight loss following laparoscopic gastric bypass leads to increased risk of internal hernia. *Surg Endosc* 2011;25:1594–8.

36. Carmody B, DeMaria EJ, Jamal M, et al. Internal hernia after laparoscopic Roux-en-Y gastric bypass. *Surg Obes Relat Dis* 2005;1:543–8.

37. Steele KE, Prokopowicz GP, Magnuson T, Lidor A, Schweitzer M. Laparoscopic antecolic Roux-en-Y gastric bypass with closure of internal defects leads to fewer internal hernias than the retrocolic approach. *Surg Endosc* 2008;22:2056–61.

38. Stenberg E, Szabo E, Agren G, et al. Closure of mesenteric defects in laparoscopic gastric bypass: a multicentre, randomised, parallel, open-label trial. *Lancet* 2016;387:1397–1404.

39. Sapala JA, Wood MH, Sapala MA, Flake TM, Jr. Marginal ulcer after gastric bypass: a prospective 3-year study of 173 patients. *Obes Surg* 1998;8:505–16.

40. Csendes A, Burgos AM, Altuve J, Bonacic S. Incidence of marginal ulcer 1 month and 1 to 2 years after gastric bypass: a prospective consecutive endoscopic evaluation of 442 patients with morbid obesity. *Obes Surg* 2009; 19:135–8.

41. Cucchi SG, Pories WJ, MacDonald KG, Morgan EJ. Gastrogastric fistulas. A complication of divided gastric bypass surgery. *Ann Surg* 1995;221:387–91.

42. Tucker ON, Szomstein S, Rosenthal RJ. Surgical management of gastro-gastric fistula after divided laparoscopic Roux-en-Y gastric bypass for morbid obesity. *J Gastrointest Surg* 2007;11:1673–9.

43. Buchwald H, Buchwald JN, McGlennon TW. Systematic review and meta-analysis of medium-term outcomes after banded Roux-en-Y gastric bypass. *Obes Surg* 2014;24:1536–51.

44. Chapman AE, Kiroff G, Game P, et al. Laparoscopic adjustable gastric banding in the treatment of obesity: a systematic literature review. *Surgery* 2004;135:326–51.

45. Chevallier JM, Zinzindohoue F, Douard R, et al. Complications after laparoscopic adjustable gastric banding for morbid obesity: experience with 1,000 patients over 7 years. *Obes Surg* 2004;14:407–14.

46. Biagini J, Karam L. Ten years experience with laparoscopic adjustable gastric banding. *Obes Surg* 2008;18:573–7.

47. Vijgen GH, Schouten R, Pelzers L, Greve JW, van Helden SH, Bouvy ND. Revision of laparoscopic adjustable gastric banding: success or failure? *Obes Surg* 2012;22:287–92.

48. Schouten R, Japink D, Meesters B, Nelemans PJ, Greve JW. Systematic literature review of reoperations after gastric banding: is a stepwise approach justified? *Surg Obes Relat Dis* 2011;7:99–109.

49. Abu-Abeid S, Szold A. Laparoscopic management of Lap-Band erosion. *Obes Surg* 2001;11:87–9.

50. Brown WA, Egberts KJ, Franke-Richard D, Thodiyil P, Anderson ML, O'Brien PE. Erosions after laparoscopic adjustable gastric banding: diagnosis and management. *Ann Surg* 2013;257:1047–52.

51. Himpens J, Dapri G, Cadiere GB. A prospective randomized study between laparoscopic gastric banding and laparoscopic isolated sleeve gastrectomy: results after 1 and 3 years. *Obes Surg* 2006;16:1450–6.

52. Chiu S, Birch DW, Shi X, Sharma AM, Karmali S. Effect of sleeve gastrectomy on gastroesophageal reflux disease: a systematic review. *Surg Obes Relat Dis* 2011;7:510–5.

53. Soricelli E, Iossa A, Casella G, Abbatini F, Cali B, Basso N. Sleeve gastrectomy and crural repair in obese patients with gastroesophageal reflux disease and/or hiatal hernia. *Surg Obes Relat Dis* 2013;9:356–61.

54. Buchwald H, Estok R, Fahrbach K, Banel D, Sledge I. Trends in mortality in bariatric surgery: a systematic review and meta-analysis. *Surgery* 2007;142:621–32; discussion 32–5.

55. Biertho L, Lebel S, Marceau S, et al. Perioperative complications in a consecutive series of 1000 duodenal switches. *Surg Obes Relat Dis* 2013;9:63–8.

56. Hamoui N, Chock B, Anthone GJ, Crookes PF. Revision of the duodenal switch: indications, technique, and outcomes. *J Am Coll Surg* 2007;204:603–8.

57. Aasheim ET, Bjorkman S, Sovik TT, et al. Vitamin status after bariatric surgery: a randomized study of gastric bypass and duodenal switch. *Am J Clin Nutr* 2009;90:15–22.

58. Sinha N, Shieh A, Stein EM, et al. Increased PTH and 1.25(OH)(2)D levels associated with increased markers of bone turnover following bariatric surgery. *Obesity (Silver Spring)* 2011;19:2388–93.

59. Slater GH, Ren CJ, Siegel N, et al. Serum fat-soluble vitamin deficiency and abnormal calcium metabolism after malabsorptive bariatric surgery. *J Gastrointest Surg* 2004;8:48–55; discussion 4–5.

60. Baltasar A, Serra C, Perez N, Bou R, Bengochea M. Clinical hepatic impairment after the duodenal switch. *Obes Surg* 2004;14:77–83.

61. Keshishian A, Zahriya K, Willes EB. Duodenal switch has no detrimental effects on hepatic function and improves hepatic steatohepatitis after 6 months. *Obes Surg* 2005;15:1418–23.

Intestines

20

Prevention and Management of Complications after Duodenal and Small Bowel Surgery

A.-K. Stadler, M. Büchler and O. Strobel

ABSTRACT

The duodenal region with its complex anatomy can be affected by multiple diseases, requiring management by a variety of technically demanding surgical procedures. Small bowel surgery is technically less demanding but frequently necessary in emergency conditions that are associated with an increased risk of complications. Most complications of duodenal and small bowel surgery are characterised by leakage of aggressive secretions that can be very difficult to manage. Unsuccessful initial management of such leakages often results in the formation of gastrointestinal and enteroatmospheric fistulae, which are associated with high morbidity, a severe reduction in the quality of life and high mortality. This chapter provides an overview of typical complications after duodenal and small bowel surgeries and summarises the options for their successful initial management and for the management of gastrointestinal fistulae.

KEYWORDS

Duodenal surgery, small bowel surgery, complication management, leakage, gastrointestinal fistulae, enterocutaneous fistula, enteroatmospheric fistula

INTRODUCTION

The duodenum, with its central location in the upper abdomen, has a complex anatomy as the site of junction of both the common bile duct and the pancreatic ducts with the gastrointestinal tract. This region can be affected by multiple neoplastic, inflammatory and functional diseases that require a broad variety of technically demanding surgical procedures that aim to cure the underlying disease while maintaining or reconstructing biliary and pancreatic drainage and gastrointestinal continuity. This variety of surgical procedures is associated with a similarly broad range of possible complications. The most frequent and, at the same time, the most difficult complications to manage are leakages after duodenal surgery. With several litres of bile, pancreatic juice, gastric juice and oral nutrition passing through this area, such leakage can result in high-flow output of aggressive secretions that can be very difficult to manage and can result in severe secondary complications. Although the surgery of the jejunum and ileum is significantly less complex, enteric leakages are frequent complications after emergency surgery for severe peritonitis or trauma, requiring several relaparotomies or leaving the abdomen open. Unsuccessful initial management of leakages after duodenal and small bowel surgery results in the formation of gastrointestinal fistulae, which have a major impact on the morbidity and mortality of patients. Morbidity from gastrointestinal fistulae includes pain, wound problems, nutritional deficiencies and recurrent septic states and represents a significant burden with respect to both the quality of life of the patients and the treatment costs.[1] As most gastrointestinal fistulae are the result of complications of surgical and medical interventions and their unsuccessful management, this important topic tends to be underrepresented in the medical literature.[1]

This chapter aims to provide an overview of typical complications that can appear after duodenal and small bowel surgery and to summarise possible options for the management of these complications. Although it is obvious that the best management for such complex problems has to be tailored on a case-specific basis, we also have tried to give some general recommendations, including which parameters need to be considered for making decisions.

OVERVIEW OF DIFFERENT SURGICAL PROCEDURES AND ASSOCIATED COMPLICATIONS

Duodenal and small bowel surgery encompasses a wide range of surgical procedures. This part of the chapter focusses on the main procedure types and their corresponding specific complications. An overview of surgical procedures and corresponding specific complications is provided in Table 20.1.

Duodenal Ulcer Surgery and Duodenal Stump Closure

Although subtotal or total gastrectomy are most frequently performed for gastric cancer and are addressed in greater detail in Chapter 17, these procedures require sufficient closure of the duodenal stump, and duodenal stump insufficiency is one of the most feared complications

Table 20.1 Surgical procedures involving the duodenum and small intestine and their specific postoperative complications

	Surgical procedures	Indications	Possible complications
Stomach and duodenum	Subtotal gastrectomy Total gastrectomy	Gastric cancer Ulcer disease	Duodenal stump insufficiency
	Pyloroplasty Excision of duodenal ulcer Duodenotomy Duodenal wedge resection	Benign stenosis, pylorospasm Ulcer disease Bleeding ulcer, tumour enucleations Small, benign tumours, gastrointestinal stromal tumours	Insufficiency/leakage
	Duodenojejunostomy Pancreas-sparing duodenectomy Subtotal duodenectomy Distal duodenectomy	Coverage procedure, e.g., ulcer Benign tumours of the duodenum	Insufficiency/leakage Insufficiency of choledocho- and pancreatojejunostomy, pancreatitis
	Pancreatoduodenectomy	Carcinoma of duodenum, pancreas or distal bile duct Complex ulcers	Postoperative pancreatic fistula and other specific complications
	Ampullectomy	Adenoma/stenosis of ampulla of Vater	Duodenal leakage, pancreatic fistula, acute pancreatitis
Small bowel	Elective segmental resection		Insufficiency Short bowel syndrome
	Surgery for Crohn's disease		Fistulas, abscess, insufficiency
	Elective or emergency surgery involving extensive adhesiolysis	Other indication requiring surgery, mechanical ileus	Deserosations: Perforation of small and large bowel
	Emergency resections for ischaemia Extended segmental resections	Acute mesenteric ischaemia	
	Emergency resections for peritonitis	Acute peritonitis	Deserosations: Perforation of small and large bowel
	Decompression laparotomy, open abdomen	Abdominal compartment	Enteroatmospheric fistulae

after these procedures.[2] Moreover, subtotal gastrectomy may be the procedure of choice for extended duodenal ulcers in which oversewing is not safe. The most frequent indication for emergency gastric and duodenal surgery remains complicated ulcer disease. Although the absolute frequency of surgery for peptic ulcer disease has decreased with the introduction of proton-pump inhibitors and eradication therapy for *Helicobacter pylori* for effective conservative management[3] and with endoscopic management of ulcer bleeding, patients now tend to present with increased comorbidities and often with more extended ulcers after conservative management. The management of such extended perforating and penetrating ulcers can be very demanding and requires an experienced surgeon, who can choose the safest option from a broad variety of procedures—ranging from simple oversewing, wedge resection, coverage procedures (e.g., by duodenojejunostomy) and subtotal gastrectomy with duodenal stump closure or with direct anastomosis to the duodenum/ulcer wall to emergency pancreatoduodenectomy.[4,5] The safest technique for closure of the duodenal stump during subtotal gastrectomy for duodenal ulcer depends on several factors including the size of the ulcer, the local extension to the neighbouring structures such as the pancreatic head and hepatoduodenal ligament, and the general condition of the patient. Although direct closure of the duodenal stump after sufficient mobilisation of the duodenum, as described by Nissen in 1933[6] and later modified by Bsteh,[6] remains the standard procedure, the rigidity of the inflamed tissue in a chronic (callous) duodenal ulcer can render such direct closure difficult or impossible. In such cases, additional coverage with serosal patches such as omentum, the falciform ligament and a rectus abdominis muscle flap may be performed. If the extent of subtotal gastrectomy allows a tension-free approximation of the remaining stomach and duodenal stump, a Billroth-I reconstruction with direct restoration of continuity by gastroduodenostomy, including the callous ulcer wall in the anastomosis, can be a safe option. Another option is the management of the duodenal stump by a duodenojejunostomy. In all cases of difficult duodenal stump closure, the placement of a T-tube in the common bile duct for diversion of bile flow is an additional option to protect the duodenal stump. It should be emphasised that there is no best 'standard management' for the difficult duodenal stump, but the choice of the best procedure has to be made on a case-by-case basis. Therefore, there are only very few noncontrolled studies comparing different techniques. One such study compared duodenojejunostomy in 62 cases with 62 matched cases

chosen from a group of 259 conventional closures.[6] In this study, duodenojejunostomy was safer, with a mortality of 4.8% versus 16.1% and a duodenal leak rate of 14.5% versus 29%, and additional biliary diversion was associated with lower duodenal leak rates after both procedures. Roux-en-Y-duodenojejunostomy is also an option for the management of duodenal perforations for other reasons (e.g., iatrogenic origin), especially if the perforation is located near the papilla of Vater.

Duodenotomy

A pyloropasty in the adult may be indicated to improve stomach emptying in patients with benign peptic stenosis of the pyloric region or pylorospasm associated with other procedures such as an oesophagectomy. The classical pyloroplasty (Heinecke-Mikulicz) consists of a longitudinal full-thickness pylorotomy reaching from the gastric antrum to the proximal duodenum with a transverse closure, resulting in a pyloric sphincterotomy and plastic extension of the gastric outlet.

A duodenotomy has to be performed to get access to the duodenal lumen in the context of several procedures. If surgical haemostasis of bleeding duodenal ulcers becomes necessary after failure of endoscopic management, access to the ulcer is usually gained by a longitudinal duodenotomy (often with pylorotomy) and transverse closure, similar to that described for pyloroplasty. Other indications for duodenotomy are small/benign duodenal tumours that can be managed by enucleation or duodenal wedge resection. A duodenotomy is also performed during surgical ampullectomy (*see* **Surgery of the Second Part of the Duodenum and Ampullary Region**).

The common complications of pyloroplasty and duodenotomy in the perioperative course are leakages by insufficient suturing. Duodenal stenosis may develop as a long-term complication.

Surgery of the Second Part of the Duodenum and Ampullary Region

Surgical procedures on the second part of the duodenum can be demanding, because this is the site of the junction of the common bile duct and major pancreatic duct at the papilla major and of the junction of the minor pancreatic duct at the papilla minor with the duodenum. Any surgical procedure necessary in this part of the duodenum has to aim for a complete cure (e.g., R0 resection of a neoplastic lesion) of the underlying pathology and a preservation or reconstruction of the biliary and pancreatic drainages. During both proximal and distal (to the papilla of Vater) partial duodenectomies, great care has to be taken to allow for safe closure (or anastomosis) of the duodenum, without compromising the papilla. A probe placed in the duodenum through the cystic duct and common bile duct after cholecystectomy usually allows the surgeon to safely locate the papilla during these procedures. A pancreas-sparing total duodenectomy is a rare operation that should be carried out in specialised centres for duodenal neoplasms, especially for premalignant multiple duodenal adenomas in the context of familial adenomatous polyposis.[7,8] Pancreas-sparing duodenectomy requires the reinsertion of the common bile duct and major pancreatic duct (or their common channel) into the jejunum (neoduodenum). The minor pancreatic duct can be reinserted or has to be closed and should be identified. Surgical ampullectomy is a good option for surgical treatment of adenomas located at the papilla of Vater, for postinflammatory stenosis and for some functional pathologies. This procedure has been widely replaced by endoscopic management in clinical practice but is underestimated, because it provides excellent long-lasting results.[9] Surgical ampullectomy requires a longitudinal duodenotomy, excision of the papilla of Vater and the reinsertion of the main pancreatic duct and common bile duct. The specific complications of these procedures are leakages of the anastomosis, resulting in biliary, postoperative pancreatic fistula (POPF),[10] combined fistula and duodenal leakage, dependent on the site of insufficiency. The POPF can also be the result of damage to the pancreatic parenchyma during mobilisation of the duodenal wall from the pancreatic head or can originate from a minor pancreatic duct that has not been properly identified. Another severe complication is the development of acute pancreatitis. If postoperative acute pancreatitis develops as a result of pancreatic ductal obstruction, it is frequently severe and associated with disruption of the anastomosis and severe secondary complications.

Pancreatoduodenectomy

The majority of duodenal, ampullary and periampullary neoplasms are malignant at the time of diagnosis and require partial pancreatoduodenectomy as an oncological adequate resection. Similarly, pancreatoduodenectomy is always an option for the conditions discussed in the paragraph above if pancreas-sparing procedures cannot be safely performed. Furthermore, emergency partial pancreatoduodenectomy (or total pancreatectomy) are backup procedures for damage-control surgery in selected complicated cases in which conservative, endoscopic and interventional managements have failed and less-invasive surgical management does not solve the problem safely, as discussed above.[4,5] Pancreatoduodenectomy is associated with a high morbidity, and POPF is certainly still the single-most important complication that dictates outcome.[10,11] The range of complications after pancreatoduodenectomy and the current evidence on how to reduce and manage these complications are a vast topic that goes far beyond the scope of this chapter and are addressed in detail in Chapters 31 to 36 of this book.

Small Bowel Surgery

We have divided small bowel surgery into five areas associated with specific risks of complications that also impact complication management. These areas are listed below.

Elective Segmental Resections

These procedures account for only a small part of bowel resections, because the main indications are mainly taking down of loop ileostomies established during previous rectal cancer surgery, rare neoplasms of the small bowel, gastrointestinal bleeding originating from the small bowel or secondary involvement of the small bowel by tumours of other organs. Such segmental small bowel resections are usually not technically demanding and require primary small intestinal anastomoses that are relatively safe, independent of the fact which technique of anastomosis is used.[12] Although rare, the main complication remains anastomotic leakage, usually requiring immediate reoperation and reresection but can result in severe courses with enteral fistulae (see below) if the initial management fails.

Surgery for Crohn's Disease

Although the most frequent procedure for Crohn's disease is ileocaecal resection, segmental small bowel resection and stricturoplasty are also frequently used in this disease. The unique pathophysiology of Crohn's disease, with the need for immunosuppressive therapy; the likely need of additional resections, with loss of small bowel length in the future; and an increased risk of complications such as anastomotic failure, abscess and fistula formation have to be kept in mind during elective surgery, emergency surgery and complication management in these patients. A detailed description of this topic is beyond the scope of this chapter and can be found in publications dedicated to this complex disease.[13,14]

Emergency or Elective Surgery Involving Extensive Adhesiolysis

If patients with extensive intestinal adhesions after previous abdominal surgery (especially after surgery for peritonitis or those who have had a complicated course after a previous operation) require emergency surgery for ileus or elective surgery for an unrelated new pathology, extensive adhesiolysis may be necessary. During such operations, utmost care has to be taken to avoid or repair serosal tears or perforations of the small bowel that will result in small bowel leaks and can result in postoperative courses, with an open abdomen and enteral fistulae (see below), if initial complication management fails.

Emergency Surgery for Small Bowel Ischaemia

Small bowel ischaemia can occur both as the consequence of adhesions or incarcerated hernias due to strangulation and prolonged bowel distension or as the consequence of mesenteric vascular ischaemia. If small bowel ischaemia has occurred as a consequence of strangulation or distension, irreversibly, ischaemic segments can usually be clearly distinguished from segments recovering after adhesiolysis and decompression. Dependent on the local conditions and the general condition of the patient, a segmental resection with primary anastomosis, generation of an anastomotic enterostomy or a discontinuity resection can be performed. When making this decision, the risk of anastomotic insufficiency has to be considered. As described above, secondary lesions by serosal tears or perforations during adhesiolysis have to be strictly avoided or thoroughly repaired.

If small bowel ischaemia results from a thrombosis or embolism to the superior mesenteric artery, the first step is to restore mesenteric perfusion, if possible, and to resect the segment that is irreversibly damaged.[15] In these cases, it can be difficult to distinguished irreversibly and reversibly damaged small bowel, and a second-look strategy may be useful.

Furthermore, the fashioning of enterostomies may offer a safer alternative, with the additional benefit of a window for mucosa evaluation compared with a primary anastomosis. The best management of patients with small bowel ischaemia is again a topic that cannot be covered in adequate detail here but is described in detail in Chapters 23 and 24 of this book. The typical complications that cannot always be avoided are the necessity for secondary resections, owing due to additional ischaemia and the high mortality associated with the underlying disease.

Emergency Resections for Peritonitis

Small bowel perforations account for only a small part of cases with secondary peritonitis. The most frequent causes for spontaneous small bowel perforations include local ischaemia due to incarceration, strangulation or prolonged distension, perforation in the context of Crohn's disease, small bowel ulcers and small bowel tumours. Small bowel perforations can also be secondary to blunt or, more frequently, to perforating abdominal trauma. However, a significant part of small bowel perforations occurs as complications of abdominal surgery. Therefore, the management of these small bowel perforations is described in more detail in the second part of this chapter devoted to the complication management. Many of such small bowel lesions that occur in the context of damage-control surgery require repeated relaparotomies or an open abdomen and result in the formation of enteroatmospheric fistulae.

Although leakages are frequently in focus as the dominant perioperative complication after small bowel surgery, the development of the short bowel syndrome is a severe long-term complication of extended small bowel resections that we always have to keep in mind. Although extensive resections of damaged small bowel may frequently be safer to avoid leakages, they harbour an increased risk of developing a subsequent short-bowel syndrome. Therefore, the surgical strategy in complex cases has to be frequently a compromise that balances the risks of leakage and of small bowel syndrome and attempts to save as much small bowel as possible.

PREVENTION OF COMPLICATIONS

Complications have a direct impact on the outcome of surgery, and the incidence of specific complications is often used as an indicator of its quality. Therefore, the prevention of complications must be our first aim. However, early detection and effective management of complications are almost equally important, because these factors define if a patient can be rescued from the complication and secondary complications or if even death can be avoided. The prevention of complications is a broad field. As described above, the broad variety of different pathologies affecting the duodenum and small bowel have to be treated with multiple different surgical procedures. Each of these procedures has its own risks of complications, and this risk is affected by multiple factors, including the underlying pathology, patient-related parameters and treatment-related parameters.

In the following section, we present some general recommendations on how complications in duodenal and small bowel surgery may be prevented or reduced. Many of these general aspects are covered in detail in Chapters 2 to 7. It is well known that morbidity and mortality after complex surgery are associated with hospital and surgeon volume[16] (*see also* Chapters 9 and 10). Therefore, the most experienced surgeons should perform or assist complex cases. Among the procedures described above, this may be especially applicable not only to duodenectomies and ampullectomy but also for the management of a difficult duodenal stump. If experience (i.e., procedure volume) for a specific procedure is not sufficient at a local hospital, the possibility of referral to a specialised centre should be considered in elective surgery cases. Most of the above-mentioned surgical complications are leakages by insufficient closure or at the anastomosis. The prerequisites to avoid leakages that have to be respected during surgery are adequate blood supply, tension-free anastomosis and sutures and meticulous suturing technique.[17] However, surgery is always team work, and one other prerequisite is the absence of severe bowel oedema. Bowel oedema must be avoided by the surgeon by careful handling and low blood loss, but it is mainly defined by perioperative volume management by the anaesthesiologists.[18] A standardised perioperative management is probably almost as important as the surgery itself, not only for prevention but also for early detection and timely management of complications. Standard operating procedures with respect to important aspects of perioperative care, including antibiotics, thrombosis and ulcer prophylaxis; patient education; early postoperative mobilisation; nutrition; timely removal of catheters and drains; postoperative laboratory controls; etc. are mandatory.

MANAGEMENT OF COMPLICATIONS

Even with the highest quality of surgery and perioperative care, complications cannot be completely avoided, and despite intensive research on improvement of surgical outcome, morbidity rates after complex abdominal surgery remain considerable. This is probably best documented for pancreatic surgery, where mortality has been reduced to well below 5%; however, morbidity rates are still as high as 40%.[19] In major surgical procedures and especially in major abdominal surgery, the postoperative course is defined by the occurrence and severity of one specific complication that will lead to subsequent complications up to a fatal outcome if not managed successfully (*see also* Chapter 6). For duodenal and small bowel surgery, the

major specific complications are enteric leakages, which may result in peritonitis and severe septic complications up to multiple organ failure and death, but even if a fatal outcome is prevented, the septic complications may also result in the formation of gastrointestinal fistulae, with a significant reduction in the quality of life in the long term.[1]

Effective management of these surgical 'pacemaker' complications is, therefore, crucial to prevent severe subsequent problems, fatalities and severe impairment in the long term. The first prerequisite for effective complication management, especially for duodenal and intestinal leaks, is early detection and intervention. Here, in-house standards with respect to the postoperative monitoring of the patient and early detection of a deviation from a normal postoperative course become important. If a complication, that is, a deviation from the normal postoperative course, is suspected, adequate diagnostic measures have to be initiated in a timely fashion, and the best management has to be defined by an experienced team based on complex information that includes the exact surgical procedure performed; the postoperative course up to date; interval between surgery and detection of the complication; the results of diagnostic imaging and laboratory tests; the current condition and the comorbidities of the patient and the availability of and expertise with the different treatment options (e.g., surgical reintervention, interventional endoscopy and interventional radiology). The importance of such expertise with complication management is highlighted by the observation that differences in mortality after complex surgical procedures between low- and high-volume hospitals are not associated with large differences in complication rates but are explained by the ability of a hospital to effectively rescue patients from complications.[20]

Presentation and Clinical Workup of Complications

Most of the above-mentioned complications after duodenal and small bowel surgery involves infections such infected fluid collections, abscesses and peritonitis. Whereas peritonitis usually presents as an acute abdomen with the development of a septic state, the clinical presentation of an abscess may be less specific with symptoms such as delayed gastric emptying and ileus. An infectious complication should be suspected if the parameters for infection after the operation stay elevated or rise again after an initial peak in their early postoperative course. Although standards for postoperative surveillance by laboratory tests differ between centres and countries, we have experience with the C-reactive protein level, which enables the early diagnosis and diagnostic workup for potential infectious complications.[21,22] If other frequent postoperative infections such as superficial wound infections, pneumonia, urinary tract infections and infected central venous catheters are ruled out, further diagnostic workup is warranted. In this case, contrast-enhanced computed tomography (CT) is the imaging modality of choice, because it will, in most cases, allow us to differentiate between a locally confined problem such as an abscess and a perforation with diffuse peritonitis. In case of a localised problem, an interventional CT-guided percutaneous drainage can be placed. Ultrasound for diagnosis and ultrasound-guided percutaneous drainage may be effective alternatives for units with experience in interventional ultrasonography. Of course, a leak can also present itself by an abnormal drain output and/or wound secretion. In case of doubt, the oral administration of the dye methylene blue can be used to prove its presence.

Management of Duodenal Leakage

The management of duodenal leakage is demanding and needs to be tailored in a case-by-case fashion, depending on several parameters. The most important parameters are (i) the interval between the operation and the diagnosis of the complication and (ii) the general condition of the patient. Potential management strategies for duodenal leakage are summarised in Table 20.2. Surgical revision is the first choice if a surgical closure appears possible and the risk to induce further damage is low. This is the case if the leakage is detected early, within the first 4 to 7 postoperative days. With an increasing interval from the initial operation and if the leakage has already persisted for several days, the success rate of a surgical closure decreases, whereas the danger to induce secondary lesions increases. If the decision for surgical reintervention is made, the revision should be performed by an experienced surgeon who is able to perform the entire spectrum of procedures listed in Table 20.2. In case of postoperative duodenal leakage, the spectrum of possible or necessary procedures is similar to that described for the management of the difficult duodenal stump, described above. If a primary suture of the duodenum was performed in the first operation and has become insufficient, an attempt to resuture the now-inflamed tissue will often result in another leak. Additional coverage procedures or management by duodenojejunostomy may increase safety. Additional biliary diversion by choledochotomy and insertion of a T-tube during surgical revision or by a percutaneous transhepatic cholangiographic drainage (PTCD) drainage after surgery may offer additional protection, as described

Table 20.2 Management options for duodenal leakages

Treatment classes	Therapy

Surgical revisions	• Direct closure of perforations
	• Coverage by duodenojejunostomy (Roux-en-Y)
	• Re-resection and reanastomosis
	• Surgical drainage
	  – Additional coverage with serosal flaps
	  – Additional T-tube for biliary diversion
	• Emergency pancreatoduodenectomy
	• Total pancreatectomy

Interventional radiology	• Percutaneous interventional drainages • Percutaneous transhepatic cholangiodrainage for biliary diversion • Angiographic interventions for arterial bleeding
Endoscopic interventions	• Duodenal stenting • Stenting of biliary and/or pancreatic ducts • Nasobiliary drainage for biliary diversion • Endoscopic drainages • Jejunal catheter (for enteral nutrition)

Pharmacological treatment	• Supportive therapy
	  – Antibiotic therapy of infection
	  – Somatostatin analogues to decrease gastrointestinal/pancreatic/bile secretions
	• Loperamide (opioids) for bowel rest
	• Parenteral nutrition or enteral nutrition (via tube aboral of fistula)
	• Wound care, skin protection

for the management of duodenal perforations above.[6] If the defect cannot be safely managed by suture or coverage or a duodenojejunostomy, the difficult decision for resection (up to emergency pancreatoduodenectomy or total pancreatectomy) versus simple catheter drainage has to be made. Emergency pancreatoduodenectomy is a demanding procedure with high morbidity and has to be considered carefully but can solve the problem.[5] Controlled surgical drainage with the placement of catheters into the duodenum (e.g., Foley catheters) during surgery or percutaneous drainage represents less-invasive alternatives that may result in successful closure of the leak[23] or in the establishment of a stable fistula that can be surgically revised after an interval of 3 months. Again, additional biliary diversion by PTCD should be considered. If surgical revision does not appear promising, radiological and/or endoscopic interventions have to be considered. Although percutaneous drainage (either CT-guided or ultrasound-guided) will then be the best choice for most patients, endoscopic treatment (e.g., stenting and placement of nasobiliary catheters) may be a valuable alternative in selected cases of duodenal leakage. In patients with leaks from the choledocho- or pancreatojejunostomy or with acute obstructive pancreatitis after ampullectomy or pancreas-sparing duodenectomy, endoscopic retrograde cholangiopancreatography (ERCP) and stenting may represent good treatment options if performed by experienced interventional endoscopists. Both surgical and interventional therapies have to be accompanied with pharmacological and supportive medical therapy (Table 20.2). Antibiotic therapy, fluid replacement and parenteral nutrition (or enteral via a jejunal catheter) have to be administered in a standardised fashion. Additional administration of somatostatin analogues for inhibition of gastrointestinal secretion may be beneficial.[24]

Management of Small Bowel Leaks

In contrast to duodenal leaks, isolated small bowel leaks after segmental resection of the jejunum or ileum are a rare complication. If detected in time, anastomotic insufficiency after small bowel segmental resection can be treated by simple additional segmental resections and reanastomosis. Small bowel anastomotic leakage is defined as a connection between the intra- and extraluminal compartments due to a defect in the intestinal wall of the anastomosis. A severity grading range from grade A, with no intervention needed, and grade B, with interventional treatment (e.g., percutaneous drainage), to grade C, with need of relaparotomy.[25]

However, most small bowel leakages occur as complications in more complex settings, such as peritonitis, multiple revisions, open abdomen and a frozen abdomen. Risk factors and strategies to prevent small bowel leakages are listed in Table 20.3. Additional risk factors identified in a retrospective study in 764 patients are chronic obstructive pulmonary disease (COPD), long-term use of corticosteroids, perioperative blood transfusion and peritonitis.[26] Further risk factors are malnutrition, obesity and arterial hypertonia with altered blood vessels.[27]

The presentation and diagnostic principles for managing small bowel leakages are very similar to what we described above for the duodenum. In the complex situations of open abdomen, enteric leaks will become obvious by suspicious looking drainage or wound secretions. Again, very similar to duodenal leaks, surgical revision is the first choice, and the success rate of surgical closure of the leak decreases with an increasing duration of leak and associated peritonitis. In contrast to duodenal

Table 20.3 Risk factors of and strategy for prevention for enteric fistulae

Risk factors	Preventive strategy
Foreign intra-abdominal material	• Avoid implantation of mesh grafts in inlay position • Avoid suture material with strong foreign material reaction • Remove drainages as soon as possible
Inflammation or infection Bacterial peritonitis	• Anti-inflammatory therapy, antibiotics
History of radiation	
Neoplasia, distal obstruction	• Resection, bypass or stoma proximal of the obstruction
Malnutrition	• Pre- and perioperative nutrition support
Extensive visceral resection	
Bowel ischaemia	• Negative-pressure wound therapy with low suction pressures
Mechanical trauma/desiccation	• Cover the bowel with great omentum or plastic sheet • Avoid direct contact between closure system and viscera • Avoid extensive and aggressive debridement • Avoid programmed relaparotomies; do them on demand
Prolonged open abdomen	• Close abdomen as fast as possible • Choose a temporal closure system preventing fascial retraction

Adapted from: Di Saverio S, Tarasconi A, Walczak DA, et al. Classification, prevention and management of entero-atmospheric fistula: a state-of-the-art review. *Langenbecks Arch Surg* 2016;401: 1–13.

complications, interventional therapy is usually no alternative for the treatment of leakages in the free small intestine. Although direct suture is often performed, resection and reanastomosis are often a safer option. Segmental resections with generation of an anastomotic enterostomy or discontinuity resections with terminal enterostomy can represent safe alternatives. However, dependent on the location of the resection, enterostomies can result in the short bowel syndrome and in complex wound problems, if combined with abdominal wall defects. However, in complex situations, with multiple enteric leakages, even the formation of a proximal deviation jejunostomy can be considered in rare cases.

In the case of recurrent enteric leaks in a 'frozen' abdomen with severe adhesions, all of these options (suture, resection and enterostomy) may be impossible. In such cases, the placement of catheters and/or the application of vacuum-assisted wound closure (VAC) systems can be used with the aim to establish stable enteric fistulae, which can then be addressed by surgical revisions after consolidation. An enterocutaneous fistula is an established fistula that extends from the intestine to the intact skin. In contrast, small bowel fistulae that occur in the setting of an open abdomen are called enteroatmospheric fistulae.

Management of Enterocutaneous and Enteroatmospheric Fistulas

Gastrointestinal fistulae are associated with high comorbidity and a severe impact on the patient's quality of life.[1] Although the first aim of complication management after small bowel surgery is the prevention of gastrointestinal fistulae, in some cases, the formation of fistulae cannot be avoided and the generation of a stable fistula may be the only way out of peritonitis and sepsis. In these cases, the optimal management of gastrointestinal fistulae becomes important.

Enterocutaneous and enteroatmospheric fistulae are associated with a variety of problems, depending on their localisation in the gastrointestinal tract and abdominal wall/open abdomen, their output and their distribution in the case of multiple fistulae. These criteria define the complexity of fistula management and can be used for a classification that has been developed for enteroatmospheric fistulae, as summarised in Table 20.4.

Therefore, the management of gastrointestinal fistulae has to address several aspects that are summarised in Table 20.5. If the attempt to directly close a gastrointestinal leak has failed and a leak persists, the first aim is to establish a 'controlled' fistula, that is, to divert fistula output from the abdominal cavity or the open abdomen. In case of a closed abdomen, this can be established by leaving surgical drains in place until a stable fistula tract has formed. In the absence of suitably located surgical drains, additional placement of interventional drains may be necessary. In the case of an enteroatmospheric fistula, the diversion of fistula output from the open abdomen can be very difficult but has to be achieved to allow for granulation and closure of the abdominal cavity. In this case, some inventive spirit is necessary, and multiple solutions have been described in the literature; these solutions have been nicely summarised with exemplary figures in a recent review.[28] Most of the techniques described are based on a principle of negative-pressure wound therapy (NPWT) or VAC to allow cleansing and granulation of the viscera, accompanied by a technique to divert fistula outflow from the surrounding wound dressing.[28–31] An example of a wound-dressing technique for enteroatmospheric fistulae used in our clinic that follows this strategy is given in Figure 20.1. For deep enteroatmospheric fistulae, diversion of the output can be generated with inflated and blocked Foley catheter or similar catheter systems. When granulation tissue with sufficient thickness has formed, skin mesh grafts can be used for faster wound closure.

With these techniques, consolidation of fistulae, which then require definitive surgical closure after an interval of several months, is achieved in the majority of cases. In a minority of 10 to 15% of cases, fistulae may close

Table 20.4   Systematic classification of enteroatmospheric fistulae

Category	Subcategory	Example
Localisation	Proximal	Oesophagus, stomach, duodenum, jejunum
	Distal	Distal ileum, large bowel
Fistula output	Low	<200 mL/24 hours
	Moderate	200–500 mL/24 hours
	High	>500 mL/24 hours
Abdominal localisation	Superficial	Draining on top of open abdomen
	Deep	Draining into the peritoneal cavity
Number and distribution of fistulae	Single	One fistula
	Multiple near fistulae	Two or more fistulae in close proximity
	Multiple distant fistulae	Two or more fistulae distant from each other

Adapted from: Di Saverio S, Tarasconi A, Walczak DA, et al. Classification, prevention and management of entero-atmospheric fistula: a state-of-the-art review. *Langenbecks Arch Surg* 2016;401:1–13.

Table 20.5 Treatment options for gastrointestinal and enteroatmospheric fistula

Therapy option	Reason/example
Drainage	To drain infected fluid collections and prevent infections/interventional radiological drainage
Wound care, cutaneous protection	To prevent and treat delayed wound healing and wound infection
Antibacterial therapy	To prevent sepsis and support the wound healing
Fluid/electrolyte management	To prevent or treat electrolyte imbalances, oedema and delayed wound healing
Nutritional support	To prevent malnutrition and delayed wound healing; in severe cases, interdisciplinary therapy strategy, together with experts of nutritional medicine
Bowel rest	Loperamide, to reduce fistula output volume. To increase transit time and to allow better entreral resorption
Pharmacological support	Somatostatin analogues, to reduce gastrointestinal secretion and fluid loss
Surgical management	To definitively close fistula and restore bowel anatomy and function

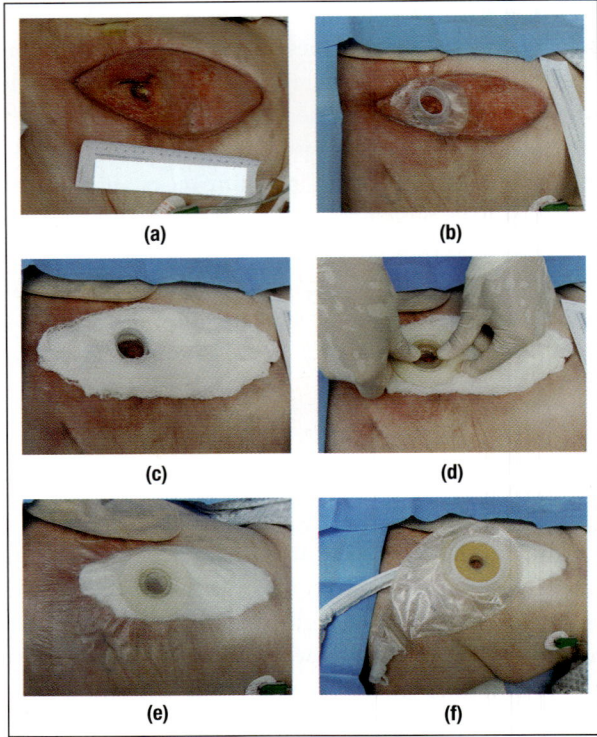

Figure 20.1 Example of a modified negative-pressure wound therapy technique using a adapter system for fistula output diversion on a superficial enteroatmospheric fistula. Wound dressings are changed at regular intervals, usually every third day or earlier when needed. (a) Situation after removal of old wound dressing and rinsing with sterile saline. (b) Positioning of a soft silicone fistula adapter on the orifice of the enteroatmospherioc fistula. The soft silicone adapter protects the fistula/bowel wall and can be cut to fit a given fistula. (c) The granulating viscera surrounding the fistula are completely covered with sterile saline-wetted wide-meshed wound compresses around the silicon adapter. (d) A plastic tube with a platform is connected with the fistula adapter. (e) Coverage of the entire wound with surrounding intact skin with a transparent adhesive foil. (f) Two separate holes for the fistula adapter outlet and for applying suction are made. A stoma bag is positioned on the platform around the fistula outlet and negative pressure is applies on the surrounding wound dressing. As a result, the entreoatmospheric fistula outflow is diverted from the surrounding granulating viscera.

Courtesy: Anna-Katharina Stadler, Markus Büchler and Oliver Strobel.

'spontaneously' with this therapy. Diversion of fistula outflow from the peritoneum and generation of a stable, controlled fistula are the prerequisites to overcome peritonitis and sepsis and to allow for consolidation of wound conditions. However, taking into account the entirety of problems associated with gastrointestinal fistulae, this 'local' fistula therapy has to be accompanied by medical and supportive therapy. Dependent on fistula location and output, the loss of fluid, electrolytes and nutritional factors has to be reduced by the medication aimed to rest bowel (e.g., loperamide) and to inhibit/reduce gastrointestinal secretions (e.g., somatostatin analogues).[24,32] Althoug there is no level 1 data for a standardised use of somatostatin in gastrointestinal fistulae, a test treatment with somatostatin, with continuation dependent on its impact on fistula output, can be recommended. Healing and consolidation of the wound conditions will work only with adequate nutritional state

of the patient. The administration of enteral nutrition (aboral of the fistula orifice) or of parenteral nutrition (in case of short bowel syndrome) has to be evaluated. In proximal, high-output gastrointestinal fistulas associated with short bowel syndrome, the implantation of a Hickman catheter for total parenteral nutrition may

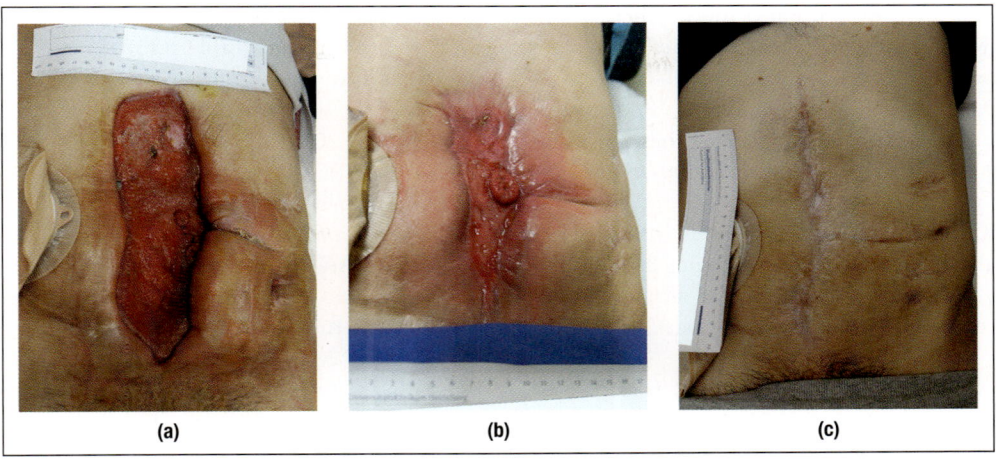

Figure 20.2 Example of a successful therapy of an enteroatmospheric fistula. A 43-year-old male patient presented with a perforated duodenal ulcer in a context of liver cirrhosis at an outside institution and was referred after two unsuccessful attempts to close the duodenum. At our institution, the severely septic patient underwent subtotal gastrectomy with proximal duodenectomy, right hemicolectomy with terminal ileostomy and biliary diversion by percutaneous transhepatic cholangiographic drainage. Although the duodenal stump remained sufficient, the patient developed an insufficiency of the gastrojejunostomy and eventually an open abdomen with enteroatmospheric fistula. (a) Situation with several enteroatmospheric fistulae on the granulating bowel. (b) Situation after several months of negative-pressure wound therapy, with partial closure of the wound and one established fistula. (c) Situation after successful surgical revision, with local fistula closure (the ileostomy remains).

Courtesy: Anna-Katharina Stadler, Markus Büchler and Oliver Strobel.

be indicated. Even if gastrointestinal fistulae appear stable, patients may present with recurrent infections and require close surveillance and antibiotic treatment to avoid the development of sepsis.

In the case of an established enterocutaneous or enteroatmospheric fistula, our recommendation is to wait for a minimum of 3 months or even longer (if acceptable to the patient) to allow adhesions to remodel and disappear and have 'optimal' conditions for the surgical revision. During this interval, adequate wound management and nutrition support (especially in the case of small bowel syndrome) are crucial for the success of a planned surgical revision. Relaparotomies for enteric fistulae can be very demanding and need to be performed with the double aim of doing a safe operation and avoiding new leaks/fistulae while preserving as much small intestine as possible to avoid short bowel syndrome. Figure 20.2 displays an example of successful fistula closure. Although most fistulae can be successfully closed by surgery, the morbidity of these operations is high. In a cohort study from a specialised centre in 153 patients with surgery for gastrointestinal fistulae closure, including 88.2% small bowel fistulae, successful closure was achieved in 83.7% patients, but the overall complication rate was 87.6%, with 3.9% 30-day mortality and 15.0% 1-year mortality.[33]

CONCLUSIONS

The duodenum and small bowel region can be affected by a broad variety of diseases that require management by a wide spectrum of different surgical procedures. Each of these surgical procedures is associated with the risk for a specific spectrum of complications. The common problem of the predominant complications after duodenal and small bowel surgery is the leakage of aggressive gastrointestinal secretions. Only early effective management of such leakages will prevent severe secondary complications and the formation of gastrointestinal and enteroatmospheric fistulae. Gastrointestinal fistulae are associated with a high morbidity and mortality but can be managed successfully by an experienced and dedicated team that addresses the entire spectrum of secondary problems described above.

REFERENCES

1. Büchler MW. Gastrointestinal fistulae. *Gut* 2001;49:iv1.
2. Aurello P, Sirimarco D, Magistri P, et al. Management of duodenal stump fistula after gastrectomy for gastric cancer: Systematic review. *World J Gastroenterol* 2015;21:7571–6.
3. Kashiwagi H. Ulcers and gastritis. *Endoscopy* 2005;37: 110–5.

4. Z'graggen K, Strobel O, Schmied BM, Zimmermann A, Büchler MW. Emergency pancreatoduodenectomy in nontrauma patients. *Pancreas* 2002;24:258–63.

5. Strobel O, Schneider L, Philipp S, et al. Emergency pancreatic surgery–demanding and dangerous. *Langenbecks Arch Surg* 2015;400:837–41. doi: 10.1007/s00423-015-1321-z.

6. Vashist YK, Yekebas EF, Gebauer F, et al. Management of the difficult duodenal stump in penetrating duodenal ulcer disease: a comparative analysis of duodenojejunostomy with "classical" stump closure (Nissen-Bsteh). *Langenbecks Arch Surg* 2012;397:1243–9.

7. de Castro SM, van Eijck CH, Rutten JP, et al. Pancreas-preserving total duodenectomy versus standard pancreatoduodenectomy for patients with familial adenomatous polyposis and polyps in the duodenum. *Br J Surg* 2008;95:1380–6.

8. Drini M, Speer A, Dow C, et al. Management of duodenal adenomatosis in FAP: single centre experience. *Fam Cancer* 2012;11:167–73.

9. Schneider L, Contin P, Fritz S, et al. Surgical ampullectomy: an underestimated operation in the era of endoscopy. *HPB (Oxford)* 2016;18:65–71. doi: 10.1016/j.hpb.2015.07.004.

10. Bassi C, Dervenis C, Butturini G, et al.; International Study Group on Pancreatic Fistula Definition. Postoperative pancreatic fistula: an international study group (ISGPF) definition. *Surgery* 2005;138:8–13.

11. Keck T, Wellner UF, Bahra M, et al. Pancreatogastrostomy versus pancreatojejunostomy for reconstruction after pancreatoduodenectomy (RECOPANC, DRKS 00000767): perioperative and long-term results of a multicenter randomized controlled trial. *Ann Surg* 2016;263:440–9.

12. Löffler T, Rossion I, Bruckner T, et al. Hand suture versus stapling for closure of loop ileostomy (HASTA trial): results of a multicenter randomized trial. *Ann Surg* 2012;256:828–35; discussion 835–6.

13. Dignass A, Van Assche G, Lindsay JO, et al. The second European evidence-based Consensus on the diagnosis and management of Crohn's disease: current management. *J Crohns Colitis* 2010;4:28–62.

14. Khanna R, Bressler B, Levesque BG, et al. Early combined immunosuppression for the management of Crohn's disease (REACT): a cluster randomised controlled trial. *Lancet* 2015;386:1825–34.

15. Tilsed JV, Casamassima A, Kurihara H, et al. ESTES guidelines: acute mesenteric ischaemia. *Eur J Trauma Emerg Surg* 2016;42:253–70.

16. Birkmeyer JD, Stukel TA, Siewers AE, Goodney PP, Wennberg DE, Lucas FL. Surgeon volume and operative mortality in the United States. *N Engl J Med* 2003; 349:2117–27.

17. Goulder F. Bowel anastomoses: the theory, the practice and the evidence base. *World J Gastrointest Surg* 2012;4: 208–13. doi: 10.4240/wjgs.v4.i9.208

18. Brandstrup B, Tønnesen H, Beier-Holgersen R. Effects of intravenous fluid restriction on postoperative complications: comparison of two perioperative fluid regimens: a randomized assessor-blinded multicenter trial. *Ann Surg* 2003;238:641–8.

19. Hartwig W, Werner J, Jäger D, Debus J, Büchler MW. Improvement of surgical results for pancreatic cancer. *Lancet Oncol* 2013;14:e476–85.

20. Ghaferi AA, Birkmeyer JD, Dimick JB. Hospital volume and failure to rescue with high-risk surgery. *Med Care* 2011;49:1076–81.

21. Welsch T, Müller SA, Ulrich A, et al. C-reactive protein as early predictor for infectious postoperative complications in rectal surgery. *Int J Colorectal Dis* 2007;22:1499–507.

22. Welsch T, Frommhold K, Hinz U, et al. Persisting elevation of C-reactive protein after pancreatic resections can indicate developing inflammatory complications. *Surgery* 2008;143:20–8.

23. Oh JS, Lee HG, Chun HJ, et al. Percutaneous management of postoperative duodenal stump leakage with foley catheter. *Cardiovasc Intervent Radiol* 2013;36:1344–9.

24. González-Pinto I, González EM. Optimising the treatment of upper gastrointestinal fistulae. *Gut* 2001;49:iv22–31.

25. Adams K, Papagrigoriadis S. Little consensus in either definition or diagnosis of a lower gastro-intestinal anastomotic leak amongst colorectal surgeons. *Int J Colorectal Dis* 2013;28:967–71. doi: 10.1007/s00384-013-1640-x.

26. Golub R, Golub RW, Cantu R Jr, et al. A multivariate analysis of factors contributing to leakage of intestinal anastomoses. *J Am Coll Surg* 1997;184:364–72.

27. Girard E, Messager M, Sauvanet A, et al. Anastomotic leakage after gastrointestinal surgery: diagnosis and management. *J Visc Surg* 2014;151:441–50. doi: 10.1016/j.jviscsurg.

28. Di Saverio S, Tarasconi A, Walczak DA, et al. Classification, prevention and management of entero-atmospheric fistula: a state-of-the-art review. *Langenbecks Arch Surg* 2016; 401:1–13. doi: 10.1007/s00423-015-1370-3.

29. Wainstein DE, Tüngler V, Ravazzola C, Chara O. Management of external small bowel fistulae: challenges and controversies confronting the general surgeon. *Int J Surg* 2011;9:198–203.

30. D'Hondt M, Devriendt D, Van Rooy F, et al. Treatment of small-bowel fistulae in the open abdomen with topical negative-pressure therapy. *Am J Surg* 2011;202:e20–4.

31. Datta V, Engledow A, Chan S, Forbes A, Cohen CR, Windsor A. The management of enterocutaneous fistula in a regional unit in the United Kingdom: a prospective study. *Dis Colon Rectum* 2010;53:192–9.

32. Hesse U, Ysebaert D, de Hemptinne B. Role of somatostatin-14 and its analogues in the management of gastrointestinal fistulae: clinical data. *Gut* 2001;49:iv11–21.

33. Owen RM, Love TP, Perez SD, et al. Definitive surgical treatment of enterocutaneous fistula: outcomes of a 23-year experience. *JAMA Surg* 2013;148:118–26.

21

Management of Complications after Laparoscopic Colon Surgery

M. Morino and M.E. Allaix

ABSTRACT

Laparoscopic colon resection for both benign and malignant diseases is associated with lower postoperative complications and better short-term outcomes than open surgery. Some postoperative complications, such as bowel perforation secondary to missed intraoperative damage and trocar site hernias, though rare, are typical for laparoscopic colon surgery. The incidence of prolonged postoperative ileus and adhesive small bowel obstruction is lower after minimally invasive surgery, whereas the rate of anastomotic leakage is similar. The last 10 years have witnessed a progressive shift towards a less-invasive approach to patients experiencing postoperative surgical morbidity. The aim of this chapter is to illustrate the different management modalities to treat surgical complications of laparoscopic colon surgery.

KEYWORDS

Laparoscopy, colon resection, morbidity, anastomotic leakage, perforation, bleeding, prolonged postoperative ileus, small bowel obstruction, trocar site hernia, relaparoscopy

INTRODUCTION

Since the first report in 1991, laparoscopic resection for colon cancer and benign diseases has increasingly gained popularity, with large randomised controlled trials (RCTs) demonstrating the short-term advantages[1–4] and similar oncological outcomes when compared with open surgery.

The minimally invasive approach to colon diseases is associated with some intraoperative complications that are unique to laparoscopy, including those related to induction of pneumoperitoneum and trocar insertion, whereas others, such as injury to intra-abdominal organs, are common to the open approach. Postoperative small bowel perforation secondary to missed intraoperative bowel injury and trocar site hernia, though rare, are typical of laparoscopic colon surgery. The rates of the most common surgical complications, such as prolonged postoperative ileus (PPI) and adhesive small bowel obstruction (SBO), are significantly lower after a minimally invasive resection than those after open surgery; however, no significant differences have been reported in anastomotic leakage and postoperative bleeding.[5,6] During the last decade, there has also been a progressive increase in the use of minimally invasive strategies for the treatment of surgical complications after laparoscopic colon resection.

This chapter discusses the mechanisms and management of complications occurring during and after laparoscopic colon resection. Indications, contraindications and outcomes of several options for the treatment of most common postoperative complications will also be reviewed.

INTRAOPERATIVE COMPLICATIONS

Organ Injuries

There is no consensus regarding the optimal method about the entry of the abdominal cavity (insertion of trocars). However, entry under direct vision is recommended in very thin patients and in those who had previous abdominal surgery; an entry site away from the prior incision is chosen, in order to minimise the risk of injury of intra-abdominal vessels and organs.

Bowel Injury

The incidence of bowel injury during laparoscopic colectomy is 1.8%, with the small bowel being the most common site of injury (55%). The insertion of the Veress needle or the first trocar represents the most common mechanism for bowel injury, followed by thermal injuries during dissection and bowel manipulation. The presence of adhesions increases the risk of bowel injury significantly.

One of the most feared complications after trocar placement is missed bowel injury, which is associated with a postoperative mortality rate of 3.6%. Therefore, extreme caution is required during both trocar insertion and removal at the end of the procedure to minimise the risk of a missed bowel injury. In case of suspected bowel injury, the bowel should be carefully and extensively explored. If a lesion is identified, it is usually possible to repair it by laparoscopic suturing. In selected cases, conversion to open surgery might be required to adequately assess the damage.

Injury to the Urinary Tract

Iatrogenic injury to the urinary tract during laparoscopic colon surgery is reported in less than 1% of patients. However, it is associated with significant morbidity. Half of the patients who experience injury to the urinary tract had undergone previous abdominal operations. The incidence of urinary tract injuries is also increased in patients with inflammatory bowel disease, diverticulitis or bulky tumours, which induce significant changes in the anatomy of the surgical planes. Mechanisms of injury include ureter ligation and transection and can be energy-induced. In addition, injury to the bladder may happen during the insertion of a trocar in the suprapubic area. A high suspicion is required to recognise this complication at the end of the operation, when the trocar is removed. If the bladder injury is confirmed, a laparoscopic suture should be performed to close the bladder wall defect and a Foley catheter should be left in place for 6 to 8 days postoperatively.

Preoperative stent placement in patients at high risk of ureteral injury might be helpful in early ureter identification, thus reducing the risk of injury. Transilluminating Foley catheters have been recently proposed. Although expensive, they could reduce the risk of ureter misidentification in selected cases. Early injury identification is key to reduce postoperative morbidity

and preserve renal function. Uretero-ureterostomy and ureteral stent positioning are the treatment modalities for intraoperatively recognised injuries to the ureter. Unfortunately, most iatrogenic ureteral injuries are detected postoperatively. The patient typically presents with flank pain, fever, abdominal pain and distention, ileus, decreased urine output or increased drainage. The management of these patients depends on the extent and site of the ureteral lesion and may include the positioning of a nephrostomy tube, followed by insertion of a ureteral stent.

Injury to Solid Organs

Intraoperative solid organ injury occurs in about 0.6% of laparoscopic colectomies, involving, most frequently, the spleen and the liver during the splenic or hepatic flexure mobilisation. The damage is self-limiting in most cases, and a splenectomy is rarely necessary.

Bleeding

Bleeding from the abdominal wall and secondary to intra-abdominal vessel injury may complicate a laparoscopic colon resection. Haemorrhage from the abdominal wall is secondary to laceration of skin vessels during trocar insertion: it can be recognised and treated intraoperatively, or it can be recognised during the postoperative course, when a haematoma appears evident. Most frequently, the injury occurs to the inferior epigastric vessels. A careful insertion of trocars lateral to the rectus sheath after transillumination of the abdominal wall helps minimise the risk of injury. When the vessel injury is diagnosed during the operation, strategies to control bleeding include suturing around the trocar site, the use of standard bipolar electrocautery and direct suture ligation of the bleeding vessel after removing the trocar.

Bleeding from intra-abdominal vessels is reported in up to 3% of laparoscopic colon resection. It is mainly due to inadvertent damage to the inferior mesenteric vessels or ileocolic vessels during dissection. Bleeding control can be achieved laparoscopically in most cases, by clamping the vessels and clipping them more proximally. When the injury occurs to vessels dissected very close to their origin from the aorta, bleeding control can be very challenging, even in very skilled hands. Most frequently, the vessel is clamped and the laparoscopic procedure converted to open surgery to achieve a definitive control of the bleeding. In our experience, bipolar coagulation is by large the most effective management strategy for small- or mid-entity bleedings, whereas clipping of a bleeding vessel should be limited to injured major vascular structures, such as inferior mesenteric vein or artery, ileocolic vessels and right colic vessels.

POSTOPERATIVE COMPLICATIONS

Most frequent postoperative complications are common for both the open and laparoscopic approaches. These include anastomotic leakage, PPI, adhesive SBO and endoluminal bleeding. Some complications, though rare, are unique to the laparoscopic approach: bowel perforation secondary to missed intraoperative injury by using energy-based devices or improper bowel manipulation and trocar site hernia.

Anastomotic Leakage

Anastomotic leakage is the most feared complication after colon surgery, since it is associated with poor function and quality of life[7] and decreased long-term survival.[8] The evidence from large RCTs shows that there are no significant differences in leakage rate after laparoscopic or open resection (3%).[6]

After laparoscopic right colectomy, a leak can occur at the level of the ileocolic anastomosis or at the sites of the enterocolotomy closure when a side-to-side anastomosis is performed (Figure 21.1). In most cases, the treatment includes the takedown of the anastomosis in combination with the creation of an end ileostomy and closure of the colonic stump or creation of a colonic mucosal fistula; however, an acute redo anastomosis is rarely performed. The main reason is that the ileocolic anastomosis is intraperitoneal, and therefore, the vast majority of patients

who develop a leakage at this level present with sepsis and diffuse faecal peritonitis.[9] Nevertheless, a minor leak could occur either from a part of the anastomosis or from the stapled bowel. In such cases, a direct suture of the hole, combined with a derivative temporary ileostomy, could be a viable choice.

On the contrary, the management of patients with left-sided colocolic or colorectal anastomotic leak is multidisciplinary and includes several strategies, depending on the patient's presentation and the location of the anastomosis (intraperitoneal vs. extraperitoneal). To date, resection of the anastomosis, combined with the creation of an end colostomy by an open approach, is the procedure performed in most circumstances. This strategy is the safest, but patients with an end stoma have reduced likelihood of stoma reversal and their quality of life is poor. The last few years have witnessed a progressive shift towards a more tailored and less invasive approach, based on the severity of the anastomotic leakage.[10] In 2010, the International Study Group of Rectal Cancer proposed a grading system of severity for anastomotic leakage after anterior resection of the rectum.[11] *Grade A* anastomotic leakage corresponds to an anastomotic leakage that is usually detected during radiological or endoscopic studies before closure of the diverting stoma and is not associated with clinical symptoms or abnormalities at laboratory tests. The postoperative course of these patients is uneventful. Although this grade of anastomotic leakage does not require therapeutic intervention, it might lead to a delay in the closure of the protective stoma. *Grade B* anastomotic leakage presents with a localised (mostly extraperitoneal)

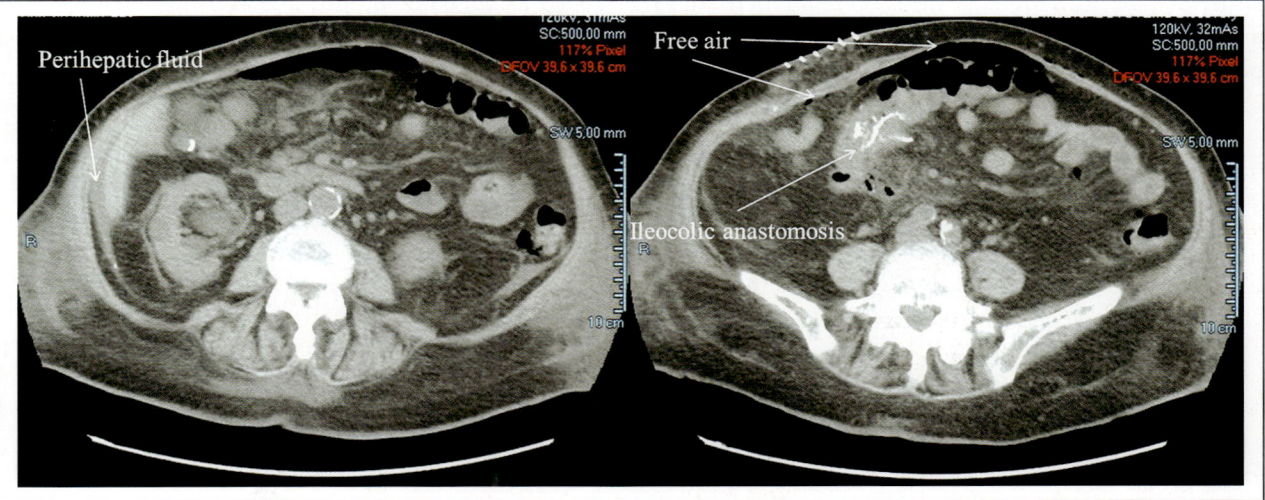

Figure 21.1 Computed tomography scan: ileocolic anastomotic leak.

Courtesy: Mario Morino and Marco E. Allaix.

abscess in a patient with mild to moderate patient's distress, abdominal pain and/or distension; laboratory tests show an increase in inflammatory markers. Treatment options in these patients include transanal or percutaneous drainage of the pelvic collection, endosponge therapy, endoscopic stenting and endoscopic clip placement.[12,13] Surgery is necessary if an interventional radiologist is not available, if the percutaneous abscess drainage is deemed not feasible or if the patient experiences deterioration of the clinical status. *Grade C* anastomotic leakage is associated with deteriorated clinical conditions of the patients who present with abdominal pain, fever and clinical signs of generalised peritonitis (Figure 21.2). Markers of infection are markedly increased. These patients require urgent reoperation after adequate resuscitation. This grading system was later validated, showing that the clinical course in patients with grade C leakage is worse than that in patients with grades A and B leakages. Most patients with colonic anastomotic leakage are categorised into grade C.

Grade C Anastomotic Leakage

Resection of the anastomosis, with exteriorisation of the descending colon to create a diverting end colostomy, is the most common surgical procedure performed in these patients. Although this strategy removes the source of sepsis, it is burdened by high postoperative morbidity rates and is associated with poor quality of life. In addition, the end colostomy is reversed in less than 50% of patients.[9] During the last few years, there has been a gradual shift in the management of selected grade C patients. Today, anastomosis takedown and creation of an end colostomy are still the standards of care in patients with diffuse bowel ischaemia, necrosis or large dehiscence of both intra- and extraperitoneal colorectal anastomoses with diffuse peritoneal contamination. Primary sutured anastomotic repair with proximal diversion might be attempted in

patients with a small anastomotic defect (less than 1 cm) in the presence of viable bowel tissues. Resection and redo anastomosis are very uncommon (Algorithm 21.1).

A less invasive approach has been proposed for the treatment of patients with leakage of an extraperitoneal anastomosis. It includes the lavage of the abdominal cavity, placement of drains into the pelvis and creation of a loop ileostomy for faecal diversion. Endoscopic procedures, such as endosponge positioning, can be added to help the leaking anastomosis heal. This strategy has proved to be safe and effective, with healing rates ranging between 54 and 100%. In addition, patients treated with peritoneal lavage, drainage and loop ileostomy have a significantly higher likelihood of stoma reversal than those who undergo resection of the anastomosis and creation of an end colostomy.

The role of the laparoscopic approach to patients with leakage of a colorectal anastomosis after laparoscopic colon resection is under debate. The current evidence shows that laparoscopy is a valid alternative to open surgery in haemodynamically stable patients who have had previous laparoscopic colorectal resection.[14,15] Lee et al[15] compared the outcomes in 16 patients undergoing open surgery after laparoscopic colorectal surgery and in 61 patients receiving laparoscopic reoperation after laparoscopic colorectal surgery. Conversion rate was 8.2% due to bowel injury, haematoma, bowel oedema, severe adhesions or difficult mobilisation of the colon. The rate of end colostomy was significantly higher in the open-surgery group (31% vs. 3%), whereas a loop ileostomy was more frequently created after laparoscopic reoperation (75% vs. 21%). Median surgical time was significantly lower in the case of laparoscopic procedures. Patients treated laparoscopically had a significantly lower rate of wound complications or intra-abdominal infection and a significantly shorter hospital stay. A significantly higher number of patients in the laparoscopic group underwent

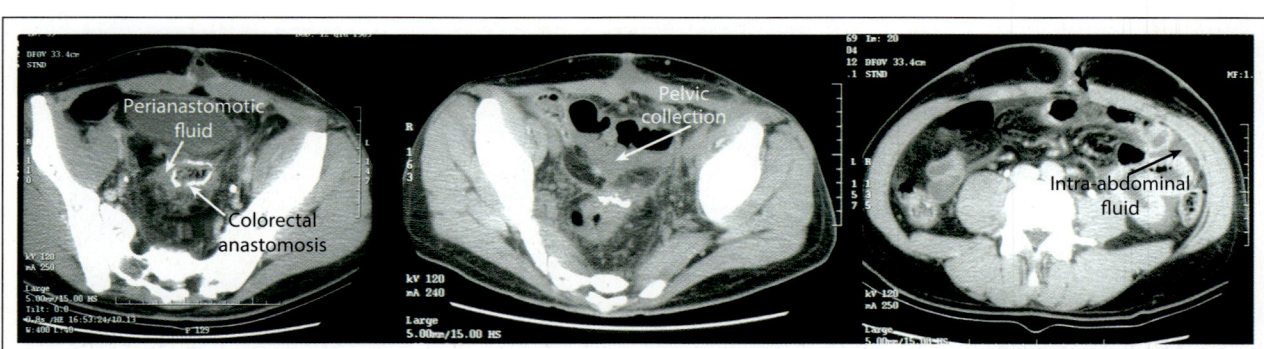

Figure 21.2   Computed tomography scan: colorectal anastomotic leak.

Courtesy: Mario Morino and Marco E. Allaix.

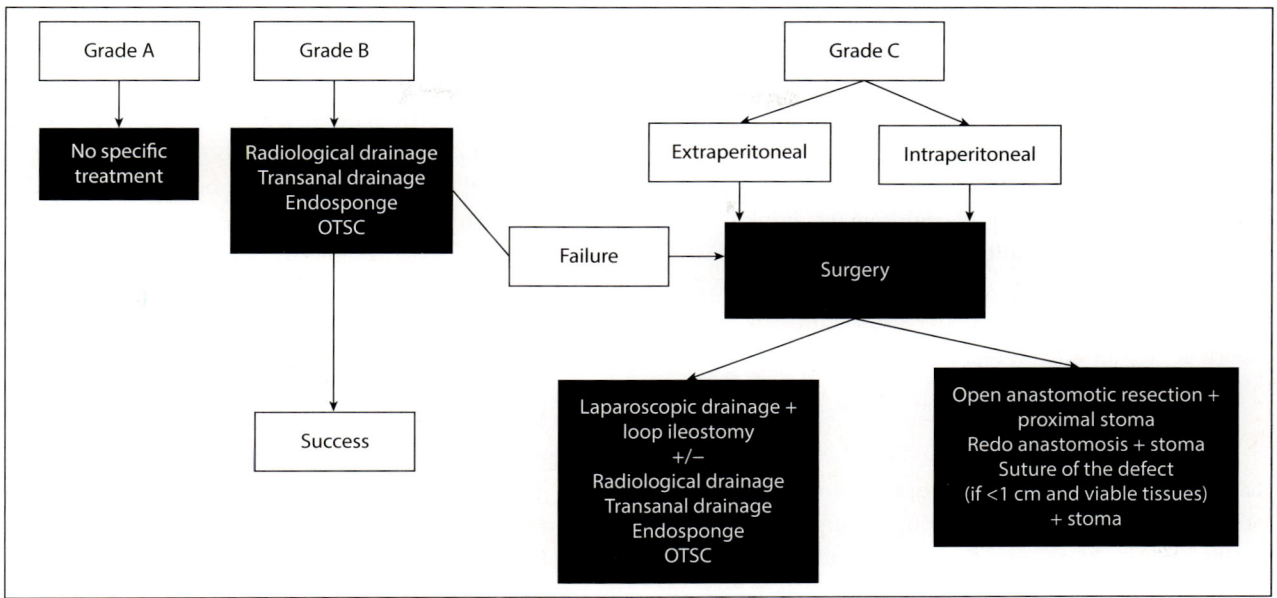

Algorithm 21.1   Treatment algorithm for colorectal anastomotic leakage.

Abbreviation: OTSC, over-the-scope clip.

Courtesy: Mario Morino and Marco E. Allaix.

stoma closure than in the open group (89% vs. 44%). Nevertheless, these are the results of highly selected patients treated in expert centres. More data are necessary to validate this approach, including a better definition of indications and contraindications.

Prolonged Postoperative Ileus

Prolonged postoperative ileus is reported in 6.5% of patients undergoing laparoscopic colon resection surgery and in 10% of patients treated by open surgery. It is associated with increased morbidity, prolonged hospital stay and increased costs.[16]

Management of PPI includes several treatment options: (a) regular assessment and correction of electrolytes, (b) reduced used of narcotics for pain relief, (c) nasogastric tube insertion in patients developing nausea and/or vomiting for gastric decompression, (d) well-balanced intravenous fluid therapy, (e) early and regular patient mobilisation, (f) parenteral nutrition, and (g) exclusion of causes such as intra-abdominal sepsis and early SBO.[17]

During the last 10 years, several studies have been focussed on the therapeutic effects of gum chewing after colon resection for both cancer and benign diseases. Current evidence shows that gum chewing, in addition to standard treatment, is associated with significantly early time to first flatus and time to first passage of faeces when compared with standard treatment alone.

The incidence of postoperative complications is similar. Length of hospital stay is slightly shorter, even though the difference does not reach statistical significance.[18] Only a few small studies have specifically assessed the impact of gum chewing on patients undergoing laparoscopic colon resection for cancer.[19,20] McCormick et al[20] randomised 51 patients with colon cancer undergoing laparoscopic colectomy to chew gum (n = 35) or to sip clear liquids (n = 16) in immediate postoperative course. Gum chewing significantly shortened the time to first bowel movement and the hospital stay. Although gum chewing seems to accelerate the return of bowel function, with early recovery from postoperative ileus, in the era of fast-track surgery and early postoperative feeding, the current level of evidence does not support the routine gum chewing. Further large studies are needed to elucidate the role of gum chewing and early resumption of oral intake.

Gastrografin® is a hyperosmolar water-soluble iodinated contrast medium that has been recently tested in the management of patients with PPI after colon surgery. It has been postulated that its hypertonicity reduces oedema-related gastrointestinal motility dysfunction, thus promoting bowel peristalsis.[21] Some RCTs[22,23] were conducted to test the hypothesis that the oral administration of Gastrografin® might shorten the duration of PPI after elective colon surgery. In an RCT comprising 80 patients with PPI after elective colon resection, Vather et al[22] reported that Gastrografin®

accelerated time to flatus or stool (18.9 vs. 32.7 hours; p = 0.047) and time to resolution of abdominal distension (52.8 vs. 77.7 hours; p = 0.013); however, it did not affect time to resolution of nausea and vomiting (64.5 vs. 74.3 hours; p = 0.404) or consumption of oral diet (75.8 vs. 90.0 hours; p = 0.297). Nasogastric tube output; analgesia, antiemetic or fluid requirement; complication rates and length of hospital stay did not differ between the two groups. Further large RCTs will shed more light on the real benefits of the use of Gastrografin® in patients experiencing PPI after colon surgery.

Small Bowel Obstruction

Rates of SBO after laparoscopic colon surgery are lower than those reported after open surgery (2–5% vs. 6–10%).[24,25] Some studies have clearly shown that the open approach is an independent risk factor for postoperative SBO.[25] The need for surgery to solve an episode of SBO is also lower after laparoscopic than after open colon resection.[26] Most common causes of SBO are trocar and extraction site hernias, internal hernias and adhesions occurring between loops of the small bowel or with the abdominal wall.[24] The diagnosis is based on symptoms and clinical examination and is confirmed by a computed tomography (CT) scan.

Trocar site and extraction site hernias are reported in less than 3% and 10% of patients, respectively. A transverse extraction incision during laparoscopic resection is associated with lower risks of hernia than a midline incision. However, these rates might be underestimated, since the onset of incisional hernia can occur months or years after surgery, and therefore, it might be missed, unless an extended follow-up has been established. In 2004, Tonouchi et al[27] proposed a classification of trocar site hernia: (1) early-onset type: dehiscence of anterior and posterior fascial plane and peritoneum, (2) late-onset type: dehiscence of the anterior and posterior fascial planes, with the peritoneum constituting the hernia sac, and (3) special type: dehiscence of the whole abdominal wall and protrusion of bowel and/or omentum. Several risk factors have been proposed, including incomplete closure of trocar fascial defects of 10 mm or greater, use of pyramidal trocars and wound infections. The onset of symptoms secondary to trocar site hernia could range from a few days to several months or years after laparoscopic colectomy; however, they generally occur within a few days postoperatively, with the characteristics of early-onset type and special type. An SBO is the main manifestation of these types of trocar site hernias but is uncommon in late-onset type

hernias. The treatment includes surgical reduction and repair of the defect in the abdominal wall.

Symptoms and treatment options in patients with extraction site hernias do not differ from those with incisional hernia after open surgery.

An internal herniation of small bowel through the defect in the mesenteric beneath the left colon, causing postoperative SBO, is reported in about 1% of patients undergoing laparoscopic colon resection. The surgical treatment, performed through a laparoscopic or an open approach, includes careful division of adhesions between the herniating small bowel and the mesocolon, reduction of the herniating jejunum loop and positioning of the small bowel in the left abdomen to the overly descending colon. The mesenteric defect is not routinely closed. The development of internal herniation after laparoscopic left colon resection is multifactorial: (1) decrease in postoperative adhesion formation after laparoscopic surgery, (2) lack of closure of the mesenteric defect created during laparoscopic surgery, and (3) tension of the left colon mesentery if the splenic flexure is not mobilised or only partially mobilised during the index laparoscopic colon resection, thus leading to increased risk of incarceration of the small bowel at this level.

The management of SBO secondary to adhesions between loops of the small bowel or with the abdominal wall is controversial. Although surgery might induce the creation of new adhesions, conservative treatment does not remove the cause of the SBO. Conservative management involves nasogastric tube placement, intravenous fluid administration and clinical observation. This strategy is recommended in patients with no clinical and radiological signs of strangulation or peritonitis and partial SBO, whereas patients presenting with complete SBO or with signs of strangulation should undergo surgical treatment.[28] Among patients who are initially managed with a conservative treatment, predicting the risk of treatment failure and progression to bowel ischaemia are challenging, since initial clinical signs such as tachycardia, fever, abdominal pain and blood tests have a relatively low specificity for intestinal ischaemia. Since a delay in surgery leads to an increased risk of clinical worsening, necrosis of the bowel and need for bowel resection, many efforts have been put to identify predictors of failure of nonoperative management. The administration of 50 to 150 mL water-soluble contrast (Gastrografin®) through the nasogastric tube at the admission in the hospital or after 48 hours of unsuccessful conservative management in the absence of clinical signs of strangulation is useful in predicting the risk for surgery, without increasing morbidity and mortality rates. The presence of Gastrografin® in the colonic lumen, detected by plain abdominal film, at 8 to 24 hours after its administration predicts resolution of SBO, thus reducing the need for surgery and shortening both time to SBO resolution and hospital stay.[29]

The need for operation in patients treated conservatively for adhesive SBO after colon resection varies between 1.4 and 20%.[30] Although open surgery is the recommended approach for the surgical treatment of patients with strangulating SBO or peritonitis, there is increasing evidence showing that the laparoscopic approach should be considered in selected patients.[31] The exclusion criteria for laparoscopy are contraindications to pneumoperitoneum, including haemodynamic instability and severe cardiopulmonary comorbidities, and to severe bowel distention. The laparoscopic approach to SBO has several potential postoperative benefits when compared with open adhesiolysis, including reduced postoperative pain, faster return of bowel function, lower medical and wound-related complication rates, lower mortality rates and shorter length of hospital stay.[32,33] In addition, some data show that laparoscopy might be associated with less (new) adhesion formation.[34] Predictors of successful laparoscopic adhesiolysis are single-band adhesion and bowel diameter less than 4 cm. Although laparoscopy appears to be a safe approach in the hands of surgeons highly experienced in laparoscopic surgery, a low threshold for open conversion should be maintained in the presence of extensive adhesions, in order to reduce the risk of intraoperative complications, such as inadvertent enterotomy.[35]

Bowel Perforation

This is a rare complication (1%) after laparoscopic colectomy. This complication is secondary to missed injury to the bowel, occurring intraoperatively during dissection. Several strategies aim to minimise the risk of bowel injury: (1) all energy-based tools (conventional electrosurgical devices, ultrasonic coagulating shears, electrothermal bipolar vessel sealers and Thunderbeat[TM]) should be used, with the tips under direct vision, in order to avoid injury secondary to lateral thermal spread, (2) these tools should be exchanged under direct visualisation, and (3) caution should be exercised during bowel manipulation by using graspers within view, thus avoiding crush or laceration.

Patients present with acute abdominal pain, clinical signs of peritonitis and fever. A CT scan shows free liquid and free air in the abdomen (Figure 21.3). A laparoscopic approach can be attempted in haemodynamically stable patients. Treatment includes suturing of the bowel wall

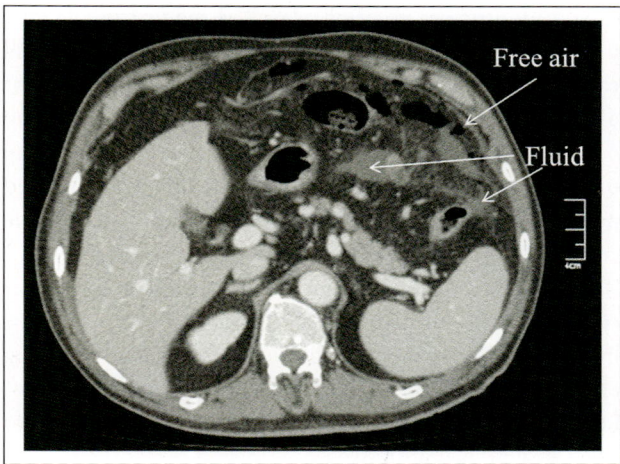

Figure 21.3 Computed tomography scan: small bowel perforation.
Courtesy: Mario Morino and Marco E. Allaix.

defect. The injured bowel segment might be exteriorised to create a stoma in the presence of a large defect in the distal ileum.

Intraluminal Bleeding

Postoperative lower-gastrointestinal bleeding from the anastomosis occurs in up to 5% of patients. Anastomotic bleeding can be managed conservatively in most cases, since it tends to stop spontaneously and severe bleeding is rare (less than 1%). Nonoperative treatment includes clinical observation, resuscitation and blood transfusion. When it fails, operative treatment modalities such as endoscopy and angiographic embolisation should be considered in haemodynamically stable patients. Endoscopic treatment is effective in detecting the site of bleeding and controlling the haemorrhage by using local adrenaline solution infusion or clips in most cases; however, it is burdened by the risk of anastomotic dehiscence. In contrast, angiographic embolisation increases the risk of bowel ischaemia.

Surgery is indicated only in unstable patients or after failure of other treatments.

Relaparoscopy in the Management of Postoperative Complications

The use of minimally invasive surgery in patients who develop complications after laparoscopic colon surgery has been recently reported, with satisfactory results. When radiological diagnostic examinations are not conclusive in patients with a suspected postoperative complication, laparoscopy should be considered as the final diagnostic examination as well as the first therapeutic tool. Laparoscopy allows to visualise the whole abdominal cavity; recognise the complication, thus making the right diagnosis and, possibly, treat it in the same session. In up to 25% of cases, relaparoscopy is negative, thus ruling out an intra-abdominal complication, with limited negative clinical impact on the following postoperative course.[36]

The most common indication for relaparoscopy after colon resection is anastomotic leakage (74%), followed by SBO and bleeding. Localisation of the site of bleeding after colon resection can be challenging; if it is not identified and controlled laparoscopically, conversion to open surgery is required.[37]

A recent systematic review of 11 studies, including 187 patients laparoscopically treated for complications after colon resections, showed that the success rate in highly selected patients is as high as 97% in the hands of surgeons skilled in advanced laparoscopic surgery. The laparoscopic approach should be considered in stable patients, whereas haemodynamically unstable patients should undergo laparotomy.[38]

Several procedures are performed to treat the anastomotic leak, based on the grade of the peritoneal contamination, the bowel viability and the entity of the anastomotic defect. In the presence of localised abdominal contamination and a small disruption of the anastomosis, the laparoscopic lavage of the peritoneal cavity with insertion of a drainage close to the anastomosis and the creation of diverting stoma should be carried out. The anastomotic leak can be sutured in selected cases. The success rate of this strategy is 90%. The study with the largest series of patients undergoing laparoscopy for suspected anastomotic leakage after elective laparoscopic colon resection was published in 2015 by Cuccurullo et al.[39] The procedure was negative in six (11%) cases, whereas the anastomotic leakage was found in 48 patients. A peritoneal lavage with creation of a loop ileostomy was the treatment of choice in most cases (91.7%), whereas a Hartmann's procedure was performed in 8.3% of patients because of large contamination of the abdomen and wide anastomotic leakage. The laparoscopic procedure was converted to open surgery because of generalised faecal peritonitis and massive colon ischaemia in 5.6% of patients. Overall, postoperative morbidity and mortality rates were 18.8% (six cases of abdominal collection, two cases of subphrenic abscess and one case of wound infection) and 8.3%, respectively.

When compared with open surgery, relaparoscopy has the advantage of reducing the surgical trauma, thus maintaining the benefits of a minimally invasive approach, including lower rates of wound infections, reduced risk of PPI and earlier hospital discharge.[40,41]

CONCLUSIONS

Although the laparoscopic approach to both benign and malignant diseases is gaining wide acceptance, a careful patient selection and high experience in laparoscopic surgery are needed to minimise the incidence of intraoperative and postoperative complications. The management of surgical complications after laparoscopic colon resection is evolving towards a minimally invasive and tailored approach.

REFERENCES

1. Lacy AM, García-Valdecasas JC, Delgado S, et al. Laparoscopy-assisted colectomy versus open colectomy for treatment of non-metastatic colon cancer: a randomised trial. *Lancet* 2002;359:2224–9.
2. Clinical Outcomes of Surgical Therapy Study Group. A comparison of laparoscopically assisted and open colectomy for colon cancer. *N Engl J Med* 2004;350:2050–9.
3. Guillou PJ, Quirke P, Thorpe H, et al; MRC CLASICC trial group. Short-term endpoints of conventional versus laparoscopic-assisted surgery in patients with colorectal cancer (MRC CLASICC trial): multicentre, randomised controlled trial. *Lancet* 2005;365:1718–26.
4. Veldkamp R, Kuhry E, Hop WC, et al; COlon cancer Laparoscopic or Open Resection Study Group (COLOR). Laparoscopic surgery versus open surgery for colon cancer: short-term outcomes of a randomised trial. *Lancet Oncol* 2005;6:477–84.
5. Schwenk W, Haase O, Neudecker J, Müller JM. Short term benefits for laparoscopic colorectal resection. *Cochrane Database Syst Rev* 2005;3:CD003145.
6. Arezzo A, Passera R, Scozzari G, Verra M, Morino M. Laparoscopy for rectal cancer reduces short-term mortality and morbidity: results of a systematic review and meta-analysis. *Surg Endosc* 2013;27:1485–502. doi: 10.1007/s00464-012-2649-x.
7. Ashburn JH, Stocchi L, Kiran RP, Dietz DW, Remzi FH. Consequences of anastomotic leak after restorative proctectomy for cancer: effect on long-term function and quality of life. *Dis Colon Rectum* 2013;56:275–80.
8. Lu ZR, Rajendran N, Lynch AC, Heriot AG, Warrier SK. Anastomotic leaks after restorative resections for rectal cancer compromise cancer outcomes and survival. *Dis Colon Rectum* 2016;59:236–44.
9. Krarup PM, Jorgensen LN, Harling H; Danish Colorectal Cancer Group. Management of anastomotic leakage in a nationwide cohort of colonic cancer patients. *J Am Coll Surg* 2014;218:940–9.
10. Phitayakorn R, Delaney CP, Reynolds HL, et al; International Anastomotic Leak Study Group. Standardized

algorithms for management of anastomotic leaks and related abdominal and pelvic abscesses after colorectal surgery. *World J Surg* 2008;32:1147–56.

11. Rahbari NN, Weitz J, Hohenberger W, et al. Definition and grading of anastomotic leakage following anterior resection of the rectum: a proposal by the International Study Group of Rectal Cancer. *Surgery* 2010;147: 339–51.

12. Arezzo A, Verra M, Passera R, Bullano A, Rapetti L, Morino M. Long-term efficacy of endoscopic vacuum therapy for the treatment of colorectal anastomotic leaks. *Dig Liver Dis* 2015;47:342–5.

13. Arezzo A, Verra M, Reddavid R, Cravero F, Bonino MA, Morino M. Efficacy of the over-the-scope clip (OTSC) for treatment of colorectal postsurgical leaks and fistulas. *Surg Endosc* 2012;26:3330–3.

14. Joh YG, Kim SH, Hahn KY, Stulberg J, Chung CS, Lee DK. Anastomotic leakage after laparoscopic protectomy can be managed by a minimally invasive approach. *Dis Colon Rectum* 2009;52:91–6.

15. Lee CM, Huh JW, Yun SH, et al. Laparoscopic versus open reintervention for anastomotic leakage following minimally invasive colorectal surgery. *Surg Endosc* 2015;29:931–6.

16. Wolthuis AM, Bislenghi G, Fieuws S, et al. Incidence of prolonged postoperative ileus after colorectal surgery: a systematic review and meta-analysis. *Colorectal Dis* 2016;18:O1–9.

17. Vather R, Bissett I. Management of prolonged postoperative ileus: evidence-based recommendations. *ANZ J Surg* 2013;83:319–24.

18. Vásquez W, Hernández AV, Garcia-Sabrido JL. Is gum chewing useful for ileus after elective colorectal surgery? A systematic review and meta-analysis of randomized clinical trials. *J Gastrointest Surg* 2009;13:649–56.

19. Asao T, Kuwano H, Nakamura J, Morinaga N, Hirayama I, Ide M. Gum chewing enhances early recovery from postoperative ileus after laparoscopic colectomy. *J Am Coll Surg* 2002;195:30–2.

20. McCormick JT, Garvin R, Caushaj P, et al. The effects of gum-chewing on bowel function and hospital stay after laparoscopic vs open colectomy: a multi-institution prospective randomized trial. *J Am Coll Surg* 2005;201: S66–7.

21. Abbas S, Bissett IP, Parry BR. Oral water-soluble contrast for the management of adhesive small bowel obstruction. *Cochrane Database Syst Rev* 2007;18:CD004651.

22. Vather R, Josephson R, Jaung R, Kahokehr A, Sammour T, Bissett I. Gastrografin in prolonged postoperative ileus: a double-blinded randomized controlled trial. *Ann Surg* 2015;262:23–30.

23. Biondo S, Miquel J, Espin-Basany E, et al. A double-blinded randomized clinical study on the therapeutic effect of Gastrografin® in prolonged postoperative ileus after elective colorectal surgery. *World J Surg* 2016;40:206–14.

24. Duepree HJ, Senagore AJ, Delaney CP, Fazio VW. Does means of access affect the incidence of small bowel obstruction and ventral hernia after bowel resection? Laparoscopy versus laparotomy. *J Am Coll Surg* 2003;197: 177–81.

25. Nakajima J, Sasaki A, Otsuka K, Obuchi T, Nishizuka S, Wakabayashi G. Risk factors for early postoperative small bowel obstruction after colectomy for colorectal cancer. *World J Surg* 2010;34:1086–90.

26. Reshef A, Hull TL, Kiran RP. Risk of adhesive obstruction after colorectal surgery: the benefits of the minimally invasive approach may extend well beyond the perioperative period. Surg Endosc. 2013;27: 1717–20.

27. Tonouchi H, Ohmori Y, Kobayashi M, Kusunoki M. Trocar site hernia. *Arch Surg* 2004;139:1248–56.

28. Di Saverio S, Coccolini F, Galati M, et al. Bologna guidelines for diagnosis and management of adhesive small bowel obstruction (ASBO): 2013 update of the evidence-based guidelines from the world society of emergency surgery ASBO working group. *World J Emerg Surg* 2013 10;8:42.

29. Ceresoli M, Coccolini F, Catena F, et al. Water-soluble contrast agent in adhesive small bowel obstruction: a systematic review and meta-analysis of diagnostic and therapeutic value. *Am J Surg* 2016;211:1114–25.

30. Jeong WK, Lim SB, Choi HS, Jeong SY. Conservative management of adhesive small bowel obstructions in patients previously operated on for primary colorectal cancer. *J Gastrointest Surg* 2008;12:926–32.

31. Jafari MD, Jafari F, Foe-Paker JE, et al. Adhesive small bowel obstruction in the United States: has laparoscopy made an impact? *Am Surg* 2015;81:1028–33.

32. Li MZ, Lian L, Xiao LB, Wu WH, He YL, Song XM. Laparoscopic versus open adhesiolysis in patients with adhesive small bowel obstruction: a systematic review and meta-analysis. *Am J Surg* 2012 ;204:779–86.

33. Saleh F, Ambrosini L, Jackson T, Okrainec A. Laparoscopic versus open surgical management of small bowel obstruction: an analysis of short-term outcomes. *Surg Endosc* 2014;28:2381–6.

34. Tittel A, Treutner KH, Titkova S, Ottinger A, Schumpelick V. Comparison of adhesion reformation after laparoscopic and conventional adhesiolysis in an animal model. *Langenbeck's Arch Surg* 2001;386:141–5.

35. Dindo D, Schafer M, Muller MK, Clavien PA, Hahnloser D. Laparoscopy for small bowel obstruction: the reason for conversion matters. *Surg Endosc* 2010;24:792–7.

36. Kirshtein B, Roy-Shapira A, Domchik S, Mizrahi S, Lantsberg L. Early relaparoscopy for management of suspected postoperative complications. *J Gastrointest Surg* 2008;12:1257–62.

37. McCormick JT, Simmang CL. Reoperation following minimally invasive surgery: are the "rules" different? *Clin Colon Rectal Surg* 2006;19:217–22.

38. Chang KH, Bourke MG, Kavanagh DO, Neary PC, O'Riordan JM. A systematic review of the role of re-laparoscopy in the management of complications following laparoscopic colorectal surgery. *Surgeon* 2016;14:287–93.

39. Cuccurullo D, Pirozzi F, Sciuto A, et al. Relaparoscopy for management of postoperative complications following colorectal surgery: ten years' experience in a single center. *Surg Endosc* 2015;29:1795–803.

40. Wind J, Koopman AG, van Berge Henegouwen MI, Slors JF, Gouma DJ, Bemelman WA. Laparoscopic reintervention for anastomotic leakage after primary laparoscopic colorectal surgery. *Br J Surg* 2007;94:1562–6.

41. Vennix S, Abegg R, Bakker OJ, et al. Surgical reinterventions following colorectal surgery: open versus laparoscopic management of anastomotic leakage. *J Laparoendosc Adv Surg Tech A* 2013;23:739–44.

22

Diagnosis and Treatment of Complications after Ileal Pouch and Rectal Surgery

W.A.A. Borstlap, G.D. Musters, P.J. Tanis, C.J. Buskens and W.A. Bemelman

ABSTRACT

Despite numerous innovations in the last decades, rectal surgery still is associated with a high rate of postoperative morbidity. The aim of this chapter is to provide a structured overview of the different surgical procedures being performed for both benign and malignant rectal diseases and their associated complications. Parallel to surgery of the colon, a shift has been made towards less-invasive treatment options for postoperative surgical complications. Early diagnosis plays an important role to increase the success of these minimally invasive techniques. Therefore, in this chapter, special attention will be paid to the minimally invasive, and so-called step-up approach of one of the most dreaded complications after rectal surgery, the anastomotic leak.

KEYWORDS

Rectal surgery, colorectal/anal anastomosis, pouch surgery, anastomotic leak, chronic sinus, presacral abscess, fistulae, carcinoma, ulcerative colitis, neorectum

INTRODUCTION

Rectal surgery can be complicated by general problems that follow any major abdominal operation, for example, haemorrhage, paralytic ileus, wound infection, herniation, respiratory insufficiency, deep venous thrombosis and pulmonary embolism. This chapter will focus on the complications that are specific to rectal surgery. The spectrum of complications differs widely, owing to the different surgical procedures currently performed for both benign and malignant rectal diseases. The technical armamentarium of the surgeon is still expanding and so are the varieties of complications that can occur. To a much greater extent than in colonic surgery, the decision to restore continuity in rectal surgery is based on many factors. Comorbidity of the patient, age, preoperative sphincter function, tumour distance from the anal verge, resection margin in relation to the sphincter complex and patients' preference, all play an important role in this, preferably shared, decision making. As a substantial part of the complications is closely related to the decision whether or not to perform a low anastomosis, this chapter differentiates between the complications after 'anastomotic surgery' and 'non-anastomotic surgery'. The dysfunctional neorectum is seen as a separate long-term complication in this chapter.

SURGERY FOR MALIGNANT DISEASE

Early in the 1980s, surgical resection of the rectum for cancer underwent a major development with the introduction of complete resection of the visceral mesentery en bloc with the rectum, the total mesorectal excision (TME). The original paper of Heald and Ryall published in 1986 showed that with the addition of TME, local recurrence rates less than 4% could be achieved.[1]

Previously, recurrence rates of up to 30 to 40% were common. For this reason, TME and clear resection margins became the basic principles of a proper resection for rectal carcinoma. The favourable early-stage rectal carcinomas, for example, those with T1, SM1, good differentiation, no lymphatic and no vascular invasions and less than 3 cm size, can be treated with local endoluminal excision. Transanal endoscopic microsurgery (TEM) or the newer transanal minimal invasive surgery (TAMIS) should be the preferred approach compared with the traditional local excision, as the former procedures are associated with lower recurrences, owing to higher rates of clear resection margins.[2]

Low Anterior Resection

Low anterior resection (LAR) is the most commonly performed procedure for the resection of rectal carcinoma. Up to 70% of the patients with rectal carcinoma who undergo surgery will receive an LAR.[3] Anterior resection is indicated for proximal rectal carcinoma. The technique involves a partial mesorectal excision, where the mesorectum is transected 5 cm below the tumour. An LAR is indicated for carcinomas located in the mid- or distal rectum (up to 10 cm from the dentate line). In these patients, the whole mesorectum is excised and the colon is anastomosed to the very distal rectum or even the upper part of the anal canal. This sphincter-saving procedure enables the formation of an anastomosis between the descending colon and the distal part of the remaining rectum. The anastomosis can be performed in a side-to-end, end-to-end, or colon-pouch fashion. Either a handsewn or a stapled anastomosis can be done, with no difference in the incidence of anastomotic leaks.[4] Local recurrence rate after LAR is around 5%.[5] The formation of a defunctioning ileo- or colostomy does not prevent anastomotic leaks but does decrease the impact of the sepsis subsequent to the leak.

Hartmann's Procedure

The Hartmann's procedure for malignant disease is traditionally being reserved for surgery in the acute setting or for patients with extensive comorbidities. Nevertheless, population-based data from the Dutch Surgical Colorectal Audit (DSCA) showed that the Hartmann's procedure is being performed in up to 27.8% of the patients who opted for a sphincter-saving procedure. This proves that, in the current practice, the Hartmann's procedure is an important alternative to abdominoperineal resection (APR) or colorectal anastomosis. Although the risk of anastomotic leakage is avoided, the Hartmann's procedure

is still associated with a substantial pelvic abscess rate of around 13%.[6,7] The majority of these pelvic abscesses originate from the rectal stump, and therefore, it is important to acquire enough length (minimally 4 cm) before suturing or stapling the distal rectum, as a short stump increases the risk of a blowout due to the increased pressure caused by the anal sphincter.

Intersphincteric Resection with Coloanal Anastomosis

In 1994, the intersphincteric resection (ISR) with a coloanal anastomosis was introduced by Schiessel et al.[8] During this procedure, the internal anal sphincter is partially or completely removed after separation from the external sphincter. Subsequently, a handsewn coloanal anastomosis is fashioned. An ISR is associated with an increased risk of anastomotic leaks and an increased risk of impaired continence, particularly in patients who have received neoadjuvant chemotherapy. However, some patients are willing to accept these risks, in order avoid a permanent colostomy.[9]

Transanal Total Mesorectal Excision

For carcinomas located between 4 cm and 10 cm from the dentate line, a new surgical procedure has been developed recently; it is the transanal TME (TaTME). The TaTME consists of an abdominal and a transanal phase. Ideally, two surgeons operate simultaneously, working towards each other until the rendezvous is made between the abdominal- and transanal planes (Figure 22.1). The basic principle of the procedure is that a SILS™ Port (e.g., GelPOINT® path) is placed in the anus, thereby creating a pneumopelvis. Especially in obese patients with a small pelvis, the pneumopelvis enables better exposure, since no structures need to be moved out of

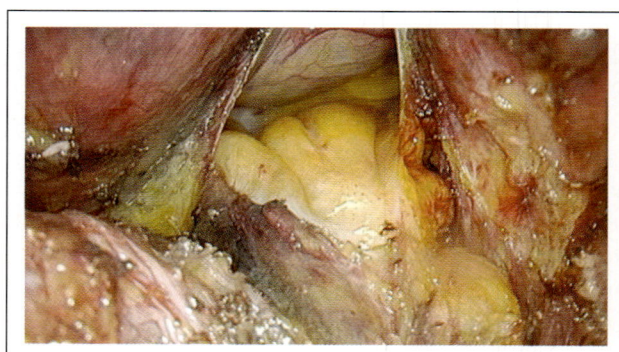

Figure 22.1 Rendez vous: bottom-up.

Courtesy: W.A.A. Borstlap, G.D. Musters, P.J. Tanis, C.J. Buskens and W.A. Bemelman.

the operation field. During TaTME, approximately 3 to 4 cm at the distal side of the carcinoma or just above the anal sphincter complex, a purse-string suture is placed to close the lumen. Subsequently, after a washout with povidone-iodine, a full-thickness, circumferential rectal transection is made up to the avascular presacral TME plane. A bottom-up approach is followed, dissecting the rectum in the TME plane beyond the level of the seminal vesicles. Laparoscopically, the left colon is fully mobilised and the rectum is dissected from above downwards, until there is a rendezvous with the bottom-up dissector. The anastomosis can be either handsewn or performed with a double-purse-string circular stapler. A stapled anastomosis is associated with a superior functional outcome compared with a handsewn one, as the remaining rectal cuff tends to be longer. A surgeon should be careful that only the anorectal wall is enclosed in the purse-string suture, as there is a risk of including the vaginal wall. An advantage of the TAMIS-TME is that the stapled anastomosis can be reinforced endoluminally.[10] Injury to the urethra should be carefully avoided as the urethra can be difficult to identify during the transanal phase, especially in the case of a hypertrophied prostate. Although the short-term outcomes seem promising, the TaTME has only been in use since 2009; therefore, it must be emphasised that the long-term oncological and functional results are still awaited, and this procedure should be performed only by experienced hands or after extensive proctoring.[11]

Abdominoperineal Resection

For some of the low rectal carcinomas (up to 5 cm from the dentate line), especially with ingrowth into the anal sphincter complex, the maintenance of bowel continuity is not an option. In these cases, an APR is advised. In about 23% of rectal carcinomas, the APR is the procedure of choice.[3] The APR that is being performed currently is not very similar to the APR that was the standard operation performed for many years before the introduction of the sphincter-saving procedures.[12] During APR, the distal colon, rectum and anal sphincter complex are removed and a permanent colostomy is constructed. Despite the fact that the APR has been applied for a long period of time, the conventional procedure still is associated with substantial rates of margin involvement and perforation of the TME specimen. Local recurrence rates after APR were around 7 to 9%.[13] To reduce these rates of local recurrences, a modification of the conventional APR has been introduced over the past years; it is called the extralevator-APR (eAPR).[14] As opposed to the conventional approach, during eAPR, the lateral

limits of the dissection are extended to the base of the levator muscle. By including the levator muscle in the specimen, more tissue remains between the carcinoma and the dissection plane, which theoretically decreases margin involvement and perforation rate.[15] The eAPR is considered one of the most complex procedures and is subsequently associated with an increased risk to perineal wound healing, because of the larger perineal defect.[16] If the margins are not threatened and the sphincter cannot be saved because of ingrowth, an intersphincteric APR is a good alternative.

Complications Related to Abdominoperineal Resection

Both the wider extent of surgical resection and the high rate of neoadjuvant therapy contribute to a perineal wound complication rates of up to 57% after APR.[17] Complications such as perineal wound infection, perineal herniation and chronic presacral sinus are associated with a high disease burden and high costs and obviously have a severe impact on the quality of life (QOL). Recently, the BIOPEX randomised trial investigated the effectiveness of a biological mesh for pelvic floor reconstruction after eAPR in terms of uncomplicated perineal wound healing. This was the first randomised controlled trial on patients undergoing APR, specifically focussing on postoperative complications. Patients were randomised either to biological mesh placement or to primary perineal wound closure. Uncomplicated perineal wound healing was reported in 66% versus 64% of the patients, respectively, at 30 days postoperatively, with no significant difference between the groups. At 12 months postoperatively, a healed perineum was reached in 95% and 98%, respectively. Perineal herniation occurred in 25% of the patients after primary closure compared with a significantly lower rate of 9% in the biological mesh group. These rates seem rather high; however, it was not specified whether these hernias were symptomatic or asymptomatic. In retrospective series, these asymptomatic hernias are not reported, explaining the discrepancy in the higher rates reported in the prospective randomised trial.

Depending on the degree of herniation, surgical repair is indicated on an individual basis, as the majority of patients are treated conservatively with supportive underwear. Surgical repair is aimed to reconstruct the pelvic floor. The approach may be abdominal or perineal. The defect can be closed using myocutaneous flaps by primary suture repair or with the use of a mesh. Current evidence on treatment options is based on case reports or small retrospective series.[18] A pooled analysis by Mjoli et al combined all the case reports and showed that the hernia recurrence rate was lowest after mesh repair (20%).[18] Owing to the radicality and extension of the operation, the sexual outcomes after APR are worse when compared with sphincter-saving procedures.[19] More than half of the patients who underwent TME (LAR/APR/Hartmann) experience a decrease in sexual function.[20] Interestingly, reported QOL does not seem to differ between LAR and APR.[21]

SURGERY FOR BENIGN DISEASE

Restorative Proctocolectomy

A restorative proctocolectomy (RP) should be considered the best definitive surgical treatment for refractory ulcerative colitis (UC) or polyposis coli. Eventually, up to a third of the patients with UC will undergo surgery during their disease course.[22] Total proctocolectomy with ileal pouch–anal anastomosis (IPAA) is a more attractive option than the traditional total proctocolectomy with a permanent end ileostomy. The RP can be performed as a single or a modified two-stage procedure. Patients with polyposis can safely have a primary RP with an ileoanal pouch anastomosis. Patients with UC are best treated with a subtotal colectomy, first followed by a completion proctectomy and later by pouch; this is named as a *modified two-stage procedure*. In the acute setting of the colitis, these patients are often malnourished and immunocompromised; these conditions are responsible for an increased risk of a complicated postoperative course. Subtotal colectomy allows the patient to recover, after which completion proctectomy can be scheduled within 3 to 6 months. The creation of an ileal reservoir with the formation of the IPAA was invented by Sir Alan Parks in 1978.[23] In his original paper, he described an S-shaped pouch composed of three 8 cm loops of small bowel and a handsewn anastomosis after mucosectomy of the remaining rectal cuff. This S-shaped pouch has the drawback of an efferent limb, which can be the cause of evacuation problems. So, Utsunomiya et al proposed the simpler J-pouch configuration.[24] Throughout the years, several reservoir types have been described (J, S, W, H and Kock pouches). Evidence from systematic reviews showed that the double-stapled J-pouch is considered superior in terms of evacuation and continence and that the J-pouch is easier to construct.[25] Both the colectomy and the proctocolectomy can be performed via an open or laparoscopic approach (totally or hand-assisted via a Pfannenstiel incision). The pouch itself is most commonly being constructed extracorporally. The bowel can be extracted through the future stoma site or via a periumbilical incision or a Pfannenstiel incision.

One of the difficulties of a laparoscopic proctectomy is the formation of the anastomosis with a cross-staple line at the distal rectum. Often, multiple staple firings are needed, which are associated with an increased anastomotic leak rate.[26] Mucosectomy before performing the anastomosis is associated not only with better disease control but also with a worse functional outcome and therefore should not be considered the standard in pouch surgery.[27] Mucosectomy should be reserved only for patients with a high risk of cuff dysplasia or recurrent inflammation in the cuff.[27] In order to prevent 'cuffitis' in the postoperative course, it is crucial that the anastomosis should be placed in a way that the rectal cuff is less than 2 cm in length. Laparoscopic ileal pouch surgery is associated with beneficial outcomes in experienced centres compared with open surgery. In terms of hospital stay, wound infection and pelvic abscess rates, laparoscopic colectomy has been shown to be superior; nevertheless, it must be stressed that the evidence for laparoscopic surgery results in severe acute UC or with perforated disease is scarce.[22,28,29]

ANASTOMOSIS-RELATED COMPLICATIONS

Anastomotic surgery of the rectum is defined as the formation of a connection between the colon or ileum on one hand and the transected rectum or anus on the other. A temporary ileo- or colostomy is often created to divert the bowel contents, in order to reduce the sequelae of anastomotic leakage; however, the leak incidence is not necessarily prevented by this diversion. The definition of an anastomotic leak has been debated through the years, owing to the wide variety of clinical symptoms with which it is associated. We recommend the definition proposed by the *International Study Group of Rectal Cancer*, which is 'A defect of the intestinal wall at the anastomotic site (including suture and staple lines of neorectal reservoirs) leading to a communication between the intra- and extraluminal compartments'.[30]

The study group also categorised the severity on the leak into three grades:

- I: Anastomotic leakage requiring no active therapeutic intervention.
- II: Anastomotic leakage requiring active therapeutic intervention but manageable without relaparotomy or relaparoscopy.
- III: Anastomotic leakage requiring relaparotomy or relaparoscopy.

In the current literature, an anastomotic leak is defined as 'symptomatic' when either grade II or III is present.[31] This definition of symptomatic leak also applies to this chapter. The rates of anastomotic leak after rectal surgery are higher (10–14%) than those after colonic surgery (2–7%).[32–35] With an associated mortality of 6% and 22%, an increased risk of having a permanent ileostomy as well as local recurrence and the need of surgical or radiological interventions leakage are the most dreaded complications after rectal surgery.[36,37]

Diagnosis of Anastomotic Leaks

The early diagnosis of an anastomotic leak is not only crucial to minimise the degree of its sequelae, but it also increases the chances of saving the anastomosis.[38,39] Clinical signs of anastomotic leaks include fever, ileus, abdominal pain, abdominal distention and even pulmonary and cardiac symptoms.[30] All these symptoms can be absent if a defunctioning ileostomy is present. Clinical evaluation and imaging can be misleading when not conducted complementarily. Therefore, adequate timing of diagnostic tests is of great importance. A contrast study performed too early increases the false-negative rate of the test.[40] However, delayed diagnosis of the leak is associated with poorer outcomes in the long term. Inflammatory markers such as C-reactive protein (CRP) and white blood cell count should be used as screening markers to augment the clinical observations. Irrespective of the signs of sepsis, patients with an elevated CRP (>150 mg/L) on days 3 to 5 postoperative should be considered for imaging. The cut-off border of a CRP level of 150 mg/L reduces the false-negative rate of both computed-tomography (CT) with rectal contrast and contrast radiography.[41] Both contrast studies and sigmoidoscopy can be used to diagnose an anastomotic leak. However, as the specificity of these imaging studies have a wide range, the decision to perform an intervention should be guided by clinical evaluation, as a negative test does not rule out an anastomotic leak.[40]

Treatment of the Anastomotic Leak

Early Anastomotic Leak

In the acute phase of a symptomatic anastomotic leak, the primary goal of the treatment is control of the sepsis. Traditionally, when continuity is not intended, the leaking anastomosis is dismantled and an end colostomy is constructed. If continuity is preferred on the long term, the anastomotic leak should be defunctioned; if not done so primarily and subsequently, drainage of the sepsis is the cornerstone of the treatment. The TME, which is being performed for malignancy, creates a large cavity behind the anastomosis. This cavity will be stuffed with pus and debris in case of a leak. The anal sphincter thereby functions as a physiological barrier, preventing drainage via the anus. Adequate and timely drainage of the abscess is of major importance. Drainage can be performed transabdominally, percutaneously or transanally. With this type of adequate drainage, the healing rate of the anastomosis is around 50%.[38] However, this could take months before the leak has closed, so the patient must be prepared for an intensive treatment period.[42] Therefore, new strategies are being investigated.[38]

Endosponge Treatment, Combined with Transanal Closure of the Defect

Weidenhagen et al was the first to describe the Endosponge® vacuum-assisted drainage.[43] An Endosponge® is placed endoscopically into the abscess cavity; by changing it twice a week and tapering the size of the Endosponge® sequentially, the cavity gradually collapses (Figure 22.2). Endosponge® treatment in this early phase shows a healing rate of 75%.[42] However, this technique is labour-intensive, expensive and could take several weeks or even months before healing of the anastomosis is achieved. Therefore, recently, a modification of this technique has been proposed, in which the Endosponge® is used to clean the cavity instead of aiming at a gradual collapse. A clean cavity that is surrounded by granulation tissue can be achieved within 1 or 2 weeks. Subsequently, the anastomotic defect is closed transanally with the use of a Lone Star® retractor (Cooper Surgical, Trumbull, US) or a SILS™ port (GelPOINT® path transanal access platform; Applied Medical, Rancho Santa Margarita, US) (Figure 22.3).[39] In patients with an IPAA for benign disease, this strategy showed high anastomotic healing rates up to 100%; however, the results after resections for malignant disease have to be awaited.[38] Leaking coloanal anastomoses might have

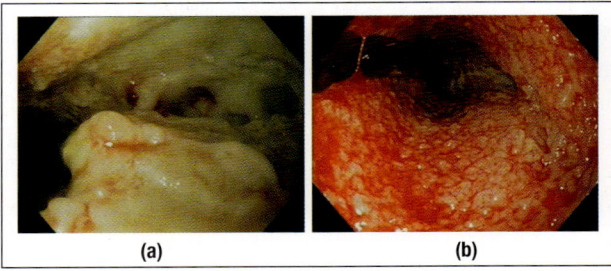

Figure 22.2 (a) Cavity with debris before endosponge treatment. (b) Granulation tissue covering cavity after endosponge treatment.

Courtesy: W.A.A. Borstlap, G.D. Musters, P.J. Tanis, C.J. Buskens and W.A. Bemelman.

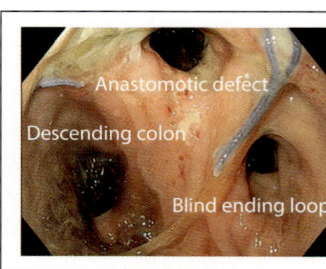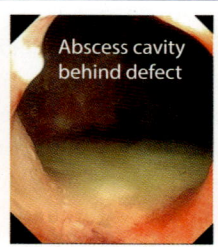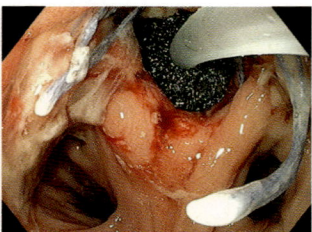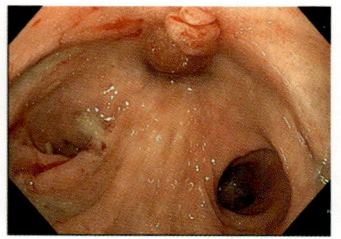

Figure 22.3   Anastomotic leak treated successfully with endosponge.
Courtesy: W.A.A. Borstlap, G.D. Musters, P.J. Tanis, C.J. Buskens and W.A. Bemelman.

a lower tendency to heal because of prior neoadjuvant radiotherapy. Technically, this anastomosis is more difficult to repair than the low colorectal anastomosis.

So, in case of an anastomotic leak diagnosed early, a step-up approach is advised, starting with minimally invasive techniques for drainage and transanal reconstruction, leaving resection of the anastomosis and the formation of an end colostomy as a last resort.[44,45]

Late Anastomotic Leakage

Late anastomotic leaks can be classified in two categories: an anastomotic defect or presacral abscess that is present for longer than 2 months after the construction of the anastomosis, including early leaks that have not been treated successfully and, secondly, the chronic presacral sinus, defined as a presacral abscess that is present more than a year after surgery. This distinction is important, as we think that both entities need different treatment strategies.

First Category: An Anastomotic Defect or Presacral Abscess that is Present More than 2 Months after the Initial Operation

The first category includes patients that present with an asymptomatic leak, which is diagnosed on imaging, classically during anastomotic assessment, before (or after) stoma reversal. Approximately 40 to 50% of the anastomotic leaks are diagnosed after the patient is discharged from the hospital.[46] The increased rates of neoadjuvant radiotherapy are probably responsible for reducing secondary healing after an anastomotic leak.[47] These late anastomotic leaks or presacral abscesses can present with a variety of symptoms such as sacral pain anal discharge, LAR syndrome, fatigue, chronic anaemia and even late evacuation of pus transanally or transvaginally. Owing to the chronic infection, the wall of the abscess, including the neorectum, becomes fibrotic and stiff. The abscess cavity cannot be filled anymore by the neorectum owing to the stiffness of the wall. Drainage alone is

therefore not enough to close the defect, particularly, in longstanding leaks.[38,44] Redo surgery with resection of the leaking coloanal or ileoanal anastomosis, followed by pull-through of a new colon loop or pouch and a new anastomosis, is a possibility in selected and motivated patients. However, this must be seen as the last option to avoid a permanent stoma. The decision to perform reconstructive surgery should be considered on individual basis. Small retrospective series have shown that redo surgery is associated with substantial complication rates and poor functional outcomes.[48,49] Therefore, it is important that the patient is closely involved in the decision-making process, and this type of surgery should be performed only in centres with extensive experience in reconstructive surgery. We would like to discuss three types of redo procedures: the conventional pull-through, the Turnbull-Cutait and the TAMIS-redo procedures.

Conventional pull-through procedure

During all operations in which the anastomosis is reconstructed, it is important to fully mobilise the left colon, ligating the inferior mesenteric pedicle, to acquire enough length for a tension-free apposition.[48] If the left colon is not available, the transverse colon should be brought down transmesenterically (Toupet procedure).[50] The reported success rate after the conventional procedure is 78.8%, with overall morbidity and reintervention rates of 32.2% and 15.6%, respectively.[48] The anastomosis is most commonly constructed in a handsewn fashion.

Turnbull-Cutait abdominoperineal pull-through procedure

The Turnbull-Cutait abdominoperineal pull-through procedure consists of rectal resection (including the leaking anastomosis) and exteriorisation of the afferent colon, followed by delayed handsewn coloanal anastomosis several days later.[51,52] The largest retrospective study showed a functioning anastomosis in 75% of the patients after this procedure.[53] A Turnbull-Cutait procedure is preferred over the conventional pull-through procedure by a small group of highly specialised surgeons. They apply it in highly selected patients who have an increased risk for a complicated course or for patients who present with a rectovaginal fistula that tracks down to the designated place of the new anastomosis. A known risk of the Turnball-Cutait is that the exteriorised colon becomes ischaemic, and therefore, the exteriorised colon should be checked carefully in the first postoperative days.

Redo transanal minimal invasive surgery

After the recent developments with the TaTME, the bottom up-approach is also applied in redo surgery.[49] The insufflation of the pelvis during TAMIS improves visualisation and surgical access and, as such, has the potential to revolutionise the approach to redo low anastomotic surgery and extensive sleeve advancement of the pouch. Furthermore, the advantage of TAMIS redo surgery is that the neorectum can be used to guide the dissection, thereby potentially minimising the chance of nerve and vascular injuries deep in the pelvis. However, the application of this technique should be investigated further before deciding on its value in redo surgery.

Second Category: Chronic Presacral Sinus

A chronic presacral sinus is defined as a presacral abscess that has been present more than a year after initial surgery and is confirmed on imaging. The sinus can be caused by an insufficiently treated anastomotic leak after a LAR or an IPAA. However, it can also occur at the top of the rectal stump after a Hartmann's procedure or in the presacral cavity after an APR.[44] Unpublished data provided by a nationwide Snapshot Audit in the Netherlands showed a presacral sinus incidence in approximately 9% of the patients after a LAR. A surprising percentage of patients with anastomotic leaks (42%) will eventually develop a presacral sinus. As mentioned earlier, a chronic sinus can cause serious long-term complications.[45] The number of patients with asymptomatic chronic sinuses is unknown; however, we believe that in the long term, the sinus will become symptomatic. Patients with a chronic sinus can present with a variety of symptoms such as a purulent anal discharge, sacral pain, difficulty in sitting or walking and urine or faecal discharge from the fistula tracts.[44,45] However, emergency presentations with osteomyelitis, hydronephrosis and necrotising fasciitis have also been described.[45]

Salvage surgery of the sinus is the only option for cure. In most patients, restoration of continuity is no longer advisable or achievable. Completion of abdominoperineal

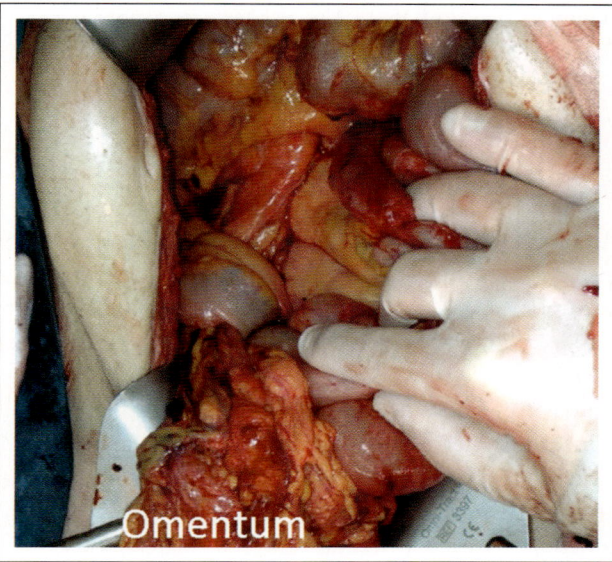

Figure 22.4 Mobilised omentum from left or right gastroepiploic artery.

Courtesy: W.A.A. Borstlap, G.D. Musters, P.J. Tanis, C.J. Buskens and W.A. Bemelman.

intersphincteric proctectomy with an end colostomy and omentoplasty in the presacral cavity is advised.[45,54] Owing to the longstanding chronic pelvic sepsis and prior irradiation in some, the cavity must be filled with healthy tissue to avoid recurrent abscesses. The omentum must be mobilised to obtain sufficient length. This can be done by pediculising the omentum on the left or right gastroepiploic artery (Figure 22.4). Alternatively, the presacral cavity can be filled by using a muscle transposition flap [vertical rectus abdominis myocutaneous (VRAM) or gracilis]. Owing to the risk of donor-site complications, for example, painful thigh wounds, sensory loss and even necrosis, omentoplasty is often preferred over the muscle flap.

NONANASTOMOSIS-RELATED COMPLICATIONS

Ureter and Urethra Lesions

Surgery deep in the pelvis puts structures such as the ureter, urethra and pelvic autonomic nerves, which are responsible for urogenital function, at risk. One of the most feared complications during rectal surgery is direct injury to the ureter; therefore, the ureter should always be identified proactively. When recognised directly, a ureter lesion can be treated, with good functional outcomes. Nevertheless, failure to detect it could lead to hydronephrosis, renal function disorders and even fistula leading to urine collection in the retroperitoneum or pelvis to the colon, abdominal wound, drain site or vagina. During the transanal phase of the TAMIS-TME, it is not so much the ureter but the urethra that should be safeguarded, as the urethra may be difficult to identify. Urethral injury is a hidden complication of this novel approach.

Urogenital Complications

Almost half of the patients that undergo rectal surgery experience a form of sexual dysfunction.[20] These mainly consist of ejaculatory and erectile dysfunctions in men (reported in 65–80%) and dyspareunia (in 53–60%) and dryness (72%) in women. Almost a third of the patients experience incontinence or retention of urine.[20] The sympathetic nerves that supply the bladder, prostate and seminal vesicles follow the branches of the internal iliac artery. These nerves are mainly involved in the ejaculatory function. During presacral and ventrolateral dissection of the mesorectum, the sympathetic nerves are at risk. The parasympathetic nerves that are located behind the endopelvic fascia and follow the ischiococcygeus and iliococcygeus muscles to the anterior genital tract are mainly responsible for the erectile function, sensation of bladder fullness and bladder emptying. The parasympathetic nerves are at risk during the deep dissection of the lateral planes.[20] Results from the Dutch-TME trial showed that difficulty in bladder emptying was significantly increased if there was a reported damage to the parasympathetic sacral splanchnic nerves and parasympathetic inferior hypogastric plexus.[20] Especially in the case of a narrow pelvis, or severe obesity, these autonomic nerves are at risk of being damaged owing to the decreased visibility. As urogenital dysfunction is a common postoperative complication, patients should be made well aware of the risk of a deterioration in urinary and sexual functions in the preoperative course.

Dysfunctional Neorectum

Urgency, constipation, incontinence of flatus and/or faeces, fragmentation, frequent bowel movements, sexual dysfunction and urinary dysfunction, all are the symptoms that can be brought under the umbrella of a 'dysfunctional neorectum'. Up to 60% of the patients undergoing rectal surgery experience disturbance in function. The height of the anastomosis directly correlates with function. In general, the lower the anastomosis, the worse the functional outcome. A recent Cochrane review showed that seven different scales can be used to assess functionality and QOL in patients with surgically treated rectal cancer.[55] The huge negative impact on the QOL, costs related to absence from work and potential social isolation have led to the consensus that there was a need for a simple, quick

and quantitative tool for the assessment of postoperative functionality and QOL. For this reason, Laurberg and coworkers developed the LARS score, which is currently being validated internationally and is being broadly supported by colorectal surgeons on an international scale.[56] It is a short five-item questionnaire that is easy to use. Hopefully, the international implementation of this questionnaire will provide the needed homogeneity in the assessment of postoperative functionality and QOL.

CONCLUSIONS

Rectal surgery is subject to a continuous development in surgical techniques and multimodulary treatment strategies. The spectrum of its complications is therefore expanding simultaneously. Early diagnosis and treatment are crucial, in order to achieve curation with minimal invasion. Patients should be closely involved in the decision-making process when striving for continuity, owing to the high morbidity associated with the redo anastomotic surgery.

REFERENCES

1. Heald RJ, Ryall RD. Recurrence and survival after total mesorectal excision for rectal cancer. *Lancet* 1986;1: 1479–82.
2. Clancy C, Burke JP, Albert MR, O'Connell PR, Winter DC. Transanal endoscopic microsurgery versus standard transanal excision for the removal of rectal neoplasms: a systematic review and meta-analysis. *Dis Colon Rectum* 2015; 58:254–61.
3. Ortiz H, Wibe A, Ciga MA, et al. Multicenter study of outcome in relation to the type of resection in rectal cancer. *Dis Colon Rectum* 2014;57:811–22.
4. Neutzling CB, Lustosa SA, Proenca IM, da Silva EM, Matos D. Stapled versus handsewn methods for colorectal anastomosis surgery. *Cochrane Database Syst Rev* 2012;2: CD003144.
5. Bonjer HJ, Deijen CL, Abis GA, et al. A randomized trial of laparoscopic versus open surgery for rectal cancer. *N Engl J Med* 2015;372:1324–32.
6. Jonker FH, Tanis PJ, Coene PL, Gietelink L, van der Harst E; Dutch Surgical Colorectal Audit Group. A comparison of low Hartmann's procedure with low colorectal anastomosis with and without defunctioning ileostomy after radiotherapy for rectal cancer: results from a national registry. *Colorectal Dis* 2016;18:785–92.
7. Sverrisson I, Nikberg M, Chabok A, Smedh K. Hartmann's procedure in rectal cancer: a population-based study of postoperative complications. *Int J Colorectal Dis* 2015; 30:181–6.
8. Schiessel R, Karner-Hanusch J, Herbst F, Teleky B, Wunderlich M. Intersphincteric resection for low rectal tumours. *Br J Surg* 1994;81:1376–8.

9. Martin ST, Heneghan HM, Winter DC. Systematic review of outcomes after intersphincteric resection for low rectal cancer. *Br J Surg* 2012;99:603–12.

10. de Lacy AM, Rattner DW, Adelsdorfer C, et al. Transanal natural orifice transluminal endoscopic surgery (NOTES) rectal resection: "down-to-up" total mesorectal excision (TME)–short-term outcomes in the first 20 cases. *Surg Endosc* 2013;27:3165–72.

11. Hompes R, Cunningham C. Extending the role of transanal endoscopic microsurgery (TEM) in rectal cancer. *Colorectal Dis* 2011;13:32–6.

12. Miles WE. A lecture on the diagnosis and treatment of cancer of the rectum: delivered at the Cancer Hospital, Brompton, on January 22nd, 1913. *Br Med J* 1913;1: 166–8.

13. den Dulk M, Marijnen CA, Putter H, et al. Risk factors for adverse outcome in patients with rectal cancer treated with an abdominoperineal resection in the total mesorectal excision trial. *Ann Surg* 2007;246:83–90.

14. Holm T, Ljung A, Haggmark T, Jurell G, Lagergren J. Extended abdominoperineal resection with gluteus maximus flap reconstruction of the pelvic floor for rectal cancer. *Br J Surg* 2007;94:232–8.

15. Nagtegaal ID, van de Velde CJ, Marijnen CA, et al; Dutch Colorectal Cancer Group. Low rectal cancer: a call for a change of approach in abdominoperineal resection. *J Clin Oncol* 2005;23:9257–64.

16. Musters GD, Sloothaak DA, Roodbeen S, van Geloven AA, Bemelman WA, Tanis PJ. Perineal wound healing after abdominoperineal resection for rectal cancer: a two-centre experience in the era of intensified oncological treatment. *Int J Colorectal Dis* 2014;29:1151–7.

17. de Bruin AF, Gosselink MP, Wijffels NA, Coene PP, van der Harst E. Local gentamicin reduces perineal wound infection after radiotherapy and abdominoperineal resection. *Tech Coloproctol* 2008;12:303–7.

18. Mjoli M, Sloothaak DA, Buskens CJ, Bemelman WA, Tanis PJ. Perineal hernia repair after abdominoperineal resection: a pooled analysis. *Colorectal Dis* 2012;14:e400–6.

19. Russell MM, Ganz PA, Lopa S, et al. Comparative effectiveness of sphincter-sparing surgery versus abdominoperineal resection in rectal cancer: patient-reported outcomes in National Surgical Adjuvant Breast and Bowel Project randomized trial R-04. *Ann Surg* 2015;261:144–8.

20. Lange MM, van de Velde CJ. Urinary and sexual dysfunction after rectal cancer treatment. *Nat Rev Urol* 2011;8: 51–7.

21. Cornish JA, Tilney HS, Heriot AG, Lavery IC, Fazio VW, Tekkis PP. A meta-analysis of quality of life for abdominoperineal excision of rectum versus anterior resection for rectal cancer. *Ann Surg Oncol* 2007;14:2056–68.

22. Buskens CJ, Sahami S, Tanis PJ, Bemelman WA. The potential benefits and disadvantages of laparoscopic surgery for ulcerative colitis: a review of current evidence. *Best Pract Res Clin Gastroenterol* 2014;28:19–27.

23. Parks AG, Nicholls RJ. Proctocolectomy without ileostomy for ulcerative colitis. *Br Med J* 1978;2:85–8.

24. Utsunomiya J, Iwama T, Imajo M, et al. Total colectomy, mucosal proctectomy, and ileoanal anastomosis. *Dis Colon Rectum* 1980;23:459–66.

25. Lovegrove RE, Heriot AG, Constantinides V, et al. Meta-analysis of short-term and long-term outcomes of J, W and S ileal reservoirs for restorative proctocolectomy. *Colorectal Dis* 2007;9:310–20.

26. Kienle P, Z'Graggen K, Schmidt J, Benner A, Weitz J, Buchler MW. Laparoscopic restorative proctocolectomy. *Br J Surg* 2005;92:88–93.

27. Chambers WM, Mc CMNJ. Should ileal pouch-anal anastomosis include mucosectomy? *Colorectal Dis* 2007; 9:384–92.

28. Bartels SA, Gardenbroek TJ, Ubbink DT, Buskens CJ, Tanis PJ, Bemelman WA. Systematic review and meta-analysis of laparoscopic versus open colectomy with end ileostomy for non-toxic colitis. *Br J Surg* 2013;100:726–33.

29. Miskovic D, Ni M, Wyles SM, Tekkis P, Hanna GB. Learning curve and case selection in laparoscopic colorectal surgery: systematic review and international multicenter analysis of 4852 cases. *Dis Colon Rectum* 2012;55:1300–10.

30. Rahbari NN, Weitz J, Hohenberger W, et al. Definition and grading of anastomotic leakage following anterior resection of the rectum: a proposal by the International Study Group of Rectal Cancer. *Surgery* 2010;147: 339–51.

31. Katsuno H, Shiomi A, Ito M, et al. Comparison of symptomatic anastomotic leakage following laparoscopic open low anterior resection for rectal cancer: a propensity score matching analysis of 1014 consecutive patients. *Surg Endosc* 2016;30:2848–56.

32. Vlug MS, Wind J, Hollmann MW, et al. Laparoscopy in combination with fast track multimodal management is the best perioperative strategy in patients undergoing colonic surgery: a randomized clinical trial (LAFA-study). *Ann Surg* 2011;254:868–75.

33. Kapiteijn E, Marijnen CA, Nagtegaal ID, et al. Preoperative radiotherapy combined with total mesorectal excision for resectable rectal cancer. *New Eng J Med* 2001;345: 638–46.

34. van der Pas MH, Haglind E, Cuesta MA, et al. Laparoscopic versus open surgery for rectal cancer (COLOR II): short-term outcomes of a randomised, phase 3 trial. *Lancet Oncol* 2013;14:210–8.

35. McDermott FD, Heeney A, Kelly ME, Steele RJ, Carlson GL, Winter DC. Systematic review of preoperative, intraoperative and postoperative risk factors for colorectal anastomotic leaks. *Br J Surg* 2015;102:462–79.

36. Snijders HS, Bakker IS, Dekker JW, et al. High 1-year complication rate after anterior resection for rectal cancer. *J Gastrointest Surg* 2014;18:831–8.

37. Arezzo A, Passera R, Ferri V, Gonella F, Cirocchi R, Morino M. Laparoscopic right colectomy reduces short-term

mortality and morbidity. Results of a systematic review and meta-analysis. *Int J Colorectal Dis* 2015;30:1457–72.

38. Gardenbroek TJ, Musters GD, Buskens CJ, et al. Early reconstruction of the leaking ileal pouch-anal anastomosis: a novel solution to an old problem. *Colorectal Dis* 2015;17:426–32.

39. van Koperen PJ, van Berge Henegouwen MI, et al. The Dutch multicenter experience of the endo-sponge treatment for anastomotic leakage after colorectal surgery. *Surg Endosc* 2009;23:1379–83.

40. Doeksen A, Tanis PJ, Wust AF, Vrouenraets BC, van Lanschot JJ, van Tets WF. Radiological evaluation of colorectal anastomoses. *Int J Colorectal Dis* 2008;23:863–8.

41. Warschkow R, Beutner U, Steffen T, et al. Safe and early discharge after colorectal surgery due to C-reactive protein: a diagnostic meta-analysis of 1832 patients. *Ann Surg* 2012;256:245–50.

42. van Koperen PJ, van der Zaag ES, Omloo JM, Slors JF, Bemelman WA. The persisting presacral sinus after anastomotic leakage following anterior resection or restorative proctocolectomy. *Colorectal Dis* 2011;13:26–9.

43. Weidenhagen R, Gruetzner KU, Wiecken T, Spelsberg F, Jauch KW. Endoscopic vacuum-assisted closure of anastomotic leakage following anterior resection of the rectum: a new method. *Surgical Endosc* 2008;22:1818–25.

44. Sloothaak DA, Buskens CJ, Bemelman WA, Tanis PJ. Treatment of chronic presacral sinus after low anterior resection. *Colorectal Dis* 2013;15:727–32.

45. Musters GD, Borstlap WA, Bemelman WA, Buskens CJ, Tanis PJ. Intersphincteric completion proctectomy with omentoplasty for chronic presacral sinus after low anterior resection for rectal cancer. *Colorectal Dis* 2016;18:147–54.

46. Floodeen H, Hallbook O, Rutegard J, Sjodahl R, Matthiessen P. Early and late symptomatic anastomotic leakage following low anterior resection of the rectum for

cancer: are they different entities? *Colorectal Dis* 2013;15:334–40.

47. den Dulk M, Smit M, Peeters KC, et al. A multivariate analysis of limiting factors for stoma reversal in patients with rectal cancer entered into the total mesorectal excision (TME) trial: a retrospective study. *Lancet Oncol* 2007;8:297–303.

48. Pitel S, Lefevre JH, Tiret E, Chafai N, Parc Y. Redo coloanal anastomosis: a retrospective study of 66 patients. *Ann Surg* 2012;256:806–10; discussion 10–1.

49. Borstlap WA, Harran N, Tanis PJ, Bemelman WA. Feasibility of the TAMIS technique for redo pelvic surgery. *Surgical Endosc* 2016;30:5364–71.

50. Toupet A. [Colonectomies with transmesenteric anastomosis]. *Mem Acad Chir (Paris)* 1963;89:628–30.

51. Cutait DE, Figliolini FJ. A new method of colorectal anastomosis in abdominoperineal resection. *Dis Colon Rectum* 1961;4:335–42.

52. Turnbull RB, Jr., Cuthbertson A. Abdominorectal pull-through resection for cancer and for Hirschsprung's disease. Delayed posterior colorectal anastomosis. *Cleve Clin Q* 1961;28:109–15.

53. Remzi FH, El Gazzaz G, Kiran RP, Kirat HT, Fazio VW. Outcomes following Turnbull-Cutait abdominoperineal pull-through compared with coloanal anastomosis. The British journal of surgery. 2009;96:424–9.

54. Wilson TR, Welbourn H, Stanley P, Hartley JE. The success of rectus and gracilis muscle flaps in the treatment of chronic pelvic sepsis and persistent perineal sinus: a systematic review. *Colorectal Dis* 2014;16:751–9.

55. Pachler J, Wille-Jorgensen P. Quality of life after rectal resection for cancer, with or without permanent colostomy. *Cochrane Db Syst Rev* 2005;2:CD004323.

56. Juul T, Ahlberg M, Biondo S, et al. International validation of the low anterior resection syndrome score. *Ann Surg* 2014;259:728–34.

23

Mesenteric Ischaemia: Decreasing Mortality by Reducing Time to Diagnosis

F. Kuehn and E. Klar

ABSTRACT

The mortality of acute mesenteric ischaemia (AMI) has remained high for decades, despite improvements in diagnostic, interventional and surgical techniques. Therefore, an AMI must be recognised as a vascular emergency requiring rapid and efficient clinical evaluation and treatment. The time to diagnosis of AMI is the most important modifiable predictor of the patient outcome. Here, focussed and specific questions, recognition of predisposing factors and clinical examination must set the course to initiate a time-saving and efficient diagnosis. The symptoms of nonocclusive mesenteric ischaemia (NOMI) are different from the ones of acute occlusive ischaemia; abdominal distension, signs of sepsis and inflammatory parameters have to be assessed carefully. Biphasic contrast-enhanced computed tomography represents the means of choice for diagnosis of arterial and venous occlusion. If there is a central occlusion of the superior mesenteric artery or signs of peritonitis, immediate surgery should be performed. However, endovascular techniques for arterial occlusion have taken on a greater importance today. If no signs of peritonitis are present, in peripheral embolism, interventional pharmacotherapy with local fibrinolysis should be instituted. The accompanying intensive care management includes volume replacement, systemic anticoagulation and antibiotic therapy, as well as close patient monitoring to exclude secondary organ failure.

KEYWORDS

Acute mesenteric ischaemia, NOMI, intestinal venous thrombosis, diagnostics, therapy, mortality

INTRODUCTION

Mesenteric ischaemia is a rare but extremely challenging clinical picture. Its outcome is strongly time-dependent, and it is still fatal in 50 to 70% of cases. A suspected mesenteric ischaemia can be the reason for a primary admission to the hospital. However, it can also occur as a complication in hospitalised and predisposed patients. It must be recognised as a vascular emergency requiring rapid and efficient clinical evaluation and treatment.

CORE STATEMENTS

Epidemiology and Mortality

- Although acute mesenteric ischaemia (AMI) applies only to approximately 1% of all patients with an 'acute abdomen', its incidence is rising in patients older than 70 years, up to 10%.
- The mortality of AMI has remained high for decades, despite improvements in diagnostic, interventional and surgical techniques.
- The time to diagnosis of AMI is the most important modifiable predictor of patient outcome.

Clinical Manifestations

- The initial clinical stage of AMI is characterised by the sudden onset of strong, spasmodic abdominal pain; after 3 to 6 hours, this phase is followed by a painless interval. Subsequently, there is a collapse of the mucosal barrier with bacterial translocation and gangrene of the intestinal wall.

- The symptoms of nonocclusive mesenteric ischaemia (NOMI) are different from the ones of acute occlusive ischaemia. The NOMI is also often more difficult to detect. Abdominal distension, signs of sepsis and inflammatory parameters have to be assessed carefully.
- The symptoms of patients with intestinal venous thrombosis depend on the extent of disease. Often, nonspecific abdominal symptoms occur, which usually last for some time before the condition is recognised.

Diagnostics

- Focussed and specific questions, recognition of predisposing factors and clinical examination must set the course to initiate a time-saving and efficient diagnosis.
- Biphasic contrast-enhanced computed tomography (CT) represents the means of choice for diagnosis of arterial and venous occlusions.

Therapy

- If there is central occlusion of the superior mesenteric artery (SMA) or signs of peritonitis, immediate surgery should be performed.
- If resection of large bowel segments becomes necessary, the critical residual lengths must be preserved in order to prevent a short bowel syndrome.
- Today, endovascular techniques for arterial occlusion have taken on a greater importance. If no signs of peritonitis are present, in peripheral embolism, interventional pharmacotherapy with local fibrinolysis should be instituted.
- For stable patients with the NOMI, interventional catheter angiography is recommended. This enables diagnosis and treatment with selective application of vasodilators into the SMA.
- Acute and chronic portal vein thrombosis should be treated interventionally with transhepatic catheter lysis. This should be done even in the absence of symptoms up to 4 weeks after the signal event, in order to prevent secondary complications of portal hypertension such as oesophageal or gastric varices.
- The accompanying intensive care management includes volume replacement, systemic anticoagulation and antibiotic therapy as well as close patient monitoring to exclude secondary organ failure.

DEFINITION AND EPIDEMIOLOGY

Acute mesenteric ischaemia is a time-critical emergency resulting in irreversible hypoperfusion of the mesenteric organs within a few hours. In Western countries, around 85% of these cases affect the functional terminal vascular bed of the SMA—running from the central collateral blood supply to the mobile convolutions of the small intestine.[1,2] The large diameter and narrow take-off angle of the SMA make it anatomically most susceptible to embolism. Although an AMI occurs only in approximately 1% of all patients with an 'acute abdomen', its incidence in patients older than 70 years is rising and has now reached 10%. Several risk factors should be considered for AME, and these risk factors include heart failure, atrial fibrillation, coronary heart disease (CHD), arterial hypertension and peripheral vascular disease.[3,4]

Despite improvements in diagnostic, interventional and surgical techniques, the mortality of AMI ranges in literature between 50 and 70%.[5] This is partly due to the rarity of the disease and the resulting associated disregard as an important differential diagnosis.[5] Secondly, often, routine diagnostic modalities are used, which are time-consuming and mostly unrewarding. In order to reduce the high mortality rate of this disease—if there is any suspicion of its existence—the appropriate diagnostic methods should be initialised straightaway; the pertinent therapeutic approach should then follow immediately. Only with vigilance, accurate evaluation of the medical history and optimal time management is there a possibility to use the short time span before irreversible ischaemia manifests and to improve outcomes of patients with AMI.

In this chapter, we will discuss separately the different forms of mesenteric ischaemia, namely acute occlusive mesenteric ischaemia, NOMI and venous thrombosis of the mesenteric–portal axis.

OCCLUSIVE MESENTERIC ISCHAEMIA

Pathophysiology and Clinical Aspects

The SMA is a single central vessel, which has a vulnerable terminal vascular zone. Owing to collateralisation, the coeliac and inferior mesenteric arteries are phylogenetically better protected against an acute occlusion of their main trunks. An acute complete circulatory disruption of the intestine leads within 6 hours to irreversible mucosal ischaemia with leucocyte infiltration and formation of oxygen radicals.[6] The mortality rate rises from 0 to 10% with swift treatment to 50 to 60% with delays of 6 to 12 hours and to 80 to 100% with delays of more than 24 hours after the onset of symptoms.[7] The initial clinical stage is characterised by a sudden onset of strong, spasmodic abdominal pain; after 3 to 6 hours, this phase is followed by a painless interval, which is explained by the elimination of the intramural pain receptors as a result of prolonged hypoperfusion of the intestinal wall. Subsequently, there is a collapse of the mucosal barrier with bacterial translocation and gangrene of the intestinal wall; the bacterial infiltration leads to peritonitis, ileus, sepsis and multiorgan failure.[1] Algorithm 23.1 illustrates

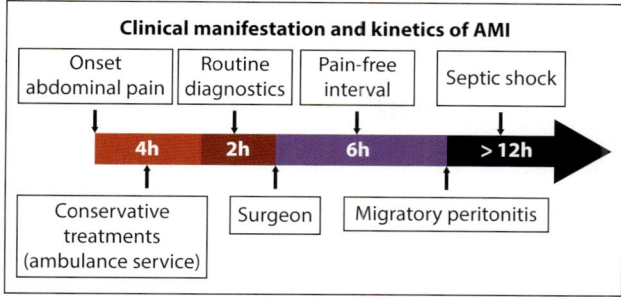

Algorithm 23.1 Kinetics of acute mesenteric ischaemia (AMI) from the onset of disease to septic shock.

Reprinted with permission from: Kuehn F, Klar E. Vaskuläre Komplikationen im Darmtrakt. *Gastroenterologie Up2date* 2014; 10:159–70. (Thieme-Verlag). doi: 10.1055/s-0034-1377490.

the timeline from the onset of symptoms until irreversible gangrene, with associated consequences.

Diagnostics

Acute mesenteric ischaemia represents a vascular emergency and must be detected as early as possible. Here, time-saving and focussed diagnostics are vital. Inflexible routine diagnostic programmes or wrong diagnostic tools can significantly extend time to diagnosis and contribute to the high mortality of AMI. The diagnostic delay—even if there is a suspicion of AMI—accounts for an average of 7.9 hours, and therapy requires another 2.5 hours before reperfusion of the mesenteric region is achieved.[7] Already within a warm ischaemia time of 6 hours, there is disintegration of the mucosal barrier with subsequent bacterial translocation, and morphological changes of the intestinal wall follow. Consequently, when acute occlusive mesenteric ischaemia is suspected, biphasic contrast-enhanced CT with three-dimensional multiplanar

reconstruction (MPR-CT) is the diagnostic tool of choice (Algorithm 23.2).

The CT scan should include the whole abdomen, in both the arterial and venous phases.[1] The venous phase is required for the diagnosis of mesenteric venous thrombosis. In order to save time and achieve even better imaging of alterations in the intestinal wall, oral contrast agents should not be used. It is essential to define and communicate to the radiologist the suspected diagnosis when requesting diagnostic imaging. Although magnetic resonance imaging (MRI) can theoretically be used for diagnosis, CT should be preferred because of the time it saves. The universal availability and the quality of multidetector CT (MDCT) allows sufficient enhancement of the mesenteric vessels (Figure 23.1).

Three-dimensional reconstruction by CT angiography (CTA) accurately depicts the mesenteric vascular anatomy. In addition to examining the wall of the intestine, the main advantages of multidetector CTA over catheter angiography are its use in ruling out other disorders during the differential diagnosis of AMI. As a result, catheter angiography is becoming less popular.[8] The sensitivity and specificity of MPR-CT are 93% and 100%, respectively; its positive and negative predictive values are between 94 and 100%.[9] Because mesenteric

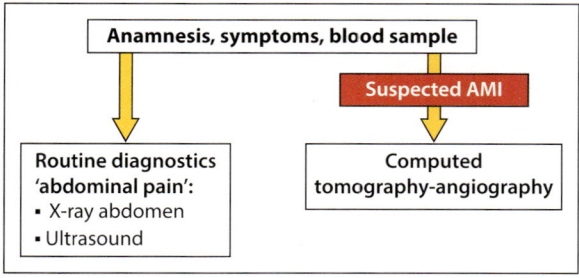

Algorithm 23.2 Diagnostic approach for suspected acute mesenteric ischaemia (AMI).

Reprinted with permission from: Kuehn F, Klar E. Vaskuläre Komplikationen im Darmtrakt. *Gastroenterologie Up2date* 2014; 10:159–70. doi: 10.1055/s-0034-1377490.

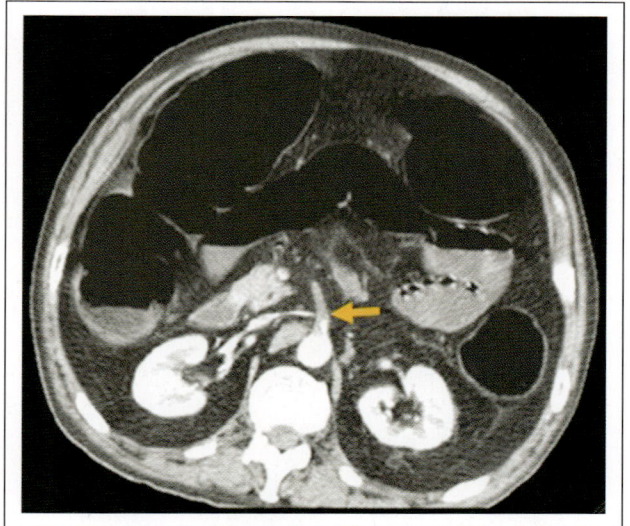

Figure 23.1 Computed tomography after intravenous contrast administration (arterial phase), with evidence of occlusion of the superior mesenteric artery close to its origin, by an embolus (arrow). Distension of the represented portions of the intestine is a sign of paralytic ileus.

Reprinted with permission from: Klar E, Rahmanian PB, Bücker A, et al. Acute mesenteric ischemia: a vascular emergency. *Dtsch Arztebl Int* 2012;109:249–56.

ischaemia generally leads to a distension of the intestinal loops, ultrasound should not be used for examination (class III recommendation, level of evidence C, according to the American College of Cardiology/ American Heart Association [ACC/AHA] guidelines). The widespread use of an initial abdominal plain X-ray does not probably lead to a significant time delay; next to a possible exclusion of free abdominal air, it can show signs of an advanced intestinal ischaemia (Figure 23.2).

Laboratory Parameters

Various serum parameters are associated with AMI. Since none of the parameters is equipped with a high sensitivity or specificity for diagnosis of AMI, they can only be regarded as supplementary information. The serum lactate level serves as a nonspecific parameter for the degree of anaerobic metabolism of the ischaemic tissue. Indeed, the lethality of AMI is associated with increased lactate serum levels; however, neither does a normal serum lactate definitely exclude an AMI, nor is an increased lactate level conclusive for AMI.[10] In correlation with clinical signs and imaging, it can be used as relatively important additional information for diagnosis and in the postoperative course. Furthermore, a pronounced leucocytosis is known as a nonspecific predictor of an unfavourable course of AMI.[11] According to a recent study, measuring procalcitonin levels can be helpful in

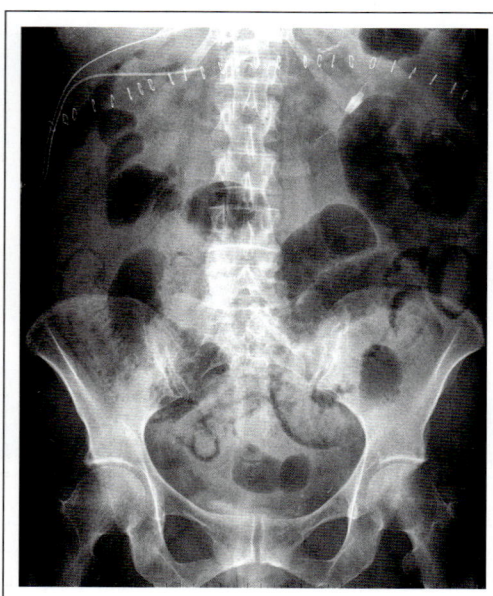

Figure 23.2 Abdominal film showing air inside the intestinal wall as a sign of advanced intestinal ischaemia.

Courtesy: Florian Kuehn and Ernst Klar.

excluding acute ischaemia.[12] However, these parameters should also be regarded as being nonspecific.

Therapy

The type of therapy on the one hand depends on the cause and localisation of AMI and on the other hand depends on the clinical status of the patient. Clinical signs of peritonitis or evidence of pre-existing gangrene—recognisable via CT scan by air in the intestinal wall or in the portal vein (portal gas)—demand urgent surgical treatment.[1]

Surgical Treatment Options

Clinical signs of peritonitis, evidence of gangrene, central occlusion of the SMA or failure of endovascular options require immediate surgical treatment.[1] The principle of treatment is to try and obtain arterial reperfusion before intestinal resection. In this scenario, surgeons must be equipped with the techniques of embolectomy and reconstruction of visceral arteries.[13] At the same time, the septic focus has to be controlled by the identification and resection of irreversibly ischaemic portions of the intestine. Often, the damage to the inner mucosal layer is much more extensive than estimated externally; for this reason, in case of doubt, discontinuous resections with or without temporay diversion should be considered. The underestimation of a relatively ischaemic segment that leads to an anastomotic leak contributes to an increased mortality in these cases.[14] The bowel segments with an 'uncertain' reperfusion require a 'second-look' operation, especially if the patient is haemodynamically unstable. If a major resection of bowel becomes necessary, the following critical residual lengths must be kept in mind[15]:

- 100 cm with a terminal jejunostomy (colon removed) (Figure 23.3)
- 65 cm in a jejunocolonic anastomosis (colon retained) (Figure 23.4)
- 35 cm in case of a jejunoileal anastomosis (Figure 23.5)

Resection beyond these critical lengths inevitably leads to short bowel syndrome, with the need for permanent parenteral nutrition or a small bowel transplantation.[15]

Extended resections in the elderly patients with relevant comorbidities have to be considered very carefully. In about 40 to 60% of patients with an AMI, only surgical exploration without resection is conducted and only palliative care has to be started.[16]

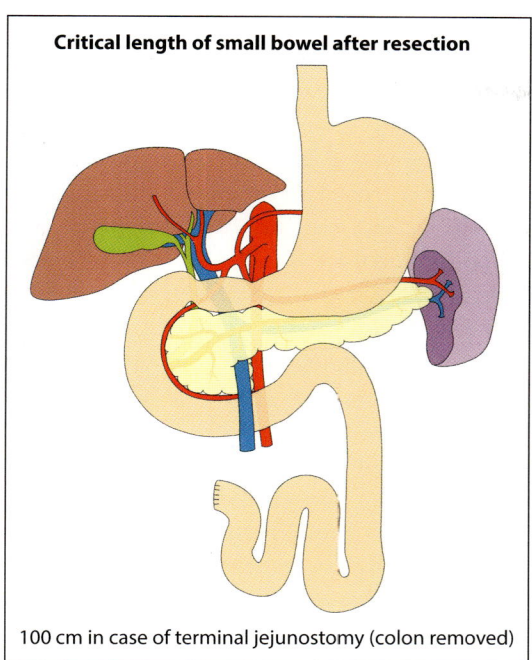

Critical length of small bowel after resection

100 cm in case of terminal jejunostomy (colon removed)

Figure 23.3 Critical lenghts in case of terminal jejunostomy (colon removed).

Reprinted with permission from: Kuehn F, Klar E. Vaskuläre Komplikationen im Darmtrakt. *Gastroenterologie Up2date* 2014; 10:159–70. doi: 10.1055/s-0034-1377490.

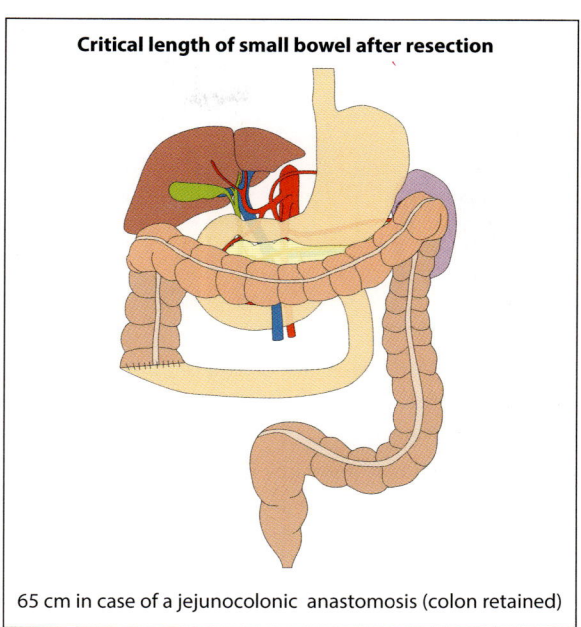

Critical length of small bowel after resection

65 cm in case of a jejunocolonic anastomosis (colon retained)

Figure 23.4 Critical lenghts in case of jejunocolonic anstomosis (colon retained).

Reprinted with permission from: Kuehn F, Klar E. Vaskuläre Komplikationen im Darmtrakt. *Gastroenterologie Up2date* 2014; 10:159–70. doi: 10.1055/s-0034-1377490.

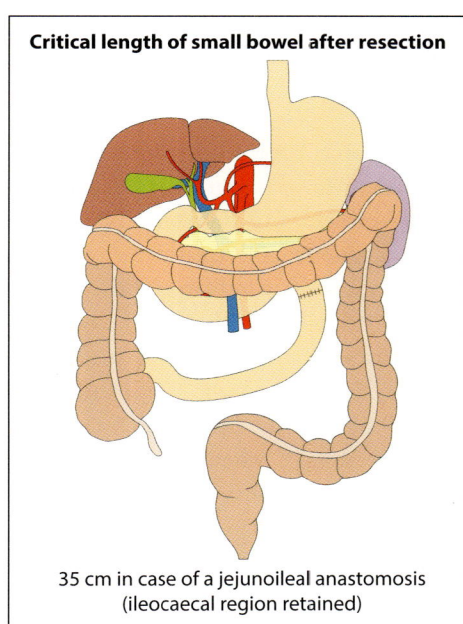

Critical length of small bowel after resection

35 cm in case of a jejunoileal anastomosis (ileocaecal region retained)

Figure 23.5 Critical lenghts in case of jejunoileal anastomosis (ileocaecal region retained).

Reprinted with permission from: Kuehn F, Klar E. Vaskuläre Komplikationen im Darmtrakt. *Gastroenterologie Up2date* 2014; 10:159–70. doi: 10.1055/s-0034-1377490.

Endovascular Techniques

If there are no signs of peritonitis and the patient is haemodynamically stable, endovascular techniques can be considered first. The endovascular approach consists of angiographically controlled catheter aspiration embolectomy and the catheter lysis with recombinant tissue plasminogen activator (rt-PA) or urokinase, or pharmacotherapy with prostaglandin E1.[17] In such cases, fractionation of the thrombus by using a guide wire increases the surface area, which comes in contact with the fibrinolytic agent and so speeds up the dissolution of the thrombus. The aim is to reopen the main arterial branches of the SMA, as this will allow the remaining occluded segments of intestine to be well compensated for as a result of good collateral growth.[1] If fibrinolysis and/or pharmacotherapy show changes of the vascular wall, percutaneous transluminal angioplasty (PTA) via the femoral artery can recanalise arteriosclerotic vascular occlusions or stenoses or at least facilitate a bridging reperfusion to this area (Figure 23.6). In case of an opened abdomen, this possibility is offered by retrograde catheterisation by using a peripheral SMA tributary to obtain access to the central segment.[18]

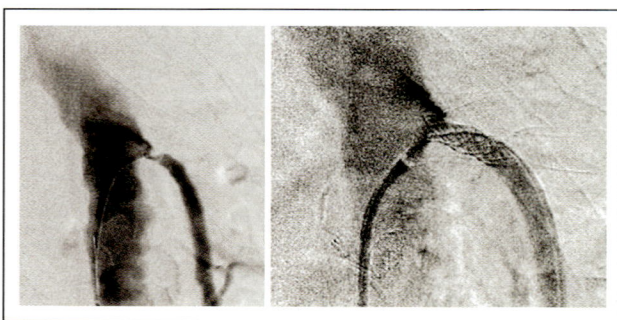

Figure 23.6 Stent percutaneous transluminal angioplasty (PTA) of the superior mesenteric artery after fibrinolysis of a thrombotic occlusion.

Reprinted with permission from: Klar E, Rahmanian PB, Bücker A, et al. Acute mesenteric ischemia: a vascular emergency. *Dtsch Arztebl Int* 2012;109:249–56.

Intensive Care

In addition to prompt diagnosis and therapy, the accompanying intensive care management plays a fundamental role in the treatment of mesenteric ischaemia. An immediate stabilisation of haemodynamics by sufficient intravenous fluid replacement is essential if there is a systemic inflammatory response syndrome (SIRS) and a shift of fluid volume into the ischaemic bowel segments. In addition, swift anticoagulation should be initialised with bolus application of 5000 IE heparin intravenously, followed by perfusor-controlled administration with an initial dose of 20.000 IU heparin/24 hours.[1] Systemic antibiotic therapy is mandatory and should be started early. Toxic ischaemic end products and bacterial translocation may cause a long-term septic clinical picture. The intensive care treatment should be continued until all organ functions are stable and the infectious parameters are at a low level. Frequent postoperative controls to exclude secondary organ failure are obligatory.[1]

NONOCCLUSIVE MESENTERIC ISCHAEMIA

Pathophysiology and Clinical Manifestations

The nonocclusive mesenteric ischaemia is a consequence of a reduction of the cardiac output or hypovolaemia and results in a reactive vasospasm in the mesenteric area. It is characterised by varying degrees of ischaemia, up to gangrene in different intestinal segments. Although the mortality rate has been reduced in recent decades by the introduction of selective angiography, with local application of vasodilators, at 50 to 70%, it is still very

high.[19] The symptoms of the NOMI are different from those of acute occlusive ischaemia; the NOMI is often more difficult to detect. However, its occurrence is concentrated in certain patient groups—one group of patients is undergoing chronic haemodialysis; hypovolaemia due to fluid removal results in intestinal vasospasm.[1] The other group includes patients after cardiac surgery with extracorporeal circulation. The NOMI is present at around 0.5 to 1% of all patients after cardiac surgery.[10,20] Pathogenetically, this can be explained by a reduction in cardiac output or a perioperative hypotonic phase, which can lead to a vascular constriction of the splanchnic area. In addition, heart–lung machines can also contribute to reduced splanchnic blood flow.[1,21] Next to surgical factors, such as duration of bypass and the need for an intra-aortic balloon pump, the patient's age, an impaired left ventricular function, peripheral vascular disease and cerebrovascular and renal insufficiency also contribute to the risk of developing the NOMI.[1,22]

Clinical examination in these patients is challenging and of limited value owing to intubation and sedation. Abdominal distension, signs of sepsis and inflammatory parameters have to be assessed carefully. Since the lactate serum levels may be increased after surgery, with extracorporeal circulation without mesenteric ischaemia, it can only serve as supplementary information.[23]

Diagnosis and Treatment

The diagnostic and therapeutic approach to NOMI depends on the patient's condition. If the patient is stable, interventional catheter angiography is recommended. This enables diagnosis and treatment of choice, with selective application of vasodilators into the SMA; for example, PGE1 alprostadil 20 µg as a bolus, followed by perfusor-controlled administration at 60 to 80 µg/24 hours; alternatively, PGI2 epoprostenol 5 to 6 ng/Kg/min heparin i.v. 20,000 IU/24 hours. This can successfully interrupt generalised vascular spasm.[1] Control angiography has to follow, in order to confirm the success of vasodilation (Figure 23.7).

The nonstable patient needs immediate surgery, with abdominal exploration and resection of irreversibly damaged ischaemic segments. Subsequently, these patients also receive an angiography, with concomitant pharmacotherapy, in order to dissolve the causative vasospasm. The indication for a 'second look' operation has to be provided generously. The diagnostic and therapeutic approach in case of suspected NOMI is illustrated in Algorithm 23.3.

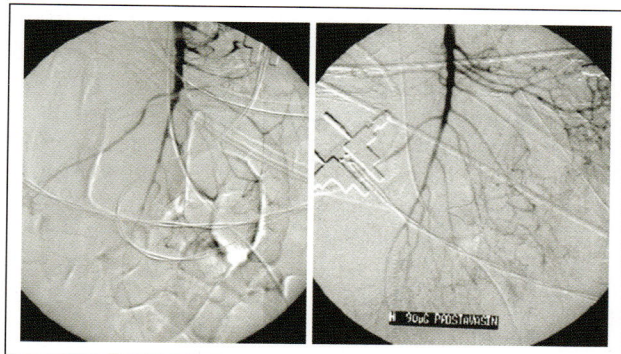

Figure 23.7 Nonocclusive mesenteric ischaemia after cardiac surgery before and after intra-arterial Prostavasin infusion.

Reprinted with permission from: Klar E, Rahmanian PB, Bücker A, et al. Acute mesenteric ischemia: a vascular emergency. *Dtsch Arztebl Int* 2012;109:249–56.

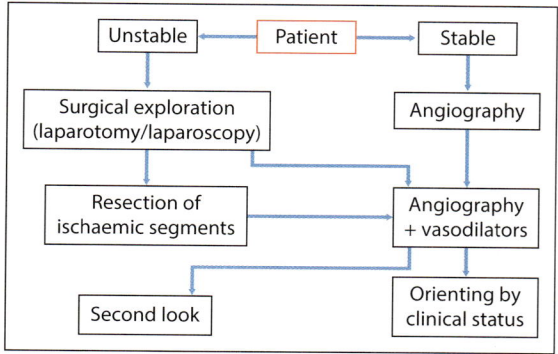

Algorithm 23.3 Algorithm for diagnosis and treatment of a suspected nonocclusive mesenteric ischaemia.

Courtesy: Florian Kuehn and Ernst Klar.

INTESTINAL VENOUS THROMBOSIS

If centrally located and affecting several areas downstream, a venous thrombosis can lead to irreversible damage to the intestinal wall.[24] However, thrombosis of the superior mesenteric vein alone is normally effectively compensated for by sufficient collateral vessel formation, even in central segments. In contrast, an additional complete thrombosis of the portal vein leads to varying venous infarction of segments of the small bowel.[1] The symptoms of the patient depend on the extent of thrombosis. Often, the patient presents with nonspecific abdominal symptoms, which usually last for some time. The biphasic contrast-enhanced CT with MPR reconstruction is the diagnostic tool of choice for the imaging of venous thrombosis, thickened intestinal walls and ascites. Here, too, if there are signs of peritonitis, surgical exploration with resection

of infarcted segments has to follow. Intraoperatively, an antegrade catheter thrombolysis (transmesenteric) can also be initiated for subsequent local lysis; rt-PA (2 mg/h) is administered for 2 to 3 days, accompanied by daily angiographic monitoring. Shortly after thrombosis, the venous endothelium already experiences inflammatory alterations. Owing to a high recurrence rate, surgical thrombectomy is done only in exceptional cases.[1] The treatment of choice in stable patients without peritonitis is the recanalisation via transjugular transhepatic access, combinable with the implantation of a stent shunt (transjugular intrahepatic portosystemic stent shunt [TIPS]).[24,25] The angiographic images of Figure 23.8a

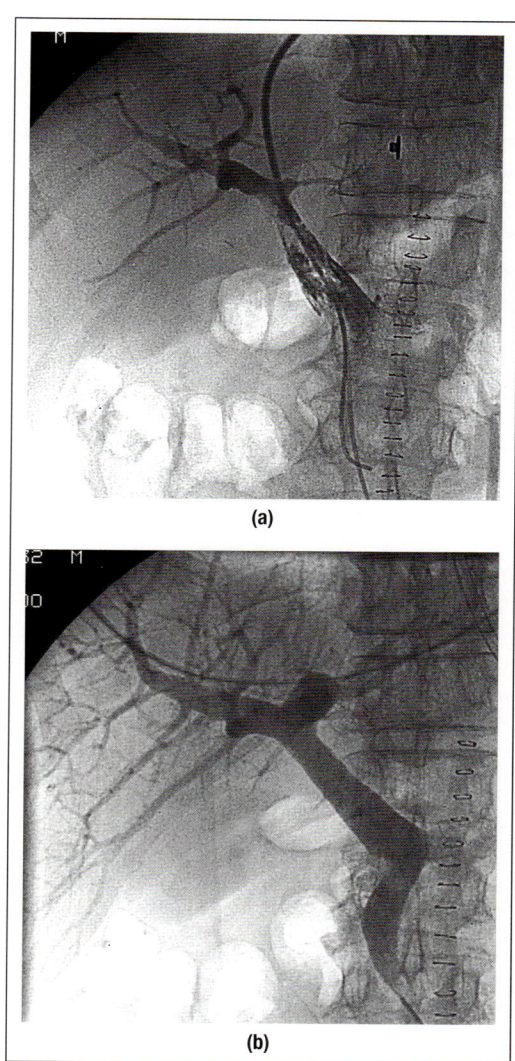

Figure 23.8 Portal vein thrombosis (a) before, and (b) 7 days after ante- and retrograde catheter lysis.

Reprinted with permission from: Kuehn F, Klar E. Vaskuläre Komplikationen im Darmtrakt. *Gastroenterologie Up2date* 2014;10:159–70. doi: 10.1055/s-0034-1377490.

and b represent the course of a portal vein thrombosis before and 7 days after ante- and retrograde catheter lyses. With involvement of the portal vein, endovascular recanalisation is recommended, even in clinically compensated patients and also after an expired time interval of up to 3 to 4 weeks. Thus, life-threatening secondary complications, such as upper gastrointestinal bleeding due to oesophageal or gastric varices, can be avoided in the further course. In case of a septic thrombosis, at first, a systemic intravenous antibiotic treatment has to be administered, since the recanalisation of the portal vein can lead to the release of bacteria within the thrombus in the bloodstream.[1]

CONCLUSIONS

Mesenteric ischaemia represents a vascular emergency, and it must be detected as early as possible. Here, time-saving diagnostics and a consequent treatment are the decisive factors in the prognosis of mesenteric ischaemia. Immediate surgery must be performed for an acute abdomen. Revascularisation of the intestine is the primary aim of treatment, and irreversibly damaged portions of the intestine have to be resected.

REFERENCES

1. Klar E, Rahmanian PB, Bücker A, et al. Acute mesenteric ischemia: a vascular emergency. *Dtsch Arztebl Int* 2012; 109:249–56.

2. Kühn F, Klar E. Vaskuläre Komplikationen im Darmtrakt. *Gastroenterologie Up2date* 2014;10:159–70 (Thieme-Verlag). doi: 10.1055/s-0034-1377490.

3. Dahlke MH, Asshoff L, Popp FC et al. Mesenteric ischemia-outcome after surgical therapy in 83 patients. *Dig Surg* 2008;25:213–9.

4. Schoots IG, Koffeman GI, Legemate DA, et al. Systematic review of survival after acute mesenteric ischaemia according to disease aetiology. *Br J Surg* 2004;91:17–27.

5. Acosta S. Epidemiology of mesenteric vascular disease: clinical implications. *Semin Vasc Surg* 2010;23:4–8.

6. Luther B. *Intestinale Durchblutungsstörungen. Mesenterialinfarkt, Angina abdominalis, Therapieoptionen, Prognosen.* Steinkopff Verlag Darmstadt; 2001.

7. Luther B, Moussazadeh K, Müller BT, et al. Die akute mesenteriale Ischämie – unverstanden oder unheilbar? *Zentralbl Chir* 2002;127:674–84.

8. Kellow ZS, MacInnes M, Kurzencwyg D, et al. The role of abdominal radiography in the evaluation of the nontrauma emergency patient. *Radiology* 2008;248:887–93.

9. Aschoff AJ, Stuber G, Becker BW, et al. Evaluation of acute mesenteric ischemia: accuracy of biphasic mesenteric multi-detector CT angiography. *Abdom Imaging* 2009; 34:345–57.

10. Filsoufi F, Rahmanian PB, Castillo JG, et al. Predictors and outcome of gastrointestinal complications in patients undergoing cardiac surgery. *Ann Surg* 2007;246:323–9.

11. Block T, Nilsson TK, Bjorck M, et al. Diagnostic accuracy of plasma biomarkers for intestinal ischemia. *Scand J Clin Lab Invest* 2008;68:242–8.

12. Markogiannakis H, Memos N, Messaris E, et al. Predictive value of procalcitonin for bowel ischemia and necrosis in bowel obstruction. *Surgery* 2011;149:394–403.

13. Park WM, Cherry KJ Jr, Chua HK, et al. Current results of open revascularization for chronic mesenteric ischemia: a standard for comparison. *J Vasc Surg* 2002;35:853–9.

14. Unalp HR, Atahan K, Kamer E, et al. Prognostic factors for hospital mortality in patients with acute mesenteric ischemia who undergo intestinal resection due to necrosis. *Ulus Travma Acil Cerrahi Derg* 2010;16:63–70.

15. Messing B, Crenn P, Beau P, et al. Long-term survival and parenteral nutrition dependence in adult patients with the short bowel syndrome. *Gastroenterology* 1999;117: 1043–50.

16. Ritz JP, Germer CT, Buhr HJ. Prognostic factors for mesenteric infarction: mutlivariat analysis with regard to patients age. *Ann Vasc Surg* 2005;19:328–34.

17. Schoots IG, Levi MM, Reekers JA, et al. Thrombolytic therapy for acute superior mesenteric artery occlusion. *J Vasc Interv Radiol* 2005;16:317–29.

18. Pisimisis GT, Oderich GS. Technique of hybrid retrograde superior mesenteric artery stent placement for acute-on-chronic mesenteric ischemia. *Ann Vasc Surg* 2011;25:132.e7–1.

19. Björck M, Wanhainen A. Nonocclusive mesenteric hypoperfusion syndromes: recognition and treatment. *Semin Vasc Surg* 2010;23:54–64.

20. Mangi AA, Christison-Lagay ER, Torchiana DF, et al. Gastrointestinal complications in patients undergoing heart operation: an analysis of 8709 consecutive cardiac surgical patients. *Ann Surg* 2005;241:895–901.

21. Benk C, Klemm R, Schaller S et al. Was der Herzchirurg schon immer über die Herz-Lungen-Maschine wissen wollte. *Zeitschrift für Herz-, Thorax- und Gefäßchirurgie* 2008;22:237–44.

22. Acosta S, Ögren M, Sternby N-H, et al. Fatal non-occlusive mesenteric ischaemia: Population-based incidence and risk factors. *J Intern Med* 2006;259:305–13.

23. Harnik IG, Brandt LJ. Mesenteric venous thrombosis. *Vasc Med* 2010;15:407–18.

24. Goykhman Y, Ben-Haim M, Rosen G, et al. Transjugular intrahepatic portosystemic shunt: current indications, patient selection and results. *Isr Med Assoc J* 2010;12:687–91.

25. Sasaki S, Ueda N, Nakano T, et al. Portal and superior mesenteric venous thrombosis treated with thrombolytic therapy via the superior mesenteric artery and vein. *Nippon Shokakibyo Gakkai Zasshi* 2011;108:59–67.

24

Acute Mesenteric Ischaemia in Developing Countries

R. Nagaraja

ABSTRACT

Acute mesenteric ischaemia (AMI) describes a heterogeneous group of disorders primarily involving mesenteric vasculature, resulting in bowel gangrene. Despite advances in diagnosis and treatment, it still remains a very morbid condition with a high mortality. Four main types of AMI are embolism and thrombosis in the superior mesenteric artery, mesenteric venous thrombosis and nonocclusive mesenteric ischaemia. The condition should always be suspected in a patient with severe abdominal pain with no or minimal abdominal signs. A multidetector row computed tomography of the abdomen with angiography is the single most important and specific test to diagnose AMI. In the majority of these patients, in the developing world, emergent resection of the gangrenous bowel may be the only treatment possible as a life-saving measure, after resuscitation. In early stages, before bowel gangrene sets in, intervention using either endovascular or open surgical techniques may be used in patients with arterial occlusion who present early in the disease course. Initial treatment should always be followed by long-term anticoagulation to prevent such catastrophic episodes in the future.

KEYWORDS

Mesenteric ischaemia, intestinal gangrene, thrombosis, embolism

INTRODUCTION

Acute mesenteric ischaemia (AMI) describes a group of disorders involving the mesenteric vasculature, which might result in bowel gangrene, unless the natural history is interfered by an early vascular intervention. It was described by Cokkinis[1] as early as 1930s as a condition in which 'diagnosis is impossible, the prognosis hopeless and the treatment almost useless'. His statement largely holds true to this date, except for slight improvements in diagnosis, treatment and even prognosis. This might probably be considered an abdominal condition that may be equated with myocardial infarction (MI) or stroke with respect to the urgency, in which diagnosis and treatment are required (time is muscle in MI is equivalent to time is bowel in AMI). Along similar lines, AMI may be termed an 'intestinal attack or an intestinal stroke'.

Despite better insights into the pathophysiology of AMI, these syndromes remain highly morbid events, with reported mortality rates exceeding 60%.[2] The reasons are manifold: the aetiology and presentation of AMI vary widely, recognition of the condition is delayed frequently, ischaemia and reperfusion are equally injurious, the resection of large lengths of gangrenous bowel is sometimes incompatible with life and translocation of bacteria results in endotoxaemia and septicaemia. Furthermore, the rarity of AMI (1–2 per 1000 hospital admissions)[3] makes it difficult to undertake randomised or case–control trials. Hence, most of our understanding of the disease process comes from the analysis of observational noncomparative studies.

A secondary clinical entity of mesenteric ischaemia occurs because of mechanical obstruction, such as internal hernia with strangulation, volvulus, intussusception, tumour compression and aortic dissection. For instance, blunt trauma may cause an isolated dissection of the superior mesenteric artery (SMA) and lead to intestinal infarction. These so-called secondary causes require only a one-time treatment for the bowel gangrene and usually do not require vascular intervention or a close postoperative follow-up. For the same reason, nonocclusive mesenteric ischaemia may be managed similarly.

ANATOMY OF MESENTERIC VASCULATURE

The intestines are supplied by branches from the coeliac axis (CA) and the SMA and the inferior mesenteric artery (IMA). The chances of developing intestinal ischaemia are determined by the systemic perfusion pressure, collateral circulation between the mesenteric vessels, the number and calibre of the splanchnic vessels that are affected and the duration of the ischaemic insult. These will be discussed separately.

Collateral Circulation

These provide substantial protection from ischaemia in the setting of a segmental vascular occlusion. The collaterals between circulations are as follows:

- CA and the SMA: Superior and inferior pancreatoduodenal arteries and the arc of Buhler.
- SMA and IMA: Middle and left colic arteries through the marginal artery of Drummond and the arc of Riolan.
- IMA and systemic circulation: Superior and middle rectal vessels.

Mesenteric Pathophysiology

The splanchnic blood flow accounts for 10 to 35% of the cardiac output, depending on the resistance of the mesenteric arterioles. Control mechanisms contributing to mesenteric vascular tone are either intrinsic or extrinsic.

Intrinsic (auto) regulation of mesenteric blood flow occurs in response to sudden decrease in perfusion pressure. The proposed mechanisms for this are direct arteriolar smooth muscle relaxation and a metabolic response to adenosine and other metabolites of mucosal ischaemia.[4]

Extrinsic regulation is via neural and hormonal mechanisms, which include the sympathetic nervous system, the renin–angiotensin axis and vasopressin. These cause mesenteric vasoconstriction and venorelaxation.

The intestine is capable of compensating for up to 75% acute reduction in mesenteric blood flow for nearly 12 hours, without substantial injury, partly by increased oxygen extraction.[5] Collateral circulation between the mesenteric vessels opens up almost immediately.

Acute mesenteric ischaemia arises primarily from the inflow or outflow problems of SMA circulation. The importance of the CA and IMA in AMI lies in the extensive collateral circulation, which may allow sufficient perfusion of the bowel. Because of its highly abundant blood supply, gastric ischaemia is rare. The SMA is anatomically the most susceptible to embolism owing to its large calibre and narrow take-off angle from the aorta. The IMA is seldom the site of lodgement of an embolus owing to its smaller lumen.[6]

Ischaemic damage is caused by both hypoxia and reperfusion injury. After a short period of ischaemia, most of the damage is due to reperfusion injury, whereas after longer periods, the detrimental effects of hypoxia predominate.[7]

The outcomes or, at least, the histological changes due to reperfusion injury of the ischaemic bowel are worse than those due to ischaemia alone.[8] Hypoxic and reperfusion injuries are mediated by arachidonic acid metabolites (prostacyclines, leukotrienes and thromboxane) and oxygen-derived free radicals.[9] The effects of hypoxic/ischaemic damage are local, but the effects of reperfusion injury are systemic, owing to the release of these mediators into the systemic circulation, causing injury to the lungs (adult respiratory distress syndrome), liver, heart and kidney.[10] The poor prognosis of AMI is probably mainly because of the development of the multiple organ failure syndrome.[11]

CLASSIFICATION OF ACUTE MESENTERIC ISCHAEMIA

Broadly, AMI may be classified into occlusive and nonocclusive types. Occlusive ones may be subdivided into arterial and venous obstructions, and arterial obstruction can further be divided into embolic and thrombotic occlusions. The importance of this classification lies in the management and prognostic differences in the four main categories mentioned in Table 24.1.

Mesenteric Arterial Embolism

Embolism to the mesenteric arteries is most commonly from a cardiac source and atheromatous plaques of the aorta. The embolus usually lodges in the SMA distal to the take-off of the middle colic artery but lodges at its origin in 15%.[12]

Mesenteric Arterial Thrombosis

This usually occurs as an acute event superimposed on chronic mesenteric ischaemia due to sudden occlusion

Table 24.1 Classification of acute mesenteric ischaemia

Broad classification
• Occlusive acute mesenteric ischaemia
– Arterial (embolic/thrombotic)
– Venous
• Nonocclusive acute mesenteric ischaemia
Simpler classification
• Mesenteric arterial embolism
• Mesenteric arterial thrombosis
• Mesenteric venous thrombosis
• Nonocclusive mesenteric ischaemia

from thrombosis over an atherosclerotic stenosis. Usually, there is no association between inherited coagulation defects and mesenteric arterial thrombosis (MAT).[13,14] Thrombosis of the mesenteric vessels usually involves the origin of the vessel, and at least two major splanchnic arteries are involved before the clinical manifestations appear, which complicate attempts at revascularisation.[15]

Mesenteric Venous Thrombosis

Most patients with mesenteric venous thrombosis (MVT) have a heritable/acquired prothrombotic disorder,[16–18] the true frequency of which is difficult to estimate, since most studies have included patients with all forms of deep vein thrombosis (DVT). Other important risk factor for this includes abdominal inflammatory conditions, such as diverticulitis and pancreatitis.

Nonocclusive Mesenteric Ischaemia

Nonocclusive mesenteric ischaemia (NOMI) is thought to occur as a result of splanchnic hypoperfusion and vasoconstriction.[19] The usual presentation is an elderly patient admitted to the intensive care unit (ICU) with a life-threatening illness and is being treated with drugs known to reduce intestinal perfusion. Other exacerbating events include sepsis, cardiac arrhythmias and administration of medications such as digoxin and alpha-adrenergic agonists. There are reports of NOMI occurring in patients after cocaine use,[20] after cardiac surgery[21,22] and after dialysis.[23]

The pathogenesis of NOMI is probably related to mesenteric vasospasm, a homoeostatic mechanism that functions to maintain perfusion to vital organs (cardiac and cerebral) at the expense of the splanchnic and peripheral circulations. Vasopressin and angiotensin are probably the neurohormonal mediators of this phenomenon.

There has been a decline in mortality due to NOMI (though still high),[15,24] owing to the widespread use of invasive haemodynamic monitoring in the ICU, prompt correction of hypotension and the use of systemic vasodilators in cardiac failure.

CLINICAL PRESENTATIONS

The median age of patients reported in the literature[2] is approximately 70 years in all aetiological subsets.

AMI can present *precipitously*, with severe abdominal pain and decompensation over hours, or *insidiously*, with symptom progression over days.

AMI due to arterial embolism usually presents with sudden-onset abdominal pain out of proportion to the signs on physical examination, gut emptying at the onset of pain and a cardiac source for embolisation.

The subacute pattern is characterised by a more gradual development of vague abdominal signs and symptoms. These include less-intense and nonspecific abdominal pain accompanied by nausea, vomiting and changes in bowel habits, with a prior history of postprandial pain. The abdomen may become distended but still have active bowel sounds. Patients with MAT and MVT usually present with this subacute form. Patients with MVT may have symptoms for weeks to months (typically 5–14 days) before diagnosis.[12,25]

A personal history of a prior embolic or cardiac event in embolic AMI or a personal or familial history of DVT or pulmonary embolism is seen in about 50% of patients with acute MVT.[26] Patients with acute MAT frequently have antecedent symptoms of chronic mesenteric ischaemia.

In the early phases, signs of peritoneal irritation such as abdominal guarding and rebound tenderness are absent. As the bowel becomes more ischaemic, resulting in full-thickness bowel infarction, obvious peritoneal signs start appearing.

INVESTIGATIONS

The routine laboratory studies are nonspecific. Although abnormal laboratory values may be helpful in accentuating suspicion for AMI, normal values do not exclude the presence of AMI. These tests usually reveal an increase in haematocrit, consistent with haemoconcentration and leucocytosis with a left shift. The renal and liver function tests may become abnormal at the advanced stages. A metabolic acidosis is a common finding, with a persistent base deficit.

A few other laboratory tests have been used to evaluate their use in the early diagnosis of AMI. Elevated levels of serum amylase,[27] lactate[28] and D-dimer[29] have been found in varying proportions in patients with AMI in different studies. Other experimental studies have assessed the utility of elevated levels of serum alpha-glutathione S-transferase[30] and intestinal fatty acid–binding protein in these patients.[31]

Plain abdominal radiography was (not anymore in Europe) the initial investigation in patients presenting with acute abdominal pain but is not diagnostic in these patients for AMI. In advanced stages of ischaemia, pneumatosis of the bowel wall can be detected. Specifically, portal vein gas on abdominal radiography up into the liver portends an extremely poor prognosis.

Intraluminal contrast evaluations of the upper and lower gastrointestinal tracts are contraindicated, because residual contrast can limit visualisation of the mesenteric vasculature during diagnostic angiography, and when used in the presence of bowel perforation, barium causes intense peritonitis.

Duplex ultrasonography may be of some benefit in visualising flow in the SMA and CA. Portal vein gas has also been noted on duplex evaluation. Unfortunately, a significant percentage of patients have dilated, air-filled loops of bowel, which make ultrasonography difficult.

Computed tomography (CT) of the abdomen and pelvis with intravenous contrast is currently, in many countries, the single most important investigation in these patients. It is rapid, noninvasive, and widely available in most hospitals, in addition to providing patient-specific information on vessel occlusion or bowel ischaemia.

Magnetic resonance angiography (MRA) and the new generation of CT angiography, known as multidetector row CT (MDCT), have a high degree of accuracy for diagnosing occlusive and nonocclusive AMIs, with an accuracy of upto 96%.[32]

Early evaluations of the role of CT in mesenteric ischaemia revealed low sensitivity of 64%.[33] The development of MDCT has greatly improved this figure to more than 90%.[32,34] A diagnosis of mesenteric ischaemia is suspected by finding bowel wall thickening, mucosal nonenhancement, intramural air, dilatation, portal venous gas and pneumatosis intestinalis.[35–37] Kirkpatrick et al[34] suggested using CT angiography findings of portal venous gas, pneumatosis or a combination of bowel wall thickening with venous thrombosis, solid organ infarction, or focal lack of enhancement of bowel wall, as criteria for the diagnosis of mesenteric ischaemia, provided sensitivity and specificity rates of 96% and 94%, respectively. The presence of pneumatosis on CT does not necessarily indicate that transmural infarction has occurred but is more likely in patients with pneumatosis and portomesenteric venous gas.[38]

Mesenteric angiography remains the definitive diagnostic study. Early and liberal use of angiography has been the major factor for decreasing the mortality in these patients over the past three decades.[15] Selective cannulation of the origins of the CA and SMA may be required to completely define the anatomy and pathophysiology. Both anteroposterior (for origins of the SMA and CA) and lateral views (distal parts) are needed for adequate visualisation of the mesenteric vasculature. Angiography is relatively less sensitive for superior mesenteric vein thrombosis.[39] Invasive angiography carries the advantage of treating the disease in patients with arterial occlusions, particularly in those presenting early (Figures 24.1 and 24.2).

TREATMENT

The overall treatment in these patients may be divided into general/systemic and specific/local (Table 24.2; Algorithms 24.1 and 24.2).

The initial treatment of patients diagnosed with AMI is systemic and includes volume resuscitation; maintenance of haemodynamics; correction of acidosis, if necessary; and administration of appropriate antibiotics. Anticoagulation with heparin should be started immediately to prevent further propagation of the occlusion. Continuous

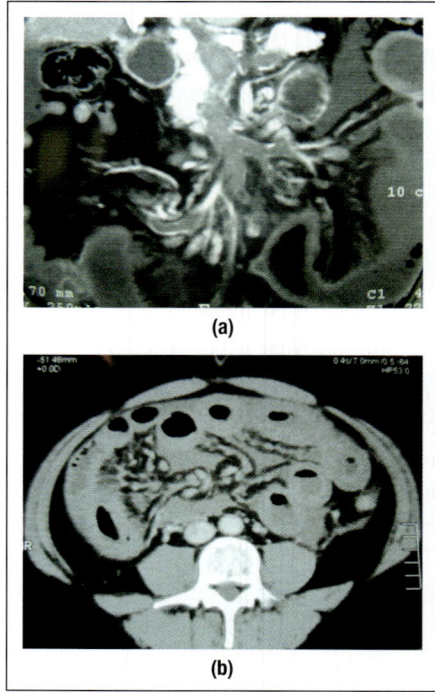

(a)

(b)

Figure 24.1 Computed tomography scan of (a) the abdomen showing extensive portal vein thrombosis (coronal section), and (b) diffuse small bowel wall thickening (axial section).

Courtesy: Raghavendra Nagaraja.

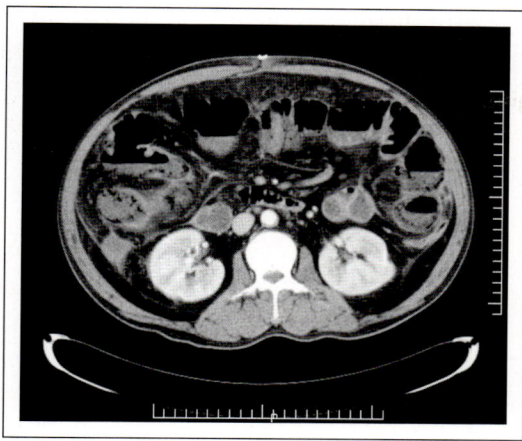

Figure 24.2 Computed tomography scan of the abdomen (axial section) showing pneumatosis involving the small bowel and right colon despite a patent superior mesenteric artery (SMA) (after SMA catheter thrombolysis and gangrenous bowel resection), probably due to continued vasospasm.

Courtesy: Raghavendra Nagaraja.

haemodynamic monitoring with invasive lines and intake/output monitoring are essential in patients who are sick at presentation.

The specific local treatment may be further subdivided into those affecting the vascular and bowel changes. In patients presenting late or in those having MVT or limited-length bowel gangrene, bowel treatment is most important. However, in patients presenting early, without peritoneal signs on examination, emergent vascular treatment alone may be sufficient. Unfortunately, the proportion of these early interventions in patients is very less.

The vascular intervention may range from clot aspiration, catheter thrombolysis and angioplasty to stent placement, depending on the disease extent and local expertise available.

Open vascular surgery may be planned if the endovascular option is not available or as per institutional policies. Open surgical procedures may include reimplantation in ostial occlusions; thrombectomy or endarterectomy in short-length and long-segment occlusions where an autogenous vein graft is not available and prosthesis cannot be used; vascular bypass in uncontaminated field, with a good distal runoff; and retrograde mesenteric stenting.

Although a decade-old systematic review[2] has not shown a significant benefit of revascularisation (open or endovascular) in arterial AMI, recent studies have revealed significant improvement in morbidity and mortality, with a reduction in bowel resection rates.[40–42]

Surgery should not be delayed in patients with peritoneal signs and those suspected of having intestinal

Table 24.2 Treatment of acute mesenteric ischaemia

- General/systemic
  - Volume resuscitation
  - Broad-spectrum antibiotics
  - Anticoagulation
  - Maintenance of haemodynamics, with monitoring
- Specific/local
  - Bowel
  - Vascular

infarction or perforation based on clinical, radiographical or laboratory parameters. The benefit of early (<12 hours of the suspected event) and liberal use of angiography has been shown to decrease mortality rates.[15]

Preserving each centimetre of viable bowel is of utmost importance in patients with extensive small bowel gangrene requiring extensive resection. Aggressive revascularisation (open/endovascular) and liberal use of second-look laparotomy to inspect bowel viability in doubtful cases, rather than aggressive resection at the first operation, are the strategies that have been found to improve outcomes.[43] One does not need to decide on the restoration of bowel continuity in the first surgery; closed ends may be left inside for inspection during the second look on the next day, in order to decide on anastomosis or creation of stoma.

Mesenteric Arterial Embolism

After the initial resuscitation and diagnosis, the next important step is to identify the source of the embolus and prevent further episodes. The heart, the most common source, needs to be evaluated for arrhythmia, vegetations, valvular disease and mural thrombus, and appropriate actions should be taken at the earliest.

The traditional treatment of mesenteric arterial embolism (MAE) is early surgical embolectomy. This is done by an arteriotomy distal to the embolus and then advancing a balloon-tipped embolectomy catheter proximally. Subsequently, SMA is palpated for pulsation and the frankly gangrenous bowel is resected. Intraoperative duplex ultrasonography and fluorescein angiography help decision making in identifying persistently ischaemic segments.[44] Postoperatively, papaverine is administered to attenuate vasospasm. A second-look laparotomy in the next 24 to 48 hours may be necessary to resect additional ischaemic or gangrenous bowel.

With the development of interventional techniques, radiological interventions have become the initial procedure in these patients. Clot aspiration and/or

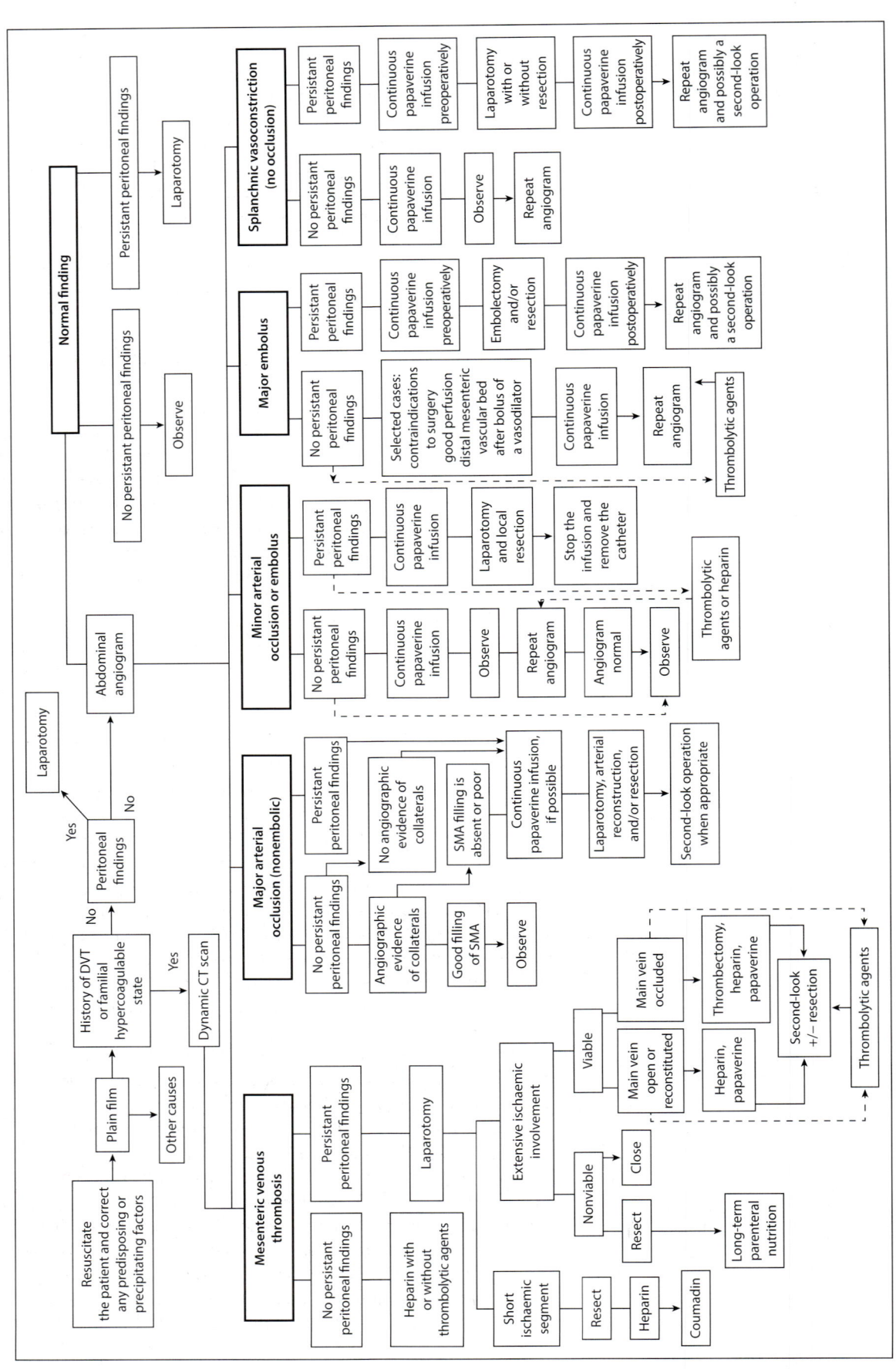

Algorithm 24.1 Diagnosis and treatment of intestinal ischaemia. Solid lines indicate accepted management plan; dashed lines indicate alternate management plan.

Abbreviations: CT, computed tomography; DVT, deep vein thrombosis; SMA, superior mesenteric artery.

Adapted from: American Gastroenterological Association medical position statement: Guidelines on intestinal ischemia. *Gastroenterology* 2000;118:951–3.

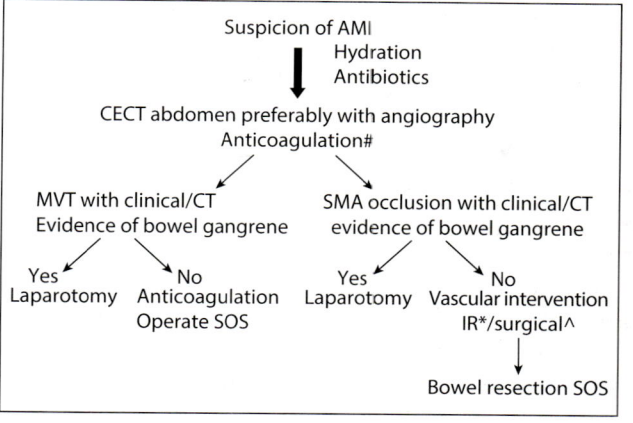

Algorithm 24.2 Simpler protocol for managing patients with acute mesenteric ischaemia.

#Anticoagulation: Unfractionated heparin 80–90 units/Kg loading dose with 15 units/Kg infusion along with 6 hourly aPTT monitoring. This may be changed to therapeutic dose of low-molecular-weight heparin after the initial phase; however, many prefer to use it from the beginning.

*IR: Interventional radiology procedures, usually involving SMA catheter placement, clot aspiration, thrombolytic and vasodilator infusion (the protocols differ; we use streptokinase 2 lakhs units stat with 50,000 units/h infusion for 6 hours and check angio after 24 hours along with papaverine 60 mg stat and 30 mg/h infusion for 24 hours), angioplasty and stenting.

^Surgical: Thrombectomy/endarterectomy/bypass/reimplantation.

Abbreviations: AMI, acute mesenteric ischaemia; CECT, contrast-enhanced computed tomography; CT, computed tomography; IR, interventional radiology; MVT, mesenteric venous thrombosis; SMA, superior mesenteric artery.

catheter-directed thrombolysis have been used, with high success rates, and have reduced the mortality rates.[45–48] It is to be considered in patients who undergo angiography within 8 hours of the onset of abdominal pain and who do not have clinical evidence of bowel infarction or other contraindications to thrombolytic therapy. A detailed review of thrombolytic therapy has reported a success rate and 30-day survival of 90%.[49] Concomitant infusion of papaverine has been advocated.[12] Surgery is indicated in patients who do not demonstrate clot lysis within 4 hours or those who develop peritoneal signs. Long-term management is aimed at the prevention of future embolic events, typically with the use of oral anticoagulants.[50]

Mesenteric Arterial Thrombosis

Treatment of acute MAT is principally surgical. Thrombectomy alone is unlikely to offer a satisfactory solution because of diffuse atherosclerotic disease. Hence, various revascularisation techniques, along with thrombectomy, and resection of non-viable segments are advocated. Mesenteric artery reconstruction is associated with good long-term patency rates and symptom-free survival (79% and 77%, respectively) but has a high perioperative mortality rate of 52%.[51] Prolonged surgery in such sick patients, though might appear preferable, may not be feasible. Successful endovascular approaches with stenting have been reported.[52–54] After recovery, antiplatelet agents such as aspirin may reduce the risk of recurrent mesenteric ischaemia (Figures 24.3–24.5).[50]

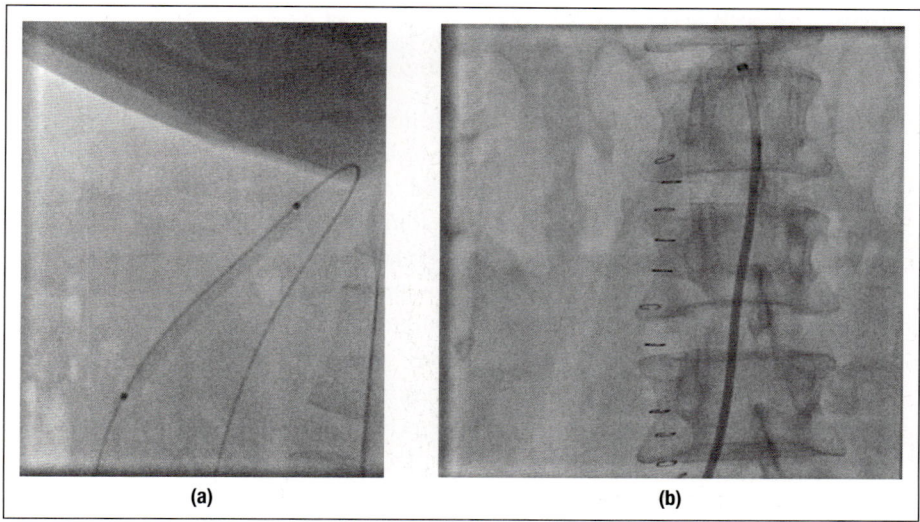

Figure 24.3 Digital subtraction angiography showing (a) balloon angioplasty (left, left anterior oblique view), and (b) stenting of the superior mesenteric artery (right, anteroposterior view).

Courtesy: Raghavendra Nagaraja.

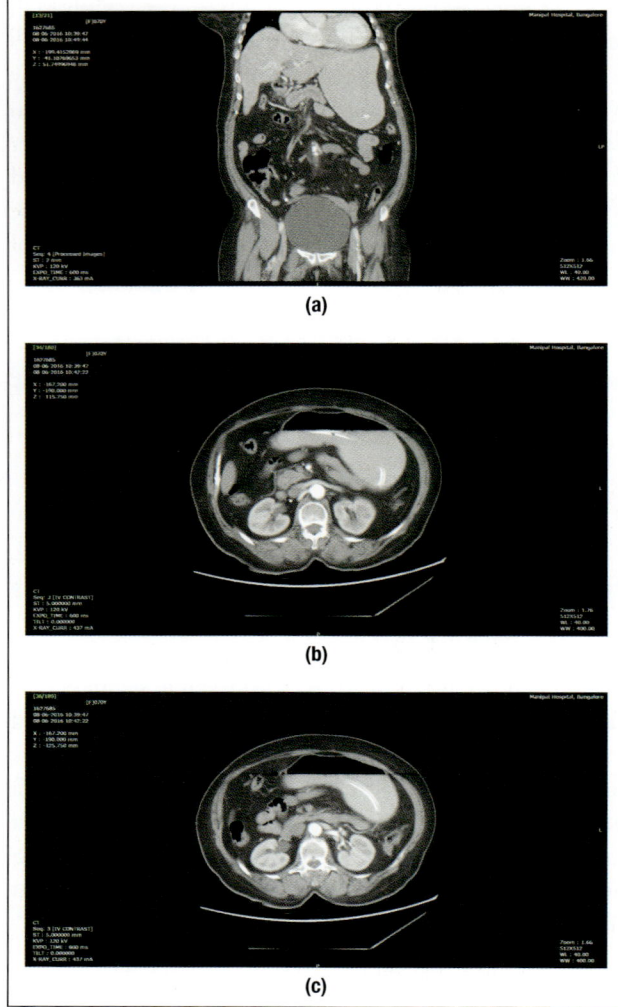

Figure 24.4 Computed tomography scan of the abdomen demonstrating (a) superior mesenteric artery (SMA) block beyond origin in coronal view, (b) patent SMA origin in an axial view, and (c) blocked SMA distally.

Courtesy: Raghavendra Nagaraja.

Mesenteric Venous Thrombosis

Treatment of acute MVT includes anticoagulation and resection of the infarcted bowel.[55] Patients who do not have peritoneal signs can be observed closely, whereas other patients should proceed directly to laparotomy. Administration of papaverine into the SMA during angiography is advocated because of concomitant arterial spasm. Prevention of recurrent venous thrombosis with warfarin is indicated for at least 6 months; however, a longer duration may be required if a thrombophilic state has been identified.[56,57] Successful venous thrombolysis has been reported in a small number of patients.[6,47,58]

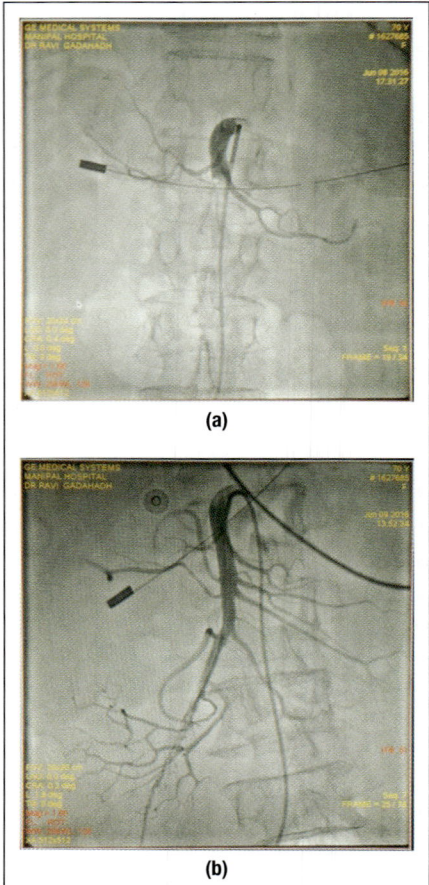

Figure 24.5 Digital subtraction angiography demonstrating superior mesenteric artery (SMA) angiography of the patient in Figure 24.4 (a) before (left, blocked SMA), and (b) after (right, recanalised SMA) catheter thrombolysis.

Courtesy: Raghavendra Nagaraja.

Nonocclusive Mesenteric Ischaemia

Primary therapy for these patients involves papaverine infusion through an angiographic catheter into SMA and an attempt to reverse the underlying condition, leading to splanchnic vasoconstriction. Some surgeons also advocate the concomitant use of intravenous heparin to prevent thrombosis in the cannulated vessel.[12] Surgical exploration should be emergent in patients with peritoneal signs. Postoperative papaverine infusion is also indicated. In patients who did require segmental bowel resection, a delay in completing the intestinal anastomosis and aggressive reexploration may improve survival.[59]

Overall, the treatment depends on the type of AMI, duration and severity of illness; extent of bowel gangrene; the socioeconomic/financial status of the patient and the medical facilities available. Arterial occlusion presenting early to a tertiary care hospital may be managed with an emergent vascular intervention, which may be accompanied/followed by bowel resection. The same patient presenting late to a secondary or tertiary care centre may be managed by an early bowel treatment with/without vascular treatment, depending on local facilities. In countries like India, where patients would have to bear their medical expenses, those from poor socioeconomic status with extensive gangrene requiring massive small bowel resection that results in short bowel would definitely go on to require home parenteral nutrition or subsequent small bowel transplantation. In such patients, surgical treatment may be curtailed/avoided.

FOLLOW-UP AND FURTHER TREATMENT

The need of subsequent follow-up and treatment depends predominantly on the extent of bowel resected and the type of AMI. The initial treatment in all these patients should include anticoagulation. The parenteral anticoagulation used perioperatively should be changed to oral before discharge. The small therapeutic range of these medications means that they will require close follow-up and monitoring, at least in the initial few weeks. Patients with short bowel with or without a stoma, manifesting the short bowel syndrome, would require antisecretory (proton-pump inhibitors and octreotide) and antimotility drugs (loperamide and codeine). The problem is obviously more difficult when the patient has a stoma, and at times, this may be a very complicated clinical scenario. The nutritional support is the next most important step in the management of these patients once they recover. The quality and quantity of stoma output, urine output, weight gain/loss and serum albumin levels are the simple parameters that would give an idea on the requirements and extent of the need of parenteral nutrition. The costs of long-term parenteral nutrition, risks of infection with recurrent hospital admission and the need of subsequent small bowel transplantation (when required) make it an expensive and unaffordable treatment option for the weaker sections of our society.

PROGNOSIS

Despite significant improvements in critical care, diagnosis and technology, AMI remains a disease that is accompanied with high morbidity and mortality. The prognosis still depends on the type of AMI (MVT having better prognosis), duration of illness, comorbid conditions, presence of organ failure at presentation, need of surgery and bowel resection and the extent of the bowel resection.[43,60–62]

IS THERE ANY DIFFERENCE IN THE PATTERN OF ACUTE MESENTERIC ISCHAEMIA IN WESTERN COUNTRIES AND INDIA?

An Indian study[60] has found MVT to be more common in patients who are at least a decade younger than those in their western counterparts and the mortality rates are slightly lower, probably because of younger patients, with less comorbidities associated with MVT.

WHAT IS THE IMPORTANCE OF CLASSIFYING ACUTE MESENTERIC ISCHAEMIA INTO DIFFERENT TYPES?

Classification is important for both management and prognosis. Embolic AMI should be investigated to look for the source of embolism, in order to tackle it at the earliest, whereas thrombotic occlusion should be investigated to decide the intervention (angioplasty/endarterectomy/bypass). Venous occlusion in early stages may be managed by only anticoagulation; surgery is required when gangrene is present. Prognostically, MVT is much better than arterial occlusions and NOMI. Long-term anticoagulation is required in patients with MVT and a few with embolic AMI.

SHOULD ALL PATIENTS WITH ACUTE MESENTERIC ISCHAEMIA BE INTERVENED/OPERATED?

Patients with MVT who present very early without peritoneal signs or evidence of bowel gangrene on imaging are probably rare exceptions and may be managed with anticoagulation alone. Even in patients without peritoneal signs, a diagnostic laparoscopy might be indicated and is not harmful. Arterial occlusions does require immediate vascular and/or bowel intervention.

The systematic review by Schoots et al[2] revealed the beneficial effect of surgery (bowel resection) on the outcome of all patients with AMI, irrespective of aetiology, with mortality rates decreasing by 22 to 55%; the maximum benefit was seen in patients with MVT and least was seen in those with MAT.

SHOULD ALL PATIENTS WITH ACUTE MESENTERIC ISCHAEMIA UNDERGO VASCULAR INTERVENTION?

A relatively old systematic review[2] demonstrated that revascularisation did not result in a significant improvement in outcome, except in patients with MVT, in which mortality decreased by 50%, but the number of such patients was small. The probable explanation was that ischaemia-reperfusion injury is more injurious than ischaemic injury. However, vascular intervention seems logical, as the disease is primarily related to the blood vessels. The recent literature is flooded with studies focussing specifically on vascular interventions in these patients (both endovascular and surgical), and some of them have found decreased mortality rates to under 30%.[40–43,45–49] Most of these studies are observational, retrospective and noncomparative.

SHOULD ALL PATIENTS WITH ACUTE MESENTERIC ISCHAEMIA UNDERGO THROMBOPHILIA EVALUATION?

Inherited hypercoagulable state is present in up to 75% of patients with MVT[16–8] and is more likely to be present in patients with isolated MVT than in those with simultaneous portal and splenic vein thrombus.[63] The Factor V Leiden (FVL) mutation is the most common cause in the current literature and was reported in 20 to 40% of cases.[14] Resistance to activated protein C also occurs from other mutations in about 10% of patients.[64,65] Prothrombin (PT) mutation, with higher plasma PT levels, is present in 8% of individuals with venous thrombosis and in 2% of healthy controls.[66] In addition to these, deficiencies of naturally occurring anticoagulant proteins, protein S, protein C and antithrombin (AT) III are the causes in about 8 to 10% of patients, whereas antiphospholipid antibodies are present in approximately 4% of patients.[13,14,64]

Usual recommendation for the evaluation of thrombophilia is to postpone laboratory testing for at least 3 months after acute thrombotic episode and for at least 2 weeks after discontinuation of oral anticoagulant therapy.[67,68] Some studies have shown that screening for thrombophilia in the acute phase after thrombosis, before anticoagulation treatment, can be used to disprove deficiencies of proteins C and S.[69] Patients may falsely be diagnosed as deficient in these proteins in the acute phase; hence, retest after termination of anticoagulation treatment is beneficial. Limited information is available on the potential problem of thrombophilia screening in the acute phase of DVT.[70]

The narrow therapeutic interval of anticoagulants and high risk of rethrombosis and bleeding, when out of this therapeutic range, underlies the importance of individualised risk stratification to justify prolonged treatment regimes.[71] Indefinite prophylaxis with anticoagulants is indicated in the high-risk groups (>1 spontaneous thrombosis, single life-threatening event, 1 thrombosis in the presence of >1 defect). Short-term prophylaxis may be useful in the moderate-risk group in the high-risk situations (asymptomatic individuals, 1 thrombosis in response to a prothrombotic stimulus).[72,73]

Acute mesenteric ischaemia, being a life-threatening event, merits the long-term anticoagulation, irrespective of the presence of procoagulant factors. This, along with the need to stop anticoagulation for 2 weeks for thrombophilia testing and the inaccuracy of these tests during an acute episode, creates more confusion on the usefulness of these tests in AMI.

IS THERE A DIFFERENCE IN THE PRESENTATION, TREATMENT AND PROGNOSIS OF PATIENTS WITH ARTERIAL AND VENOUS DISEASES?

Patients with MVT are at least a decade younger, have a longer duration of symptoms, lesser extent of bowel gangrene or shorter length of bowel resected and infrequent involvement of the colon.[60,63]

CONCLUSIONS

Acute mesenteric ischaemia is still a very morbid condition with a high mortality, despite technological advances in diagnosis and treatment.

Four main types of AMI are SMA embolism, SMA thrombosis, MVT and nonocclusive mesenteric ischaemia.

Multidetector row CT of the abdomen with angiography is the single most important and specific test to diagnose AMI.

The condition should preferably be treated in a dedicated, multidisciplinary 'intestinal stroke' centre.

Emergent resection of the gangrenous bowel is the most important and may be the only treatment possible as a life-saving measure, after resuscitation in the majority of these patients, particularly in those presenting late to a secondary care centre.

Vascular intervention, either endovascular or open surgical, must be employed in patients presenting early.

Second-look operations should be used liberally, and small bowel length should be saved as much as possible.

Follow-up treatment to reduce chances of further episodes of occlusion, either in the abdomen or elsewhere, is as important as the initial intervention.

REFERENCES

1. Cokkinis AJ. *Mesenteric Vascular Occlusion*. Bailliere, Tindall and Cox: London; 1926. pp. 1–93.
2. Schoots IG, Koffeman GI, LegemateDA, LeviM, van GulikT M. Systematic review of survival after acute mesenteric ischaemia according to disease aetiology. *Br J Surg* 2003;91:17–27.

3. Stoney RJ, Cunningham CG. Acute mesenteric ischemia. *Surgery* 1993;114:489–90.

4. Rosenblum JD, Boyle CM, Schwartz LB. The mesenteric circulation. Anatomy and physiology. *Surg Clin North Am* 1997;77:289–306.

5. Boley SJ, Frieber W, Winslow PR, et al. Circulatory responses to acute reduction of superior mesenteric arterial flow. *Physiologist* 1969;12:180.

6. Cappell MS. Intestinal (mesenteric) vasculopathy. I. Acute superior mesenteric arteriopathy and venopathy. *Gastroenterol Clin North Am* 1998;27:783.

7. Zimmerman BJ, Granger DN. Reperfusion injury. *Surg Clin North Am* 1992;72:65.

8. Parks DA, Granger DN. Contributions of ischemia and reperfusion to mucosal lesion formation. *Am J Physiol* 1982;250:G749–53.

9. Zimmerman BJ, Grisham MB, Granger DN. Mechanism of oxidant-mediated microvascular injury following reperfusion of the ischemic intestine. *Basic Life Sci* 1986;49:881–6.

10. Oldham KT, Guice KS, Turnage RH, et al. The systemic consequences of intestinal ischemia/reperfusion injury. *J Vasc Surg* 1993;93:136–7.

11. YasuharaH. Acute mesenteric ischemia: the challenge of gastroenterology. *Surg Today* 2005;35:185–95.

12. McKinsey JF, Gewertz BL. Acute mesenteric ischemia. *Surg Clin N Am* 1997;77:307–18.

13. Martinelli I, Mannucci PM, De Stefano V, et al. Different risks of thrombosis in four coagulation defects associated with inherited thrombophilia: a study of 150 families. *Blood* 1998;92:2353–8.

14. Thomas DP, Roberts HR. Hypercoagulability in venous and arterial thrombosis. *Ann Intern Med* 1997;126:638–44.

15. Boley SJ, Brandt LJ, Sammartano RJ. History of mesenteric ischemia. The evolution of a diagnosis and management. *Surg Clin North Am* 1997;77:275–88.

16. Acosta S, Alhadad A, Svensson P, Ekberg O. Epidemiology, risk and prognostic factors in mesenteric venous thrombosis. *Br J Surg* 2008; 95:1245–51.

17. Rhee RY, Gloviczki P. Mesenteric venous thrombosis. *Surg Clin North Am* 1997;77:327–38.

18. Amitrano L, Brancaccio V, Guardascione MA, et al. High prevalence of thrombophilic genotypes in patients with acute mesenteric vein thrombosis. *Am J Gastroenterol* 2001;96:146–9.

19. Wilcox MG, Howard TJ, Plaskon LA, et al. Current theories of pathogenesis and treatment of nonocclusive mesenteric ischemia. *Dig Dis Sci* 1995;40:709–16.

20. Endress C, Gray DG, Wollschlaeger G. Bowel ischemia and perforation after cocaine use. *AJR Am J Roentgenol* 1992;159:73–5.

21. Gennaro M, Ascer E, Matano R, et al. Acute mesenteric ischemia after cardiopulmonary bypass. *Am J Surg* 1993; 166:231–6.

22. Garofalo M, Borioni R, Nardi P, et al. Early diagnosis of acute mesenteric ischemia after cardiopulmonary bypass. *J Cardiovasc Surg (Torino)* 2002; 43:455–9.

23. Diamond SM, Emmett M, Henrich WL. Bowel infarction as a cause of death in dialysis patients. *JAMA* 1986;256:2545–7.

24. Deehan DJ, Heys SD, Brittenden J, Eremin O. Mesenteric ischaemia: prognostic factors and influence of delay upon outcome. *J R Coll Surg Edinburgh* 1995;40:112–5.

25. Font VE, Hermann RE, Longworth DL. Chronic mesenteric venous thrombosis: difficult diagnosis and therapy. *Cleve Clin J Med* 1989;56:823–8.

26. Harward TR, Green D, Bergan JJ, et al. Mesenteric venous thrombosis. *J Vasc Surg* 1989;9:328–33.

27. Wilson C, Imrie CW. Amylase and gut infarction. *Br J Surg* 1986;73:219–21.

28. Lange H, Jäckel R. Usefulness of plasma lactate concentration in the diagnosis of acute abdominal disease. *Eur J Surg* 1994;160:381–4.

29. Block T, Nilsson TK, Björck M, Acosta S. Diagnostic accuracy of plasma biomarkers for intestinal ischaemia. *Scand J Clin Lab Invest* 2008; 68:242–8.

30. Gearhart SL, Delaney CP, Senagore AJ, et al. Prospective assessment of the predictive value of alpha glutathione S-transferase for intestinal ischemia. *Am Surg* 2003;69:324–9.

31. Kanda T, Fujii H, Tani T, et al. Intestinal fatty acid-binding protein is a useful diagnostic marker for mesenteric infarction in humans. *Gastroenterology* 1996;110:339–43.

32. Ofer A, Abadi S, Nitecki S, et al. Multidetector CT angiography in the evaluation of acute mesenteric ischemia. *Eur Radiol* 2009;19:24.

33. Taourel PG, Deneuville M, Pradel JA, et al. Acute mesenteric ischemia: diagnosis with contrast-enhanced CT. *Radiology* 1996;199:632–6.

34. Kirkpatrick D, Kroeker MA, Greenberg HM. Biphasic CT with mesenteric CT angiography in the evaluation of acute mesenteric ischemia: initial experience. *Radiology* 2003;229:91–8.

35. Horton KM, Fishman EK. Multi-detector row CT of mesenteric ischemia: can it be done? *Radiographics* 2001;21:1463–73.

36. Chou CK, Mak CW, Tzeng WS, et al. CT of small bowel ischemia. *Abdom Imaging* 2004;29:18–22.

37. Zandrino F, Musante F, Gallesio I, et al. Assessment of patients with acute mesenteric ischemia: multi-slice computed tomography signs and clinical performance in a group of patients with surgical correlation. *Minerva Gastroenterol Dietol* 2006;52:317–25.

38. Kernagis LY, Levine MS, Jacobs JE. Pneumatosis intestinalis in patients with ischemia: correlation of CT findings with viability of the bowel. *AJR Am J Roentgenol* 2003;180:733–6.

39. Bakal CW, Sprayregen S, Wolf EL. Radiology in intestinal ischemia. Angiographic diagnosis and management. *Surg Clin North Am* 1992;72:125–41.

40. Roussel A, Castier Y, Nuzzo A, et al. Revascularization of acute mesenteric ischemia after creation of a dedicated multidisciplinary center. *J Vasc Surg* 2015;62:1251–6.

41. Raupach J, Lojik M, Chovanec V, et al. Endovascular management of acute embolic occlusion of the superior mesenteric artery: a 12-year single center experience. *Cardiovasc Intervent Radiol* 2016;39:195–203.

42. Karkkainen JM, Lehtimaki TT, Saari P, et al. Endovascular therapy as a primary revascularization modality in acute mesenteric ischemia. *Cardiovasc Intervent Radiol* 2015;38: 1119–29.

43. Park WM, Gloviczki P, Cherry KJ (Jr), et al. Contemporary management of acute mesenteric ischaemia: factors associated with survival. *J Vasc Surg* 2002;35:445–52.

44. Reinus JF, Brandt LJ, Boley SJ. Ischemic diseases of the bowel. *Gastroenterol Clin North Am* 1990;19:319–43.

45. Puippe GD, Suesstrunk J, Nocito A, Pfiffner R, Glenck M, Pfammatter T. Outcome of Endovascular revascularisation in patients with acute obstructive mesenteric ischaemia—a single centre experience. *VASA* 2015;44:363–70.

46. McBride KD, Gaines PA. Thrombolysis of a partially occluding superior mesenteric Artery thromboembolus by infusion of streptokinase. *Cardiovasc Intervent Radiol* 1994; 17:164–6.

47. Rivitz SM, Geller SC, Hahn C, Waltman AC. Treatment of acute mesenteric venous thrombosis with transjugular intramesentericurokinase infusion. *J Vasc Intervent Radiol* 1995;6:219–23.

48. Simó G, Echenagusia AJ, Camúñez F, et al. Superior mesenteric arterial embolism: local fibrinolytic treatment with urokinase. *Radiology* 1997;204:775–9.

49. Schoots IG, Levi MM, Reekers JA, et al. Thrombolytic therapy for acute superior mesenteric artery occlusion. *J Vasc Interv Radiol* 2005;16:317–29.

50. Klempnauer J, Grothues F, Bektas H, Pichlmayr R. Long-term results after surgery for acute mesenteric ischemia. *Surgery* 1997;121:239–43.

51. Cho JS, Carr JA, Jacobsen G, et al. Long-term outcome after mesenteric artery reconstruction: a 37-year experience. *J Vasc Surg* 2002;35:453–60.

52. Demirpolat G, Oran I, Tamsel S, et al. Acute mesenteric ischemia: endovascular therapy. *Abdom Imaging* 2007; 32: 299–303.

53. Wyers MC, Powell RJ, Nolan BW, Cronenwett JL. Retrograde mesenteric stenting during laparotomy for acute occlusive mesenteric ischemia. *J Vasc Surg* 2007;45: 269–75.

54. Yoon YW, Choi D, Cho SY, Lee DY. Successful treatment of isolated spontaneous superior mesenteric artery dissection with stent placement. *Cardiovasc Intervent Radiol* 2003; 26: 475–8.

55. Kumar S, Sarr MG, Kamath PS. Mesenteric venous thrombosis. *N Engl J Med* 2001;345:1683–8.

56. Petitti DB, Strom BL, Melmon KL. Duration of warfarin anticoagulant therapy and the probabilities of recurrent thromboembolism and hemorrhage. *Am J Med* 1986; 81: 255–9.

57. Abdu RA, Zakhour BJ, Dallis DJ. Mesenteric venous thrombosis—1911 to 1984. *Surgery* 1987;101:383–8.

58. Poplausky MR, Kaufman JA, Geller SC, Waltman AC. Mesenteric venous thrombosis treated with urokinase via the superior mesenteric artery. *Gastroenterology* 1996;110: 1633–5.

59. Ward D, Vernava AM, Kaminski DL, et al. Improved outcome by identification of high-risk nonocclusive mesenteric ischemia, aggressive re-exploration, and delayed anastomosis. *Am J Surg* 1995;170:577–81.

60. Nagaraja R, Rao P, Kumaran V, et al. Acute mesenteric ischaemia—an Indian perspective. *Indian J Surg* 2015; 77:843–9. doi: 10.1007/s12262-014-1034-5.

61. Kougias P, Lau D, El Sayed HF, et al. Determinants of mortality and treatment outcome following surgical interventions for acute mesenteric ischemia. *J Vasc Surg* 2007; 46:467–74.

62. Gupta PK, Natarajan B, Gupta H, et al. Morbidity and mortality after bowel resection for acute mesenteric ischemia. *Surgery* 2011;150:779–87.

63. Kumar S, Kamath PS. Acute superior mesenteric venous thrombosis: one disease or two? *Am J Gastroenterol* 2003; 98:1299–304.

64. Provan D, O'Shaughnessy DF. Recent advances in haematology. *BMJ* 1999; 318:991–4.

65. de Visser MC, Rosendaal FR, Bertina RM. A reduced sensitivity for activated protein C in the absence of factor V Leiden increases the risk of venous thrombosis. *Blood* 1999; 93:1271–6.

66. Margaglione M, Brancaccio V, Giuliani N, et al. Increased risk for venous thrombosis in carriers of the prothrombin G—>A20210 gene variant. *Ann Intern Med* 1998; 129:89–93.

67. Tripodi A, Mannucci PM. Laboratory investigation of thrombophilia. *Clin Chem* 2001;47:1597–606.

68. Tripodi A. Issues concerning the laboratory investigation of inherited thrombophilia. *Mol Diagn* 2005;9:181–6.

69. Munster AMB, Sidelmann JJ, Gram J. Thrombophilia screening in the acute phase of deep venous thrombosis. *Scand J Clin Lab Invest* 2009;69:633–5.

70. Kovacs MJ, Kovacs J, Anderson J, et al. Protein C and protein S levels can be accurately determined within 24 hours of diagnosis of acute venous thromboembolism. *Clin Lab Haematol* 2006;28:9–13.

71. Ansell J, Hirsh J, Poller L, Bussey H, et al. The pharmacology and management of the vitamin K antagonists: the Seventh ACCP Conference on Antithrombotic and Thrombolytic Therapy. *Chest* 2004;126:204S–33S.

72. Bauer KA. Management of patients with hereditary defects predisposing to thrombosis including pregnant women. *Thromb Haemost* 1995;74:94–100.

73. Bauer K. Hypercoagulable states. In: Hoffman R, Benz EJ, Shattil SJ, Furie B, Cohen HJ, editors. *Hematology: Basic Principles and Practice.* 2nd ed. Churchill Livingstone; 1991.

Liver, Gallbladder and Bile Ducts

25

Liver Failure

G. Györi, M. Lesurtel and P.-A. Clavien

ABSTRACT

Despite the development in surgical technique and perioperative care, posthepatectomy liver failure (PHLF) is still observed in up to 9% of patients after liver resection and is associated with up to 75% of mortality. Current strategies aim at improving the assessment of liver function and accurately predicting future liver remnant size, as well as augmenting growth after resection. Until today, the treatment of PHLF is limited to symptomatic support. Besides the established goal-directed approach to enhance circulatory, ventilatory and renal functions in PHLF, recent developments showed promising preclinical data for functional therapy. This chapter focusses on the pre- and postoperative aspects of the management of liver failure after extensive liver surgery.

KEYWORDS

Posthepatectomy liver failure, PHLF, liver resection, future liver remnant, FLR, liver regeneration

INTRODUCTION

Liver resection for primary or nonprimary liver tumours has become routine practice and is mostly inevitable for a curative treatment.[1] Extensive resection is possible owing to the liver's unique ability to regenerate and restore its function even after removal of a substantial part of the organ. Nevertheless, posthepatectomy liver failure (PHLF) is seen in up to 9% of patients and remains the main cause of postoperative mortality.[2,3]

Insufficient function of the future liver remnant (FLR) plays a major role in the aetiology of PHLF and is expressed by decreased secretory, synthetic and detoxifying capacities, manifesting in the triad of hyperbilirubinaemia, coagulopathy and hepatic encephalopathy.[4]

COMMON DEFINITIONS OF POSTHEPATECTOMY LIVER FAILURE

The 50–50 criteria predict a 59% risk of perioperative mortality in patients with bilirubin levels >50 μmol/: and a prothrombin time <50% on postoperative day 5.[5] Mullen et al proposed that a peak serum bilirubin level more than 7 mg/dL was the most powerful predictor of 90-day overall or major complications and overall or liver-related mortality after major hepatectomy, with a 33% risk of death.[6] The International Study Group of Liver Surgery (ISGLS's) definition uses bilirubin elevation on or after postoperative day 5 and grades PHLF based on international normalised ratio (INR) derangement, with a postoperative mortality of more than 50% in patients with an INR >2.0.[7] In a recent analysis of 680 hepatectomies comparing the three definitions, ISGLS was found to be the least stringent, and overall, their value in clinical decision making is yet to be determined.[8]

LIVER REGENERATION

The human response to major tissue loss after liver resection is a complex process involving interplay between parenchymal and nonparenchymal cells and is driven by multiple signals aimed at restoring liver volume.[9–12] The initiation and synchronisation of replications in different types of hepatic cells depend on the extent of the resection, tissue damage or both. After a massive resection, 90% of the hepatocytes appear to replicate.[9,10] Briefly, the process of liver regeneration involves mediators similar to those found in acute inflammation. Normally, hepatocytes are in the quiescent G0 phase. After resection, the remaining hepatocytes enter the G1 phase. Cytokines derived predominantly from Kupffer cells prime hepatocytes, tumour necrosis factor alpha (TNF-α) and, subsequently, interleukin-6 are released, contributing to the initiation of the cell cycle.[9] Mitogenic factors are required for the regenerative process to enter the S phase; primarily growth factors such as hepatocyte growth factor (HGF), vascular endothelial growth factor (VEGF), epidermal growth factor (EGF), thrombospondin-1 (TSP-1), serotonin (5-HT) and transforming growth factor beta (TGF-β) are crucially involved in this process.[1,13,14] Growing experimental and clinical evidence further suggests a central role of platelets and platelet-derived factors in liver regeneration.[1]

DEVELOPMENT OF POSTHEPATECTOMY LIVER FAILURE

Despite the complexity, fortunately, only a small amount of liver is necessary to maintain liver function and regeneration. More than a decade ago, Schindl et al showed the correlation between liver remnant size and PHLF. Half of the patients with a liver remnant less than 26% developed severe hepatic failure when compared with 1.2% of patients who had a larger volume remaining.[3]

To this day, an FLR of 25% is currently used as the lower limit in patients with normal liver function. This needs to be adapted accordingly in patients with impaired liver function.[15]

A recent review identified five important factors contributing to the development of PHLF: (i) haemodynamic imbalance, (ii) disturbed bile salt homeostasis, (iii) impaired liver innate immune defense, (iv) gut microbiota and (v) impaired liver function.[4]

Haemodynamic Imbalance

Posthepatectomy liver failure is comparable to 'small for size' (SFS) syndrome in the setting of liver transplantation, where portal hyperperfusion and arterial hypoperfusion have a deleterious effect on the recovery of liver function.[16] In noncirrhotic patients, increased portal flow and pressure increased the risk for PHLF.[17]

Bile Salt Homeostasis

Excessive intracellular accumulation of bile due to the damage of canalicular transporters causes damage to the hepatocytes and results in apoptosis.[18] Experimental animal models show that altered bile homeostasis negatively affects liver regeneration.[19,20]

Impaired Liver Innate Immune Defence

The liver's innate immune system is activated during liver regeneration.[21] After resection, cytokine release by Kupffer cells is shown to be impaired.[22] In addition, phagocytic activity of the reticuloendothelial system after major resection is lower, contributing to the increased infection risk.[3,23]

Microbiota: Gut–Liver Axis

In the recent literature, there have been reports on gut microbiota modulating the liver's regenerative ability through interference with bile salt physiology and effects on bacterial endotoxins.[24,25]

Impaired Liver Function

Quality of the liver parenchyma plays a key role in liver regeneration and can be altered for various reasons, such as cholestasis, steatosis, cirrhosis and damage from preoperative chemotherapy.[4]

RISK ASSESSMENT AND PREVENTION OF LIVER FAILURE

Accurate assessment of liver volume and function is required in order to achieve a proper estimate of the functional reserve. The measurement of the volume of the FLR is usually performed with 2D volumetry on computed tomography (CT) or magnetic resonance imaging (MRI) scans.[26,27] Currently, an FLR of 25% is considered as the lower threshold in full-functioning livers and needs to be adapted to up to 40% in the presence of impaired liver function.[15]

Liver function is evaluated using a combination of preoperative biochemistry (bilirubin for secretory function and INR for synthetic function) and metabolic function tests, as well as certain imaging techniques.[4] Function testing can be performed using the LiMAx test, measuring ^{13}C-labelled methacetin in the exhaled breath, or the indocyanine green (ICG) clearance, measuring the retention rate of intravenous ICG at 15 minutes. The latter is a readily available test that, in combination with volumetry, provides accurate estimates of liver function. Further refinements use intraoperative ICG clearance to estimate the function of the FLR. This is especially useful for risk avoidance in two-stage procedures.[28,29] Imaging techniques include gadolinium-enhanced MRI,[30,31] which shows a good correlation with regional liver function, with its added advantage of simultaneous operative planning. Liver fat content in this setting could help identify patients at risk for insufficient FLR growth when planned for a two-stage procedure.[32] In addition (Tc^{99m})-labelled hepatobiliary iminodiacetic acid (HIDA) scintigraphy might be used to estimate the metabolic liver function.[33] Preliminary reports propose HIDA scanning as a potential assessment tool in complex two-stage liver resections, but this has to be validated in large cohorts.[34,35]

Future Liver Remnant Enlargement

As mentioned above, the induction of hypertrophy should be performed if the FLR is expected to be less than 25% in patients without liver disease or 40% in patients with a reduced hepatic reserve.[15] Portal vein embolisation (PVE) and portal vein ligation (PVL) show comparable preoperative hypertrophic responses and postoperative morbidity.[36] Overall, the FLR is expected to grow by about 40% compared with baseline and expands the pool of resectable patients by 20%.[2] However, results are limited, as the progression of disease occurs in one-third of patients due to increased arterial flow to the embolised lobe and long waiting times to surgery.[37] If PVE or PVL do not lead to adequate hypertrophy, this has to be interpreted as a contraindication for major liver resection.[4,38] In patients with bilobar tumours that are not resectable in one attempt, a two-staged hepatectomy is an excellent approach that increases and clears the FLR for a curative treatment attempt.[4,15]

Further refinement of the two-staged approach led to the development of the associating liver partition and portal vein ligation for staged hepatectomy (ALPPS), combining PVL clearance of the remaining lobe and split of the liver in situ and the removal of the ligated lobe 7 days later.[39,40] Its major advantage is the significantly increased hypertrophy rate of up to 80% within the first week.[41] First reports showed somewhat higher morbidity and mortality rates, and the there is some evidence that the second step should not be performed in case of major complications after the first step or insufficient function of the FLR.[34,42,43]

Preoperative Optimising

There have been data suggesting that reduction of chemotherapy-associated portal hypertension by splenic artery ligation has a beneficial effect on postoperative morbidity.[44] In a rodent model, this has also shown to result in increased arterial flow and enhanced liver regeneration and function.[45]

In cases of patients with steatosis, effects of a very-low-calorie diet have been shown to improve outcomes in a liver transplant setting[46]; however, this has yet to be confirmed in the setting of oncological liver resection.

Further administration of unsaturated omega-3 fatty acids might improve the postoperative risk profile after major liver resection[47]—the definitive results of this prospective randomised trial are expected soon. There have been promising data on the role of platelets and thrombopoietin in liver regeneration; thus, platelet infusion or administration of thrombopoietin might provide an option for cirrhotic patients, but this has yet to be confirmed in human trials.[4,48]

Although there have been reports on beneficial outcomes for preoperative internal biliary drainage,[49] drainage-related complications are seen in up to a third of patients, and the definitive role of routine drainage in optimising patients remains inconclusive.[49–52]

Perioperative Optimising

There is some evidence that blood transfusion increases postoperative morbidity and tumour recurrence through transfusion-related inflammatory response.[53] Blood loss can be reduced by hepatic preconditioning[54]; however, prolonged clamping should be avoided.[55]

There is no benefit for routine drain placement after major liver resection; it might even be associated with an increased rate of complications and PHLF.[56,57] Further, there is no evidence for a beneficial effect of routine antibiotic prophylaxis in major hepatectomies.[58,59]

MANAGEMENT OF POSTHEPATECTOMY LIVER FAILURE

Unfortunately, data on treatment of PHLF are scare, and especially, large randomised controlled trials are missing. In addition, few treatments for acute or acute-on-chronic liver failure have been validated for PHLF.

Goal-Directed Therapy

As PHLF, in most cases, is strongly associated with multiorgan dysfunction, it requires a systemic treatment approach, resembling principles applied in acute liver failure and sepsis.[60–62]

Although there is no evidence of a benefit from prophylactic antibiotic treatment after liver resection,[58] some data suggest that, as long as systemic inflammatory response syndrome (SIRS) is present after resection or when patients are at the stage of liver failure,[63] administration of antibiotics seems to be useful.[64] Goal-directed therapy should aim at treating circulation, renal and ventilatory dysfunction, coagulation abnormalities, hepatic encephalopathy and nutritional status.[2]

Functional Therapy

Although there have been promising results for the Molecular Absorbent Recirculation System (MARS®)—it reduces toxicity by removing albumin-bound and water-soluble toxins from plasma—in the setting of acute or chronic hepatic failure, it has been validated for PHFL only in small, uncontrolled and nonrandomised trials. In the unfortunate setting of septic multiorgan failure and PHLF, MARS® has not shown a positive influence on patient survival.[65–67] Preclinical reports for the newly developed University College London–Liver Dialysis Device show a survival benefit in acute liver failure, but its clinical validation is pending.[68] Further, there have been promising results in patients with acute or acute-on-chronic liver failure who undergo extracorporeal haemodialysis and albumin dialysis (Prometheus) and plasma replacement with fresh frozen plasma (high-volume plasmapheresis); however, these have yet to be confirmed for PHLF.[4,69,70]

CONCLUSIONS

Liver failure after hepatic resection remains a great challenge in modern surgical practice. New imaging techniques and preoperative assessment tools, effective preventive measures, active surgical modelling of the FLR and improved perioperative care stand in opposition to the urge to push further the limits of resectability and curability. Despite promising preliminary results for functional therapies, to this date, the main management after development of PHLF consists of goal-directed support.

Patients should be managed in specialised centres with the ability to utilise all the latest developments for improved outcomes.

REFERENCES

1. Starlinger P, Assinger A. Importance of platelet-derived growth factors in liver regeneration. *Expert Rev Gastroenterol Hepatol* 2016;10:557–9.

2. van den Broek MA, Olde Damink SW, Dejong CH, et al. Liver failure after partial hepatic resection: definition, pathophysiology, risk factors and treatment. *Liver Int* 2008;28:767–80.

3. Schindl MJ, Redhead DN, Fearon KC, et al. The value of residual liver volume as a predictor of hepatic dysfunction and infection after major liver resection. *Gut* 2005;54:289–96.

4. van Mierlo KM, Schaap FG, Dejong CH, Olde Damink SW. Liver resection for cancer: new developments in prediction, prevention and management of postresectional liver failure. *J Hepatol* 2016;65:1217–31.

5. Balzan S, Belghiti J, Farges O, et al. The "50–50 criteria" on postoperative day 5: an accurate predictor of liver failure and death after hepatectomy. *Ann Surg* 2005;242:824–8, discussion 8–9.

6. Mullen JT, Ribero D, Reddy SK, et al. Hepatic insufficiency and mortality in 1,059 noncirrhotic patients undergoing major hepatectomy. *J Am Coll Surg* 2007;204:854v62; discussion 62–4.

7. Rahbari NN, Garden OJ, Padbury R, et al. Posthepatectomy liver failure: a definition and grading by the International Study Group of Liver Surgery (ISGLS). *Surgery* 2011;149:713–24.

8. Skrzypczyk C, Truant S, Duhamel A, et al. Relevance of the ISGLS definition of posthepatectomy liver failure in early prediction of poor outcome after liver resection: study on 680 hepatectomies. *Ann Surg* 2014;260:865–70; discussion 70.

9. Clavien PA, Petrowsky H, DeOliveira ML, Graf R. Strategies for safer liver surgery and partial liver transplantation. *N Engl J Med* 2007;356:1545–59.

10. Taub R. Liver regeneration: from myth to mechanism. *Nat Rev Mol Cell Biol* 2004;5:836–4v7.

11. Fausto N, Campbell JS, Riehle KJ. Liver regeneration. *J Hepatol* 2012;57:692–4.

12. Michalopoulos GK. Principles of liver regeneration and growth homeostasis. *Compr Physiol* 2013;3:485–513.

13. Michalopoulos GK. Liver regeneration. *J Cell Physiol* 2007;213:286–300.

14. Clavien PA. Liver regeneration: a spotlight on the novel role of platelets and serotonin. *Swiss Med Wkly* 2008;138:361–70.

15. Vauthey JN, Abbott DE. Commentary on "Feasibility study of two-stage hepatectomy for bilobar liver metastases". *Am J Surg* 2012;203:698–9.

16. Eipel C, Abshagen K, Vollmar B. Regulation of hepatic blood flow: the hepatic arterial buffer response revisited. *World J Gastroenterol* 2010;16:6046–57.

17. Allard MA, Adam R, Bucur PO, Termos S, Cunha AS, Bismuth H, et al. Posthepatectomy portal vein pressure predicts liver failure and mortality after major liver resection on noncirrhotic liver. *Ann Surg* 2013;258:822–9; discussion 9–30.

18. Perez MJ, Briz O. Bile-acid-induced cell injury and protection. *World J Gastroenterol* 2009;15:1677–89.

19. Uriarte I, Fernandez-Barrena MG, Monte MJ, et al. Identification of fibroblast growth factor 15 as a novel mediator of liver regeneration and its application in the prevention of post-resection liver failure in mice. Gut. 2013;62:899–910.

20. Fan M, Wang X, Xu G, Yan Q, Huang W. Bile acid signaling and liver regeneration. *Biochim Biophys Acta* 2015;1849:196–200.

21. Fausto N, Campbell JS, Riehle KJ. Liver regeneration. *Hepatology* 2006;43:S45–53.

22. Prins HA, Meijer C, Boelens PG, et al. Kupffer cell-depleted rats have a diminished acute-phase response following major liver resection. *Shock* 2004;21:561–5.

23. Schindl MJ, Millar AM, Redhead DN, et al. The adaptive response of the reticuloendothelial system to major liver resection in humans. *Ann Surg* 2006;243:507–14.

24. Liu HX, Keane R, Sheng L, Wan YJ. Implications of microbiota and bile acid in liver injury and regeneration. *J Hepatol* 2015;63:1502–10.

25. Liu HX, Rocha CS, Dandekar S, Wan YJ. Functional analysis of the relationship between intestinal microbiota and the expression of hepatic genes and pathways during the course of liver regeneration. *J Hepatol* 2016;64: 641–50.

26. van der Vorst JR, van Dam RM, van Stiphout RS, et al. Virtual liver resection and volumetric analysis of the future liver remnant using open source image processing software. *World J Surg* 2010;34:2426–33.

27. Dello SA, van Dam RM, Slangen JJ, et al. Liver volumetry plug and play: do it yourself with ImageJ. *World J Surg* 2007;31:2215–21.

28. Uchida Y, Furuyama H, Yasukawa D, et al. Hepatectomy based on future liver remnant plasma clearance rate of indocyanine green. *HPB Surg* 2016;2016:7637838. doi: 10.1155/2016/7637838.

29. Lau L, Christophi C, Nikfarjam M, et al. Assessment of liver remnant using ICG clearance intraoperatively during vascular exclusion: early experience with the ALIIVE Technique. *HPB Surg* 2015;2015:757052. doi: 10.1155/2015/757052.

30. Verloh N, Haimerl M, Zeman F, et al. Assessing liver function by liver enhancement during the hepatobiliary phase with Gd-EOB-DTPA-enhanced MRI at 3 Tesla. *Eur Radiol* 2014;24:1013–9.

31. Bastati N, Wibmer A, Tamandl D, et al. Assessment of orthotopic liver transplant graft survival on gadoxetic acid-enhanced magnetic resonance imaging using qualitative and quantitative parameters. *Invest Radiol* 2016;51: 728–34.

32. Barth BK, Fischer MA, Kambakamba P, Lesurtel M, Reiner CS. Liver-fat and liver-function indices derived from Gd-EOB-DTPA-enhanced liver MRI for prediction of future liver remnant growth after portal vein occlusion. *Eur J Radiol* 2016;85:843–9.

33. de Graaf W, van Lienden KP, Dinant S, et al. Assessment of future remnant liver function using hepatobiliary scintigraphy in patients undergoing major liver resection. *J Gastrointest Surg* 2010;14:369–78.

34. Truant S, Baillet C, Deshorgue AC, et al. Drop of Total Liver function in the interstages of the new associating liver partition and portal vein ligation for staged hepatectomy technique: analysis of the "Auxiliary Liver" by HIDA scintigraphy. *Ann Surg* 2016;263:e33–4.

35. Petrowsky H. Does volume translate in function in interstage associating liver partition and portal vein ligation for staged hepatectomy?: commentary on "drop of total liver function in the interstages of the new associating liver partition and portal vein ligation for staged hepatectomy technique: analysis of the auxiliary liver by hepatobiliary iminodiacetic acid scintigraphy". *Ann Surg* 2016;263:e35.

36. Pandanaboyana S, Bell R, Hidalgo E, et al. A systematic review and meta-analysis of portal vein ligation versus portal vein embolization for elective liver resection. *Surgery* 2015;157:690–8.

37. Hoekstra LT, van Lienden KP, Doets A, Busch OR, Gouma DJ, van Gulik TM. Tumor progression after preoperative portal vein embolization. *Ann Surg* 2012;256:812–7; discussion 7–8.

38. Farges O, Belghiti J, Kianmanesh R, et al. Portal vein embolization before right hepatectomy: prospective clinical trial. *Ann Surg* 2003;237:208–17.

39. de Santibanes E, Clavien PA. Playing Play-Doh to prevent postoperative liver failure: the "ALPPS" approach. *Ann Surg* 2012;255:415–7.

40. Schnitzbauer AA, Lang SA, Goessmann H, et al. Right portal vein ligation combined with in situ splitting induces rapid left lateral liver lobe hypertrophy enabling 2-staged extended right hepatic resection in small-for-size settings. *Ann Surg* 2012;255:405–14.

41. Schadde E, Ardiles V, Slankamenac K, et al. ALPPS offers a better chance of complete resection in patients with primarily unresectable liver tumors compared with conventional-staged hepatectomies: results of a multicenter analysis. *World J Surg* 2014;38:1510–9.

42. Schadde E, Ardiles V, Robles-Campos R, et al. Early survival and safety of ALPPS: first report of the International ALPPS Registry. *Ann Surg* 2014;260:829–36; discussion 36–8.

43. Truant S, Scatton O, Dokmak S, et al. Associating liver partition and portal vein ligation for staged hepatectomy (ALPPS): impact of the inter-stages course on morbi-mortality and implications for management. *Eur J Surg Oncol* 2015;41:674–82.

44. Schwarz L, Faitot F, Soubrane O, Scatton O. Splenic artery ligation for severe oxaliplatin induced portal hypertension: a way to improve postoperative course and allow adjuvant chemotherapy for colorectal liver metastases.: Letter to editor: comment about "Nodular regenerative hyperplasia (NRH) complicating oxaliplatin chemotherapy in patients undergoing resection of colorectal liver metastases". *Eur J Surg Oncol* 2014;40:787–8.

45. Ren YS, Qian NS, Tang Y, Liao YH, Liu WH, Raut V, et al. Beneficial effects of splenectomy on liver regeneration in a rat model of massive hepatectomy. *Hepatobiliary Pancreat Dis Int* 2012;11:60–5.

46. Doyle A, Adeyi O, Khalili K, Fischer S, Dib M, Goldaracena N, et al. Treatment with Optifast® reduces hepatic steatosis and increases candidacy rates for live donor liver transplantation. *Liver Transpl* 2016;22:1295–300.

47. Linecker M, Limani P, Botea F, et al. "A randomized, double-blind study of the effects of omega-3 fatty acids (Omegaven) on outcome after major liver resection". *BMC Gastroenterol* 2015;15:102.

48. Haegele S, Offensperger F, Pereyra D, et al. Deficiency in thrombopoietin induction after liver surgery is associated with postoperative liver dysfunction. *PLoS One* 2015;10:e0116985.

49. Farges O, Regimbeau JM, Fuks D, et al. Multicentre European study of preoperative biliary drainage for hilar cholangiocarcinoma. *Br J Surg* 2013;100:274–83.

50. Ferrero A, Lo Tesoriere R, Vigano L, Caggiano L, Sgotto E, Capussotti L. Preoperative biliary drainage increases infectious complications after hepatectomy for proximal bile duct tumor obstruction. *World J Surg* 2009;33: 318–25.

51. Hochwald SN, Burke EC, Jarnagin WR, Fong Y, Blumgart LH. Association of preoperative biliary stenting with increased postoperative infectious complications in proximal cholangiocarcinoma. *Arch Surg* 1999;134:261–6.

52. Kloek JJ, van der Gaag NA, Aziz Y, et al. Endoscopic and percutaneous preoperative biliary drainage in patients with suspected hilar cholangiocarcinoma. *J Gastrointest Surg* 2010;14:119–25.

53. Miki C, Hiro J, Ojima E, Inoue Y, Mohri Y, Kusunoki M. Perioperative allogeneic blood transfusion, the related cytokine response and long-term survival after potentially curative resection of colorectal cancer. *Clin Oncol (R Coll Radiol)* 2006;18:60–6.

54. Simillis C, Robertson FP, Afxentiou T, Davidson BR, Gurusamy KS. A network meta-analysis comparing perioperative outcomes of interventions aiming to decrease ischemia reperfusion injury during elective liver resection. *Surgery* 2016;159:1157–69.

55. Datta G, Fuller BJ, Davidson BR. Molecular mechanisms of liver ischemia reperfusion injury: insights from transgenic knockout models. *World J Gastroenterol* 2013;19:1683–98.

56. Squires MH, 3rd, Lad NL, Fisher SB, et al. Value of primary operative drain placement after major hepatectomy: a multi-institutional analysis of 1,041 patients. *J Am Coll Surg* 2015;220:396–402.

57. Olthof PB, Coelen RJ, Wiggers JK, Besselink MG, Busch OR, van Gulik TM. External biliary drainage following major liver resection for perihilar cholangiocarcinoma: impact on development of liver failure and biliary leakage. *HPB (Oxford)* 2016;18:348–53.

58. Hirokawa F, Hayashi M, Miyamoto Y, et al. Evaluation of postoperative antibiotic prophylaxis after liver resection: a randomized controlled trial. *Am J Surg* 2013;206:8–15.

59. Zhou YM, Chen ZY, Li XD, Xu DH, Su X, Li B. Preoperative antibiotic prophylaxis does not reduce the risk of postoperative infectious complications in patients undergoing elective hepatectomy. *Dig Dis Sci* 2016;61:1707–13.

60. Kimura F, Shimizu H, Yoshidome H, et al. Circulating cytokines, chemokines, and stress hormones are increased in patients with organ dysfunction following liver resection. *J Surg Res* 2006;133:102–12.

61. Rivers E, Nguyen B, Havstad S, et al. Early goal-directed therapy in the treatment of severe sepsis and septic shock. *N Engl J Med* 2001;345:1368–77.

62. Jalan R, Olde Damink SW, Hayes PC, Deutz NE, Lee A. Pathogenesis of intracranial hypertension in acute liver failure: inflammation, ammonia and cerebral blood flow. *J Hepatol* 2004;41:613–20.

63. Togo S, Tanaka K, Matsuo K, et al. Duration of antimicrobial prophylaxis in patients undergoing hepatectomy: a prospective randomized controlled trial using flomoxef. *J Antimicrob Chemother* 2007;59:964–70.

64. Rolando N, Gimson A, Wade J, Philpott-Howard J, Casewell M, Williams R. Prospective controlled trial of selective parenteral and enteral antimicrobial regimen in fulminant liver failure. *Hepatology* 1993;17:196–201.

65. Heemann U, Treichel U, Loock J, et al. Albumin dialysis in cirrhosis with superimposed acute liver injury: a prospective, controlled study. *Hepatology* 2002;36:949–58.

66. Rittler P, Ketscher C, Inthorn D, Jauch KW, Hartl WH. Use of the molecular adsorbent recycling system in the treatment of postoperative hepatic failure and septic multiple organ dysfunction–preliminary results. *Liver Int* 2004;24:136–41.

67. van de Kerkhove MP, de Jong KP, Rijken AM, de Pont AC, van Gulik TM. MARS treatment in posthepatectomy liver failure. *Liver Int* 2003;23:44–51.

68. Lee KC, Baker LA, Stanzani G, et al. Extracorporeal liver assist device to exchange albumin and remove endotoxin in acute liver failure: results of a pivotal pre-clinical study. *J Hepatol* 2015;63:634–42.

69. Rifai K, Ernst T, Kretschmer U, et al. Prometheus–a new extracorporeal system for the treatment of liver failure. *J Hepatol* 2003;39:984–90.

70. Larsen FS, Schmidt LE, Bernsmeier C, et al. High-volume plasma exchange in patients with acute liver failure: An open randomised controlled trial. *J Hepatol* 2016;64:69–78.

26

Prevention and Management of Complications after Laparoscopic Liver Resection

C.-W. Lin and D. Cherqui

ABSTRACT

Laparoscopic liver resection had been proved to be a feasible and safe procedure for the treatment of hepatic tumours. The outcome and complication rate after laparoscopic liver resection is not different compared with open hepatectomy. Although the result is same or even better, a whole new set of surgical techniques is required for laparoscopic liver resection, because the traditional open techniques may not be feasible under laparoscopic approach. The prevention and principle of management for complications after liver resection are the same, but special techniques may be needed in laparoscopic liver resection. In this chapter, the prevention and management of the complications after laparoscopic liver resection will be discussed.

KEYWORDS

Laparoscopic liver resection, hepatectomy, complication, HCC, bile leakage, bleeding

INTRODUCTION

After Gagner et al reported the first laparoscopic partial hepatectomy in 1992,[1] the feasibility and safety of laparoscopic liver resection (LLR) have been increasingly demonstrated in literature publications.[2–6] Nevertheless, LLR remains a challenging and complicated procedure.– Performing LLR requires substantial technical experience in both hepatobiliary and advanced laparoscopic surgery. Two consensus conferences were organised in 2008[7] and 2014.[8] In 2008, the first LLR international consensus conference was held in Louisville, Kentucky. There, it was concluded that LLR was attainable for tumours less than 5 cm and located in the peripheral parts of the liver. Moreover, laparoscopic lateral sectionectomy should be considered a standard procedure. Ever since the consensus meeting, the number of cases of LLR have increased worldwide. Laparoscopic liver resection has become a field of surgical innovation, especially at highly specialised

centres. The most recent LLR international consensus conference was held in Japan in 2014. The panel included an independent jury, who reviewed the available expert literature and elaborated a new set of recommendations. While emphasising the limited evidence available, the new recommendations validated that minor resections may be set as a standard practice. However, major resections and/or complex anatomical resections still remain at the evaluation stage.[8]

For a stand-alone liver resection procedure, that is, without reconstruction or anastomosis, the laparoscopic approach may be considered excellent.[2,9] However, laparoscopic liver procedures have met a great deal of resistance for several years, which is why they have been adopted much slower than other procedures. The reasons for this were the perceptions that there would be uncontrollable bleeding and inadequate oncological outcomes, such as tumour seeding and/or involvement of the resection margins. The lack of advanced training in laparoscopic techniques in established liver surgeons may have also contributed to the reluctance of adoption of LLR. It is certainly a difficult procedure that requires expertise in both the liver surgery and the advanced laparoscopic techniques. Mastery in simple laparoscopic procedures, such as cholecystectomy, is clearly insufficient for the advanced skills needed in LLR. Thus, 'open' liver surgeons need to adapt to a whole new set of techniques. Likewise, an expert laparoscopic surgeon with no surgical background on the indications and techniques of liver resection is unsuitable to perform LLR.

Several comparative studies have showed that LLR is associated with fewer postoperative complications than open operations.[10–12] A recent comprehensive review of the literature of over 9000 cases by Ciria et al[13] reported a cumulative mortality rate of 0.4%. This is a favourable comparison with the rate of 0 to 5.4% reported in the open-resection experience of high-volume centres. The causes of the 37 reported deaths were bleeding, sepsis and liver failure. There were no deaths during operation. A 10.5% morbidity rate was reported, with a range of 0 to 50% across studies. Liver-specific complications accounted for 4% and included bile leaks, transient liver failure, transient ascites and abdominal collections. The remaining 6% were complications common to all operations, including haemorrhage, wound infection, hernia, bowel injury, intra-abdominal fluid accumulation and respiratory or urinary tract infections. This chapter will focus on the prevention and management of complications after LLR.

INDICATIONS AND PATIENT SELECTION FOR LAPAROSCOPIC LIVER RESECTION

The careful selection of patients for LLR is crucial for a successful LLR and for a good outcome. A new scoring system predicting the difficulty of an LLR was proposed by Ban et al. This scoring system included the extent of liver resection, liver function, tumour size, tumour location and tumour proximity to the major vessels.[14] In this study, a significant predictor for major operative events, by univariate and multivariate analyses, is the location of tumours in difficult areas (segments IVa, VII and VIII). Despite the fact that these tumours are increasingly being managed laparoscopically in experienced centres[15–17], they still necessitate challenging and complicated procedures, which require a long period of training. Presently, the vast majority of hepatopancreatobiliary (HPB) centers practice laparoscopic minor resection, including left lateral sectionectomy and peripheral

wedge resections. A smaller number of teams are using the laparoscopic approach for formal right or left hemihepatectomy. Finally, even smaller number of teams, mainly from Asia, have reported complex anatomical resection, including difficult locations such as segmentectomy VII or VIII and anterior or posterior sectionectomy.[18–20]

Categorising LLRs is no different than open liver resections. Based on the Couinaud's segmentation and Brisbane 2000 terminology of liver anatomy and resections[21], the most laparoscopically amenable segments are II, III, IVb, V and VI[7] (Figure 26.1). Isolated resection of posterior-superior liver tumours (segments I, IVa, VII and VIII) and major hepatectomy have been reported[16,18,19,22]; however, these are technically more challenging and should be reserved for expert surgeons who are able to expand their limits beyond safely mastering the laparoscopic resections of segments II to VI. In the comprehensive review by Ciria et al[13] the majority (70%) were minor resections (two segments or less), including nonanatomic wedge resections and left lateral sectionectomies (20% each). Anatomical segmentectomies and sectionectomies, classified as minor by the amount of resected liver, are indeed very complex resections that were reported mainly by Asian surgeons and account for 13% and 5% of the cases, respectively. Major resections of three or more segments accounted for 24% of the cases, with right and left hemihepatectomies representing 13% and 11%, respectively. When deciding the appropriateness of LLR, the major determinants

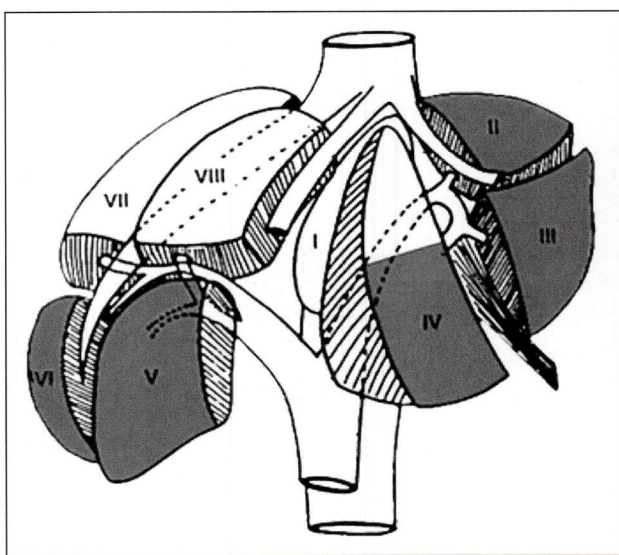

Figure 26.1 The most favourable lesions for laparoscopic resection are solitary tumours less than 5 cm and located in peripheral liver segments II to VI.

Table 26.1 The indication and difficulty of laparoscopic liver resection

		Easy	Difficult
Tumour	Size	<5 cm	>5 cm
	Depth	Superficial/pedunculated	Deep
	Location	Segment II, III, IVb, V, VI	Segment I, IVa, VII, VIII
	Number	Single	Multiple
Distance from hepatic hilum, proximal hepatic veins or IVC		>1 cm	<1 cm
Surgeon experience[27]		<25 cases	>25 cases
Liver background		Normal	Injured
Extent of resection		Lateral sectionectomy Peripheral wedge resection	Right/left hemihepatectomy Anatomic segmentectomy Sectionectomy (two segments) Extended resection Donor hepatectomy

Abbreviation: IVC, inferior vena cava.

are the extent of resection, size, location and number of lesions and the proximity to the major vessels (Table 26.1).

Indications According to Tumour Size and Location

For LLR, the most favourable lesions are solitary tumours less than 5 cm and located in the periphery, that is, segments II to VI[7] (Figure 26.1). Such cases are recommended as initial procedures when initiating an LLR program. Pedunculated tumours located at the inferior or left lateral surface, which are even greater than 5 cm in diameter, are also suitable for laparoscopic resection. The laparoscopic approach should be considered the standard for left lateral sectionectomy.[7,23] Peripheral wedge resections are also considered easy procedures.

Laparoscopic major resections are now well-standardised.[22,24,25] Before they gain wider acceptance, they will require a higher level of training and experience. Finally, more difficult cases include lesions located in the posterior-superior liver (segments I, IVa, VII and VIII) and lesions in proximity to the major vessels or the hepatic hilum. These cases should be restricted to experienced centres but are being increasingly reported.[16,18,19]

Indications According to Tumour Pathology and Underlying Liver Disease

The main indications for LLR are, as in open surgery, primary and secondary liver cancers. Obviously, principles of oncological resection are essential. Surgical margins should not be different between open and laparoscopic liver tumour resections. If an inadequate margin for a tumour becomes a concern in the laparoscopic approach, an open technique should be adopted if an adequate margin is deemed feasible for the same tumour by using an open approach.

The status of the underlying liver should also be taken into account. Patients with benign disease have an underlying normal liver, whereas patients with malignant disease usually have some degree of liver injury. Obviously, 90% of patients with hepatocellular carcinoma (HCC) have underlying chronic liver injury, chronic hepatitis B or C infection, and alcoholic and nonalcoholic steatohepatitis as the most common causes. In addition, nowadays, a significant proportion of patients with colorectal liver metastases have some degree of liver disease due to chemotherapy-induced injury. Nearly 50% of our laparoscopic experience has been associated with patients who have chronic liver diseases.[26,27] Despite longer operative time and more pedicle clamping cycles, patients who undergo laparoscopic resection generally have a better recovery than their open-resection counterparts.[13,26] Tranchart et al evaluated the risk factors for postoperative complications after LLR, by multivariate analysis; they concluded that resection for malignant tumours is one of the independent predictors of postoperative morbidity.[28] This should be taken into account when considering to proceed with a laparoscopic approach.

THE LEARNING CURVE

The level of surgical difficulty for any LLR varies from case to case and is highly dependent on not only tumour characteristics and patient factors but also the surgeon's experience. Gradually, acquainting oneself with the skills required for higher-level LLR is important before moving on to more complex procedures.

During a 12-year period, Cherqui et al analysed 174 LLRs. They determined that, by comparing the incidence of conversion to open procedures in three different time frames[29], a learning curve of 60 cases was required for LLR. Surgical techniques and energy device utilisation in LLR have significantly improved in the past two decades, making LLR for tumours a reproducible and feasible method of treatment. Shortening of the LLR learning period is expected in the near future, as standardised surgical procedures are followed, advanced surgical instruments and energy devices are used and more training programmes become available. Lin et al analysed a series since 2008 and proposed a learning number of 22 cases for minor LLR, which is substantially lesser than the numbers reported previously.[27] Surgeons embarking on LLR should start with minor resections for peripherally located liver tumours. After adequate learning process and experience accumulation, LLR attempts may be extended to include major hepatectomies for tumours that are located in difficult areas. For the learning period of laparoscopic major liver resection, Nomi et al proposed that a learning curve of 45 cases was needed in order to reduce the operative time and to enter the stable phase of laparoscopic major hepatectomy.[30] However, the operations in this series were performed by an expert surgeon (Brice Gayet), so the result may not be applicable to those with less experience. Further evaluation for the learning period of laparoscopic major liver resection is required.

PERIOPERATIVE BLEEDING

The progress and popularity of LLR have been slower than other laparoscopic abdominal procedures because of persistent concerns regarding difficulties in liver mobilisation and transection, the laparoscopic management of intraoperative complications and the risks of perioperative bleeding. A whole new set of surgical techniques is required for a successful LLR. More than 40 studies in the review by[13] had concluded that there was less blood loss after LLR compared with that after open hepatectomy.[13] This lower blood loss is most likely to be due to the intra-abdominal pressure by the pneumoperitoneum[31] and haemostatic procedures through the magnified view, which enables precise manipulation. However, bleeding control during LLR is technically demanding compared with that during open procedures, Thus making bleeding control one of the most common causes for conversion to open surgery.[7,32–34]

Liver Mobilisation

The liver is the largest organ in the abdomen and is very bulky and fragile. Complete mobilisation of the liver and the area to be resected is crucial, as it provides space for surgical manipulation. In contrast to open hepatectomy, where the mobilisation of the liver is performed by holding and moving it with the surgeon's hand, there is still no surgical instrument that has a similar ability. The instruments used for LLR are somehow rigid and traumatic, carrying the risk of injury to the liver. A cholecystectomy is usually performed first in the LLR; however, the gallbladder may be left partially attached to the liver on purpose, so that it may be used as a 'handle' to move the liver around. The round ligament is also a good handle of the liver and can be grasped and retracted. The surrounding ligaments around the liver should be divided before moving the liver, in order to prevent the tear of its capsule during mobilisation (Figure 26.2). The table can also be tilted to the right or left; moving the liver by gravity helps create space necessary during the various stages of the operation.

Special attention should be paid to the short bridging veins, which directly drain towards the inferior vena cava (IVC) (Figure 26.3). The right adrenal gland is very fragile and has a rich blood supply. Dissection between, it and the liver should be done carefully (Figure 26.4), because injury to the adrenal gland might lead to bleeding, which is difficult to control.

If the liver capsule is injured during the procedure, even small oozing haemorrhage should be stopped quickly; otherwise, it will obstruct the view of the laparoscope. The bleeding from the liver surface can be managed by

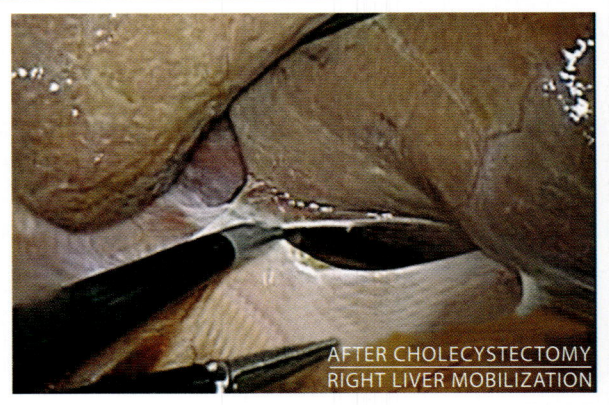

AFTER CHOLECYSTECTOMY
RIGHT LIVER MOBILIZATION

Figure 26.2 The surrounding ligaments around the liver should be divided before moving the liver, to prevent the tear of liver capsule during mobilisation.

Courtesy: Chung-Wei Lin and Daniel Cherqui.

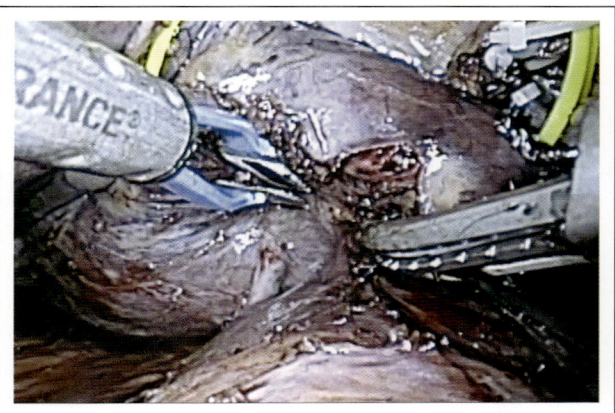

Figure 26.3 Special attention should be paid to the short bridging veins that directly drain towards inferior vena cava.

Courtesy: Chung-Wei Lin and Daniel Cherqui.

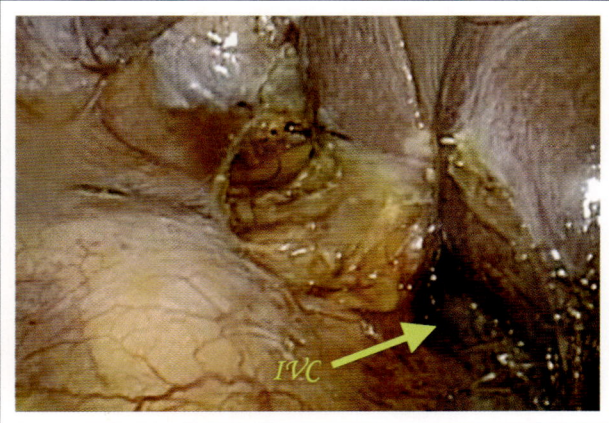

Figure 26.4 Dissection between liver and right adrenal gland should be very careful to prevent bleeding.

Abbreviation: IVC, inferior vena cava.

Courtesy: Chung-Wei Lin and Daniel Cherqui.

monopolar diathermy or bipolar electrocautery. Direct compression with gauze and absorbable haemostat matrix (i.e., Surgicel®, Ethicon Endo-Surgery, US, and Floseal®, Baxter BioSurgery, US) is usually effective in stopping the bleeding from the liver surface.

Hand-assisted laparoscopy can be used for lesions in the areas that are difficult to approach for the purpose of facilitating liver mobilisation or to aid in haemostasis. A gas-tight hand port is needed, and the port-site incision is later used for specimen extraction. Some experts suggest introducing the hand port in advance at the site of the future extraction site, so that, in case of bleeding, the surgeon can put a hand inside to fix the problem without delay.

Hepatic Inflow Control: Pringle's Manoeuvre and Hilum Dissection

One of the most important parts of LLR is to prevent or control bleeding during hepatic parenchymal transection. Successful hepatic inflow control is effective in decreasing perioperative bleeding from the hepatic arteries and portal veins. If hepatic hilum occlusion is planned, first open the pars flaccida and then encircle the hepatoduodenal ligament with a tape by passing an instrument behind the ligament and pulling the tape around it. Then, extracorporeally, the tape is guided through a short 16-Fr rubber tube to serve as a tourniquet and is returned into the abdomen in preparation for the Pringle's manoeuvre. If bleeding occurs, inflow occlusion is obtained by locking the tourniquet with a clip (Figure 26.5).

The right or left Glissonian pedicle can be dissected and looped at the junction of the hepatoduodenal ligament and liver capsule, with preserving and following

the plane of the hilar plate to encircle the whole right/left Glissonian pedicle—a step that can usually be performed without parenchymal dissection (Figure 26.6).[35] If pedicle clamping is necessary, cycles of clamping for 15 minutes, followed by 5-minute release, are undertaken. Although clamping the pedicle is not routinely employed, this procedure should be regarded as a safety precaution for surgeons, because however minimal the bleeding may be, visual obscuration poses a serious threat when

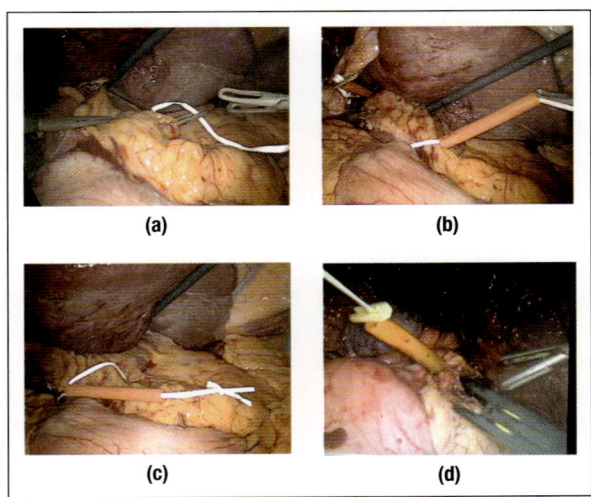

Figure 26.5 Pringle's manoeuvre in laparoscopic liver resection. a–c: Preparation of tourniquet (a): umbilical tape passed behind hepatic pedicle from the right side port; (b): rubber tube used to prepare tourniquet; (c): tourniquet ready; (d): inflow occlusion is obtained by locking the tourniquet with a locked clip.

Courtesy: Chung-Wei Lin and Daniel Cherqui.

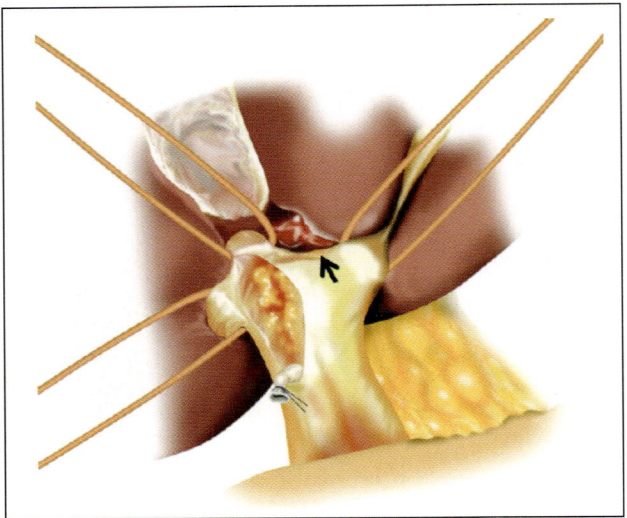

Figure 26.6 Extra-Glissonian approach for dissection of right/left pedicle.

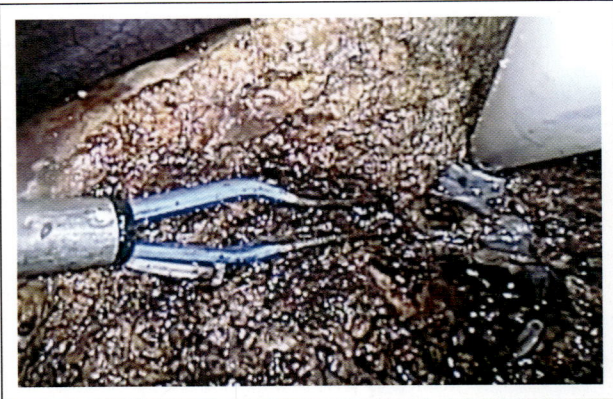

Figure 26.7 Identification of venous branches during hepatic parenchymal dissection.

Courtesy: Chung-Wei Lin and Daniel Cherqui.

attempting to control parenchymal bleeding. On-demand and intermittent inflow occlusion, meticulous liver parenchymal dissection technique, pneumoperitoneum pressure control and a low central venous pressure (CVP) level are the effective methods for limiting blood loss during LLR.

Parenchymal Dissection

Hepatic parenchymal transection is a critical step in both open and laparoscopic resections but possibly more in the latter. Consequently, prevention, rather than treatment of bleeding, is of paramount importance in laparoscopic surgery. The same principles that are crucial apply to both open and laparoscopic hepatectomies. Surgeons need to be familiar with the anatomy of liver (i.e., hepatic arteries, portal vein, biliary ducts and hepatic veins), review the recent computed tomography/magnetic resonance (CT/MR) images carefully before operation to identify the correlation of the tumour and adjacent major vessels and perform meticulous parenchymal dissection to identify and ligate vessels or bile ducts properly during transection. The superficial 2 cm of the liver parenchyma contains only small vessels that can be managed safely by using energy devices. The larger vessels are located deeper, especially the hepatic veins, which are very fragile, whereas the inflow pedicles are more solid and surrounded by a Glissonian sheath. Therefore, deeper transection requires identification of the large vessels and avoidance of blind manoeuvres (Figure 26.7).

Based on hepatic anatomy, preoperative imaging and the use of laparoscopic ultrasonography or demarcation lines seen during inflow occlusion, the liver transection line is marked by a monopolar diathermy on the liver capsule. Laparoscopic ultrasound manoeuvring and familiarity with liver anatomy under both B-mode and Doppler ultrasonography are mandatory for performing accurate LLRs.[36]

In open liver surgery, the clamp-and-crush method is an efficient and inexpensive transection technique, but newer technologies, including energy devices and staplers, are required for laparoscopic operations. There are several instruments available, and individual surgeons have developed preferences and habits with specific instruments, owing to their history and access to one or the other. There is no evidence that one device is better, and this should left to the surgeons' preference. The energy devices are mainly divided into three spectrums: (1) ultrasonic shears: Harmonic ACE® (Ethicon Endo-Surgery, Cincinnati, OH, US) and Sonicision® (Covidien, Mansfield, MA, US), (2) bipolar vessel sealant: LigaSure® (Covidien, Mansfield, MA, US) and Enseal® (Ethicon Endo-Surgery, Cincinnati, OH, US), and (3) combined ultrasonic and bipolar device: Thunderbeat® (Olympus, Tokyo, Japan). These energy devices are effective in transecting the superficial 2 cm of the liver parenchyma. Nevertheless, for dissecting deeper liver parenchyma, prior identification and selective haemostasis of the larger vessels are recommended. We use an ultrasonic aspirator (e.g., CUSA®, Integra, Plainsboro, NJ, US) (Figure 26.7). Vascular and biliary structures less than 5 mm are coagulated and/or transected by using energy devices or bipolar diathermy and are closed by clips. Vessels and bile ducts 5 to 10 mm in size are ligated with plastic locking clips (Hem-o-lok®, Teleflex Medical, Research Triangle Park, NC, US, and Lapro-Clip®, Covidien, New Heaven,

CT, US) and then divided. Laparoscopic linear staplers (Endo GIA®, Covidien, Mansfield, MA, US, and Echelon Endopath®, Ethicon Endo-Surgery, Cincinnati, OH, US) are used for larger vessels and bile ducts. The stapler can be applied to segmental portal pedicles or to isolated large portal or hepatic veins. It can also be used for division of the right or left bile duct, surrounded by the hilar plate during hemihepatectomy. The stapler should never be forced closed over thick tissue, nor should it ever be squeezed in with excessive tissue length between the jaws. Such manoeuvres risk misfiring and can lead to serious bleeding, which is hard to control. Instead, we dissect further into the liver parenchyma until the tissue fits effortlessly within the stapler. Before finally stapling the right or left portal vein branch near the bifurcation, flow in the opposite pedicle needs be confirmed (Figure 26.8). Some surgeons perform parenchymal transection with repeated application of linear staplers. We do not favour this technique because, though quicker, it lacks precision and may lead to severe bleeding. Meticulous parenchymal dissection to completely visualise intrahepatic vessels and bile ducts is preferred. Blind application of the linear stapler is considered a risky technique.

Bleeding control by compression or suture is more technically demanding in LLR than in open surgery. Continuous suction interferes with pneumoperitoneum pressure, obscures the laparoscopic view and increases the bleeding from the hepatic veins. Special surgical techniques are required when performing LLR to control perioperative haemorrhage (i.e., to identify the source of bleeding, to temporally control it by vessel clamps and to use an intracorporeal suture to close the bleeding vessel).

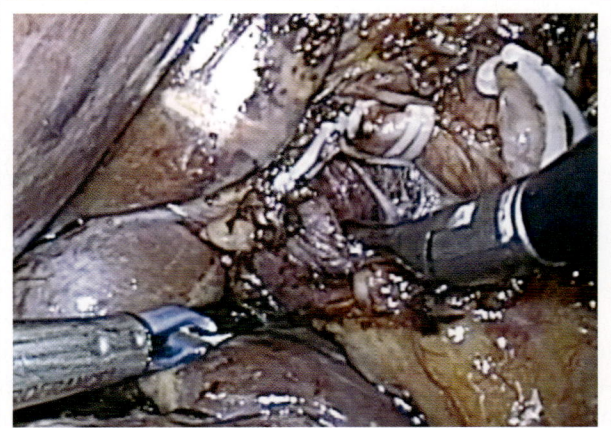

Figure 26.8 Before closing the right or left portal vein near the bifurcation, flow to the opposite lobe should be confirmed for safety. *Courtesy*: Chung-Wei Lin and Daniel Cherqui.

Intraoperative ultrasound is very useful to identify the vessel from which bleeding has occurred. If the bleeding comes from proximal hepatic veins or portal branches, sutures may be needed to manage its source. Mastering the techniques of intracorporeal suturing is very important for a successful LLR.

Intraoperative haemorrhage may be vigorous or may be insidious. Arterial bleeding is usually easily controlled with instrumental compression or by grasping the vessel when clips or sutures are applied. Hepatic venous branches are the most common sites of haemorrhage, and bleeding from these veins may be hard to manage, owing to vessel fragility and retraction.[27] Injury to the IVC may lead to massive bleeding. Although this is a more resistant vessel that can be sutured, excellent visualisation is required before attempting IVC dissection. In circumstances of significant IVC bleeding, the haemorrhage should at least be temporarily controlled by the laparoscopic method initially, because shock may quickly ensue by the time a laparotomy is performed. Surgeons, in collaboration with anaesthesiologists, must make an urgent decision on the steps needed to control bleeding. Above all, mastery of advanced laparoscopic techniques, such as intracorporeal suturing, is required to deal with IVC bleeding.

As in open surgery, low-CVP anaesthesia is recommended to reduce hepatic vein bleeding during transection. This requires close surgeon–anaesthesiologist collaboration. An advantage of the laparoscopic approach is the haemostatic effect of the pneumoperitoneum, which has a pressure that is usually higher than the CVP. Temporally elevating the pneumoperitoneum pressure and decreasing the tidal volume of ventilation have been proposed by some authors to decrease the bleeding from hepatic veins; this provides time and a clear view to control the bleeding point.[20] The threat of gas embolism has not been apparent in the literature because CO_2 used to create a pneumoperitoneum is highly soluble. However, surgeons and anaesthesiologists should remain vigilant, especially in the context of a low CVP.

Coagulation using a bipolar forceps is the primary bleeding-control method for LLR. Technical tips for bleeding control with bipolar electrocautery are described in detail.

Preservation of Intra-Abdominal Pressure

The pressure of the pneumoperitoneum is usually higher than the CVP, and this helps decrease the bleeding from the hepatic veins. Continuous suction decreases pneumoperitoneum pressure, obscures the laparoscopic view, decreases the working space and causes a burst of bleeding, resulting in even more difficult haemostatic control. The source of bleeding is identified when aspirating the blood gently and slowly to minimise the drop of pneumoperitoneal pressure. Some surgeons suggest that the pneumoperitoneum pressure should be increased up to 16 to 20 mmHg temporarily when bleeding occurs. This may slow down the bleeding from the vein and enable the source to be identified accurately.

Removal of Bipolar Forceps While Continuously Activating the Coagulation Energy

Bipolar forceps should be removed from a bleeder simultaneously during continuation of coagulation energy activation. The coagulated tissue will be torn off from the bleeder with bipolar tips when it is removed after interrupting coagulation energy, and this causes rebleeding. Saline irrigation during bipolar coagulation enhances the effect of the cautery and decreases the adhesion between the bipolar tips and tissue.

Compression with Haemostat Matrix

Direct compression of the bleeding point with gauze and absorbable haemostat matrix after bipolar cautery helps stop the bleeding (i.e., Surgicel®, Ethicon Endo-Surgery, US, and Floseal®, Baxter BioSurgery, US).

The Inflow Occlusion Technique (Pringle's Manoeuvre)

The inflow occlusion system should be prepared before liver parenchymal dissection. In case of massive and/or persistent bleeding, inflow occlusion is obtained by clamping the hepatoduodenal ligament interruptedly, with 15 minutes of clamping of the pedicle flow, interrupted by 5-minute release.

Introducing a Hand Port at the Beginning of the Procedure

A hand port can be introduced at the beginning for potentially high-risk procedures. When dealing with bleeding that is difficult to manage laparoscopically, the surgeon's hand inserted into the abdomen through the hand port helps control the haemorrhage quickly.

BILE LEAKAGE

Bile leakage is still one of the most common complications of liver resection. Over the years, the incidence of bile leakage has not declined and has been described in 1 to 14% of patients after liver resection.[37,38] Risk factors for bile leakage are high-risk procedures, with exposure of the

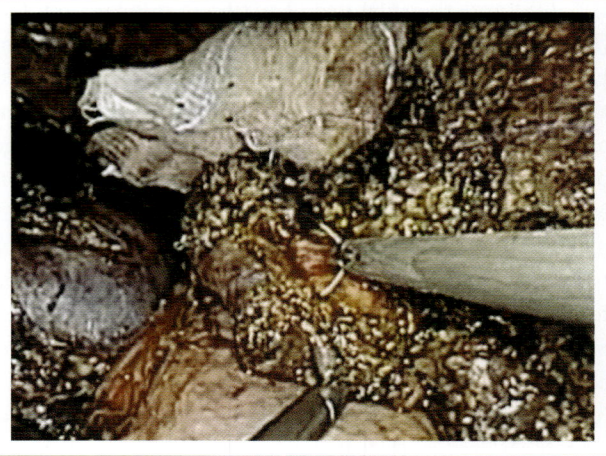

Figure 26.9   When a suspicious bile leakage is identified, the defect of bile duct should be repaired carefully by applying clips or sutures. *Courtesy*: Chung-Wei Lin and Daniel Cherqui.

major Glissonian sheath[37–39]; size of resection plane[38]; the patient's age and a prolonged operation time.[39]

The principles of prevention and management of bile leakage are not different for laparoscopic and open liver resections. Small biliary branches in the superficial layer of the liver parenchyma should be closed by using energy devices or clips. Segmental/lobar branches of the bile ducts should be identified clearly with careful parenchymal dissection, closed with locking clips or a linear stapler and then divided. When performing right/left hemihepatectomy, the patency of the contralateral bile duct should be confirmed before transection. After completion of the liver parenchymal dissection, routine inspection for a bile leak is always performed by placing a white gauze over the liver transection surface or over the cut end of the bile duct. Intraoperative cholangiography or bile leakage tests, such as injecting saline or isotonic dye (e.g., methylene blue) through the cystic stump and then clamping the distal common bile duct, may be performed selectively in patients who are suspected of having bile duct injury. When a suspicious bile leakage is identified, the defect of bile duct should be repaired carefully by applying clips or sutures (Figure 26.9).

FIBRIN SEALANT

In liver surgery, fibrin sealants are now widely used. Several studies were performed to analyse the efficacy of fibrin sealant in liver surgery on haemostasis, postoperative drainage amount and resection surface-related complications such as bile leakage, bleeding and abscess formation.[40,41] In general, these studies have shown that fibrin sealants use reduced time to haemostasis, but no strong evidence is seen in the reduction of the incidences of bile leakage after liver resections. A new type of sealant consisting of a solid matrix (TachoSil®, Takeda Nycomed, Austria) is claimed to have a better adhesive strength than other liquid fibrin sealants; however, only few studies have shown a benefit of decreasing bile leakage. Future studies are needed to further analyse the lysis of different fibrin sealants (fibrin glues vs. solid matrix fibrin sealants) by human bile. Since no evidence is noted on the efficacy of fibrin sealants on reducing resection cut surface–related complications, use of fibrin sealants routinely in liver surgeries cannot be recommended.

EXTRACTION, DRAINAGE AND CLOSURE

All resected specimens should be extracted by using a protecting plastic bag to prevent tumour spreading or wound site seeding. Small tumour specimens can be removed through trocar incisions by extending the wounds. Larger specimens are usually removed through a 5 to 8 cm suprapubic Pfannenstiel incision. Other methods of specimen removal can be performed through a pre-existing McBurney's or midline incision or through a hand-port incision. The extraction incision should fit the size of the specimen to ensure successful retrieval. Wound size should not be underestimated, in order to allow easy extraction and avoid rupture of the protecting bag. Then, the fascia layers are reapproximated and the pneumoperitoneum is reintroduced. Lavage of the operative field, examination for haemostasis and possible bile leakage are carried out. All major portal vein/bile duct branches should be secured with double clips to prevent dislocation of the clips that might lead to bleeding or bile leakage.

The use of abdominal drainage depends on the surgeons' preference. It is often used in case of major resections and should be avoided in cirrhotic patients. Irrigation of the peritoneal cavity, especially around the liver, can be performed and need to suctioned clear. The fascia of the port sites greater than 10 mm in diameter should be closed. If intercostal transpleural trocars are used, the defect in the diaphragm should be closed carefully. The pneumothorax is usually minimal and self-limited, because CO_2 is highly soluble; pleural drainage is seldom needed. The skin of the extraction wounds and port-site incisions are closed layer by layer with absorbable sutures subcutaneously to prevent fluid accumulation.

CONVERSION IS NOT A FAILURE

In the past literature, conversion rates of LLR ranged from 0 to 55%. The most cited causes for conversion are haemorrhage, poor progress of the operation, oncological or margin uncertainty, adhesions and anatomical difficulties.[4] Bleeding is the most common cause. The rate of conversion is reduced with proper patient selection, and it decreases with time and experience.[29] Conversion should not be considered a surgical failure and should be executed without hesitation when a patient's safety is being compromised.

During parenchymal transection, slow and continuous bleeding may occur, perhaps due to an elevated CVP, fragile liver parenchyma or inappropriate technique. Nonetheless, visualisation is often obscured, and the resection procedure slows down. In such a situation, intermittent portal triad clamping (total or hemi-Pringle's manoeuvre) is recommended. However, if conservative measures are ineffective in managing the bleeding, conversion to laparotomy should be performed immediately.

A few of the reported hindrances in the progression of procedure are insufficient exposure, proximity to major vessels and inability to obtain appropriate margins. Then again, failure to progress during surgery may simply be the result of an unanticipated difficult or dangerous dissection. Failure to progress or oncological uncertainty should lead to early conversion to avoid futile lengthening of surgery.

CONCLUSIONS

Laparoscopic liver resection is a safe and feasible procedure when performed on appropriately selected patients and by adequately trained surgeons. In well-selected patients, there are considerable perioperative benefits compared with open hepatectomy. In addition, oncological outcomes and survival for HCC and colorectal liver metastases have been demonstrated to be equivalent for both laparoscopic and open methods, in nonrandomised trials. Careful selection of patients amenable for LLR is crucial for successful and smooth procedures. Although the indications for the laparoscopic approach are somewhat restricted to lesion size and location, with more experience and newer technology, the possibilities of this procedure may continue to expand. As for every innovative procedure, adequate learning and proper training are fundamental. Surgeons should select easy cases in the initial stage of developing LLR, especially for the first 25 cases. Laparoscopic left lateral sectionectomies and limited resections of the peripheral-lateral segments of the liver are safe and well-received procedures and are now considered a standard practice.[8] Laparoscopic major hepatectomies are now better standardised, and anatomic segmentectomies or sectionectomies involving segments I, IVa, VII and VIII are being increasingly reported, but they remain at the evaluation stage and require higher levels of expertise. The postoperative outcomes and morbidity rate of LLR are comparable with open hepatectomy; however, a whole new set of surgical techniques is required to prevent and manage the bleeding or bile leakage for LLR and have been described above.

In liver surgery, laparoscopic resection is an excitingly flourishing field and will likely play an increasing role in the multidisciplinary approach to primary and secondary liver cancers.

REFERENCES

1. Gagner M, Rheault M, Dubuc J. Laparoscopic partial hepatectomy for liver tumor [abstract]. *Surg Endosc* 1993; 6:99.

2. Cherqui D, Husson E, Hammoud R, et al. Laparoscopic liver resections: a feasibility study in 30 patients. *Ann Surg* 2000;232:753–62.

3. Cherqui D, Laurent A, Tayar C, et al. Laparoscopic liver resection for peripheral hepatocellular carcinoma in patients with chronic liver disease: midterm results and perspectives. *Ann Surg* 2006;243:499–506.

4. Nguyen KT, Gamblin TC, Geller DA. World review of laparoscopic liver resection-2,804 patients. *Ann Surg* 2009;250:831–41.

5. Koffron AJ, Auffenberg G, Kung R, Abecassis M. Evaluation of 300 minimally invasive liver resections at a single institution: less is more. *Ann Surg* 2007;246:385–392; discussion 392–394.

6. Buell JF, Thomas MT, Rudich S, et al. Experience with more than 500 minimally invasive hepatic procedures. *Ann Surg* 2008;248:475–86.

7. Buell JF, Cherqui D, Geller DA, et al. The International Position on Laparoscopic Liver Surgery. *Ann Surg* 2009;250:825–30.

8. Wakabayashi G, Cherqui D, Geller DA, et al. Recommendations for laparoscopic liver resection: a report from the Second International Consensus Conference held in Morioka. *Ann Surg* 2015;261:619–29.

9. Cherqui D. Laparoscopic liver resection. *Br J Surg* 2003;90:644–6.

10. Dagher I, O'Rourke N, Geller DA, et al. Laparoscopic major hepatectomy: an evolution in standard of care. *Ann Surg* 2009;250:856–60.

11. Belli G, Fantini C, D'Agostino A, Cioffi L, Langella S, Russolillo N, Belli A. Laparoscopic versus open liver resection for hepatocellular carcinoma in patients with histologically proven cirrhosis: short- and middle-term results. *Surg Endosc* 2007;21:2004–11.

12. Nguyen KT, Marsh JW, Tsung A, Steel JJ, Gamblin TC, Geller DA. Comparative benefits of laparoscopic

vs open hepatic resection: a critical appraisal. *Arch Surg* 2011;146:348–56.

13. Ciria R CD, Geller D, Briceno J, Wakabayashi G. Comparative Short Term Benefits of Laparoscopic Liver Resection: 9,000 Cases and Climbing. *Ann Surg* 2016;263:761–77.

14. Ban D, Tanabe M, Ito H, et al. A novel difficulty scoring system for laparoscopic liver resection. *J Hepatobiliary Pancreat Sci* 2014;21:745–53. doi: 10.1002/jhbp.166.

15. Cho JY, Han HS, Yoon YS, Shin SH. Feasibility of laparoscopic liver resection for tumors located in the posterosuperior segments of the liver, with a special reference to overcoming current limitations on tumor location. *Surgery* 2008;144:32–8.

16. Ishizawa T, Gumbs AA, Kokudo N, et al. Laparoscopic segmentectomy of the liver: from segment I to VIII. *Ann Surg* 2012;256:959–64.

17. Yoon Y-S, Han H-S, Cho JY, et al. Total laparoscopic liver resection for hepatocellular carcinoma located in all segments of the liver. *Surg Endosc* 2010;24:1630–7.

18. Han HS, Cho JY, Yoon YS. Techniques for performing laparoscopic liver resection in various hepatic locations. *J Hepatobiliary Pancreat Surg* 2009;16:427–32.

19. Yoon YS, Han HS, Cho JY, et al. Laparoscopic liver resection for centrally located tumors close to the hilum, major hepatic veins, or inferior vena cava. *Surgery* 2013;153:502–9.

20. Honda G, Kurata M, Okuda Y, et al. Totally laparoscopic hepatectomy exposing the major vessels. *J Hepatobiliary Pancreat Sci* 2013;20:435–40.

21. Belghiti J, Clavien P, Gadzijev E, et al. The Brisbane 2000 terminology of liver anatomy and resections. *HPB* 2000;2:333–9.

22. Dagher I, Gayet B, Tzanis D, et al. International experience for laparoscopic major liver resection. *J Hepatobiliary Pancreat Sci* 2014;21:732–6.

23. Chang S, Laurent A, Tayar C, et al. Laparoscopy as a routine approach for left lateral sectionectomy. *Br J Surg* 2007;94:58–63.

24. Soubrane O, Schwarz L, Cauchy F, et al. A conceptual technique for laparoscopic right hepatectomy based on facts and oncologic principles: the caudal approach. *Ann Surg* 2015;261:1226–31.

25. Belli G, Gayet B, Han HS, et al. Laparoscopic left hemihepatectomy a consideration for acceptance as standard of care. *Surg Endosc* 2013;27:2721–6.

26. Bryant R, Laurent A, Tayar C, et al. Laparoscopic liver resection-understanding its role in current practice: the Henri Mondor Hospital experience. *Ann Surg* 2009;250:103–11.

27. Lin CW, Tsai TJ, Cheng TY, et al. The learning curve of laparoscopic liver resection after the Louisville statement 2008: will it be more effective and smooth? *Surg Endosc* 2016;30:2895–903.

28. Tranchart H, Gaillard M, Chirica M, et al. Multivariate analysis of risk factors for postoperative complications

after laparoscopic liver resection. *Surg Endosc* 2015;29: 2538–44.

29. Vigano L, Laurent A, Tayar C, et al. The learning curve in laparoscopic liver resection: improved feasibility and reproducibility. *Ann Surg* 2009;250:772–82.

30. Nomi T, Fuks D, Kawaguchi Y, et al. Learning curve for laparoscopic major hepatectomy. *Br J Surg* 2015;102: 796–804.

31. Eiriksson K, Fors D, Rubertsson S, et al. High intra-abdominal pressure during experimental laparoscopic liver resection reduces bleeding but increases the risk of gas embolism. *Br J Surg* 2011;98:845–52.

32. Vibert E, Perniceni T, Levard H, Denet C, Shahri NK, Gayet B. Laparoscopic liver resection. *Br J Surg* 2006;93: 67–72.

33. Nguyen KT, Laurent A, Dagher I, et al. Minimally invasive liver resection for metastatic colorectal cancer: a multi-institutional, international report of safety, feasibility, and early outcomes. *Ann Surg* 2009;250:842–8.

34. Nguyen KT, Marsh JW, Tsung A, et al. Comparative benefits of laparoscopic vs open hepatic resection: a critical appraisal. *Arch Surg* 2011;146:348–56.

35. Takasaki K. *Glissonean Pedicle Transection Method for Hepatic Resection*. Tokyo, Japan: Springer Science & Business Media; 2007.

36. Vigano L, Ferrero A, Amisano M, et al. Comparison of laparoscopic and open intraoperative ultrasonography for staging liver tumours. *Br J Surg* 2013;100:535–42.

37. Capussotti L, Ferrero A, Vigano L, et al. Bile leakage and liver resection: where is the risk? *Arch Surg* 2006;141:690–4.

38. Nagano Y, Togo S, Tanaka K, et al. Risk factors and management of bile leakage after hepatic resection. *World J Surg* 2003;27:695–8.

39. Lo CM, Fan ST, Liu CL, et al. Biliary complications after hepatic resection: risk factors, management, and outcome. *Arch Surg* 1998;133:156–61.

40. Marieke T, Joost M, Cornelis V, et al. Fibrin sealant for prevention of resection surface-related complications after liver resection: a randomized controlled trial. *Ann Surg* 2012;256:229–34.

41. Figueras J, Llado L, Miro M, et al. Application of fibrin glue sealant after hepatectomy does not seem justified: results of a randomized study in 300 patients. *Ann Surg* 2007;245:536–42.

27

Complications after Surgery for Perihilar Cholangiocarcinoma

E. Roos, R.J.S. Coelen and T.M. van Gulik

ABSTRACT

Cholangiocarcinoma is a heterogeneous group of malignancies that originates from the biliary tract. Perihilar cholangiocarcinoma is the most frequent form and represents 50 to 70% of all bile duct tumours. The majority of patients present with unresectable tumours at the time of diagnosis, and ultimately, only 20% of all patients are eligible to undergo curative resection. Partial hepatectomy with concomitant extrahepatic bile duct resection is the preferred treatment to achieve tumour-free margins, but this aggressive and technically challenging approach is associated with severe morbidity. This chapter deals with the specific operative risks and postoperative complications that frequently occur after resection of perihilar cholangiocarcinoma. Strategies for the management of these events are provided. Tailored preoperative care is the key to lowering the risk of postoperative complications.

KEYWORDS

Perihilar cholangiocarcinoma, hemihepatectomy, extrahepatic bile duct resection, bleeding, anastomotic leakage, biliary leakage, liver failure, multiorgan failure

INTRODUCTION

Cholangiocarcinoma is a clinically heterogeneous group of malignancies that originate in the epithelial cells of the bile ducts. Worldwide, bile duct tumours account for 3% of all gastrointestinal cancers and form the second most common hepatic malignancy.[1] Cholangiocarcinoma is commonly divided into intrahepatic, perihilar and distal tumours.[2] In the past few years, it has become more and more clear that these tumours are, clinically and biologically, separate entities, each requiring a tailored approach. The perihilar type represents the most complex type of cholangiocarcinoma, demanding an aggressive surgical approach to obtain a radical resection and, therefore, optimal preoperative preparation. This chapter focusses on the surgical treatment of perihilar cholangiocarcinoma (PHC) and its specific postoperative complications and pitfalls.

PERIHILAR CHOLANGIOCARCINOMA

Perihilar cholangiocarcinoma or Klatskin tumour arises from the hilum of the biliary tree and represents 50 to 70% of all bile duct tumours.[3,4] The aetiology of PHC remains obscure. Known risk factors account for only a minority of cases and differ between continents. In Asian populations, parasitic infections have a strong association with PHC. In the Western population, primary sclerosing cholangitis is the commonest known predisposing condition.[1] Whatever the location or origin, the only cure for cholangiocarcinoma remains an R0 resection.

Patients face many obstacles, such as cholestasis, cholangitis and difficulties in the confirmation of malignancy, in the diagnostic work-up and often require additional interventions when the future liver remnant (FLR) is too small or cholestatic (Figure 27.1). Although presentation with the sequelae of biliary obstruction

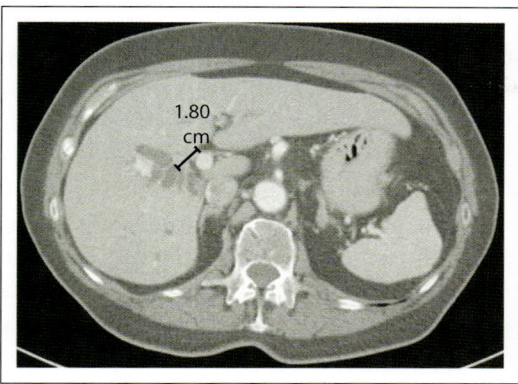

Figure 27.1 Perihilar cholangiocarcinoma (Bismuth IIIA type) with dilated biliary branches of the right system.

Courtesy: Thomas M. van Gulik.

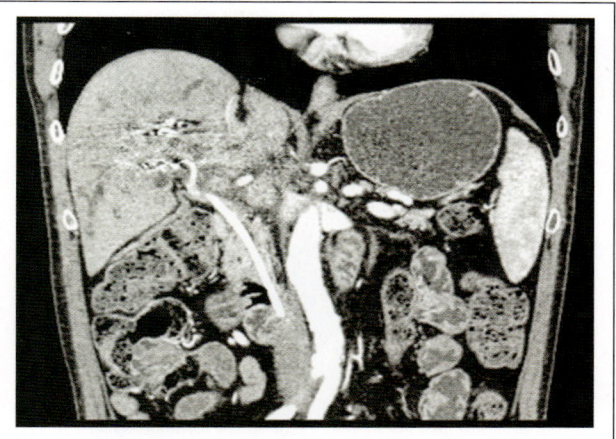

Figure 27.2 Placement of a percutaneous transhepatic biliary drainage in the left and right biliary system in a patient with perihilar cholangiocarcinoma (Bismuth IV type).

Courtesy: Thomas M. van Gulik.

is common, early symptoms are often not specific, and when jaundice develops due to local tumour progression, curative therapy is frequently not an option anymore. In 50% of patients, the tumour is not resectable at the time of diagnosis, mainly because of extensive hepatic artery and portal vein involvement or distant lymph node metastases.[5]

Differentiation of malignant and benign strictures at the liver hilum presents an additional diagnostic dilemma. Inflammatory lesions such as IgG4-related sclerosing cholangitis and primary sclerosing cholangitis show imaging characteristics mimicking PHC, and up to 15% of patients undergoing resection for PHC are ultimately diagnosed to have a benign tumour.[6,7] Extensive preoperative assessment of patients with a suspicion of PHC is thus required.

Imaging modalities are essential for diagnosis and treatment planning. Ultrasonography is the first step in diagnosing intrahepatic biliary tract dilatation. Multiphase contrast-enhanced computed tomography (CT) is used to assess vascular and lymph node involvement,[8] whereas magnetic resonance imaging provides better insight into proximal biliary branch involvement.[6] When patients present with jaundice, it is of vital importance that drainage of the FLR is performed, especially when a major liver resection is planned, leaving a small FLR.[9–11] Biliary drainage creates a safer environment for liver surgery in PHC, as it reduces jaundice and cholestasis, improves nutritional status and liver function, reduces bacterial translocation and improves the ability of the liver to regenerate after resection. Currently, there are insufficient data to support routine preoperative biliary drainage for liver resections, with FLR volumes >50%, as the risk of cholangitis and complications due to biliary

instrumentation may outweigh the benefits of biliary decompression in these patients.[9,10] Biliary drainage and stenting are performed through endoscopic retrograde cholangiopancreatography (ERCP) or the percutaneous approach, depending on local preference and expertise (Figures 27.2 and 27.3). However, after endoscopic stenting, patients often require additional percutaneous transhepatic biliary drainage (PTBD) to achieve adequate biliary decompression.[12] Preoperative biliary drainage with both ERCP and PTBD are associated with cholangitis, but unrelieved biliary obstruction runs the risk of development of liver failure due to decreased functional capacity in the event of cholestasis.[3]

The volume and function of the FLR are important parameters in risk assessment of patients with resectable PHC. Volume of FLR is measured using CT-volumetry. In postcholestatic livers, a FLR volume of 35 to 45% is

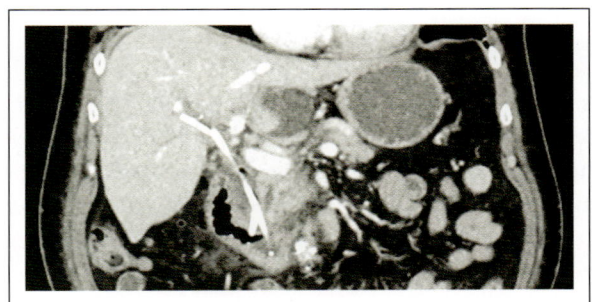

Figure 27.3 Endoprosthetic and percutaneous stenting in a patient with perihilar cholangiocarcinoma (Bismuth type IIIA).

Courtesy: Thomas M. van Gulik.

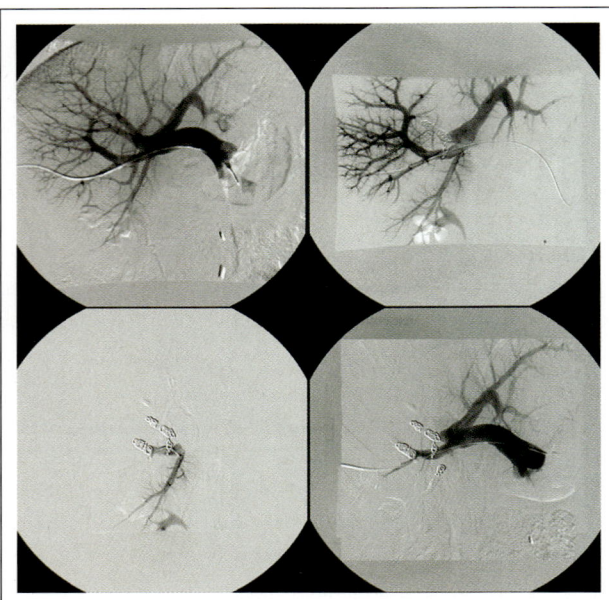

Figure 27.4 Portal vein embolisation of the right portal vein. *Courtesy*: Thomas M. van Gulik.

preferred, as parenchymal function remains compromised even after complete biliary drainage. Among the quantitative liver function tests, hepatobiliary scintigraphy provides segmental information on the actual function of the FLR.[13,14] If the functional remnant liver is insufficient, which is especially the case in patients who require an extended hemihepatectomy, selective ipsilateral portal vein embolisation (PVE) allows a safe resection (Figure 27.4). Portal vein embolisation results in the induction of compensatory hypertrophy of the FLR and reduces the risk of postresectional liver dysfunction.[15] The ALPPS (associating liver partition and portal vein ligation for staged hepatectomy) procedure for PHC is currently not advised, since the procedure for this indication is associated with high morbidity and mortality.[16]

SURGICAL RESECTION AND OPERATIVE RISKS

As mentioned above, surgical resection of the tumour is the only curative treatment for PHC. Of all patients who undergo explorative laparotomy, 40 to 70% ultimately have resectable disease.[17,18] Depending on the extent of the tumour, complete removal of the tumour can be obtained by hilar resection with en bloc (extended) hemihepatectomy, including the caudate lobe in most cases. Excision of the portal vein bifurcation, with reconstruction of the left or right veins, is performed when it is involved by the tumour. Complete lymphadenectomy of the hepatoduodenal ligament is routinely performed

along with resection. For biliary reconstruction, end-to-side anastomoses of the segmental ducts with a Roux-en-Y jejunal loop are constructed. In selected patients with Bismuth type I or II tumours, only an extrahepatic bile duct resection, without liver resection, may suffice. Frozen sections of the proximal and distal bile duct margins are routinely performed to check on tumour-free margins. This aggressive approach ensures control of the hepatic parenchymal infiltration and extension of the disease along the bile ducts and so increases the chance of an R0 resection, thereby reducing the chance of local recurrence and improving disease-free survival.[19,20]

Long-term survival depends critically on complete tumour resection. Whereas overall survival of patients receiving palliative treatment only is short (median 12 months),[21] patients with an R0 resection show median overall survival times of 30 to 46 months, and their 5-year overall survival rates range from 25 to 40%.[22,23] The best results have been reported in patients treated with neoadjuvant chemoradiotherapy and liver transplantation; however, these treatments are an option only in a carefully selected group of patients and do not apply to the majority of patients with local disease.[24]

The downside of an aggressive surgical approach for curative intent in PHC is significant postoperative morbidity and mortality. These are particularly high in patients requiring extended liver resection (five or more Couinaud segments). Reported mortality ranges from 5 to 18%, even in high-volume centres,[8,15,22,25] and morbidity is as high as 60 to 70%, with around 50% of severe complications (Clavien-Dindo grade III or higher).[26] In this chapter, we will further elaborate on typical complications and treatment of patients after partial hepatectomy for PHC. An overview of the incidence of severe complications is provided in Table 27.1.

Bleeding Complications

The risk of intraoperative bleeding in liver resection for PHC is substantial, with a reported median blood

Table 27.1 Complications and reported incidence in a selection of literature reports

Complication type	Incidence (%)
Liver failure	3–25[7,9,29,36]
Biliary leakage	6–29[7,9,29,36]
Bleeding	4–9[17,29,32]
Multiorgan failure	1–3[7,17,29]
Infections	23–66[7,17,32]
Mortality	5–18[9,15,21,29]

loss of 2 L. In other tumour types, perioperative blood transfusion is reported to be associated with an increased risk of tumour recurrence and decreased long-term survival; however, this is not as apparent in PHC, as results vary from a negative influence on survival to having no clear effect.[27,28] Intermittent vascular inflow occlusion (Pringle's manoeuvre) is recommended to reduce intraoperative blood loss during parenchymal transection, whereas control of blood loss outweighs possible ischaemic injury of the FLR.[29]

Postoperative haemorrhage according to the International Study Group of Liver Surgery (ISGLS's) guidelines entails a 4.8 mmol/L (3 g/dL) drop of haemoglobin compared with the baseline postoperative level[30] (Table 27.2). As with biliary leakage and liver failure, postoperative haemorrhage is divided into three categories according to the need of clinical management. Grade A can be managed with minimal transfusion requirements. Grade B requires a transfusion of more than two units of packed red blood cells, and coagulation products might be required. Patients with grade C are in life-threatening condition and require radiological intervention or relaparotomy to stop the bleeding. Especially in patients with a small FLR and liver failure, the synthetic capacity of the liver is diminished, resulting in coagulopathy.[31] The combination of extensive resection involving major vascular structures with decreased synthetic function of the liver results in a high risk of postoperative haemorrhage, with a reported incidence of 8% (Figure 27.5).[32,33] Patients who develop acute liver failure might have severe decrease in procoagulant and anticoagulant factors. It is important that their international normalised ratio (INR)/prothrombin time (PT) and activated partial thromboplastin time (aPTT) are monitored postoperatively. Clinically evident coagulopathy can then be corrected by administration of fresh frozen

Table 27.2 The International Study Group of Liver Surgery (ISGLS) guidelines for the definition of posthepatectomy complications

ISGLS complication grade	ISGLS definition
PHH	
Grade A	PHH requiring transfusion of up to 2 units of RBCs
Grade B	PHH requiring transfusion of >2 units of RBCs but manageable without invasive intervention
Grade C	PHH requiring radiological interventional treatment (e.g., embolisation) or relaparotomy
PHLF	
Grade A	PHLF resulting in abnormal laboratory parameters but requiring no change in the clinical management of the patient
Grade B	PHLF resulting in a deviation from the regular clinical management but manageable without invasive treatment
Grade C	PHLF resulting in a deviation from the regular management and requiring invasive treatment (e.g., haemodialysis, intubation and mechanical ventilation, extracorporeal liver support, rescue hepatectomy and transplantation)
Biliary leakage	
Grade A	Bile leakage requiring no or little change in patient's clinical management
Grade B	Bile leakage requiring a change in patient's clinical management (e.g., additional diagnostic or interventional procedures) but manageable without relaparotomy, or a grade A bile leakage lasting for >1 week
Grade C	Bile leakage requiring relaparotomy

Abbreviations: ISGLS, International Study Group of Liver Surgery; PHH, posthepatectomy haemorrhage; PHLF, posthepatectomy liver failure; RBC, red blood cell.

Adapted from: Rabhari NN, Garden JO, Padbury R, et al. Post-hepatectomy haemorrhage: a definition and grading by the International Study Group of Liver Surgery (ISLGS). *HPB* 2011;12:528–35.

Rabhari NN, Garden JO, Padbury R, et al. Posthepatectomy liver failure: a definition and grading by the International Study Group of Liver Surgery. *Surgery* 2011;149:713–24.

Koch M, Garden JO, Padbury R, et al. Bile leakage after hepatobiliary and pancreatic surgery: a definition and grading of severity by the International Study Group of Liver Surgery. *Surgery* 2011;149:680–8.

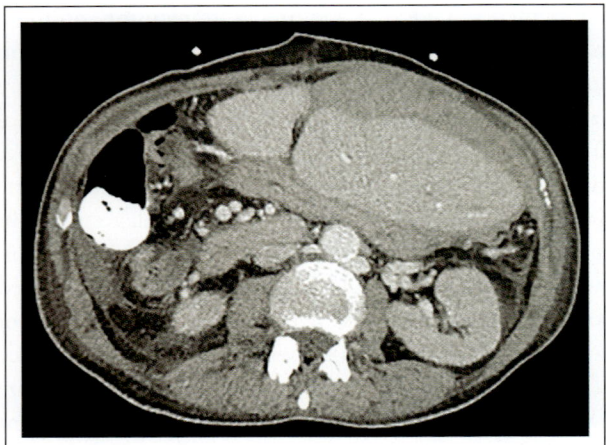

Figure 27.5 Haemorrhage after right hemihepatectomy. A haematoma is seen around the liver on computed tomography imaging.

Courtesy: Thomas M. van Gulik.

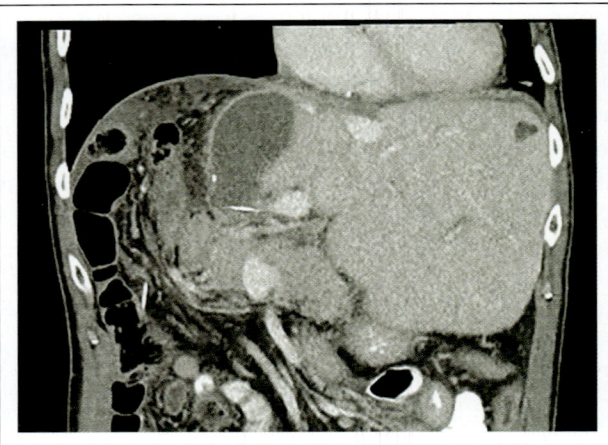

Figure 27.6 Computed tomography showing a biloma after right hemihepatectomy.

Courtesy: Thomas M. van Gulik.

plasma or other substitutes. Types of bleeding differ from postoperative development of an intra-abdominal haematoma to delayed bleeding from a pseudoaneurysm or septic bleeding due to an intra-abdominal abscess secondary to leakage of the hepaticojejunostomy. Computed tomography-angiography is advised to establish the source of bleeding. If a blush is visible, optimisation of the coagulation status and percutaneous coiling of the vessel are usually the first-line treatment.

Liver Failure

Postoperative liver failure is a dreaded complication after extensive hepatectomy and is a major cause of mortality in patients with PHC.[34] The risk of postoperative liver failure is increased due to the combination of intra-operative blood loss, a small FLR and preoperative cholestasis. Furthermore, when performing a left-sided hemihepatectomy, there is a risk of ischaemia of segments 5 and 8 due to interruption of the central ramifications of the right hepatic artery. This results in ischaemia of the said segments and will augment the risk of dysfunction of the FLR. The same applies to a right-sided hemihepatectomy, in which the arterial branch of the left hepatic artery perfusing segment 4 may be sacrificed. However, this may be a minor problem, as segment 4 is often additionally resected (extended right hemihepatectomy) (Figure 27.6). The reported incidence of liver ischaemia is 2.5 to 29%.[8,33]

There are several definitions of posthepatectomy liver failure (PHLF). The 50–50 criteria by Balzan state that a PT index <50% and a serum bilirubin >50 μg/L occurring at day 5 are strong prognostic factors.[35] This,

however, does not allow grading of different stages of liver failure. Postoperative liver failure according to ISGLS's guidelines is a postoperative deterioration in the ability of the liver remnant to maintain its synthetic, excretory and detoxifying functions, characterised by an increased INR and concomitant hyperbilirubinaemia on or after postoperative day 5. Preoperative assessment of liver function is therefore of vital importance.

According to the ISGLS's guidelines, PHLF is divided into three categories (Table 27.2).[34] It may present as a transient impairment of liver function that recovers spontaneously when the liver remnant regenerates after surgery and usually does not require a change of management (grade A). However, when by day 5, patients need fresh frozen plasma, albumin and/or other noninvasive interventions to maintain homeostasis, this is considered to be grade B liver failure. It is important that other manageable causes such as biliary obstruction are excluded and additional imaging is necessary to detect vascular complications leading to parenchymal infarction. Patients with liver failure are highly susceptible to infections, especially after previous episodes of cholangitis, in which the biliary system is infected and the function of the Kupffer cell system is depressed. Infectious parameters should therefore be monitored judiciously. When invasive treatments such as dialysis, intubation and mechanical ventilation are necessary, liver failure is classified as grade C. Mortality is reported to be 54% in these patients. Although there are liver-assist devices that aim to bridge liver function until full regeneration has occurred, a clear benefit has not been shown in the context of postresection liver failure.[36] Salvage liver transplantation is usually not an option either, as PHC in most protocols is not accepted as an indication for liver transplantation.

Biliary Leakage and Leakage of the Hepaticojejunostomy

Biliary leakage is one of the main causes of postoperative morbidity after liver surgery. It is the most common complication in patients with PHC, with an incidence of 11 to 29%.[32,33,37] One can divide biliary leakage into leakage from the cut surface of the liver and leakage of one or more of the hepaticojejunostomies; however, differentiation between the two may be difficult. The ISGLS's guideline states that bile leakage is the discharge of fluid, with an increased bilirubin concentration in the intra-abdominal drain of three times as high as the serum bilirubin on day 3, or is measured in intra-abdominal collections after reintervention at any time (Table 27.2).[38] It is divided into three stages based on the need for change in the clinical management of the patient. When biliary leakage is suspected due to biliary discharge in the abdominal drain that is usually left after a hemihepatectomy or because the patient postoperatively shows infectious symptoms, imaging is the next step. Imaging with ultrasound or contrast-enhanced CT usually reveals an intra-abdominal collection. If bile leakage originates from the cut surface of the liver, continuation of abdominal drainage or percutaneous drainage is the treatment of choice. The same approach is the initial step in the treatment of anastomotic leakage. If the leak persists for more than 5 days, a PTBD can be placed to bridge the anastomosis or to relieve leakage from one of the side braches of the biliary tract (Figure 27.7). This policy has reported success

rates of 91 to 100% after one or more attempts.[39,40] After successful PTBD placement, the abdominal drains usually cease to produce biliary fluid. This process of percutaneous drainage of a biliary leak often takes several weeks and can increase hospital stay; however, patients can often go home with the external drains. Reoperation for drainage is rarely required and should be performed only when a patient's vital parameters are severely altered and stabilisation is not possible. There is no evidence for preventive postoperative biliary drainage of the liver remnant. However, many surgeons will leave the PTBD drain(s) that was placed preoperatively across the hepaticojejunostomies in an effort to decrease pressure over the biliary-enteric anastomoses. There is no reported beneficial effect of transanastomotic drainage on the incidence of postoperative biliary leakage.[41]

Multiorgan Failure

Multiorgan failure in patients with PHC usually results from sepsis or liver failure and its sequelae. Circulatory dysfunction and hypotension are multifactorial. Low oral intake, vomiting and fluid shifts due to ascites can result in hypovolaemic shock. Management is not different from other causes of hypovolaemic shock and is based on administering fluids. Endotracheal intubation is sometimes necessary. This is often not because of respiratory failure but because of a reduced level of consciousness caused by hepatic encephalopathy. In the event of liver failure, the serum levels of ammonia are increased due to impaired detoxification of ammonia by conversion into urea. There is evidence that not only circulating neurotransmitters such as ammonia but also systemic and local inflammations play crucial roles.[31] Cerebral permeability is altered and, in combination with altered cerebral blood flow, leads to cerebral oedema and encephalopathy. Neurological management focusses on the maintenance of stable cerebral perfusion and the control of circulating ammonia. Renal dysfunction occurs in more than 50% of all patients with liver failure, and some patients may require renal replacement therapy. Renal function often normalises when liver function recovers.[31]

Infectious Complications

As in any other type of gastrointestinal surgery, infectious complications may occur after liver resection. These range from infections of the wound to those of intra-abdominal fluid collections such as bilomas, haematomas and seromas. In PHC, the frequency of infectious complications is increased because of the primary infection

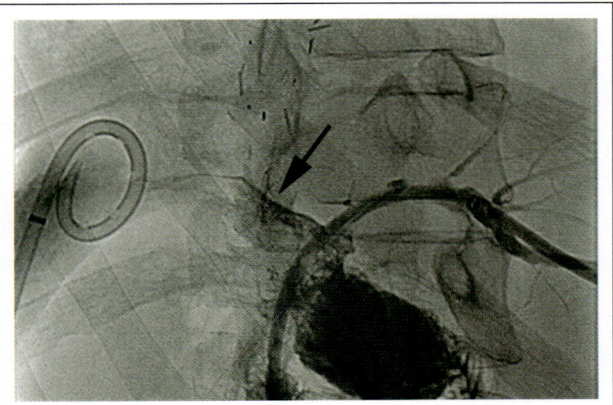

Figure 27.7 Biliary leak of the hepaticojejunostomy.
Courtesy: Thomas M. van Gulik.

of the obstructed bile ducts or the secondary infection related to the preoperative biliary stenting of the ducts. Perioperative prophylactic administration of antibiotics (e.g., a combination of gentamicin and ceftriaxone) is recommended. Infectious complications in PHC comprise 50 to 80% of all postoperative complications.[22,32] Cholangitis may occur when the biliary tract is not adequately drained preoperatively and should be treated with biliary drainage and antibiotics. Postoperative hepatic fluid collections may develop late and are usually adjacent to the resection area. These should also be treated with ultrasound-guided percutaneous drainage, as for any other abdominal fluid collections. Pneumonia is also frequent because of the location of the surgical site being close to the diaphragm and the fact that patients are often bedbound the first days after surgery. Optimal analgesia and physiotherapy can reduce the risk of pneumonia. Patients may present with a solitary liver abscess for years after resection. This usually is a sequel of a localised, low-grade cholangitis with late manifestation but may also indicate segmental biliary obstruction due to a stricture of (one of the) hepaticojejunostomies or due to local tumour recurrence. The abscess usually responds well to percutaneous drainage in combination with antibiotic treatment.

CONCLUSIONS

Since morbidity and mortality rates after liver resection for PHC are higher than those after hepatic surgery for other indications, it is important to pay attention to risk factors before surgery. Both patient-related factors and surgical parameters contribute to operative risks, resulting in a high incidence of postoperative complications. These risk factors include preoperative cholangitis,[9,25,33] small functional liver remnant volume and the extent of the liver resection,[9,25] portal vein reconstruction,[15] intraoperative blood loss,[25] old age[9] and low skeletal muscle mass.[42] However, several of these factors can be determined only intraoperatively. It is important for the care team that careful risk assessment is performed preoperatively and that attention is paid to shared decision making by identifying high-risk patients. Patients with multiple risk factors such as old age, cholangitis and the need for extended resection with vascular reconstruction clearly carry a high risk of mortality and morbidity and should receive thorough preoperative counselling. Since morbidity and mortality rates are high even in specialised units, liver surgery for PHC should be performed only in these centres. Referral to a tertiary facility is recommended at an early stage for adequate assessment and preoperative optimisation of the patient.

In conclusion, resection for PHC is a high-risk surgery with significant morbidity and mortality rates. Awareness of the several types of complications is essential for adequate monitoring and treatment of complications after hemihepatectomy. The challenge in the near future is to decrease operative risk through intensive preoperative assessment and proper preparation of patients before surgery.

REFERENCES

1. Aljiffry M, Abdulelah A, Walsh M, Peltekian K, Alwayn I, Molinari M. Evidence-based approach to cholangiocarcinoma: a systematic review of the current literature. *J Am Coll Surg* 2009;208:134–47.

2. Nakeeb A, Pitt HA, Sohn TA, et al. Cholangiocarcinoma. A spectrum of intrahepatic, perihilar, and distal tumors. *Ann Surg* 1996;224:463–73; discussion 473–5.

3. Khan SA, Thomas HC, Davidson BR, Taylor-Robinson SD. Cholangiocarcinoma. *Lancet* 2005;366:1303–14.

4. Razumilava N, Gores GJ. Cholangiocarcinoma. *Lancet* 2014;383:2168–79.

5. Ruys AT, Busch OR, Rauws EA, Gouma DJ, van Gulik TM. Prognostic impact of preoperative imaging parameters on resectability of hilar cholangiocarcinoma. *HPB Surg* 2013; 2013:657309.

6. Engelbrecht MR, Katz SS, van Gulik TM, Lameris JS, van Delden OM. Imaging of perihilar cholangiocarcinoma. *AJR Am J Roentgenol* 2015;204:782–91.

7. Kloek JJ, van Delden OM, Erdogan D, et al. Differentiation of malignant and benign proximal bile duct strictures: the diagnostic dilemma. *World J Gastroenterol* 2008;14: 5032–8.

8. Hemming AW, Reed AI, Fujita S, Foley DP, Howard RJ. Surgical management of hilar cholangiocarcinoma. *Ann Surg* 2005;241:693–702.

9. Wiggers JK, Groot Koerkamp B, Cieslak KP, et al. Postoperative mortality after liver resection for perihilar cholangiocarcinoma: development of a risk score and importance of biliary drainage of the future liver remnant. *J Am Coll Surg* 2016;223:321–31.e1.

10. Ribero D, Zimmitti G, Aloia TA, et al. Preoperative cholangitis and future liver remnant volume determine the risk of liver failure in patients undergoing resection for hilar cholangiocarcinoma. *J Am Coll Surg* 2016;223:87–97.

11. Farges O, Regimbeau JM, Fuks D, et al. Multicentre European study of preoperative biliary drainage for hilar cholangiocarcinoma. *Br J Surg* 2013;100:274–83.

12. Wiggers JK, Groot Koerkamp B, Coelen RJ, et al. Preoperative biliary drainage in perihilar cholangiocarcinoma: identifying patients who require percutaneous drainage after failed endoscopic drainage. *Endoscopy* 2015;47:1124–31.

13. Mansour JC, Aloia TA, Crane CH, Heimbach JK, Nagino M, Vauthey JN. Hilar Cholangiocarcinoma: expert consensus statement. *HPB (Oxford)* 2015;17:691–9.

14. Clavien PA, Oberkofler CE, Raptis DA, Lehmann K, Rickenbacher A, El-Badry AM. What is critical for liver surgery and partial liver transplantation: size or quality? *Hepatology* 2010;52:715–29.

15. de Jong MC, Marques H, Clary BM, et al. The impact of portal vein resection on outcomes for hilar cholangiocarcinoma: a multi-institutional analysis of 305 cases. *Cancer* 2012;118:4737–47.

16. Oldhafer KJ, Stavrou GA, van Gulik TM, Core G. ALPPS—Where do we stand, where do we go?: eight recommendations from the First International Expert Meeting. *Ann Surg* 2016;263:839–41.

17. Matsuo K, Rocha FG, Ito K, et al. The Blumgart preoperative staging system for hilar cholangiocarcinoma: analysis of resectability and outcomes in 380 patients. *J Am Coll Surg* 2012;215:343–55.

18. Coelen RJ, Ruys AT, Wiggers JK, et al. Development of a risk score to predict detection of metastasized or locally advanced perihilar cholangiocarcinoma at staging laparoscopy. *Ann Surg Oncol* 2016;30:4163–73.

19. Kosuge T, Yamamoto J, Shimada K, Yamasaki S, Makuuchi M. Improved surgical results for hilar cholangiocarcinoma with procedures including major hepatic resection. *Ann Surg* 1999;230:663–71.

20. van Gulik TM, Kloek JJ, Ruys AT, et al. Multidisciplinary management of hilar cholangiocarcinoma (Klatskin tumor): extended resection is associated with improved survival. *Eur J Surg Oncol* 2011;37:65–71.

21. Valle J, Wasan H, Palmer DH, et al. Cisplatin plus gemcitabine versus gemcitabine for biliary tract cancer. *N Engl J Med* 2010;362:1273–81.

22. Ito F, Cho CS, Rikkers LF, Weber SM. Hilar cholangiocarcinoma: current management. *Ann Surg* 2009;250:210–8.

23. Groot Koerkamp B, Wiggers JK, Gonen M, et al. Survival after resection of perihilar cholangiocarcinoma-development and external validation of a prognostic nomogram. *Ann Oncol* 2016;27:753.

24. Gores GJ, Darwish Murad S, Heimbach JK, Rosen CB. Liver transplantation for perihilar cholangiocarcinoma. *Dig Dis* 2013;31:126–9.

25. Nagino M, Ebata T, Yokoyama Y, et al. Evolution of surgical treatment for perihilar cholangiocarcinoma: a single-center 34-year review of 574 consecutive resections. *Ann Surg* 2013;258:129–40.

26. Coelen RJ, Olthof PB, van Dieren S, Besselink MG, Busch OR, van Gulik TM. External validation of the Estimation of Physiologic Ability and Surgical Stress (E-PASS) risk model to predict operative risk in perihilar cholangiocarcinoma. *JAMA Surg* 2016;151:1132–8.

27. Dekker AM, Wiggers JK, Coelen RJ, van Golen RF, Besselink MG, Busch OR, et al. Perioperative blood transfusion is not associated with overall survival or time to recurrence after resection of perihilar cholangiocarcinoma. *HPB (Oxford)* 2016;18:262–70.

28. Kimura N, Toyoki Y, Ishido K, et al. Perioperative blood transfusion as a poor prognostic factor after aggressive surgical resection for hilar cholangiocarcinoma. *J Gastrointest Surg* 2015;19:866–79.

29. van Riel WG, van Golen RF, Reiniers MJ, Heger M, van Gulik TM. How much ischemia can the liver tolerate during resection? *Hepatobiliary Surg Nutr* 2016;5:58–71.

30. Rahbari NN, Garden OJ, Padbury R, et al. Post-hepatectomy haemorrhage: a definition and grading by the International Study Group of Liver Surgery (ISGLS). *HPB (Oxford)* 2011;13:528–35.

31. Bernal W, Wendon J. Acute liver failure. *N Engl J Med* 2013; 369:2525–34.

32. Jarnagin WR, Fong Y, DeMatteo RP, et al. Staging, resectability, and outcome in 225 patients with hilar cholangiocarcinoma. *Ann Surg* 2001;234:507–17; discussion 517–9.

33. Dumitrascu T, Brasoveanu V, Stroescu C, Ionescu M, Popescu I. Major hepatectomies for perihilar cholangiocarcinoma: Predictors for clinically relevant postoperative complications using the International Study Group of Liver Surgery definitions. *Asian J Surg* 2016;39:81–9.

34. Rahbari NN, Garden OJ, Padbury R, et al. Posthepatectomy liver failure: a definition and grading by the International Study Group of Liver Surgery (ISGLS). *Surgery* 2011;149:713–24.

35. Balzan S, Belghiti J, Farges O, et al. The "50-50 criteria" on postoperative day 5: an accurate predictor of liver failure and death after hepatectomy. *Ann Surg* 2005;242:824–8; discussion 828–9.

36. van de Kerkhove MP, de Jong KP, Rijken AM, de Pont AC, van Gulik TM. MARS treatment in posthepatectomy liver failure. *Liver Int* 2003;23:44–51.

37. Regimbeau JM, Fuks D, Le Treut YP, et al. Surgery for hilar cholangiocarcinoma: a multi-institutional update on practice and outcome by the AFC-HC study group. *J Gastrointest Surg* 2011;15:480–8.

38. Koch M, Garden OJ, Padbury R, et al. Bile leakage after hepatobiliary and pancreatic surgery: a definition and grading of severity by the International Study Group of Liver Surgery. *Surgery* 2011;149:680–8.

39. Hoekstra LT, van Gulik TM, Gouma DJ, Busch OR. Posthepatectomy bile leakage: how to manage. *Dig Surg* 2012;29:48–53.

40. de Jong EA, Moelker A, Leertouwer T, Spronk S, Van Dijk M, van Eijck CH. Percutaneous transhepatic biliary drainage in patients with postsurgical bile leakage and nondilated intrahepatic bile ducts. *Dig Surg* 2013;30:444–50.

41. Olthof PB, Coelen RJ, Wiggers JK, Besselink MG, Busch OR, van Gulik TM. External biliary drainage following major liver resection for perihilar cholangiocarcinoma: impact on development of liver failure and biliary leakage. *HPB (Oxford)* 2016;18:348–53.

42. Coelen RJ, Wiggers JK, Nio CY, et al. Preoperative computed tomography assessment of skeletal muscle mass is valuable in predicting outcomes following hepatectomy for perihilar cholangiocarcinoma. *HPB (Oxford)* 2015;17:520–8.

28

How to Prevent, Diagnose and Treat Major Biliary and Vasculobiliary Injuries after Cholecystectomy

S.M. Strasberg

ABSTRACT

Biliary injury is a very morbid and costly complication of gallbladder surgery. It increased in frequency after the introduction of laparoscopic cholecystectomy. This chapter deals with the pathogenesis of biliary injury, strategies to avoid biliary injury, the presentation of biliary injury, and its medical and surgical management. A concluding section discusses the complex problem of vasculobiliary injuries, in which the vascular component may be of greater consequence than the biliary injury.

KEYWORDS

Biliary injury, bile duct injury, vasculobiliary injury, laparoscopic cholecystectomy, cholecystectomy, critical view of safety, infundibular technique

INTRODUCTION

Biliary injury is the most common severe complication of cholecystectomy. It is always morbid, increases cost and often leads to litigation. Although the likelihood of sustaining a major biliary injury as a result of cholecystectomy is low, that is, in the order of 3 to 4 per 1000 procedures, cholecystectomy is such a common procedure that bile duct injuries are fairly common. In the United States, where 700,000 cholecystectomies are performed per year, about 2500 major injuries occur annually; however, the exact data are missing. This chapter will deal with the prevention, diagnosis and treatment of major biliary injuries, including vasculobiliary injuries (VBIs). Our classification of biliary injuries is shown in Figure 28.1.[1] There is no general agreement on what constitutes a major biliary injury; most authorities consider type A injuries to be 'minor', even though they can be associated with considerable morbidity. Type D injuries are sometimes also considered minor. Conversely, all type E injuries are major. Injuries to aberrant ducts, that is, types B and C injuries, are usually intermediate in morbidity but will be included in this discussion of major injuries.

PATHOGENESIS OF BILIARY INJURIES

Several types of factors may contribute to biliary injury. These may be classified as patient-, procedure- and surgeon/hospital-related factors. Awareness of these will help prevent injury.

Patient-Related Factors

The main patient-related factors are inflammation and congenital anomalies of the bile ducts.

Inflammation

Acute cholecystitis

Acute cholecystitis may be mild, moderate or severe, as per Tokyo Guidelines 2013 (TG13).[2] The difficulty

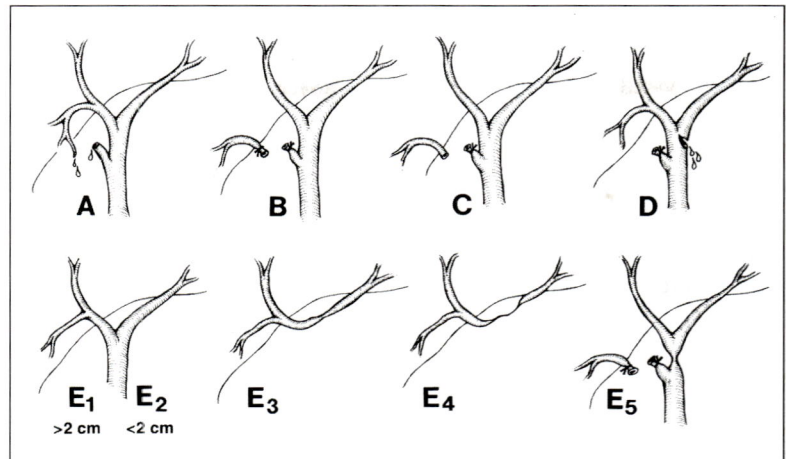

Figure 28.1 A classification of injuries to the biliary tract. The injury types A to E are illustrated. Type A injuries may originate from small bile ducts that are entered in the liver bed or from the cystic duct. Types B and C injuries usually involve aberrant right hepatic ducts. The notations >2 cm and <2 cm in type E1 and type E2 indicate the length of common hepatic duct remaining.

Reprinted with permissions from: Journal of the American College of Surgeons.

of cholecystectomy is not increased when mild acute cholecystitis is present, but it often does increases when it is moderately severe, and this is manifested by increased conversion rates.[3] The criteria for moderate severity include elapse of more than 72 hours between onset of symptoms and surgery, a palpable inflammatory mass and white blood cell count of more than 18,000 cells/mm.[3] Under these conditions, the inflammatory mass may effectively obliterate the hepatocystic triangle and increase difficulty of exposure of the cystic duct and artery (Figure 28.2).

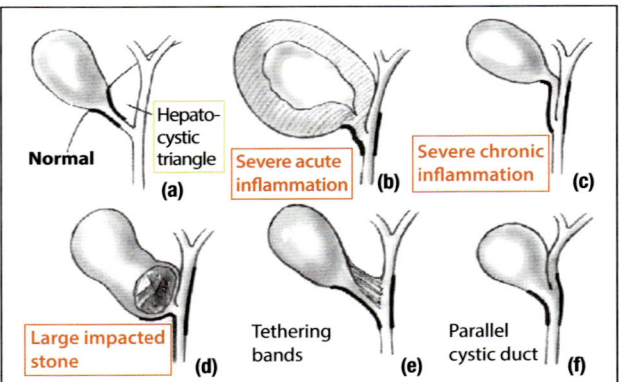

Chronic inflammation

Chronic inflammation is present in the majority of patients undergoing cholecystectomy for cholelithiasis and usually does not present major difficulty. In a minority of patients, the chronic inflammation may be severe, with dense scarring and tissue contraction due to repeated bouts of acute cholecystitis. Fibrotic contraction may shrink the gallbladder and bind it to the common hepatic duct and right hepatic artery and effectively obliterate the hepatocystic triangle (Figure 28.2). It also may result in strong adhesion to surrounding structures such as omentum, duodenum and colon or even fistulisation to the duodenum. Such inflammation may make dissection very difficult, contribute to misidentification and rarely be associated with 'extreme VBIs'[4] when certain identification techniques are used.

Figure 28.2 Conditions that predispose to the deception that the common bile duct is the cystic duct, especially when the infundibular techniques is used. (a): Condition of minimal inflammation in which the hepatocystic triangle is open and the funnel shape of the junction between the gallbladder and cystic duct (heavy line) is readily apparent. The infundibular technique is effective under these conditions. (b–f): Conditions that may give a misleading funnel shape (heavy lines) because of obliteration or concealment of the hepatocystic triangle. In these cases, the common bile duct is dissected because it appears to be the cystic duct widening into the gallbladder (b): severe acute cholecystitis, with obliteration of the hepatocystic triangle; (c): severe chronic inflammation with the same effect; (d): parallel cystic duct insertion; (e): congenital bands; (f): large impacted stone).

Rerinted with permission from: Swanstrom LL, Soper NJ. Mastery of Endoscopic and Laparoscopic Surgery. 4th ed. Philadelphia, PA: LWW; 2014.

Congenital Abnormalities

Aberrant right hepatic duct

This is the main anomaly associated with biliary injury. The aberrant low-lying right hepatic duct is a well-recognised risk factor for biliary injury and is present in 2 to 3% of patients. The most perilous situation occurs when the aberrant right duct actually joins the cystic duct and the united duct then joins with the common hepatic duct (Figure 28.3). The appearance of the junction of the united duct with the common hepatic duct is identical to that of a normal union of the cystic duct with the common hepatic duct. Consequently, there is a great potential for misidentification injury.

Other congenital abnormalities

Other congenital abnormalities may contribute to biliary injury but are of less importance. The parallel union cystic duct (Figure 28.2) occurs in about 20% of individuals. It was a well-described risk factor for biliary injury, even in the era of open cholecystectomy. The cystic duct may also insert into the biliary tree at any point from the right hepatic duct to the termination of the common bile duct. Congenital adhesions between the gallbladder and common hepatic duct may exist. Such adhesions are prominent in some individuals. They obscure the hepatocystic triangle and may fix the common hepatic duct to the side of the gallbladder (Figure 28.2). There is considerable variation in the size of bile duct from person to person. The internal diameter of the cystic duct

is normally 2 to 3 mm, which would make the external diameter about 3 to 5 mm. The normal external diameter of the supraduodenal common bile ducts ranges from 4 to 13 mm, but the normal internal diameter, measured by ultrasound, is considered to be 3 to 8 mm. Rarely, duct size may be less than these norms, and this may expose the ducts to injury. Length of the cystic duct is highly variable. A congenitally absent cystic duct is rare. An absent cystic duct is usually due to effacement of the cystic duct by a stone and is usually accompanied by severe inflammation. Rarely, a hepatic duct may actually enter the gallbladder. These are usually small accessory ducts, often referred to as ducts of Luschka. These are usually 1 mm or less in diameter. An injury to a duct of Luschka is difficult to recognise. In about 10% of individuals, a right hepatic duct measuring 2 to 3 mm in diameter lies immediately deep to the cystic plate. It is in danger of injury if the cystic plate is penetrated when dissecting the gallbladder. Sometimes, the gallbladder is intrahepatic, with only a small portion of the wall evident. Such gallbladders are hard to grasp and indirectly contribute to injury by making it difficult to expose the cystic duct.

Large Impacted Gallstones

These are often mentioned in operative notes of cholecystectomies in which biliary injuries have occurred. They tend to impair retraction and hide the cystic duct (Figure 28.2).

Obesity and Body Habitus

Obesity is common in patients undergoing cholecystectomy. Morbid obesity and large body size, in general, contribute to difficulty in operative exposure. The same is true of skeletal deformities.

Procedure-Related Factors

Most major bile duct injuries are due to misidentification of bile ducts. Therefore, the most important procedure-related factor is the use of techniques that are sometimes misleading to the surgeon in respect to the identity of bile ducts.

Misidentification: A Concept Problem

There are two main types of bile duct misidentification: misidentification of the common bile duct as the cystic duct (Figure 28.4) and misidentification of an aberrant right hepatic duct as the cystic duct (Figure 28.3).

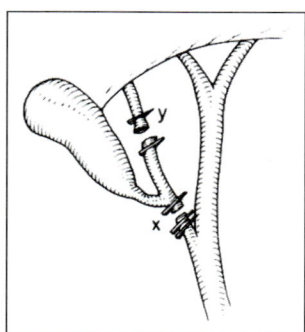

Figure 28.3 Aberrant right duct, which unites with the cystic duct before joining the common hepatic duct. The united cystic/aberrant duct at point X looks just like the cystic duct to the surgeon. To get the gallbladder out, the duct must be cut again at point Y. If it is clipped, as shown, a B injury will occur. If it is just cut, a C injury will result.

Reprinted with permissions from: Journal of the American College of Surgeons.

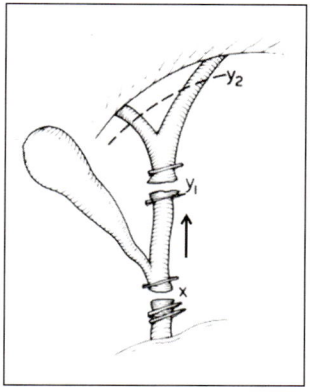

Figure 28.4 Patterns of biliary injury due to misidentification. A: The 'classical' type E injury in which the common duct is divided between clips at point x. The dissection is then carried up the left side of the common hepatic duct (arrow) and the ductal system is later divided again to remove the gallbladder either at point y1, producing E1 or E2 injury, or at point y2, producing E3 or E4 injuriy. The right hepatic artery is often injured at the second division of the biliary tree at point y1.

Reprinted with permissions from: Journal of the American College of Surgeons.

Misidentification of the common bile duct occurs when the surgeon identifies the common bile duct as the cystic duct and then clips and divides it. After transection of the common bile duct, the dissection is carried along the left side of the common hepatic duct in the belief that the dissection is proceeding along the underside of the gallbladder. Finally, to get to the cystic plate on which the gallbladder rests, the common hepatic duct is divided (Figure 28.4). The right hepatic artery is often injured at the same time (*see* **Vasculobiliary Injuries**). This is the so-called 'classical injury.'[5]

The type of injury produced may be E1 to E4 and depends upon the level of the second transection. Higher levels of transection may result from traction on the gallbladder, pulling the hepatic ducts down into the field where they are divided (Figure 28.4). In operative notes of such procedures, it is not unusual to find references to a 'second cystic duct' or an 'accessory cystic duct', which really is the common hepatic duct or higher-level biliary duct.

The second type of misidentification leads to an injury to an aberrant right hepatic duct (types B and C injuries). The piece of the aberrant hepatic duct, between entry of cystic duct and junction with the common hepatic, is mistaken to be the cystic duct (Figure 28.3). The misidentified section is clipped and usually cut. To remove the gallbladder, the aberrant duct must be cut again at a higher level.

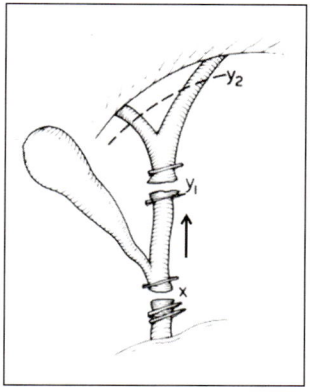

Identification Techniques

The key to understanding why misidentification occurs requires examining the rationale for identification of the cystic structures during cholecystectomy. There are five techniques in general use. These are the 'infundibular technique', cholangiography, dissection of the cystic duct to the confluence with the common hepatic duct and the common bile duct, the 'critical view of safety' (CVS) technique and the 'fundus down' (or 'top down' or 'antegrade') technique.

Infundibular technique

This technique depends on the display of the funnel-shaped junction of the lower end of the gallbladder with the cystic duct (funnel = infundibulum) (Figure 28.2). In the infundibular method, the surgeon is instructed to follow the putative cystic duct up to the gallbladder or the gallbladder down to the cystic duct, at which point, after circumferential dissection of these structures, the funnel-shaped union of cystic duct with the gallbladder is displayed. It is this flaring that was believed to provide conclusive identification of the infundibulocystic junction and, therefore, safe identification of the cystic duct. However, we have collected numerous operative notes of biliary injuries in which the surgeon describes following what was thought to be the cystic duct (actually the circumferentially dissected common bile duct) to a point that it seemed to flare into the gallbladder. In retrospect, the mistaken 'flare' occurred when the common bile duct was followed up to an inflammatory mass within which the cystic duct was hidden (hidden cystic duct syndrome).[6] This visual deception is most likely to occur when one or more factors described above are present—severe acute or chronic inflammation, a large stone in the Hartmann's pouch, adhesive bands, intrahepatic gallbladder and a short cystic duct (Figure 28.2).

Intraoperative cholangiography

Intraoperative cholangiography (IOC) reduces the severity of biliary injury, and it may reduce the incidence of injuries. Unfortunately, operative cholangiograms are sometime misinterpreted. The most common misinterpretation is the failure to recognise that when only the lower part of the biliary tree is seen, the common bile duct rather than the cystic duct has been incised and cannulated. In addition, IOC is not effective at detecting aberrant right ducts, which unite with the cystic duct before joining the common duct. The aberrant duct appears to be the cystic duct visually and on cholangiograms. Since the

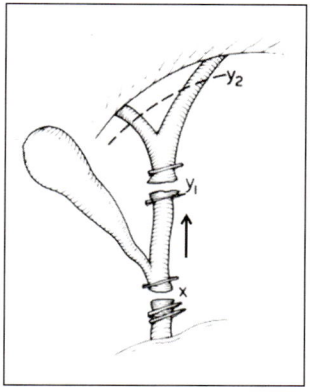

aberrant duct is usually a segmental or sectional duct, other right-sided hepatic ducts can still fill, and these are taken to represent the entire right-sided system. Since it is not unusual to obtain only partial filling of the right hepatic ducts by IOC, this is taken as a normal pattern.

Dissection of the cystic duct to the confluence with the common hepatic duct and the common bile duct

This was a common and usually safe technique when performing open cholecystectomy. There is reason to believe that its use during laparoscopic cholecystectomy has been associated with an increase in lateral injuries to the common hepatic duct (type D).

The 'critical view technique'

This technique recommends clearing the hepatocystic triangle of fat and fibrous tissue and taking the gallbladder off the lower part of its attachment to the gallbladder bed (cystic plate). Only two structures will be connected to the lower end of the gallbladder once this is done. Raising the gallbladder off the lower part of the cystic plate is an important step, equivalent in the open technique to taking the gallbladder completely off the cystic plate.[7] No attempt is made to expose the common bile duct or the common hepatic duct. A picture of the critical view is shown in Figure 28.5. This view provides conclusive and convincing demonstration that the two structures entering the gallbladder are the cystic duct and artery.[7] Taking a photo

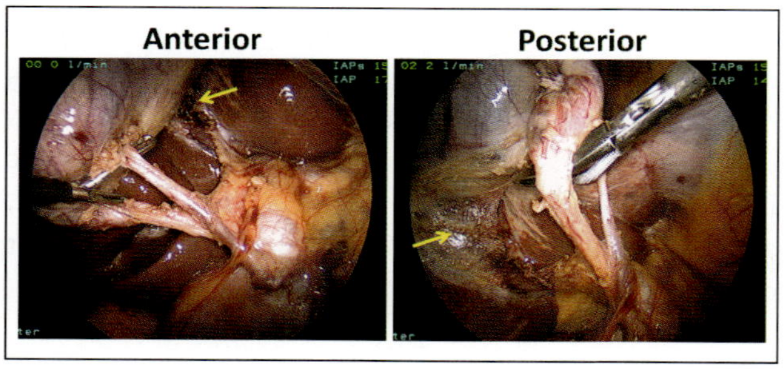

Figure 28.5 A doublet view of the 'critical view of safety'. The hepatocystic triangle has been dissected free of all tissue, except for cystic duct and artery, and the base of the cystic plate has been exposed (yellow arrows). When this view is achieved, the two structures entering the gallbladder can only be the cystic duct and artery. It is not necessary to see the common bile duct.

Reprinted with permission from: Sanford DE, Strasberg SM. A simple effective method for generation of a permanent record of the Critical View of Safety during laparoscopic cholecystectomy by intraoperative "doublet" photography. *J Am Coll Surg* 2014;218:170–8.

from the front and a photo from the back of the hepatocystic triangle, which we have named 'doublet photography' results in a good recording of the critical view.[8]

Fundus-down (or 'top-down') cholecystectomy

In this technique, the cholecystectomy is started at the fundus, taking the gallbladder off the cystic plate before any dissection or identification of structures in Calot triangle. The 'fundus-down' method seeks to pedunculate the gallbladder on the cystic artery and the cystic duct, thus making secure identification. Although it may be an effective technique of identification in most instances, our experience is that it may lead to serious biliary and vascular injuries in the presence of severe inflammation[4] (*see* **Vasculobiliary Injuries**).

Other Procedural Issues that May Contribute to Misidentification

Direction of traction

When the Hartmann's pouch is pulled superiorly rather than laterally, the cystic and common bile ducts appear to be a single continuous structure. This may contribute to the illusion that the common bile duct is the cystic duct.

Single-incision laparoscopic cholecystectomy

This technique has recently been introduced into the clinical practice. It adds to the technical difficulty of laparoscopic cholecystectomy. Although it is possible to obtain the critical view with the single-incision technique, it is more difficult. The future of the technique is uncertain at this time, given the lack of convincing clinical benefit and the possibility of increased risk of bile duct injury.

Technical Problems

Thermal injuries

Thermal injuries are more likely to occur in the presence of severe inflammation, because haemorrhage is more common when dissecting in the face of acute inflammation, and higher power settings may be used to control haemorrhage. These injuries are often not recognised at surgery and usually result in bile duct stenosis rather than loss of continuity. Division of adhesions with cautery may lead to bowel or bile duct injury if the adhesion is connected to these structures by a narrow isthmus, along which all the electrical energy must pass.

Injury to a bile duct in the course of dissection

Bile ducts may be injured in the course of dissection much in the same way as an enterotomy occurs in the course of dissecting adhesions. Inflammation, aberrant anatomy and large body habitus contribute to the likelihood of this occurrence. This will often lead to bile leakage during the procedure.

Failure to obtain secure closure of the cystic duct

The cystic duct is normally occluded with metallic clips. These are not as reliable as ligatures or suture ligatures, which were the standard methods of cystic duct closure during open cholecystectomy. When the duct is thick, rigid or wide, clips may fail and their use should usually be avoided under these circumstances. Endoloops or staplers may be used instead. Clips may cross or 'scissor' during application, resulting in poor closure, or be loosened by subsequent dissection.

Tenting injuries

The junction of the common bile duct and hepatic bile ducts may be occluded when clipping the cystic duct, while pulling up forcefully on the gallbladder. This is a very uncommon laparoscopic injury, perhaps due to the magnification afforded by laparoscopy.

Surgeon/Hospital-Related Factors

Learning Curve Effect

Inexperience with laparoscopic cholecystectomy was a well-documented cause of bile duct injuries in the first few years of the introduction of laparoscopic cholecystectomy. The likelihood of biliary injury was much greater during the early experience of a surgeon than subsequently. Cholecystectomy during the attack of acute cholecystitis is a more difficult and less commonly performed operation than elective cholecystectomy. It is possible that inexperience in the procedure during acute cholecystitis is still contributing to injury.

The lack of experience with difficult open cholecystectomy may already be a problem, as few graduating residents have much experience with this type of surgery.

Equipment

Laparoscopic equipment must be regularly maintained. Focal loss of insulation on instruments used to cauterise tissues can result in arcing and thermal injuries to bile ducts or bowel.

AVOIDANCE OF BILIARY INJURIES

Biliary injuries are best avoided by understanding the circumstances in which biliary injuries are likely to occur and the mechanisms of injuries under these circumstances. Biliary injuries cannot be completely eliminated. They may occur even in the hands of highly skilled surgeons when operative conditions are difficult.

General

Only surgeons trained and proctored in laparoscopic cholecystectomy should perform the procedure. Since laparoscopic cholecystectomy for acute cholecystitis is more difficult, it should not be attempted until experience is gained. When inflammation is severe and mandates conversion, the open procedure may also be very difficult, especially for the surgeon inexperienced in difficult open cholecystectomy. Therefore, effective 'bailout' strategies need to be available to the surgeon when conditions do not permit cholecystectomy.

Misidentification Injuries

Although still in widespread use, the author believes that the infundibular technique ought to be discarded as a sole means of ductal identification.[6] It is an error trap, that is, it works well in most circumstances and seems to be very reliable, but it is actually prone to failure under particular circumstances, which are occasionally present in patients requiring cholecystectomy. The author favours the identification of biliary anatomy by the CVS technique, since this method is good at identifying the cystic duct, even when aberrant ducts are present. If this method is not used, then routine-use cholangiography is recommended. Operative cholangiography provides a permanent record, but this can also be obtained by intraoperative photography.[8] Taking one photo of the CVS from an anterior view and another from a posterior view (doublet photography) provides an accurate record of the CVS.

There will never be a randomised trial of CVS, because to detect a difference between a bile duct injury rate of 0.1%, which was the rate in the era of open cholecystectomy, and a bile duct injury rate of 0.4%, at 95% confidence limit, it would take a trial of 4500 patients per arm. However, the utility of CVS in preventing injury has been supported by a number of observational studies.[9–13] The CVS technique works because it reproduces a time-tested method of identification in open cholecystectomy, in which the cystic duct and artery are identified but not divided until the gallbladder is free of the liver and hanging only by these two structures. In CVS, only part of the gallbladder is freed from the cystic plate but enough is freed so that it is clear that once the cystic structures are divided, the only step that will be needed to complete the resection will be to take the gallbladder off the rest of the cystic plate.

The infundibular technique, in which the funnel-shaped infundibular–cystic duct junction is the rationale for identification, is much easier to achieve than CVS. However, biliary inflammatory fusion and contraction can make the common bile duct resemble the cystic duct when this technique is used,[6] and this increases the chance of biliary injury. The CVS method protects against injury, because when the CVS has not been achieved after a reasonable trial of dissection, the surgeon is more likely to realise that conditions are too difficult to proceed in the usual manner and opt for a different approach before a biliary injury occurs. It is good that the CVS method prevents biliary injury, but if there is to be an effective and safe method of dealing with difficult gallbladders, it must include the safe and effective bailout technique, when CVS cannot be attained. By safe, we mean without bile duct injury, and by effective, we mean without need for a second operation. Otherwise, the surgeon will be tempted to push on with a risky dissection in the hepatocystic triangle, in order to avoid a second procedure or perform a cholecystostomy, which will usually necessitate a second operation. Stated otherwise, it is a good thing when surgeons reach this point in the operation, but obviously, there should be a good way to proceed when it is time to abandon the thought to do a total cholecystectomy.

Technical Problems

Injury to a Bile Duct in the Course of Dissection

Avoidance depends on the principles of careful dissection and experience, as well as recognition of circumstances in which the potential hazard in continued dissection may outweigh the benefit of completing a cholecystectomy, as outlined above.

Failure to Obtain Secure Closure of the Cystic Duct

The tips of clips should be noted to project beyond the cystic duct and to be free of any extraneous material. Clips should not be manipulated in the subsequent dissection. Preformed ligature loops should be used for closure of the cystic duct if the cystic duct is thick, rigid or wide.

Thermal Injuries

Cautery should be used with great care in the porta hepatis. The surgeon must be sure that low cautery settings are used, that only small 1- to 2-mm pieces of tissue are divided at one time and that the coagulating surfaces of instruments are not contacting adjacent tissues. Low cautery settings are essential, characteristically 30 W or less. The cystic duct should not be divided by diathermy, since this can lead to thermal necrosis of the cystic duct stump or adjacent bile duct. Attempts to stop haemorrhage by blind application of cautery clamps or by clips is very unwise. Brisk bleeding usually requires conversion. Adhesions should be divided sharply or with minimum application of power.

Tenting Injuries

The injury is avoided by not lifting the gallbladder forcefully when applying clips to the cystic duct. The lowest clip on the cystic duct should be applied first and in such a way that a portion of the cystic duct can be seen between the clip and the presumed site of the common bile duct.

Bailout Options

When after a trial of dissection the CVS cannot be obtained, the surgeon should consider abandoning the attempt to perform a laparoscopic cholecystectomy. Options include conversion to an open cholecystectomy, cholecystostomy or subtotal cholecystectomy. The latter two procedures may be done laparoscopically or open, depending upon laparoscopic skills. Rarely, the inflammation may be so severe that even the dome of the gallbladder cannot be securely identified. The best approach in these circumstances may be to enlist the help of a hepatopancreatobiliary (HPB) surgeon, even if that means discontinuance of the procedure and referral to another hospital.

Subtotal Fenestrating Cholecystectomy and Subtotal Reconstituting Cholecystectomy

These operations have been used for many years.[14,15] However, there is a lot of confusion in this area, because the terms partial cholecystectomy and subtotal cholecystectomy have been used interchangeably. 'Partial' and 'subtotal' are imprecise, because they fail to encompass an essential element in these operations, which is whether a functional remnant gallbladder may result as a consequence of performing these procedures. Therefore, a new terminology has been introduced recently to cover this aspect of the procedures.[16] In the 'subtotal fenestrating cholecystectomy', the peritonealised gallbladder wall is removed but the part of the wall on the cystic plate is left behind or only partially removed (Figure 28.6). The cystic duct is left open or sutured from

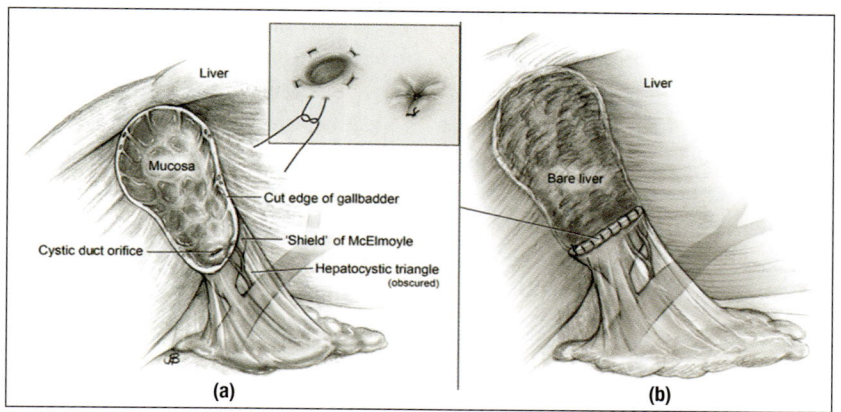

Figure 28.6 Different forms of subtotal cholecystectomy. (a) Fenestrating subtotal cholecystectomy. The free, peritonealised portion of the gallbladder has been excised, except for a lip at the lowest portion of the gallbladder. This acts as a shield to protect against inadvertently entering the hepatocystic triangle ('Shield' of McElmoyle). The portion of the gallbladder adherent to the liver has been left in situ. Stones have been extracted. The cut edge of the gallbladder may be oversewn. The mucosa is usually ablated. The cystic duct may be closed from the inside with a purse-string suture (inset). The cystic duct may be very short, and attempts to ligate the cystic duct outside the gallbladder may result in injury to the common bile duct. (b) Subtotal reconstituting cholecystectomy. The free, peritonealised portion of the gallbladder has been excised. The lowest portion of the gallbladder is closed with sutures or staples reconstituting an intact lumen, in which stones may reform. Whether the subtotal cholecystectomy is 'fenestrating' or 'reconstituting' depends on whether the lowest part of the gallbladder is left open (fenestrating) or closed (reconstituting) and not on the amount of gallbladder that is left attached to the liver.

Reprinted with permission from: Strasberg SM, Pucci MJ, Brunt LM, Deziel DJ. Subtotal cholecystectomy "fenestrating" vs "reconstituting" subtypes and the prevention of bile duct injury: definition of the optimal procedure in difficult operative conditions. *J Am Coll Surg* 2016;222:89–96.

the inside, so that no closed gallbladder remnant remains. In the reconstituting type, a small closed gallbladder remnant remains behind. Further details are beyond the scope of this chapter, and the reader is referred to the cited literature (Figure 28.6).

PRESENTATION AND INVESTIGATION

About 30% of the more serious injuries are diagnosed during surgery. Most of the rest of injuries are identified within 30 days of surgery but some appear years after laparoscopic cholecystectomy. Intraoperative diagnosis may be made by cholangiography, by observation of bile in the field or, more rarely, by seeing the lacerated or divided duct. Sometimes, the diagnosis is made after conversion for bleeding or inability to proceed in case of a difficult dissection.

Postoperative presentations are influenced by the type of injury and whether a drain has been left. The commonest presentations are pain and sepsis, with or without jaundice; jaundice without other symptoms; and biliary fistula. Some patients present only with malaise and distension. The latter is usually due to bile ascites. It is a particularly insidious presentation, which may lead to delayed diagnosis. In evaluating a biliary injury, the entire biliary tree must be accounted for. In addition, a vascular component of injury should always be suspected. Therefore, a computed tomography (CT) or magnetic resonance imaging (MRI) examining the vasculature of the porta hepatis is indicated, except in simple injuries such as cystic duct stump leak.

Pain and Sepsis

In those patients presenting with pain and sepsis, a CT scan or MRI is indicated to look for fluid collections, which may then be aspirated to determine if they are bilious. Usually, a drain is placed in the biloma and an endoscopic retrograde cholangiopancreatography (ERCP) follows. Many patients presenting with pain and sepsis but without jaundice have type A or D injuries, and definitive treatment is possible at the time of endoscopy. These scans may also detect dilated bile ducts and vascular injuries.

Jaundice

Jaundice is usually indicative of the more severe type E injuries. If jaundice is the only symptom, duct occlusion alone, for example, by clips, is likely. Transections are often accompanied by pain and sepsis due to accumulation of bile in the peritoneal cavity. In either case, ERCP is the first-line investigation. The duct may be found to be partially or completely occluded. Often, clips are seen at the point at which the dye column stops. If the ducts are only partly occluded, the entire extent of injury may be diagnosed by ERCP. Next, a CT scan is performed. In patients with complete occlusion of the bile duct(s), the bile ducts will be dilated and no biloma will be seen. Next, percutaneous transhepatic cholangiography (PTC) is performed to delineate the proximal ducts and to provide external drainage of bile. In patients with transection of the bile duct without occlusion, the ducts will be decompressed and a biloma or bile ascites is usually present. For these patients, our routine is to drain the biloma and wait for several weeks to perform the PTC. During this time, the biloma cavity will contract around the drain. Then, retrograde injection through the drain will display the biliary tree, and this facilitates PTC when ducts are decompressed. Generally, bilomas are associated with a rise in the serum bilirubin level, but serum alkaline phosphatase concentrations are normal, whereas obstruction results in high levels of both tests.

Bile Fistula

The first-line investigation is a fistulogram. Subsequent management depends upon findings of the fistulogram, which may show a stricture or a complete occlusion.

Other Symptoms

Occasionally, patients with bile ascites may complain only of vague symptoms such as malaise, constipation and distension. This is because hepatic bile is relatively nonirritating. Patients with injury to the right portal vein and the right hepatic artery (extreme VBI) may present with infarction of the right liver (pain, sepsis and hypotension). Haematobilia or bleeding from the abdominal drain due to an arterial pseudoaneurysm is a rare but very dangerous presentation.

MANAGEMENT OF BILIARY INJURIES

Management of Biliary Injuries Recogniaed at the Initial Operation

Intraoperative recognition of biliary injury is usually an indication for conversion. The following guidelines are suggested when laparotomy is undertaken for suspected injury: (1) Repair should be attempted only if the required techniques of reconstruction are commonly used by the

operating team. (2) The injury should not be increased by dissection solely for the purpose of making an exact diagnosis. When the appropriate level of expertise is not available, closed suction drains should be placed in the right upper quadrant laparoscopically and the patient referred, without performing a laparotomy. If conversion is required to control bleeding, care should be taken not to damage structures by blind clipping, clamping or suturing. A Pringle manoeuvre should be applied with an atraumatic vascular clamp or vascular tourniquet. This permits precise placement of clips, clamps or sutures on bleeding vessels, without injuring surrounding strictures. The Pringle manoeuvre should not be maintained in excess of 15 minutes. In many cases, bleeding can be controlled by direct pressure for 10 to 15 minutes, supplemented by haemostatic agents. It is advisable to obtain the assistance of a second experienced surgeon when blood loss is substantial.

Type A injuries are repaired by suture of the cystic duct and drainage. If the anatomy has been clearly demonstrated through dissection or cholangiography, laparoscopic repair by ligature loop or suture is sometimes possible. Type D injuries are treated by closure of the defect by using fine absorbable sutures over a T-tube and placement of a closed suction drain. This often requires conversion to an open procedure. The T-tube should exit through a separate incision in the duct, if possible. When type D injury is thermal in origin, or when the injury involves more than 50% of the circumference of the duct, the preferred treatment is Roux-en-Y hepaticojejunostomy. Type E injuries recognised intraoperatively should be repaired by hepaticojejunostomy. In the author's opinion, choledochocholedochotomy should be avoided, because problems related to blood supply and tension often lead to postrepair strictures. Choledochoduodenostomy has the theoretical disadvantage of tension on the anastomosis, as does loop hepaticojejunostomy.

Management of Biliary Injuries Diagnosed Postoperatively

The approach depends on complexity of injury, on whether the injury is vasculobiliary, on type of initial management and its result and on time elapsed since the cholecystectomy or a prior repair was performed.

Type A Injuries

The treatment of type A injuries is endoscopic sphincterotomy, with placement of a stent or a nasobiliary catheter. Intraperitoneal bile collections may require percutaneous drainage. Operative repair is rarely needed.

Type B Injuries

Type B injuries may remain asymptomatic or present after many years with right upper-quadrant discomfort, attacks of pain or cholangitis. Symptomatic patients require hepaticojejunostomy or hepatic resection if biliary-enteric anastomosis is not feasible. In asymptomatic patients, treatment is not recommended when the volume of liver affected is small or if the injury is remote and the isolated portion of liver parenchyma has atrophied. When the injury is recent and the section of liver is large (e.g., the whole right liver), repair is recommended.

Type C Injuries

Type C injuries usually require drainage of the bile collections and biliary-enteric anastomosis, hepatic resection or ligation of the duct. If the duct is of small diameter, for example, <2 mm, observation is advisable, as drainage may cease after several weeks. Essentially, this converts the problem from a type C to a type B injury, and usually, such patients remain asymptomatic. If drainage persists, then resection of the affected segment(s) or ligation is preferable, since attempts to repair ducts less than 2 mm in diameter may result in stricture. With ducts of larger diameter, reconstruction by hepaticojejunostomy is possible. Insertion of a transhepatic catheter before biliary reconstruction is a useful aid. It also may be used to control bile drainage and to drain the subhepatic bile collection preoperatively.

Type D Injuries

Treatment by endoscopic sphincterotomy and stent is the treatment of choice in the postoperative period. When operation is required, the technique of repair is the same as that when the problem is discovered at time of initial surgery. Again, if the injury is thermal or involves more than 50% of the duct diameter, hepaticojejunostomy is probably a better choice.

Type E Injuries

The best chance for lasting repair is the initial repair. Strictures and, sometimes, clip occlusions may be treated by dilatation and stents, placed either by ERCP or transhepatically. In our experience, nonsurgical therapy is most likely to be successful when the strictures are mild, appear months to years after surgery or are of short length. Pitt et al reported 76% success rate with interventional techniques.[17] Failures tend to occur when E3 or E4 lesions are treated, when a fistula is present or when a stricture occurs shortly after a hepaticojejunostomy

has been done. Nonsurgical therapy is most likely to be successful in patients in which operative repair is rather easy and nonsurgical treatment often requires multiple endoscopic procedures. The age and health of the patient as well as the likelihood of good long-term outcome should be considered when choosing therapy for a stricture. Operation is required for failure of stent therapy and when there is ductal discontinuity.

Timing of Surgery

Factors favouring immediate repair are early referral, stable patient, lack of right upper-quadrant bile collections, absence of vascular injury and less complex injury, which can be diagnosed rapidly. Many patients are referred between 1 week and 6 weeks after the primary operation, when local inflammation may be expected to be great. In these patients, percutaneous tubes are inserted to relieve obstruction from affected segments, to drain subhepatic collections and to control sepsis. Repair is performed when inflammation has settled, usually about 3 months after the last operation; that is, it is not done in the intermediate period. This delayed approach is sometimes used even when the patient is referred within the first week, especially in complex injuries and in those with a thermal aetiology. The delayed approach is also advisable in the presence of an associated vascular injury because of the risk of performing an anastomosis to a portion of the bile duct that is ischaemic (*see* **Vasculobiliary Injuries**). Immediate repair may also be undertaken when the injury is diagnosed months after surgery, for instance, after failure of stenting of a stenosis or after late failure of a biliary-enteric anastomosis.

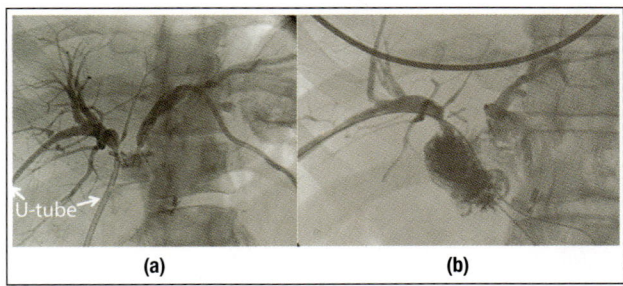

Figure 28.7 Patient with high E4 injury. (a): The U-tube was placed in the right hepatic ducal system after referral. The tube in the left duct was placed 3 months later on the day before surgery. These tubes are very helpful guides to the ducts at the time of surgery. (b): Completed double-barrelled anastomosis seen several days after surgery.

Courtesy: Steven M. Strasberg.

Preoperative Preparation

The complete extent of the injury or biliary tract must be diagnosed preoperatively. Failure to do so may result in exclusion of bile ducts from the repair. Our policy is to perform conciliation between CT and PTC studies to be sure that all ducts are accounted for. The percutaneous transhepatic tubes placed to ensure biliary drainage from all liver segments also serve as guides to the position of the injured ducts at surgery (Figure 28.7). Usually, only one PTC tube is required to decompress the biliary system between the time of referral and repair if the end of the tube rests in or traverses the subhepatic biloma. Therefore, the additional guide tubes, for instance, as shown in Figure 28.7, may be placed on the day before surgery.

Operative Technique

The procedure consists of two parts: display of the ducts and biliary enteric anastomosis. A generous midline or 'J' incision is used, and adhesions are taken down. The inferior face of segment 4 is dissected until the guide tubes are exposed. The peritoneum at the base of segment 4 is incised and the dissection continued directly on liver substance until the hilar plate is exposed and lowered. The guide tube in the left hepatic duct should now be readily palpable. The left hepatic duct is opened directly over the tube. The principles of anastomosis are that it must be tension free, with good blood supply and mucosa-to-mucosa contact and of adequate calibre. Fine absorbable sutures should be used. Most experts in this field recommend Roux-en-Y hepaticojejunostomy in preference to either choledochocholedochotomy or choledochoduodenostomy, since a tension-free anastomosis is always possible with

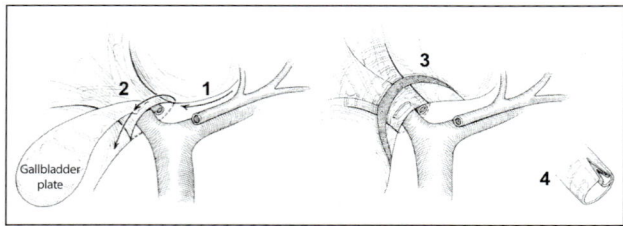

Figure 28.8 Four-step technique for identifying isolated right hepatic ducts. (1) Identify left duct by Hepp–Couinaud technique. (2) Find right portal pedicle and divide gallbladder plate. (3) Core or lift the liver off the right portal pedicle. (4) Open bile duct on the anterior surface.

Reprinted with permission from: Strasberg SM, Picus DD, Drebin JA. Results of a new strategy for reconstruction of biliary injuries having an isolated right-sided component. *J Gastrointest Surg* 2001;5:266–74.

hepaticojejunostomy. Whenever possible, we prefer to construct side-to-side anastomoses to avoid dissection behind bile ducts, which may affect their blood supply.[18] For E1 to E3 lesions, the anastomosis may be done to the extrahepatic portion of the left hepatic duct after it is lowered by dividing the liver plate (Hepp–Couinaud approach).[19] E4, E5, B and C lesions have an isolated right hepatic duct that must be repaired. We described an approach to isolated right hepatic duct injuries (Figure 28.8).[20] Dissection of the left duct first provides a guide to the coronal plane in which the intrahepatic right hepatic ducts will be found, and these may be exposed by removing liver tissue. Exposure is also facilitated by dividing the bridge of tissue between segments 3 and 4, by fully opening the gallbladder fossa, which often collapses with adherence of it walls. If these manoeuvres are not sufficient, resecting part of segments 4b and/or 5 will open the upper porta hepatis, as described by Mercado et al.[21]

The use of anastomotic stents is controversial. There is no evidence that they are helpful if a large-calibre mucosa-to-mucosa anastomosis can be made. We use them when very small ducts have been anastomosed. In cases in which a primary repair has failed, it is not always necessary to perform a fresh hepaticojejunostomy. Stenting (and balloon dilatation) can sometimes be successful if the strictures are short. Occasionally, biliary reconstruction is not possible or advisable. When ductal reconstruction to a part of the liver is impossible, then resection should be performed.[22,23]

OUTCOME OF TREATMENT

Most surgical series of biliary reconstruction cite very good short-term results.[17,18,22,24,25] However, it is well established from older literature describing ductal injury during open cholecystectomy that there is a progressive restenosis rate. Two-thirds of recurrences are diagnosed in the first 2 years after repair, but postrepair stenosis has been described after 10 years or more. The restenosis rate varies from 5 to 28%. There is a recent indication that the results in the laparoscopic era may not be as good as these, perhaps because of increased severity of injury.

Comparison among surgical series is not easily done because of lack of standard reporting and effect of differences in the severity of injuries treated in different series. Injuries above the confluence of the right and left hepatic ducts that involve several bile ducts have a worse prognosis than injuries of the common hepatic duct, and the proportion of severe injuries in a series will affect the outcome. Reporting of treatment failure is not uniform. Length of follow-up is another obvious variable that

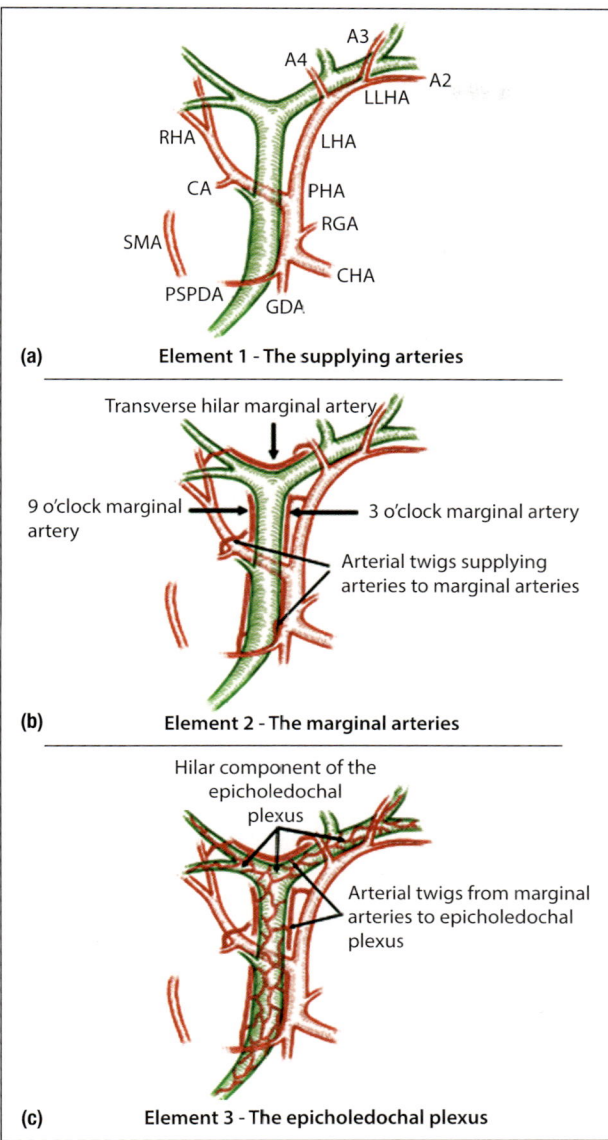

(a) Element 1 - The supplying arteries

(b) Element 2 - The marginal arteries

(c) Element 3 - The epicholedochal plexus

Figure 28.9 Blood supply to the bile ducts. (a) The supplying arteries. The supplying arteries shown give branches to the marginal arteries. PSPD: posterior superior pancreatoduodenal artery, the most important and constant artery; CHA: common hepatic artery; PHA: proper hepatic artery; GDA: gastroduodenal artery; RHA: right hepatic artery; LHA: left hepatic artery; CA: cystic artery; LLSA: left lateral sectional artery; A2, A3 and A4: arteries to segments 2, 3 and 4. Replaced arteries arising from the superior mesenteric artery can also supply the bile ducts (b) Marginal arteries. Marginal arteries are disposed at 3 o-clock and 9 o-clock positions on the common bile duct/common hepatic duct. The hilar marginal artery runs across the top of the confluence of the right and left hepatic ducts. (c) Epicholedochal plexus. The epicholedochal plexus is supplied by the marginal arteries.

Reprinted from: HPB (Oxford), Vol. 13, Strasberg SM, Helton WS, An analytical review of vasculobiliary injury in laparoscopic and open cholecystectomy. Pages 1-14, Copyright (2011), with permission from Elsevier.

affects outcome and is not uniform among series. Some authors have reported that quality of life and life span are adversely affected by a biliary injury, but others have found minimal effect on quality of life.

VASCULOBILIARY INJURIES

Blood Supply to the Bile Ducts

The blood supply to the ducts has three elements: afferent vessels, marginal arteries and an epicholedochal plexus. These are illustrated in Figures 28.9. The marginal artery labelled 'hilar marginal artery' in Figure 28.9 can function as an arterial shunt between the two sides of the liver.

Definition of Vasculobiliary Injury

A VBI is defined as a combined injury to a bile duct and a hepatic artery and/or portal vein; the bile duct injury may be due to operative trauma, be ischaemic in origin or both and may or may not be accompanied by various degrees of hepatic ischaemia.[26] Vasculobiliary injuries may be divided into two types. In the common variety, the right hepatic artery and a bile duct are injured. This variant accounts for about 90% of VBIs. The uncommon type involves a bile duct, a major hepatic artery and a major portal vein. The consequences of the second type of injury are usually much more severe, and they are called 'extreme VBIs'.[4]

Right Hepatic Artery Vasculobiliary Injury

Pathogenesis of Right Hepatic Artery Vasculobiliary Injury

About 20% of major bile duct injuries also involve an injury to the right hepatic artery. The right hepatic artery is injured more commonly than other arteries, because it lies closer to the common hepatic duct. In the 'classical' injury referred to previously, the common bile duct is mistaken to be the cystic duct, usually due to the use of the infundibular technique of ductal identification. After transection of the common bile duct, the dissection is carried along the left side of the common hepatic duct in the belief that the dissection is proceeding along the underside of the gallbladder. Finally, to get to the cystic plate on which the gallbladder rests, the common hepatic duct is divided. The point at which the common hepatic duct is transected is often exactly where the right hepatic artery usually passes under the duct. Consequently, the artery is injured by direct mechanical or thermal trauma or is clipped, thinking that it the cystic artery. The injury is frequently associated with brisk bleeding, and the diagnosis of a VBI is made. The principles of avoidance of this injury are the same principles as discussed above under 'Avoidance of Biliary Injuries: Misidentification Injuries'.

Effect of Right Hepatic Artery Injury on Outcome of an Accompanying Biliary Injury

The chief consequence of the right hepatic artery injury is ischaemia of the part of the common hepatic duct lying between the site of transection of the common hepatic duct and the confluence of the right and left hepatic ducts. This has been determined from the fact that although the mechanical injury to the common hepatic duct is in its mid portion, the actual level of injury identified at the time of definitive repair is at the confluence. This suggests that ischaemic 'die-back' has occurred to the confluence.[26] The progression of ischaemia may take weeks to occur. As a result, it could be predicted that early repairs to the common hepatic duct will tend to fail when there has been an injury to the right hepatic artery due to ischaemia to the duct. Recurrent stricture is much less likely to occur if reconstruction is delayed, either by intention or by late referral for repair, or if the repair is performed at a higher level in the biliary tree. An important inference is that assessment of the hepatic arteries should be part of the investigation of all major biliary injuries. In addition, in the face of a right hepatic artery injury, consideration should be given to delaying repair for about 3 months.

Effect of Bile Duct Injury on Collateral Blood Flow to the Right Hemiliver in the Presence of a Right Hepatic Artery Injury

Isolated right hepatic artery injury without a biliary injury (or injury to the portal vein) rarely results in clinically important hepatic ischaemia, because preformed arterial shunts running along the bile ducts supply enough blood to the right liver to avoid infarction. If the VBI is high, then the hilar communicating artery, which shunts blood between the left and right hepatic arteries, may be injured. In such cases, when the right hepatic artery is occluded and blood cannot be shunted from left to right through the hilar communicating artery, the right liver may become ischaemic. The consequence of such ischaemia may be atrophy of the right liver or the slow development of patchy infarction. These areas of infarction may become abscesses with secondary infection.

Repair of the Right Hepatic Artery in Right Hepatic Artery Vasculobiliary Injury

Immediate repair of the right hepatic artery has been performed either by end-to-end anastomosis or with a graft—usually taken from the inferior mesenteric vein (IMV). The opportunity for repair is limited, both because the procedure has to be done in close proximity to the injury, ideally within hours, and because the injury is frequently too extensive for repair. Since only 10% of patients with a right hepatic artery or bile duct injury develop clinically significant hepatic ischaemia, the alternate strategy of allowing slow infarction to take place in a minority of patients and treating it by resection, if necessary, might result in better overall outcomes than routine early reconstruction.

Extreme Vasculobiliary Injuries

These injuries usually involve both a major hepatic artery, including the proper hepatic artery and one of its primary branches, and the main portal vein or one of its primary branches.[4] Occasionally, only the proper hepatic artery is involved. Extreme injuries account for only about 5% of VBIs. Although uncommon, they are important since their consequences are so serious. Hepatic infarction is frequent, often with rapid onset and frequently necessitating emergency right hepatectomy or urgent liver transplantation. Death has occurred in about 50% of such cases.

Pathogenesis and Treatment of Extreme Vasculobiliary Injuries

The pathogenesis of the injury has been understood from study of operative notes.[4] The operations were started laparoscopically and converted to an open procedure because of severe chronic or acute inflammation. At open surgery, 'fundus-down' cholecystectomy was attempted. Severe bleeding was encountered due to injury to a major portal vein and/or hepatic artery. The two common aetiological features were severe inflammation necessitating conversion to an open procedure and the decision to perform the cholecystectomy by the fundus-down technique.

The gallbladder rests on the cystic plate, which inserts into the front of the right portal pedicle (Figure 28.10). If the plane of dissection in a cholecystectomy is behind rather than in front of the cystic plate and the dissection is continued downwards in this plane, the sheath of the right portal pedicle containing the major vascular and biliary structures supplying the right liver will be incised, exposing the structures to injury (Figure 28.10). Injury to the contents of the sheath is much more likely to occur when there is severe chronic inflammation with contractive fibrosis, since the cystic plate may become

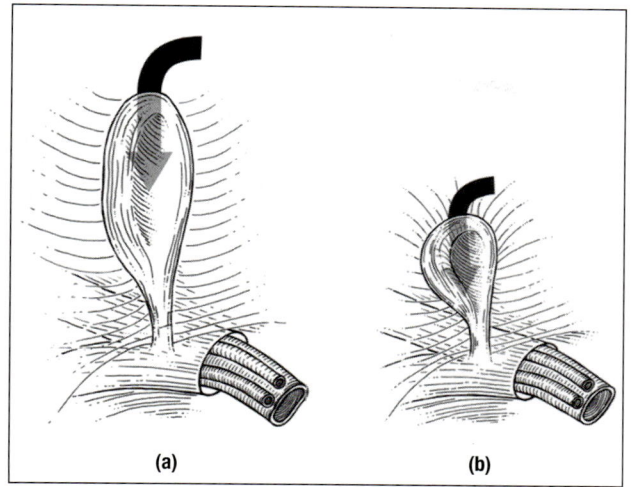

Figure 28.10 The relationship between cystic plate and right portal pedicle (a) under normal circumstances, and (b) in the presence of severe contractive inflammation. The cystic plate inserts into the surface of the right portal pedicle. Dissection downwards in the plane behind or within the cystic plate (arrow) will lead down to the portal pedicle, with potential injury to vessels and bile duct. When inflammation is mild (a) entry into the plane behind the plate is usually readily detected by visualisation of liver tissue. When there is contractive inflammation, the cystic plate is thickened (b) and determining the position of the dissection in relation to the plate is difficult. In addition, the plate is foreshortened, so the distance from the top of the plate to the pedicle may only be 2 to 3 cm. Both of these factors greatly increase the likelihood of injury to the pedicle.

Reprinted from: HPB (Oxford), Vol. 14, Strasberg SM, Gouma DJ, 'Extreme' vasculobiliary injuries: association with fundus-down cholecystectomy in severely inflamed gallbladders. Pages 1–8, Copyright (2012), with permission from Elsevier.

short and thick (Figure 28.10). To prevent extreme VBI, there should be awareness that fundus-down cholecystectomy in the face of severe inflammation will tend to bring the dissection onto the right portal pedicle, with predicable consequences. The desire to complete a cholecystectomy should be very secondary to completing the operation safely—an attitude that we refer to as the 'culture of cholecystectomy.'[1,27,28]

Treatment depends upon the type of injury and its effects. At the mildest end of the spectrum, a portion of the liver will undergo ischaemic atrophy, with no long-term consequences. In these cases, the accompanying biliary injury may be repaired after a delay of several months to allow hepatic regeneration in the ischaemic portion of the liver. In most cases, there is rapid infarction of the affected portion of the liver, usually the right hemiliver. Early vascular repair, with prevention

of hepatic infarction, is the ideal treatment but is rarely possible, because the liver deprived of both portal vein and arterial supply will infarct within an hour or so. Thus, most patients require hepatic resection, usually of the right hemiliver, or immediate or delayed orthotopic liver transplantation.

ORTHOTOPIC LIVER TRANSPLANTATION FOR BILIARY INJURIES

Orthotopic liver transplantation for biliary injuries is well described.[29,30] It has usually been performed for end-stage liver disease, that is, secondary biliary cirrhosis. The usual sequence of events is biliary injury, followed by multiple repairs—usually not at expert centres—with repeated attacks of cholangitis, which damage the liver and the bile ducts. Hepatic fibrosis and hepatic abscesses are common in these cases. The combination of liver injury and high unreconstructable biliary strictures necessitates transplantation. Occasionally, transplantation has been performed for acute ischaemia associated with extreme VBIs.[29,30] Good results have been reported, especially in the chronic cases. The fact that transplantation may be the consequence of a cholecystectomy gone wrong stands as a stark reminder of the importance of prevention of biliary injuries.

CONCLUSIONS

Major biliary injuries are morbid. Usually, they are caused by misidentification of bile ducts. Prevention depends upon use of dependable means of identification such as CVS and cholangiography. Stenoses may sometimes be treated by stenting. Hepaticojejunostomy is the mainstay of operative treatment. Results of repair of complex injuries in expert centres are good.

REFERENCES

1. Strasberg SM, Hertl M, Soper NJ. An analysis of the problem of biliary injury during laparoscopic cholecystectomy [see comments]. *J Am Coll Surg* 1995;180: 101–25.

2. Yokoe M, Takada T, Strasberg SM, et al. TG13 diagnostic criteria and severity grading of acute cholecystitis (with videos). *J Hepatobiliary Pancreat Sci* 2013;20:35–46.

3. Ibrahim S, Hean TK, Ho LS, Ravintharan T, Chye TN, Chee CH. Risk factors for conversion to open surgery in patients undergoing laparoscopic cholecystectomy. *World J Surg* 2006;30:1698–704.

4. Strasberg SM, Gouma DJ. 'Extreme' vasculobiliary injuries: association with fundus-down cholecystectomy in severely inflamed gallbladders. *HPB* 2012;14:1–8.

5. Branum G, Schmitt C, Baillie J, et al. Management of major biliary complications after laparoscopic cholecystectomy. *Ann Surg* 1993;217:532–40.

6. Strasberg SM, Eagon CJ, Drebin JA. The "hidden cystic duct" syndrome and the infundibular technique of laparoscopic cholecystectomy—the danger of the false infundibulum. *J Am Coll Surg* 2000;191:661–7.

7. Strasberg SM, Brunt LM. Rationale and use of the critical view of safety in laparoscopic cholecystectomy. *J Am Coll Surg* 2010;211:132–8.

8. Sanford DE, Strasberg SM. A simple effective method for generation of a permanent record of the Critical View of Safety during laparoscopic cholecystectomy by intraoperative "doublet" photography. *J Am Coll Surg* 2014;218:170–8.

9. Heistermann HP, Tobusch A, Palmes D. Prevention of bile duct injuries after laparoscopic cholecystectomy. "The critical view of safety". *Zentralblatt fur Chirurgie* 2006;131:460–5.

10. Avgerinos C, Kelgiorgi D, Touloumis Z, Baltatzi L, Dervenis C. One thousand laparoscopic cholecystectomies in a single surgical unit using the "critical view of safety" technique. *J Gastrointest Surg* 2009;13:498–503.

11. Misra M, Schiff J, Rendon G, Rothschild J, Schwaitzberg S. Laparoscopic cholecystectomy after the learning curve: what should we expect? *Surg Endosc* 2005;19:1266–71.

12. Yegiyants S, Collins JC. Operative strategy can reduce the incidence of major bile duct injury in laparoscopic cholecystectomy. *Am Surg* 2008;74:985–7.

13. Sanjay P, Fulke JL, Exon DJ. 'Critical view of safety' as an alternative to routine intraoperative cholangiography during laparoscopic cholecystectomy for acute biliary pathology. *J Gastrointest Surg* 2010;14:1280–4.

14. Elshaer M, Gravante G, Thomas K, Sorge R, Al-Hamali S, Ebdewi H. Subtotal cholecystectomy for "difficult gallbladders": systematic review and meta-analysis. *JAMA Surgery* 2015;150:159–68.

15. Henneman D, da Costa DW, Vrouenraets BC, van Wagensveld BA, Lagarde SM. Laparoscopic partial cholecystectomy for the difficult gallbladder: a systematic review. *Surg Endosc* 2013;27:351–8.

16. Strasberg SM, Pucci MJ, Brunt LM, Deziel DJ. Subtotal cholecystectomy: "fenestrating" vs. "reconstituting" subtypes and the prevention of bile duct injury: definition of the optimal procedure in difficult operative conditions. *J Am Coll Surg* 2016;222:89–96.

17. Pitt HA, Sherman S, Johnson MS, et al. Improved outcomes of bile duct injuries in the 21st century. *Ann Surg* 2013;258:490–9.

18. Winslow ER, Fialkowski EA, Linehan DC, et al. "Sideways": results of repair of biliary injuries using a policy of side-to-side hepatico-jejunostomy. *Ann Surg* 2009;249:426–34.

19. Hepp J. Hepaticojejunostomy using the left biliary trunk for iatrogenic biliary lesions: the French connection. *World J Surg* 1985;9:507–11.

20. Strasberg SM, Picus DD, Drebin JA. Results of a new strategy for reconstruction of biliary injuries having an isolated right-sided component. *J Gastrointest Surg* 2001;5:266–74.

21. Mercado MA, Orozco H, de la Garza L, Lopez-Martinez LM, Contreras A, Guillen-Navarro E. Biliary duct injury: partial segment IV resection for intrahepatic reconstruction of biliary lesions. *Arch Surg* 1999;134:1008–10.

22. Laurent A, Sauvanet A, Farges O, Watrin T, Rivkine E, Belghiti J. Major hepatectomy for the treatment of complex bile duct injury. *Ann Surg* 2008;248:77–83.

23. Pekolj J, Yanzon A, Dietrich A, Del Valle G, Ardiles V, de Santibanes E. Major liver resection as definitive treatment in post-cholecystectomy common bile duct injuries. *World J Surg* 2015;39:1216–23.

24. Thomson BN, Parks RW, Madhavan KK, Wigmore SJ, Garden OJ. Early specialist repair of biliary injury. *Br J Surg* 2006;93:216–20.

25. de Reuver PR, Rauws EA, Bruno MJ, et al. Survival in bile duct injury patients after laparoscopic cholecystectomy: a multidisciplinary approach of gastroenterologists, radiologists, and surgeons. Surgery. 2007;142:1–9.

26. Strasberg SM, Helton WS. An analytical review of vasculobiliary injury in laparoscopic and open cholecystectomy. *HPB* 2011;13:1–14.

27. Strasberg SM, Strasberg SM. Biliary injury in laparoscopic surgery: part 1. Processes used in determination of standard of care in misidentification injuries. *J Am Coll Surg* 2005;201:598–2603.

28. Strasberg SM. A teaching program for the "culture of safety in cholecystectomy" and avoidance of bile duct injury. *J Am Coll Surg* 2013;217:751.

29. Thomson BN, Parks RW, Madhavan KK, Garden OJ. Liver resection and transplantation in the management of iatrogenic biliary injury. *World J Surg* 2007;31:2363–9.

30. Ardiles V, McCormack L, Quinonez E, et al. Experience using liver transplantation for the treatment of severe bile duct injuries over 20 years in Argentina: results from a National Survey. *HPB* 2011;13:544–50.

29

Complications of Surgery for Portal Hypertension

R. Panwar, S. Pal and P. Sahni

ABSTRACT

Patients with portal hypertension require surgery only to deal with complications like variceal bleeding. The availability of endoscopic therapy and minimally invasive transjugular intrahepatic portosystemic shunt procedure has limited the role of surgery in patients with portal hypertension, especially in patients with cirrhosis. However, surgery still remains an attractive option in patients without cirrhosis. Many surgical procedures, including nonselective shunts, partial shunts, selective shunts and devascularisation procedures, have been described, and each one of these has its own advantages and problems. The choice of procedure depends on both the clinical scenario and the local expertise. The surgery is technically demanding, and there is a long list of potential short- and long-term complications. The presence of collaterals throughout the abdomen makes dissection difficult and results in blood loss. The vascular adhesions and continuous oozing of blood obscure the surgical field and increase the risk of injury to adjacent organs. In patients with cirrhosis, the postoperative course may get further complicated by the compromised function of the liver. However, with experience and careful selection of patients, surgery may still be performed safely for managing complications of portal hypertension.

KEYWORDS

Portal hypertension, portosystemic shunt surgery, devascularisation, complications, cirrhosis, extrahepatic portal venous obstruction, noncirrhotic portal fibrosis

INTRODUCTION

In 1945, Whipple reported the first series of portacaval shunts in patients with portal hypertension.[1] Thereafter, a number of randomised controlled trials (RCTs) were done to assess the portacaval shunt in patients who had cirrhosis and portal hypertension.[2–5] Although the portacaval shunt was effective in controlling variceal bleeding, there was an increase in the number of long-term deaths due to liver failure. Most of these studies were biased in favour of medical management, as surgery was offered as 'salvage' for patients who failed to respond to medical management. Nevertheless, a few centres, for example, Orloff et al,[6] continued to report good immediate and long-term results with portacaval shunts in patients with cirrhosis. Moreover, in the Indian subcontinent, we and others have continued to offer nonselective shunt surgery (proximal lienorenal shunt and its variants) to patients with noncirrhotic portal hypertension due to extrahepatic portal venous obstruction (EHPVO) and noncirrhotic portal fibrosis (NCPF), with good long-term outcomes.[7–10]

To decrease the rates of liver decompensation, the techniques of partial and selective shunting were described by Inokuchi and Kobayashi[11] and Warren et al.[12] Again, selective and nonselective shunts were compared in multiple randomised trials.[13–15] In general, the results were similar, as the selectivity of shunts was lost with time.[16] During the same period, some centres described excellent results with nonshunt procedures, for example, devascularisation procedures by Hassab[17] and Sugiura and Futagawa.[18] The devascularisation techniques (modified Hassab's procedure) have also been adopted by us successfully for managing noncirrhotic patients with bleeding varices and nonshuntable anatomy.[19]

The advent of endoscopic therapy, the availability of liver transplantation and the development of transjugular intrahepatic portosystemic shunt (TIPSS) have limited the role of surgery in patients with cirrhosis. Randomised trials comparing surgery with endoscopic management found that surgery was associated with lower rebleed rates, higher encephalopathy rates and similar mortality rates.[20] There was no difference in rebleeding rate, incidence of encephalopathy and survival in a randomised trial comparing distal splenorenal shunt (DSRS) with TIPSS.[21] Thus, in patients with portal hypertension due to cirrhosis, endoscopic therapy and TIPSS have become the preferred treatment options, as these are less invasive, easy to administer and do not make future transplant surgery more difficult. However, in patients with portal hypertension due to noncirrhotic causes, where the liver function is well preserved, surgery remains a better treatment option. Transjugular intrahepatic portosystemic shunt is not an option in patients with EHPVO, and its use in NCPF is also not well documented.

HAEMODYNAMICS OF PORTAL HYPERTENSION

Portal hypertension is defined as portal venous pressure more than 10 mmHg. Direct measurement of the portal venous pressure is difficult and may be hazardous. Measurement of hepatic venous pressure gradient (HVPG) is easier and more practical and hence is the more commonly used parameter in the clinical setting. Although portal hypertension is defined as HVPG more than 5 mmHg, the complications of portal hypertension usually occur after the HVPG is more than 10 mmHg and the threshold for variceal bleeding is 12 mmHg.[22]

Hepatic venous pressure gradient is raised only in the sinusoidal and postsinusoidal obstructions. Thus, it does not have any role in the diagnosis of portal hypertension caused by presinusoidal obstruction, for example, EHPVO, NCPF and schistosomiasis. In presinusoidal obstruction, the portal pressure can be measured directly by cannulation of a portal venous tributary. However, the presence of oesophageal varices itself indicates increased portal pressure. Thus, rather than using the difficult and

Table 29.1 Classification of the causes of portal hypertension

Site of block	Examples
Prehepatic	Extrahepatic portal venous obstruction
	Portal vein thrombosis

Hepatic	• Presinusoidal
	  – Noncirrhotic portal fi brosis;
	  – Schistosomiasis
	• Sinusoidal
	  – Cirrhosis
	• Postsinusoidal
	  – Veno-occlusive disease

Posthepatic	Hepatic venous outflow tract obstruction

risky method of direct cannulation, portal hypertension can be diagnosed by endoscopic visualisation of oesophageal varices.

The portal venous system carries venous blood from the intestine to the liver via the portal vein. The nutrient-rich portal blood then reaches the hepatic sinusoids via the small branches of the portal veins. The hepatic sinusoids facilitate the exchange of substances between the liver and the portal blood. From the sinusoids, the blood drains into the hepatic veins through the central veins and small hepatic veins. The hepatic veins ultimately return the blood back to the systemic circulation through the inferior vena cava. During this process, the liver metabolises gut-derived toxins, clears the bacteria and also removes and stores excess nutrients. Any obstruction to blood flow in the portal venous system increases pressure in the vascular channels downstream to the obstruction, resulting in portal hypertension. The obstruction can be prehepatic, intrahepatic or posthepatic. Intrahepatic obstruction can be presinusoidal, sinusoidal or postsinusoidal (Table 29.1 and Figure 29.1).

INDICATIONS FOR SURGERY IN PORTAL HYPERTENSION

Variceal bleeding and ascites are the major complications of portal hypertension. A patient with portal hypertension may require a surgical intervention for the prevention or treatment of these complications. Liver transplantation is the treatment of choice for patients who have portal hypertension in the setting of decompensated cirrhosis. However, we will discuss only the complications of nontransplant procedures for portal hypertension.

The following is a list of various conditions associated with portal hypertension that may require surgical treatment.

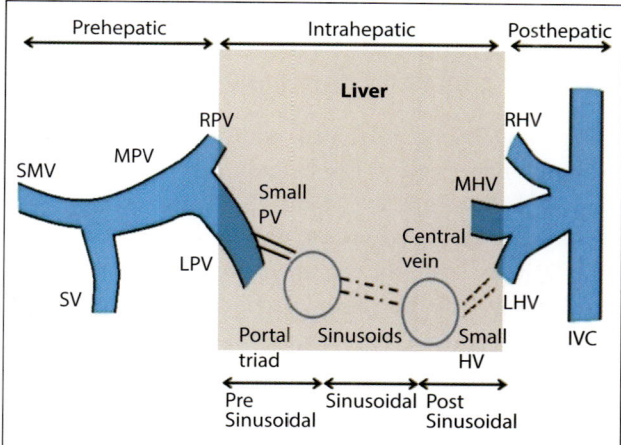

Figure 29.1 Schematic representation of sites of obstruction to portal blood flow in portal hypertension.

Abbreviations: SMV, superior mesenteric vein; SV, splenic vein; MPV, main portal vein; RPV, right portal vein; LPV, left portal vein; PV, portal veins; HV, hepatic veins, MHV, middle hepatic vein; LHV, left hepatic vein; RHV, right hepatic vein; IVC, inferior vena cava.

Courtesy: Rajesh Panwar, Sujoy Pal and Peush Sahni.

- Emergency
  - Uncontrolled variceal bleeding from oesophageal, gastric and/or ectopic varices
  - Complications of uncontrolled ascites, for example, ruptured umbilical hernia
  - Liver failure
- Elective
  - Primary prophylaxis for variceal bleeding
  - Secondary prophylaxis for variceal bleeding
  - Symptomatic hypersplenism
  - Intractable ascites
  - Portal biliopathy
  - Growth retardation in children with EHPVO
  - Umbilical hernia
  - Progressive liver dysfunction

ROLE OF SURGERY IN VARICEAL BLEEDING

Variceal haemorrhage is responsible for a large proportion of deaths in patients with portal hypertension. Prevention or control of variceal bleeding is an important and, probably, the most common indication for surgery in these patients. The various shunt and nonshunt procedures that have been described for the control or prevention of variceal bleeding include the following:

- Portosystemic shunt procedures
  - Nonselective: Portacaval (side-to-side or end-to-side), proximal splenorenal with splenectomy, side-to-side splenorenal, mesocaval and mesoatrial

  - Partial: Sarfeh's shunt (portacaval shunt using a synthetic interposition graft)
  - Selective: Distal splenorenal (Warren et al)[12] and coronary caval (Inokuchi and Kobayashi)[11]
- Portoportal shunt, for example, Rex shunt
- Nonshunt procedures
  - Devascularisation: Hassab's procedure[17] and its modifications, and Sugiura and Futagawa[18] procedure and its modifications.
  - Transection procedures: Oesophageal transection and gastric transection.
  - Resection procedures: Total gastrectomy and partial oesophagogastrectomy with jejunal or colonic interposition.
  - Direct ligation of varices: Crile's procedure and Boerema's procedure.

Portosystemic shunt procedures decompress the high-pressure portal system into the low-pressure systemic venous circulation through an artificially created channel. The nonshunt procedures directly tackle the bleeding areas by disconnecting them from the high-pressure portal system. Thus, the portal hypertension persists, but the areas prone to bleeding are shielded from its effects.

Although the role of surgery in patients with cirrhosis and portal hypertension is decreasing, in patients with noncirrhotic portal hypertension, surgery is a one-time treatment option that provides long-lasting relief from variceal bleeding, without some of the long-term complications seen in patients with cirrhosis.

The choice of surgical procedure is based on the following principles:

- The functional status of liver: Patients with deranged liver function may be offered a selective or partial shunt, whereas those with normal liver function may be treated by a nonselective shunt. A DSRS or partial portacaval shunt with H-graft is generally offered to patients with cirrhosis (usually Child's A status), whereas a proximal splenorenal shunt suits patients with EHPVO and NCPF well.
- Availability of shuntable vessels: The commonly used shuntable vessels on the portal venous side are the portal vein, the splenic vein and the superior mesenteric vein, with the coronary vein being used less frequently. On the systemic venous side, the inferior vena cava and the left renal vein are used commonly. The nonavailability of any of these veins may limit the options, for example, a portacaval shunt cannot be offered to patients with EHPVO. Thrombosis of all the shuntable veins on the portal venous side precludes any shunt surgery and becomes an indication for devascularisation procedures.

- Presence of massive or symptomatic splenomegaly: Shunts that include splenectomy may be chosen over others if the spleen is massively enlarged (as in NCPF) or symptomatic (if patients have splenic infarcts and have pain) or if the patients have clinically important hypersplenism (menorrhagia, gum bleeds, epistaxis and anaemia), as is the case in nearly half of the patients with noncirrhotic portal hypertension.[8]
- Presence of uncontrolled ascites: A selective shunt does not relieve ascites and thus should be avoided in patients who have ascites.
- Candidates for liver transplant in the near future: Portacaval shunt is avoided in these patients, as it requires dissection in the hepatoduodenal ligament and thus makes future transplant surgery difficult. Sarfeh's interposition portacaval shunt, on the other hand, is better, as it is easy to dismantle during transplantation and, in fact, can facilitate the anhepatic phase by maintaining portosystemic flow.

Transjugular Intrahepatic Portosystemic Shunt

Transjugular intrahepatic portosystemic shunt is a minimally invasive nonselective portosystemic shunt that behaves like a side-to-side portacaval shunt. It decreases the portal pressure and thus controls the variceal bleeding and ascites. It can be used in the elective and emergency settings. It has replaced emergency surgical shunts for the management of refractory acute variceal bleeding in patients with cirrhosis. It is also a first-line option as a 'bridge' to transplantation, as it avoids the risks of general anaesthesia and a difficult surgery. Transjugular intrahepatic portosystemic shunt is relatively safe, with a procedure-related mortality of around 1 to 2%, and successfully arrests bleeding in more than 90% of patients.[23–25]

SYMPTOMATIC HYPERSPLENISM AND OTHER INDICATIONS FOR SPLENECTOMY

Patients with portal hypertension usually have an enlarged spleen and other features of hypersplenism such as anaemia, thromobocytopenia and leucopenia. Symptomatic hypersplenism occurs in around 33% of patients with cirrhotic portal hypertension[26] and in around 25% of patients with noncirrhotic portal hypertension[27] and may manifest with spontaneous bleeding, weakness, dyspnoea and recurrent infections. Splenectomy is indicated for symptomatic hypersplenism and usually restores the blood counts. Splenectomy is also considered for patients with asymptomatic hypersplenism, which interferes with the treatment of the primary disease, for example, interferon therapy cannot be given for the treatment of hepatitis C if the platelet count is less than 50,000/mm^3.[28]

COMPLICATIONS OF SPLENECTOMY, PORTOSYSTEMIC SHUNT AND DEVASCULARISATION PROCEDURES

The complications associated with surgical procedures for portal hypertension can be grouped according to the time of their occurrence (Table 29.2). The management would also vary based on the timing and severity of the complication. All the complications associated with splenectomy have not been described here, as these are available in standard text books. Only those complications of splenectomy that are related to the presence of portal hypertension are discussed.

Intraoperative Complications

Haemorrhage

Surgery in patients with portal hypertension is difficult and is associated with a much higher risk of intraoperative bleeding. In a study by Prasad et al,[7] the mean (standard deviation [SD]) blood loss during proximal splenorenal shunt surgery in children with EHPVO was 735 (315) mL. Increased portal pressure results in the opening up of portosystemic

Table 29.2 Complications of surgery for portal hypertension

Timing	Complications
Intraoperative	Haemorrhage Injury to adjacent organs: gastric fundus, splenic flexure of colon, tail of pancreas, oesophagus, diaphragm, bile duct, etc.
Early postoperative	Haemorrhage Respiratory: atelectasis, pneumonia and pleural effusion Postoperative hepatic decompensation Ascites Surgical site infections Thrombocytosis Gastroparesis Thrombotic complications Gastric, colonic, oesophageal, pancreatic or biliary leak/fistula Acute pancreatitis
Long-term	Rebleeding Hepatic encephalopathy: overt or subclinical Thrombocytosis OPSI Nephropathy Myelopathy

Abbreviations: OPSI, overwhelming postsplenectomy infections.

collaterals in the abdominal wall, peritoneal cavity and retroperitoneum. The collaterals develop even in areas that are usually considered avascular, for example, the splenorenal ligament, splenophrenic attachments and the left triangular ligament. Sometimes, even entering the abdomen is difficult because of the presence of the collaterals in the subcutaneous and preperitoneal tissues. In the abdominal cavity, there may be vascular adhesions of the organs or the omentum to the parietal wall, especially if there has been a prior surgical procedure. The collaterals have very thin walls and lack a tunica media, owing to their origin from very small veins, and they rupture with minimal trauma. The walls of these collaterals are friable, and injury to a single collateral may result in rapid blood loss. The bleeding may be controlled by applying pressure; however, attempted suture ligation may further accentuate the bleeding from these friable vessels. The best strategy is to prevent bleeding by careful and meticulous dissection and liberal use of ligatures. Often, it is a good idea to pack the bleeding site and move to dissection in another area. However, one should not have more than two bleeding sites at any time, as these patients can quickly loose a large amount of blood from the high-pressure portal circulation. If bleeding occurs at the second site, it should be packed, and one should move back to the initial bleeding site to achieve haemostasis. Rarely, the bleeding may be difficult to control by suture ligation, and massive blood loss and multiple transfusions may result in coagulopathy and hypothermia. In such a scenario, it is best to pack the bleeding site effectively with laparotomy pads to maintain tamponade, ensure haemostasis and abandon the procedure. The patient can be re-explored after 48 hours after stabilisation and correction of hypothermia and coagulopathy. In our experience of 955 procedures for noncirrhotic portal hypertension, uncontrolled intraoperative bleeding occurred in 6 (0.6%) patients, resulting in mortality.

Hypotensive anaesthesia with nitroprusside has been found to significantly decrease the mean (SD) intraoperative blood loss (from 1286 [523] to 517 [220] mL) and transfusion requirement (from 3.0 [1.2] to 0.9 [0.9] units) in patients undergoing surgery for portal hypertension.[29] The use of energy sources, for example, a vessel-sealing device, may also help minimise the blood loss during surgery.[30]

Injury to Adjacent Organs

Organs in close relation to the spleen such as the fundus of the stomach, splenic flexure of the colon and tail of the pancreas can be injured during surgery. The fundus of the stomach lies in close relation to the upper pole of the spleen. The gastrosplenic ligament at this site may have large collaterals and may be too short for safe division between ligatures. In addition, when glue has been used by the endoscopist for sclerotherapy, the fundus and the greater curvature are often densely adherent to the splenic pole and hilum. The glue (intravascular or extravasated) causes intense fibrosis and dense adhesions. In addition, presence of the hardened glue in the stomach wall makes it brittle and thus prone to injury. In such cases, this step may be left till the last and the gastrosplenic ligament may be divided close to the splenic capsule. If injury to the stomach occurs and is recognised during surgery, it may be repaired in two layers. Rarely, en bloc resection of the gastric fundus with the mobilised spleen may be required. Similarly, injury to the splenic flexure of colon may also be repaired primarily, taking care to avoid faecal contamination.

Injury to the pancreatic tail may cause bleeding and may require resection of a small part of the tail of pancreas. The left renal artery and renal pelvis may be injured during dissection of the renal vein for a splenorenal shunt. This usually occurs when there is aberrant anatomy, for example, branch of the renal artery lying anterior to the renal vein. Injury to a renal artery branch results in ischaemic infarct of the supplied area, as renal arteries are end arteries. This should be avoided by looping the aberrant artery and keeping it out of the field during the renal vein dissection and clamping.

A portacaval procedure requires dissection in the hepatic hilum, which may result in iatrogenic injury to the bile duct. A replaced hepatic artery from the superior mesenteric artery is especially at risk during portacaval shunt surgery and should always be identified by palpation before starting the dissection.

Early Postoperative Complications

Bleeding

Postoperative intra-abdominal bleeding is a dreaded and life-threatening complication of surgery for portal hypertension. Postoperative bleeding can present in many ways. Slow bleeding manifesting as continuous low-volume sanguineous drain output, without any haemodynamic consequences, is usually due to inadequate haemostasis of the retroperitoneum during the surgery. We overrun the cut edge of the retroperitoneum by using interlocking nonabsorbable sutures at the time of primary surgery to prevent postoperative bleeding. The initial management includes monitoring of the drain output and the vital parameters and correction of hypothermia and coagulopathy. Conservative management may be continued if patient remains haemodynamically stable and has no or minimal drop in haemoglobin over a period of time, and the drain output decreases or becomes light in colour. Re-exploration should be considered if the drain output remains high, despite normal coagulation parameters, or if the patient becomes haemodynamically unstable.

Sudden high-volume haemorrhagic drain output with haemodynamic compromise is a life-threatening complication and suggests bleeding from a larger vessel such as the splenic vein, splenic artery or the shunt. It may occur in the early postoperative period due to a slipped ligature or later if an abscess or infectious collection erodes into a vessel. This may present with hypotension and abdominal distension if there is no drain or the drain is blocked. The abdominal cavity can accommodate a large volume of blood, and thus, distension is a late sign. Intra-abdominal bleeding should be suspected and ruled out even in the absence of abdominal distension if there is unexplained haemodynamic instability. The management includes rapid resuscitation, re-exploration and suture ligation of the bleeding vessel. If there is bleeding from the shunt, an attempt should be made to control the bleeding by using reinforcing sutures. Sometimes, the bleeding is due to partial disruption of the shunt. In such an event, it is better to dismantle the anastomosis and do it afresh. Rarely, the vessels may be so friable that it is not possible to redo the anastomosis. In such a scenario, the only option is to ligate the splenic vein and attempt a repair of the renal vein (an autologous/prosthetic graft may be rarely required).

In a study of 562 devascularisation procedures for portal hypertension,[31] intra-abdominal bleeding occurred in 32 (5.7%) patients, of which 8 could not be salvaged, resulting in a high case fatality rate of 25%. In our experience of 855 procedures for EHPVO (unpublished data), intra-abdominal bleeding occurred in 23 (2.7%) patients. Of these, 12 (52%) patients required re-exploration.

Respiratory Complications

Surgery for portal hypertension is usually done through a thoracoabdominal, subcostal or upper midline incision. Inadequate pain management in the early postoperative period may result in poor inspiratory effort and basal atelectasis. This may be managed by providing good pain relief and incentive spirometry. However, if not properly managed, basal atelectasis may progress to basal pneumonitis, which requires treatment with intravenous antibiotics. Mild pleural effusion is a common complication but usually does not require any specific treatment. Rarely, the effusion might require ultrasound-guided drainage

if the patient develops respiratory distress. Respiratory complications occurred in around 17% of patients in a series of modified Suguira procedure reported by Mathur et al.[32]

Ascites

Ascites is a common early and a long-term complication of surgery for portal hypertension. Surgery causes disruption of lymphatic pathways in the abdominal wall and the retroperitoneum, resulting in the formation of ascites, which presents as increased serous output from the abdominal drain. Any postoperative liver dysfunction can further increase the ascites. Although ascites usually resolves spontaneously in patients with normal liver function, it may require diuretics for a short duration. However, in patients with cirrhosis, it is a troublesome complication, is difficult to treat and prolongs the postoperative hospital stay. The incidence of postoperative ascites depends on the type of procedure performed. In a randomised trial, ascites occurred in 11 of 27 patients who underwent a devascularisation procedure, whereas none of the 27 patients who underwent a nonselective shunt developed ascites.[33] Selective shunts worsen the ascites and are usually avoided in patients who have ascites or who are at a risk for this complication.

Manifestations of Inadvertent Injuries to Adjacent Organs

Although rare, inadvertent injuries can occur to adjacent organs such as stomach, colon and tail of pancreas, resulting in gastric, colonic and pancreatic leaks, respectively. Hollow viscus leaks may present with fistula if the contents find the way to the outside through the drain or the surgical wound and may be managed conservatively, especially if the patient does not have features of peritonitis or sepsis and if fistula output is low. These patients may develop subphrenic or other intra-abdominal collections, which may be managed by percutaneous drainage. Uncontrolled intra-abdominal leaks present with features of peritonitis and require surgical intervention in the form of lavage and drainage. In addition, an uncontrolled gastric leak would require repair of the defect after freshening of margins along with a tube gastrostomy and a feeding jejunostomy.

An uncontrolled colonic leak would require either a resection anastomosis or exteriorisation of the injury site as a colostomy or a proximal ileostomy, depending upon the clinical situation. Injury to the pancreatic tail may result in pancreatic fistula or formation of a pseudocyst. Pancreatic fistulae are usually managed conservatively. Pseudocysts may require internal drainage if they persist, increase in size and become symptomatic. In a retrospective series of

155 Sugiura and Futagawa procedures,[34] postoperative peritonitis occurred in 6 (3.9%) patients and subphrenic collection occurred in 3 (1.9%) patients. The incidences of pancreatic pseudocyst and pancreatic fistula in the same series were 1.9% and 0.6%, respectively. Liu et al[31] reported only 1 gastric fistula in a series of 562 Hassab's procedures. In our experience, there was only 1 gastric, oesophageal and pancreatic fistula each in 855 procedures for noncirrhotic portal hypertension.

The lower thoracic oesophagus is at risk for injury during devascularisation procedures. Oesophageal transection may result in a leak, stricture or fistula formation. Controlled leaks can be managed conservatively for spontaneous closure, whereas uncontrolled leaks require either a percutaneous or a surgical intervention. Oesophageal strictures usually respond to endoscopic dilatation. Sugiura and Futagawa[35] reported 39 (6%) leaks in their series of 636 devascularisation procedures. Of these, five patients who had major leaks died. The rest of the 34 patients had minor leaks and were successfully managed conservatively. Strictures developed in 16 patients, and all were successfully managed by either bougie or endoscopic dilatation. Mathur et al[32] reported an oesophageal leak rate of 6%; all the patients improved with conservative management. The rate of oesophageal stricture in the same series was 15%.

Injury to pancreatic parenchyma during dissection of the splenic vein can result in acute pancreatitis in the postoperative period. This is a life-threatening complication and occurs more commonly after DSRS, which requires complete dissection of the splenic vein from the pancreas for splenoportal disconnection. Jin et al[36] reported 11 (7%) patients with acute pancreatitis after 154 DSRS procedures; 6 of these patients died. In another series of 111 DSRS procedures reported by Elwood et al,[37] 2 patients developed acute pancreatitis in the postoperative period.

Postoperative Liver Decompensation

This complication occurs mainly in patients with cirrhosis. The stress of surgery may precipitate liver failure in patients who already have a compromised liver function. Patients with well-compensated liver dysfunction, for example, Child–Pugh class A, usually develop transient decompensation, which presents as worsening of ascites, and require only supportive care and diuretics. However, patients with poor liver function may develop progressive liver failure, which manifests as hepatic encephalopathy after surgery, especially if there is an added insult such as sepsis in the postoperative period. Management is

essentially supportive, including admission to an intensive care unit and treatment of the precipitating factors such as infection. Patients with high-grade encephalopathy or hepatic coma may require ventilatory support. Renal function if deranged (hepatorenal syndrome) may require dialysis. The prognosis is poor if multiorgan failure ensues. In a study by Liu et al,[31] the rates of hepatic encephalopathy and hepatorenal syndrome after 562 devascularisation procedures in patients with cirrhosis were 3.2% and 3.0%, respectively, with mortality rates of 33.3% and 23.5%, respectively.

Infectious Complications

Infectious complications occur more commonly if surgery requires entry into a hollow viscus, for example, gastrotomy to control bleeding from varices. Superficial surgical site infection presents with pain, erythema and purulent discharge from the wound site and usually resolves once the wound is opened and drained. Deep infections, although rare, are dangerous and may cause necrosis of the sheath and leak of ascitic fluid from the wound and may further progress to burst abdomen with evisceration, if not diagnosed early. The necrotic sheath should be debrided and abdominal closure should be done by using the Bogota bag technique. If possible, the Bogota bag should be fixed to the healthy margins of the sheath rather than the skin.

Other infectious complications include intra-abdominal collections and infected loculated ascites. These are suspected if a patient develops fever in the postoperative period and can be diagnosed by an ultrasound or a computed tomography (CT) scan. These require percutaneous drainage and treatment with antibiotics based on the culture and sensitivity pattern.

The rate of infectious complications was around 1.6% in a large series of elective devascularisation procedures, out of which 0.5% were incision site infections and 1.1% were infected subphrenic collections.[31]

Thrombotic Complications

Early thrombotic complications include shunt thrombosis and portal vein thrombosis. Early shunt thrombosis is usually related to technical issues such as a kink or compression. Shunt thrombosis may go unnoticed initially or may present with worsening ascites. If diagnosed early, it may respond to anticoagulation or an endovascular procedure. If shunt thrombosis is not diagnosed early, it may present later with rebleeding. In a study of partial portacaval shunts by Collins et al,[38] the rate of early shunt thrombosis was 8% (in 6 out of 72 patients). All shunts with early thrombosis in these series were salvaged, either by catheter-directed thrombolysis or by reoperation.

Portal vein thrombosis usually occurs due to extension of a thrombus from a tributary that has been ligated during surgery. The thrombus that forms at this site can extend proximally into the portal vein. Acute portal vein thrombosis occurred in 3% of patients in a series of 562 devascularisation procedures.[31] The symptoms of portal vein thrombosis depend on the adequacy of the collateral circulation. The clinical presentation can range from asymptomatic to worsening of ascites to mesenteric ischaemia. The thrombotic complications may also be related to the pre-existing hypercoagulable state or postsplenectomy thrombocytosis.

Others

A few patients develop gastroparesis, which presents as vomiting or high nasogastric tube output. It may be a consequence of vagotomy or a fluid collection in relation to the stomach. It usually responds to conservative management and prokinetic drugs. Acute gastric dilatation, which used to be a dreaded complication of splenectomy, has now become extremely rare with the routine use of nasogastric drainage.

Reactive thrombocytosis is a common finding after splenectomy. In one study, 75% of patients developed thrombocytosis after splenectomy.[39] Platelet counts peak at 7 to 20 days after surgery. A cytokine-driven process resulting in increased interleukin-6 and tumour necrosis factor-alpha levels has been implicated in the pathogenesis of postsplenectomy thrombocytosis.[40] The condition is usually self-limited and does not require any specific treatment. However, some patients are at increased risk of thrombotic complications after splenectomy, for example, those with a pre-existing thrombophilic disorder or those with autonomous thrombocytosis. In a study, thrombotic complications occurred in around 5% of patients after splenectomy, and platelet counts above 650,000/mm^3 were associated with increased risk of thrombotic complications.[41] Hence, treatment with antiplatelet drugs may be justified in patients who develop severe thrombocytosis (platelet count >1,000,000/mm^3) after splenectomy. Patients with a known thrombophilic disorder should receive anticoagulation perioperatively and, possibly, life long after the shunt surgery. Treatment with cytoreductive agents, for example, hydroxyurea and anagrelide, may be justified if platelet counts rise above 1,400,000/mm^3.

Some patients develop unexplained fever, usually low to moderate grade, without any identifiable cause, even after extensive work-up. These patients possibly have postsplenectomy fever, which remits after a few weeks. Most of these patients are treated with empirical oral antibiotics, even though no source of infection can be found.

Long-Term Complications

The most important long-term complications of the surgical procedures done for prevention or treatment of variceal bleeding are rebleeding and hepatic encephalopathy.

Rebleeding

Rebleeding is essentially a failure of therapy rather than a complication. Rebleeding occurs more commonly after nonshunt procedures as compared with shunt procedures. Rebleeding after a shunt is usually because the shunt is thrombosed. Shunt thrombosis may occur because of technical reasons, for example, compression and kink, or because of a hypercoagulable state. Using a small-size portal tributary for shunt also increases the chances of shunt thrombosis. In a study by Mishra et al,[10] only the size of the splenic vein had a significant impact on the long-term patency of proximal splenorenal shunts. The long-term shunt patency in this series was only 43%. We evaluated shunt patency in 212 of our nearly 1000 patients and found the long-term patency of proximal lienorenal shunts to be around 84%, as assessed by direct visualisation of shunt (72%) or by the presence of dilated renal vein (12%) on ultrasonogram. There was indirect evidence of shunt patency (regression of varices on oesophagoscopy) in another 7% patients (unpublished data). However, it should be noted that rebleeding does not occur in all patients who develop shunt thrombosis.

Nonshunt procedures only disconnect the areas prone to bleeding from the high-pressure portal circulation. With time, new connections may develop that cause reappearance of varices and the risk of rebleeding. Bleeding can also occur from severe portal hypertensive gastropathy.

Patients with rebleeding should be managed initially with endoscopic therapy. After initial control of bleeding, patients may be offered a second shunt surgery or endoscopic variceal eradication, with life-long endoscopic follow-up. The choice between a second shunt and endoscopic therapy depends on the aetiology of portal hypertension, availability of another shuntable vein and the clinical situation. A second shunt surgery, usually a mesocaval shunt, is offered to patients who have noncirrhotic portal hypertension and a shuntable vein. A second shunt is also desirable in patients who have ectopic varices (which are not amenable to endoscopic therapy) or portal biliopathy (may be curative in some and may facilitate a subsequent biliary procedure in others).

Hepatic Encephalopathy

Hepatic encephalopathy is a symptom of worsening liver function. It is considered to be a consequence of the accumulation of gut-derived toxins due to their decreased hepatic clearance. Portosystemic shunts divert the blood away from the liver and thus may accelerate the development of encephalopathy in patients with already compromised liver function. Selective and partial shunts preserve some of the blood flow to the liver and have a lower incidence of hepatic encephalopathy than nonselective shunts in the initial period, but this advantage may be lost with time, as the shunt loses selectivity. Nonshunt procedures do not decrease hepatic blood flow and thus are associated with lower rates of hepatic encephalopathy.

Some patients who otherwise do not have any clinical features of hepatic encephalopathy are detected to be having subtle changes on electroencephalography (EEG) or on psychometric tests such as reverse counting, construction of a five-pointed star and number connection test. This condition is known as 'subclinical' or 'minimal hepatic' encephalopathy.[46] Overt or subclinical hepatic encephalopathy frequently occurs in patients with cirrhosis, especially after portosystemic shunts. Patients with NCPF (10–30%, depending on the type of test) also develop features of subclinical encephalopathy after nonselective shunt procedures, and overt encephalopathy occurs in 7 to 10% of the cases.[47] There is also some evidence (based on retrospective analysis) that in patients with NCPF, the shunt size should be limited to less than 1.3 cm, so as to prevent or decrease the occurrence of postshunt encephalopathy in these patients.[48] On the other hand, patients with idiopathic EHPVO do not develop overt or subclinical encephalopathy after portosystemic shunts.[49] This is because these patients have normal liver function.

Subclinical encephalopathy usually does not require any treatment; however, patients may be advised to avoid activities such as driving and handling machinery that requires fine judgement. Medical management, for example, lactulose, may be tried initially for overt encephalopathy. The initial dose is 30 mL every 8 hours, which is later adjusted to achieve three semiformed stools per day. Sodium benzoate given at a dose of 5 g twice daily is a cheaper alternative, which is equally effective as lactulose.[50] A baseline clinical and mental status examination should be done before starting medical management, and the patients should be reassessed at regular intervals thereafter for improvement in mental status. Assessment should be done hourly or 2 hourly for patients with high-grade encephalopathy. The interval may be increased if the patient improves. The baseline ammonia level should be measured, and it should be repeated at 72 hours. Ammonia levels do not correlate with grade of encephalopathy, but the demonstration of decrease in levels of ammonia from the baseline levels may be used as a marker for success of therapy. Psychometric tests are not useful for monitoring treatment, as they are too sensitive and may remain abnormal for a long time. If the symptoms are not controlled by medical management, surgical ligation or radiological occlusion of the shunt may be required.

Splenectomy-Related Complications

Overwhelming postsplenectomy infection (OPSI) is a rare but life-threatening complication that is usually caused by encapsulated bacteriae, for example, *Streptococcus pneumoniae*, *Neisseria meningitidis* and *Haemophilus influenzae*. Overwhelming postsplenectomy infection is uniformly fatal without treatment and has a mortality rate of 40 to 70%, even after treatment with antibiotics. Although the risk of infection remains life long, most OPSIs occur within the first few years after splenectomy and the risk is highest in patients with haematological disorders.[51] In order to prevent OPSI, routine polyvalent vaccine is recommended 2 weeks before the planned splenectomy. However, in our experience of more than 1500 splenectomies over the past 40 years with or without shunt procedures in patients with noncirrhotic portal hypertension, the incidence of OPSI was negligible (three documented patients). We do not vaccinate all our patients before shunt surgery.[8]

Rare Shunt-Related Complications

Shunt myelopathy

Shunt myelopathy or portosystemic myelopathy[52] is a rare long-term complication of portosystemic shunt surgery and has been described only in case reports. It usually presents with spastic paraparesis, with brisk reflexes and an extensor plantar response. The upper limbs are usually spared. Sensations, cerebellar function and sphincter reflexes are usually normal. It is a diagnosis of exclusion and requires extensive investigation to rule out other diagnoses. A magnetic resonance imaging (MRI) scan should be done to rule out spinal cord compression or myelitis; vitamin B_{12} and folate level tests should be done to rule out deficiency; and electromyography should be done to rule out secondary motor neuron involvement. Human immunodeficiency virus infection and autoimmune disorders should also be considered in the differential diagnosis.[53]

Shunt myelopathy is usually associated with hyperammonaemia and hepatic encephalopathy, which generally co-exist, and predates the onset of myelopathy in most instances. Hypoproteinaemia and abnormal EEG are other important markers for diagnosis. Pathogenesis is poorly understood, but the portosystemic shunting is considered responsible for the disease by allowing gut-derived neurotoxins or nitrogenous breakdown products to bypass the liver. Portosystemic myelopathy has been reported after total as well as partial shunts, but the interval between the shunt surgery and onset of myelopathy is significantly shorter after total shunts, thus implicating the volume of shunted blood as a risk factor.[52] Liver transplant is the treatment of choice for patients with cirrhosis and should be offered early in the course of illness.[54] In the early stages, there is only demyelination of the spinal cord, which can be reversed with transplant. The damage becomes irreversible once the axonal loss sets in.[53]

Portosystemic myelopathy has also been reported after portosystemic shunts in patients with NCPF.[55] As the liver function is preserved in these patients, the portosystemic shunting is considered the primary pathology, and shunt blockade, either surgical or radiological, should be offered as treatment. In our study of prophylactic proximal splenorenal shunts in patients with NCPF,[9] 3 of 38 patients (8%) developed myelopathy on long-term follow-up. Two patients were managed with surgical shunt ligation, whereas the third one was managed with angiographic embolisation of the shunt.

Glomerulopathy

There are reports of some patients developing renal dysfunction (nephrotic range proteinuria and renal failure) after portosystemic shunts. In a study by Pal et al,[9] 4 of 38 patients (10.5%) who underwent prophylactic proximal splenorenal shunt for NCPF developed renal dysfunction on long-term follow-up. Some studies have reported the findings of renal biopsies in these patients, which have shown features of membranoproliferative glomerulonephritis, with deposition of IgA and variable deposition of complement, IgG and IgM in the capillaries. [56–58] Portosystemic shunts have been implicated in the pathogenesis of this renal disease, as they divert the blood away from the liver, thereby reducing the clearance of immune complexes formed in the portal circulation, which can ultimately result in immune complex–induced glomerulonephritis. This hypothesis is based on the premise of a single renal biopsy done at the time of renal dysfunction, and none of these reported cases had a baseline renal biopsy before or at the time of construction of the shunt. There is enough evidence that the patients with cirrhosis and NCPF may have glomerular involvement, even before the shunt surgery. In a study by Callard et al,[59] glomerular lesions were detected in 9 of 10 (90%) patients with cirrhosis who underwent renal biopsy at the time of portacaval shunt procedures. These changes were called 'cirrhotic glomerulosclerosis'. In another study,[60] glomerular lesions were detected in 12 of 23 (52%) patients with cirrhosis who underwent renal biopsy at the time of liver transplantation.

Renal lesions have also been observed in patients with NCPF. Kumar et al[61] performed renal biopsy, renal function tests and urinalysis in 10 patients with NCPF at the time of splenorenal shunt surgery. Four patients with NCPF were found to have significant deposition of IgA and C3, all of whom had abnormal creatinine clearance (<80 mL/min) and increased urinary protein (>250 mg/24 hours). Renal function tests and urinalysis done at 6 months after the shunt surgery did not show any deterioration.

Thus, there is no evidence to suggest the role of shunt surgery in the renal dysfunction that develops in some patients after these procedures. This may actually be a part of the disease process itself.

The rates of complications after surgery for portal hypertension vary widely, depending on the expertise and the type of procedure. Table 29.3 lists the early and long-term results of some of the larger series of surgical operations done for the management of variceal bleeding. We have listed the incidence of various complications in our experience of surgery for portal hypertension in Tables 29.4 and 29.5 (unpublished data). In the following discussion, we have tried to highlight the effects of the type of procedure on the incidence of postoperative complications.

SHUNT VERSUS DEVASCULARISATION PROCEDURES

Devascularisation procedures require more extensive dissection and may require division and anastomosis of hollow viscus. Thus, early complications such as ascites, gastroparesis and oesophageal leaks occur more frequently after devascularisation procedures.

Table 29.3 Early and long-term results of some large series of various surgical procedures performed for the control of variceal bleeding

Author (Year)	Diagnosis	Procedure	Groups	n	Mortality (30-day) (%)	Shunt thrombosis (%)	Rebleed (%)	Encephalopathy (%)	Percent long-term survival (years of follow-up)
Orloff[42] (1995)	Cirrhosis	Portacaval (unselected patients, surgery within 8 hours of initial contact)	1963–1978	180	42			9	30 (15 y)
			1978–1990	200	15	0.5	1	8	57 (15 y)
Prasad[7] (1994)	EHPVO	Proximal splenorenal shunt (children)	Elective	140	0.7	Not mentioned	11	0	95 (15 y)
			Emergency	20	10	Not mentioned			
Livingstone[43] (2006)	Cirrhosis	Distal splenorenal shunt	Nil	507	4.6	Not mentioned	12	13.9	34.4 (10 y)
Paquet[44] (1989)	Cirrhosis	Mesocaval, good liver function	Nil	100	10	10	5.5	12.2	35.1 (10 y)
Collins[38] (1998)	Cirrhosis	Sarfeh's shunt, good liver function	Nil	72	7.7	Early: 8.3 (all salvaged) Late: 5	8	Not mentioned	54 (7 y)
Raia[45] (1994)	Schistosomiasis	Proximal splenorenal shunt	Nil	32	6.2	23.5	28.6	39.3	57.1
		Distal splenorenal shunt	Nil	30	0	14.3	22.2	14.8	85.2
		Devascularisation	Nil	32	0	Not applicable	21.4	0	92.9
Sugiura[35] (1984)	73% cirrhotic	Oesophageal transections with paraoesophagogastric devascularisation	Prophylactic	185	4.3	Not applicable		Not mentioned	72: cirrhotic, 96: noncirrhotic (10 y)
			Elective	349	3.2	Not applicable	6	Not mentioned	72: cirrhotic, 95: noncirrhotic (10 y)
			Emergency	102	13.7	Not applicable		Not mentioned	55: cirrhotic, 90: noncirrhotic (10 y)
Mathur[32] (1999)	EHPVO and NCPF	Modified Sugiura	Nil	68	4	Not applicable	11	0	88 (5 y)
Liu[31] (2013)	Cirrhosis	Modified Hassab	Nil	562	4.6	Not applicable	9.7	Not mentioned	Not mentioned

Abbreviations: EHPVO, extrahepatic portal venous obstruction; NCPF, noncirrhotic portal fibrosis.

Table 29.4 Early outcomes of surgery for extrahepatic portal venous obstruction

Procedure	Mortality (%)	Morbidity (%)
Overall	2.1 (n = 965)	12.2 (n = 855)
Portosystemic shunt (proximal lienorenal shunt in 98%)	1.2 (n = 831)	10.1 (n = 759)
Devascularisation	9.2 (n = 109)	28.1 (n = 96)
Elective	1.3 (n = 912)	9.3 (n = 690) (PSRS only)
Emergency	15.1 (n = 53)	27.8 (n = 41) (PSRS only)

Abbreviation: PSRS, proximal splenorenal shunt.

Table 29.5 Incidence of various postoperative complications after surgery for extrahepatic portal venous obstruction-related portal hypertension (n = 855)

Postoperative complications	Incidence, n (%)
Re-explorations	19 (2.2)
Intra-abdominal bleeding	23 (2.7)
Respiratory complications	21 (2.5)
Wound infections	13 (1.5)
Intra-abdominal collections	13 (1.5)
Sepsis	2 (0.2)
Pancreatitis	1 (0.1)
Pancreatic fistula	1 (0.1)
Gastric fistula	1 (0.1)
Oesophageal fistula	1 (0.1)

Among long-term complications, devascularisation procedures are associated with higher rebleeding rates because of previously discussed reasons. Hepatic encephalopathy occurs less frequently, as these procedures do not decrease the hepatic blood flow. A recent meta-analysis that compared portosystemic shunt surgery with devascularisation procedures in patients with cirrhotic portal hypertension (two studies included patients with schistosomiasis) found significantly higher rate of rebleeding (20.2% vs. 9.6%) and significantly lower rate of hepatic encephalopathy (8.3% vs. 12.7%) with devascularisation procedures. However, there was no significant difference in the operative mortality (5.3% vs. 3.4%) and long-term survival (88% vs. 87%).[62] Table 29.6 shows the differences between shunt procedures and devascularisation procedures.

NONSELECTIVE VERSUS SELECTIVE SHUNTS

The selective and partial shunts maintain some hepatic blood flow and thus are associated with a lower incidence of hepatic encephalopathy. However, for the same reason, selective shunts may worsen the ascites. A selective shunt, for example, distal splenorenal shunt, may lose selectivity over time, thus resulting in a similar incidence of hepatic encephalopathy on long-term follow-up.

In a meta-analysis of RCTs of selective versus nonselective shunts (Table 29.7), there was no significant difference in the rates of rebleeding (9.6% vs. 11.2%; four RCTs, including around 100 patients in each group; heterogeneity 0%), encephalopathy (22.4% vs. 32.1%; five RCTs, including around 140 patients in each group;

Table 29.6 Studies comparing results of shunt and devascularisation procedures

Author (year)	Type of study	Procedure	n	Diagnosis	Rebleed, n (%)	p-value	Encephalopathy, n (%)	p-value
Borgonovo[33] (1996)	RCT	Shunt	27	Cirrhosis	3 (11)	NS	15 (56)	0.002
		Devasc	27		9 (33)		6 (22)	
Da Silva[63] (1986)	RCT	Shunt	62	Schistosomiasis	6 (10)	NS	10 (16)	<0.05
		Devasc	32		4 (12)		0 (0)	
Orozco[64] (1994)	Retrospective	Shunt	101	Cirrhosis	13 (13)	NS	Not mentioned	–
		Devasc	55		8 (15)		Not mentioned	
Xu[65] (2005)	Retrospective	Shunt	356	Cirrhosis (98%)	30 (8)	–	19 (5)	–
		Devasc	229		54 (24)		10 (4)	
Ezzat[66] (1990)	Retrospective	Shunt	123	Cirrhosis or schistosomiasis	9 (7)	<0.05	23 (19)	<0.05
		Devasc	96		30 (31)		7 (7)	

Abbreviations: RCT, randomised controlled trial; devasc, devascularisation; NS, not significant.

Table 29.7 Randomised trials comparing selective and nonselective shunts

Author (year)		n	Diagnosis	Rebleed, n (%)	p-value	Encephalopathy, n (%)	p-value
Da Silva[63] (1986)	Selective	29	Schistosomiasis	2 (7)	NS	2 (7)	–
	Nonselective	31		4 (13)		8 (26)	
Conn[13] (1981)	Selective	24	Cirrhosis	3 (16)	NS	6 (32)	NS
	Nonselective	29		2 (9)		5 (23)	
Fischer[15] (1981)	Selective	24	Cirrhosis	2 (8)	NS	1 (4)	NS
	Nonselective	19		2 (11)		2 (11)	
Millikan[14] (1985)	Selective	27	Cirrhosis	3 (11)	NS	7 (27)	<0.01
	Nonselective	28		4 (14)		22 (75)	

Abbreviation: NS, not significant.

heterogeneity 66%) and late mortality (19.2% vs. 20.6%; four RCTs, including around 100 patients in each group; heterogeneity 36%).[16]

COMPLICATIONS OF TRANSJUGULAR INTRAHEPATIC PORTOSYSTEMIC SHUNT

The creation of TIPSS is associated with a number of complications (Table 29.8) that may be related to the procedure itself or to the creation of a portosystemic shunt. Overall procedure-related morbidity is around 15 to 20%.[25]

Procedure-Related Complications

Access to the hepatic vein from a neck vein may cause puncture-site bleeding or haematoma, inadvertent puncture of the carotid artery or trachea, pneumothorax, cardiac arrhythmias and puncture of the inferior vena cava

Table 29.8 Complications of transjugular intrahepatic portosystemic shunt in a series of 100 consecutive patients[23]

Complication	Incidence (%)
• Procedure-related	
– Mortality	1
– Intraperitoneal haemorrhage	6
– Biliary haemorrhage	4
– Liver capsular haematoma	3
– Shunt dislocation	2
– Shunt migration	2
• Shunt-related: hepatic encephalopathy	Increased from 10 to 25%
• Stent-related	
– Shunt stenosis	22
– Shunt occlusion	11
– Variceal bleeding	11

or atrial wall.[25] The liver capsule may be punctured during the creation of the intrahepatic tract, which may result in haemoperitoneum. Injury to the biliary radicals during the creation of the intrahepatic tract may result in the formation of a fistula. This may present as haemobilia or lead to thrombosis of the TIPSS. Extrahepatic puncture of the portal vein may result in exsanguinating haemorrhage during dilatation of the tract.[25] The incidence of procedure-related deaths is less than 2%, and most of the deaths occur either due to intraprocedure myocardial infarction or intraperitoneal bleeding.[25]

Stent-Related Complications

The most important stent-related complications are stenosis and occlusion of the stent. The bare metal stents that were used initially for TIPSS had a high stenosis rate of about 75% at 12 months.[67] Shunt stenosis or occlusion may clinically present as rebleeding and/or reappearance or worsening of ascites. The introduction of covered stents has significantly improved patency rates.[68] Shunt patency can be monitored using a Doppler ultrasound, and any stenosis can be managed by angiographic intervention. Other stent-related complications are misplacement, migration, infection and thrombosis.[25] In addition, haemolytic anaemia may occur because of the bare metallic wires of the stent.[69]

Shunt-Related Complications

Portosystemic encephalopathy occurs in around 30% of patients after TIPSS,[70–72] and its incidence is similar to that of nonselective surgical shunts. Using a smaller-diameter stent is thought to decrease the incidence of encephalopathy. However, in a randomised trial of 8 mm and 10 mm stents, there was no difference in the encephalopathy rates.[73] The patients receiving the 8 mm stent had significantly higher incidence of portal hypertension-related complications at 1 year. Portosystemic myelopathy, which is a rare complication of portosystemic shunt surgery, has been reported after TIPSS as well.[74] Generalised coagulopathy, a life-threatening complication, has been reported in around 3% of patients after the TIPSS procedure. Possible reasons for development of coagulopathy after TIPSS include worsening of hepatic synthetic function, destruction of platelets by the stent and rapid reabsorption of fibrinolytic substances from the ascites.[25]

SURGERY FOR COMPLICATIONS OF ASCITES

Although ascites is a troublesome complication, it is usually treated medically with diuretics, with or without large-volume paracentesis. Ascites alone is almost never an indication for elective surgery in patients with portal hypertension. The presence of ascites may have a bearing on the choice of surgery when it is being performed for another indication such as variceal bleeding. Selective shunts do not relieve ascites, and devascularisation procedures may actually aggravate it. Thus, nonselective shunts should be preferred in patients with uncontrolled ascites.

Umbilical hernias occur more frequently in patients with cirrhosis, with a 20% risk of developing these in patients with ascites and cirrhosis. Umbilical hernias may be repaired electively, but because of a higher operative risk owing to their deranged liver function, there is a tendency to manage them conservatively and offer surgery only if complications develop. In a retrospective study,[75] the proportion of emergency operations for umbilical hernia was significantly higher in patients with portal hypertension (37.7% vs. 4.9%). The complications occurred more commonly after emergency repair than after elective repair (20.8% vs. 8.3%; Table 29.9), but there was no statistically significant difference in the mortality rates (7.4% vs. 3.7%). Age more than 65 years, model for end-stage liver disease (MELD) score >15, albumin level <3 g/dL and sepsis at presentation were predictors of postoperative mortality. In another retrospective study,[76] the success rate of conservative management was only 23% and elective repair was found to be safer. The patients on conservative management can develop incarcerated hernia, which may require emergency surgery. In some patients, tense ascites may cause pressure necrosis of the skin overlying the hernia, resulting in ruptured umbilical hernia. A ruptured umbilical hernia requires immediate surgical repair, as ascitic fluid can easily get infected, resulting in bacterial peritonitis. Thus, an elective repair may be a better choice in good-risk patients with preserved

Table 29.9 Incidence of postoperative complications after elective and emergency repair of umbilical hernia in patients with portal hypertension, as described in a retrospective study[75] of 390 patients

Complication	Incidence in elective surgery (%) (n = 241)	Incidence in emergency surgery (%) (n = 149)
• Surgical site infection		
– Superficial	0.8	1.3
– Deep	0.4	1.3
– Organ space infection	0.4	2.7
• Sepsis	2.9	10.7
• Prolonged ventilation	1.7	8.7
• Pneumonia	0.8	3.4
• Bleeding	0.4	2.0
• Re-exploration	3.3	8.1

liver function, whereas conservative management may be offered to high-risk patients (old age and high MELD) or patients who are expected to undergo liver transplantation in the near future.

The common early postoperative complications of umbilical hernia repair in patients with portal hypertension include wound infections, sepsis, respiratory complications and liver decompensation. Emergency surgery is associated with significantly higher incidence of sepsis, prolonged ventilation and re-exploration. In the long term, survival depends on the functional status of the liver; however, the increased abdominal pressure due to uncontrolled ascites may result in recurrence. In a prospective study,[77] elective repair of umbilical hernia was done for 30 patients with cirrhosis and ascites (median MELD of 12; interquartile range 8–16). There was no operative mortality, and only two patients developed complications (one hepatic decompensation and one pneumonia). There were two deaths on long-term follow-up, and neither was related to the repair of the umbilical hernia. Two patients developed recurrence of the hernia.

SURGERY FOR PORTAL BILIOPATHY

Patients with portal hypertension may develop biliary obstruction due to enlarged collaterals within and around the walls of the bile duct. This phenomenon is known as portal biliopathy. The biliary obstruction may be the result of direct compression by enlarged collaterals or may be due to ischaemic strictures of the bile duct as a result of chronic venous congestion. Portal biliopathy is more commonly seen in the patients with EHPVO but may also occur in patients with NCPF and cirrhosis. Surgical treatment is indicated in patients with EHPVO and NCPF and may require two stages. The first stage is a nonselective portosystemic shunt (proximal splenorenal shunt) that decreases the portal pressures and decompresses the collaterals around the bile duct. The first stage alone relieves the biliary obstruction in some patients. In others, it facilitates the second-stage surgery (Roux-en-Y hepaticojejunostomy) by decreasing the portal pressure and periportal collaterals. Thus, the surgical procedures for portal biliopathy include a nonselective portosystemic shunt and Roux-en-Y hepaticojejunostomy. The complications of shunt procedures have already been discussed.

Bile leak may occur from the liver biopsy site and may require endoscopic intervention to relieve the distal obstruction. If portal biliopathy persists after the shunt surgery, a side-to-side Roux-en-Y hepaticojejunostomy may be required. The most important intraoperative complication is bleeding because there are numerous collaterals in the hepatoduodenal ligament, the gallbladder wall, the gallbladder bed and the wall of the bile duct. Sometimes, it is difficult to even identify the bile duct. The specific postoperative complications include bile leak, ascites and cholangitis.[78]

ELECTIVE VERSUS EMERGENCY SURGERY

Emergency surgery for portal hypertension is associated with a higher mortality rate. Emergency surgery is done only for controlling variceal bleeding after all other measures have failed. Most of these patients would already have failed at least two attempts of endoscopic therapy and would have received multiple transfusions. Many would have a Sengstaken–Blakemore tube placed to temporarily stop the bleeding. There is a risk of aspiration, because these patients are usually in altered sensorium, with the stomach full of blood. The surgery also needs to be done briskly, as the aim is to arrest the bleeding as soon as possible. This increases the chances of intraoperative bleeding and inadvertent injury to adjacent organs.

In a study by Prasad et al,[7] the mortality rate in children for emergency proximal splenorenal shunt was 10% compared with 0.7% for elective shunts. In a series of patients with EHPVO undergoing the modified Hassab's procedure,[19] the mortality and morbidity rates were 36.4% and 63.6%, respectively, for emergency surgery compared with 4.4% and 18.5%, respectively, for elective surgery. In a series of devascularisation procedures by Sugiura and Futagawa,[35] the mortality rate for emergency surgery was 13.7% compared with 3.2% for elective procedures.

Emergency surgery in patients with cirrhosis and bleeding varices is only done as a salvage therapy. Although the success rate for control of bleeding is up to 95%, the mortality rates are high. These patients usually have liver decompensation and hepatic encephalopathy and also are at increased risk of infections, for example, spontaneous bacterial peritonitis, pneumonia and urinary tract infection.[79] Emergency control of bleeding varices usually requires entry into a hollow viscus, for example, gastrotomy, which may predispose these patients to infectious complications. The risk of aspiration, need for mechanical ventilation and massive blood transfusion may predispose these patients to respiratory complications. Even emergency surgery for other indications in patients with cirrhosis, such as umbilical hernia, has a much higher risk of complications, especially the infectious and respiratory complications.[75]

CIRRHOTICS VERSUS NONCIRRHOTICS

Surgery is associated with much higher mortality rate in patients with cirrhosis. In general, the risk increases with increasing Child status (10% in Child's A to 82% in Child's C). Patients with cirrhosis and portal hypertension who undergo abdominal surgery are at increased risk for developing refractory ascites, leak of ascitic fluid and infectious complications.[80]

Among the long-term complications, patients with cirrhosis have a higher incidence of hepatic encephalopathy, especially after the shunt surgery (around 30%). Encephalopathy may also occur in patients with NCPF after shunt surgery, but its incidence is much lower and is usually controlled with medical management. However, in some patients with refractory encephalopathy, the shunt may need to be blocked.[9] In patients with cirrhosis, the liver function may deteriorate with time, resulting in hepatic failure and death. In a study by Sugiura and Futagawa,[35] the 10-year survival after devascularisation procedures was only 72% in patients with cirrhosis compared with 95% in those with noncirrhotic portal hypertension.

NONCIRRHOTIC PORTAL FIBROSIS VERSUS EXTRAHEPATIC PORTAL VENOUS OBSTRUCTION

There is not much difference in the incidence of early postoperative complications between EHPVO and NCPF. However, some long-term complications occur more often in patients with NCPF. Although the liver function is preserved in both these disorders, patients with NCPF may have mild liver dysfunction, which gets unmasked once the blood is shunted away from the liver by portosystemic shunt, resulting in hepatic encephalopathy. Patients with EHPVO, on the other hand, do not develop encephalopathy unless they have transfusion-related viral hepatitis, which progresses to cirrhosis with time. In a study of prophylactic surgery for prevention of variceal bleeding in patients with EHPVO, none of the 89 patients developed hepatic encephalopathy on long-term follow-up and 90% were asymptomatic. A similar study in 39 patients with NCPF resulted in 18% incidence of encephalopathy and 47% long-term morbidity, including encephalopathy (7/39), myelopathy (3/39), glomerulonephritis (3/39) and ascites (5/39).[9]

CONCLUSIONS

Surgery in patients with portal hypertension can be performed safely. The presence of liver dysfunction, the choice of surgical procedure and the experience of the surgeon, all have a bearing on the incidence and severity of complications.

REFERENCES

1. Whipple AO. The problem off portal hypertension in relation to the hepatosplenopathies. *Ann Surg* 1945;122:449–75.

2. Jackson FC, Perrin EB, Smith AG, Dagradi AE, Nadal HM. A clinical investigation of the portacaval shunt. II. Survival analysis of the prophylactic operation. *Am J Surg* 1968;115:22–42.

3. Conn HO, Lindenmuth WW. Prophylactic portacaval anastomosis in cirrhotic patients with esophageal varices and ascites. Experimental design and preliminary results. *Am J Surg* 1969;117:656–61.

4. Resnick RH, Chalmers TC, Ishihara AM, et al. A controlled study of the prophylactic portacaval shunt. A final report. *Ann Intern Med* 1969;70:675–88.

5. Jackson FC, Perrin EB, Felix WR, Smith AG. A clinical investigation of the portacaval shunt. V. Survival analysis of the therapeutic operation. *Ann Surg* 1971;174:672–701.

6. Orloff MJ. Fifty-three years' experience with randomized clinical trials of emergency portacaval shunt for bleeding esophageal varices in cirrhosis: 1958-2011. *JAMA Surg* 2014;149:155–69.

7. Prasad AS, Gupta S, Kohli V, Pande GK, Sahni P, Nundy S. Proximal splenorenal shunts for extrahepatic portal venous obstruction in children. *Ann Surg* 1994;219:193–6.

8. Pal S, Mangla V, Radhakrishna P, et al. Surgery as primary prophylaxis from variceal bleeding in patients with extrahepatic portal venous obstruction. *J Gastroenterol Hepatol* 2013;28:1010–4.

9. Pal S, Radhakrishna P, Sahni P, Pande GK, Nundy S, Chattopadhyay TK. Prophylactic surgery in non-cirrhotic portal fibrosis: is it worthwhile? *Indian J Gastroenterol* 2005;24:239–42.

10. Mishra PK, Patil NS, Saluja S, Narang P, Solanki N, Varshney V. High patency of proximal splenorenal shunt: a myth or reality? A prospective cohort study. *Int J Surg* 2016;27:82–7.

11. Inokuchi K, Kobayashi Y. Selective shunt method for portal hypertension–our method of the left gastric venous-caval shunt. *Shujutsu* 1969;23:138–50.

12. Warren WD, Salam AA, Hutson D, Zeppa R. Selective distal splenorenal shunt. Technique and results of operation. *Arch Surg* 1974;108:306–14.

13. Conn HO, Resnick RH, Grace ND, et al. Distal splenorenal shunt vs. portal-systemic shunt: current status of a controlled trial. *Hepatology* 1981;1:151–60.

14. Millikan WJ, Jr, Warren WD, Henderson JM, et al. The Emory prospective randomized trial: selective versus nonselective shunt to control variceal bleeding. Ten-year follow-up. *Ann Surg* 1985;201:712–22.

15. Fischer JE, Bower RH, Atamian S, Welling R. Comparison of distal and proximal splenorenal shunts: a randomized prospective trial. *Ann Surg* 1981;194:531–44.

16. Yin L, Liu H, Zhang Y, Rong W. The surgical treatment for portal hypertension: a systematic review and meta-analysis. *ISRN Gastroenterol* 2013;2013:464053.

17. Hassab MA. Gastroesophageal decongestion and splenectomy. A method of prevention and treatment of bleeding from esophageal varices associated with bilharzial hepatic fibrosis: preliminary report. *J Int Coll Surg* 1964;41:232–48.

18. Sugiura M, Futagawa S. A new technique for treating esophageal varices. *J Thorac Cardiovasc Surg* 1973;66:677–85.

19. Mangla V, George J, Pal S, et al. Long-term results of modified Hassab's procedure in patients with extrahepatic portal venous obstruction. *Trop Gastroenterol* 2011;32:S49.

20. Khan S, Tudur Smith C, Williamson P, Sutton R. Portosystemic shunts versus endoscopic therapy for variceal rebleeding in patients with cirrhosis. *Cochrane Database Syst Rev* 2006;4:CD000553.

21. Henderson JM, Boyer TD, Kutner MH, et al. Distal splenorenal shunt versus transjugular intrahepatic portal systematic shunt for variceal bleeding: a randomized trial. *Gastroenterology* 2006;130:1643–51.

22. Kumar A, Sharma P, Sarin SK. Hepatic venous pressure gradient measurement: time to learn! *Indian J Gastroenterol* 2008;27:74–80.

23. Rossle M, Haag K, Ochs A, et al. The transjugular intrahepatic portosystemic stent-shunt procedure for variceal bleeding. *N Engl J Med* 1994;330:165–71.

24. LaBerge JM, Ring EJ, Gordon RL, et al. Creation of transjugular intrahepatic portosystemic shunts with the wallstent endoprosthesis: results in 100 patients. *Radiology* 1993;187:413–20.

25. Freedman AM, Sanyal AJ, Tisnado J, et al. Complications of transjugular intrahepatic portosystemic shunt: a comprehensive review. *Radiographics* 1993;13:1185–210.

26. Liangpunsakul S, Ulmer BJ, Chalasani N. Predictors and implications of severe hypersplenism in patients with cirrhosis. *Am J Med Sci* 2003;326:111–6.

27. Rajalingam R, Javed A, Sharma D, et al. Management of hypersplenism in non-cirrhotic portal hypertension: a surgical series. *Hepatobiliary Pancreat Dis Int* 2012;11:165–71.

28. Kedia S, Goyal R, Mangla V, et al. Splenectomy in cirrhosis with hypersplenism: improvement in cytopenias, Child's status and institution of specific treatment for hepatitis C with success. *Ann Hepatol* 2012;11:921–9.

29. Sood S, Jayalaxmi TS, Vijayaraghavan S, Nundy S. Use of sodium nitroprusside induced hypotensive anaesthesia for reducing blood loss in patients undergoing lienorenal shunts for portal hypertension. *Br J Surg* 1987;74:1036–8.

30. Yao HS, Wang WJ, Wang Q, et al. Randomized clinical trial of vessel sealing system (LigaSure) in esophagogastric devascularization and splenectomy in patients with portal hypertension. *Am J Surg* 2011;202:82–90.

31. Liu Y, Li Y, Ma J, Lu L, Zhang L. A modified Hassab's operation for portal hypertension: experience with 562 cases. *J Surg Res* 2013;185:463–8.

32. Mathur SK, Shah SR, Nagral SS, Soonawala ZF. Transabdominal extensive esophagogastric devascularization with gastroesophageal stapling for management of noncirrhotic portal hypertension: long-term results. *World J Surg* 1999;23:1168–74; discussion 1174–5.

33. Borgonovo G, Costantini M, Grange D, Vons C, Smadja C, Franco D. Comparison of a modified Sugiura procedure with portal systemic shunt for prevention of recurrent variceal bleeding in cirrhosis. *Surgery* 1996;119:214–21.

34. Mercado MA, Morales Linares JC, Gomez Mendez TJ, Granados J, Prado E, Orozco H. Complications of splenectomy in the Sugiura-Futagawa procedure. *Rev Gastroenterol Mex* 1995;60:145–8.

35. Sugiura M, Futagawa S. Results of six hundred thirty-six esophageal transections with paraesophagogastric devascularization in the treatment of esophageal varices. *J Vasc Surg* 1984;1:254–60.

36. Jin G, Murayama KM, Thompson JS, Rikkers LF. Pancreatic complications after distal splenorenal shunt. *Liver Transpl Surg* 1995;1:26–9.

37. Elwood DR, Pomposelli JJ, Pomfret EA, Lewis WD, Jenkins RL. Distal splenorenal shunt: preferred treatment for recurrent variceal hemorrhage in the patient with well-compensated cirrhosis. *Arch Surg* 2006;141:385–8; discussion 388.

38. Collins JC, Ong MJ, Rypins EB, Sarfeh IJ. Partial portacaval shunt for variceal hemorrhage: longitudinal analysis of effectiveness. *Arch Surg* 1998;133:590–2; discussion 592–4.

39. Boxer MA, Braun J, Ellman L. Thromboembolic risk of postsplenectomy thrombocytosis. *Arch Surg* 1978;113:808–9.

40. Chuncharunee S, Archararit N, Hathirat P, Udomsubpayakul U, Atichartakarn V. Levels of serum interleukin-6 and tumor necrosis factor in postsplenectomized thalassemic patients. *J Med Assoc Thai* 1997;80:S86–91.

41. Stamou KM, Toutouzas KG, Kekis PB, et al. Prospective study of the incidence and risk factors of postsplenectomy thrombosis of the portal, mesenteric, and splenic veins. *Arch Surg* 2006;141:663–9.

42. Orloff MJ, Orloff MS, Orloff SL, Rambotti M, Girard B. Three decades of experience with emergency portacaval shunt for acutely bleeding esophageal varices in 400 unselected patients with cirrhosis of the liver. *J Am Coll Surg* 1995;180:257–72.

43. Livingstone AS, Koniaris LG, Perez EA, Alvarez N, Levi JU, Hutson DG. 507 Warren-Zeppa distal splenorenal shunts: a 34-year experience. *Ann Surg* 2006;243:884–92; discussion 892–4.

44. Paquet KJ, Mercado MA, Kalk JF, Koussouris P, Siemens F, Muting D. 100 meso-caval interposition-shunts for recurrent variceal hemorrhage in portal hypertension. A prospective study. *Rev Invest Clin* 1989;41:309–17.

45. Raia S, da Silva LC, Gayotto LC, Forster SC, Fukushima J, Strauss E. Portal hypertension in schistosomiasis: a long-term follow-up of a randomized trial comparing three types of surgery. *Hepatology* 1994;20:398–403.

46. Rikkers L, Jenko P, Rudman D, Freides D. Subclinical hepatic encephalopathy: detection, prevalence, and relationship to nitrogen metabolism. *Gastroenterology* 1978;75:462–9.

47. Sarin SK, Nundy S. Subclinical encephalopathy after portosystemic shunts in patients with non-cirrhotic portal fibrosis. *Liver* 1985;5:142–6.

48. Pal S, Desai P, Rao G, Sahni P, Nundy S, Chattopadhyay T. Non-cirrhotic portal fibrosis: results of surgery in 317 consecutive cases over a 25-year period from an Indian center (abstract). *Gastroenterology* 2002;123:T1454–88.

49. Mohapatra MK, Mohapatra AK, Acharya SK, Sahni P, Nundy S. Encephalopathy in patients with extrahepatic obstruction after lienorenal shunts. *Br J Surg* 1992;79:1103–5.

50. Sushma S, Dasarathy S, Tandon RK, Jain S, Gupta S, Bhist MS. Sodium benzoate in the treatment of acute hepatic encephalopathy: a double-blind randomized trial. *Hepatology* 1992;16:138–44.

51. Waghorn DJ. Overwhelming infection in asplenic patients: current best practice preventive measures are not being followed. *J Clin Pathol* 2001;54:214–8.

52. Conn HO, Rossle M, Levy L, Glocker FX. Portosystemic myelopathy: spastic paraparesis after portosystemic shunting. *Scand J Gastroenterol* 2006;41:619–25.

53. Rao PK, Sheth KA, Nadig R, Patil M, Channagiri AK. Portosystemic myelopathy: a rare neurological

presentation of portosystemic shunts. *J Clin Exp Hepatol* 2012;2:393–5.

54. Koo JE, Lim YS, Myung SJ, et al. Hepatic myelopathy as a presenting neurological complication in patients with cirrhosis and spontaneous splenorenal shunt. *Korean J Hepatol* 2008;14:89–96.

55. Anand BA, Agarwala S, Nundy S. Encephalomyelopathy following portocaval shunt in noncirrhotic portal fibrosis: a case report. *Trop Gastroenterol* 1992;13:152–4.

56. Soma J, Saito T, Sato H, Ootaka T, Abe K. Membranoproliferative glomerulonephritis induced by portosystemic shunt surgery for non-cirrhotic portal hypertension. *Clin Nephrol* 1997;48:274–81.

57. Karashima S, Hattori S, Nakazato H, et al. Membranoproliferative glomerulonephritis in congenital portosystemic shunt without liver cirrhosis. *Clin Nephrol* 2000;53:206–11.

58. Smet AD, Kuypers D, Evenepoel P, et al. 'Full house' positive immunohistochemical membranoproliferative glomerulonephritis in a patient with portosystemic shunt. *Nephrol Dial Transplant* 2001;16:2258–62.

59. Callard P, Feldmann G, Prandi D, et al. Immune complex type glomerulonephritis in cirrhosis of the liver. *Am J Pathol* 1975;80:329–40.

60. Axelsen RA, Crawford DH, Endre ZH, et al. Renal glomerular lesions in unselected patients with cirrhosis undergoing orthotopic liver transplantation. *Pathology* 1995;27:237–46.

61. Kumar A, Bhuyan UN, Nundy S. Glomerulonephritis complicating non-cirrhotic portal fibrosis. *J Gastroenterol Hepatol* 1989;4:271–5.

62. Zong GQ, Fei Y, Liu RM. Comparison of effects of devascularization versus shunt on patients with portal hypertension: a meta-analysis. *Hepatogastroenterology* 2015;62:144–50.

63. da Silva LC, Strauss E, Gayotto LC, et al. A randomized trial for the study of the elective surgical treatment of portal hypertension in mansonic schistosomiasis. *Ann Surg* 1986;204:148–53.

64. Orozco H, Mercado MA, Takahashi T, Rojas G, Hernandez J, Tielve M. Survival and quality of life after portal blood flow preserving procedures in patients with portal hypertension and liver cirrhosis. *Am J Surg* 1994;168:10–4.

65. Xu XB, Cai JX, Leng XS, et al. Clinical analysis of surgical treatment of portal hypertension. *World J Gastroenterol* 2005;11:4552–9.

66. Ezzat FA, Abu-Elmagd KM, Aly MA, et al. Selective shunt versus nonshunt surgery for management of both schistosomal and nonschistosomal variceal bleeders. *Ann Surg* 1990;212:97–108.

67. Casado M, Bosch J, Garcia-Pagan JC, et al. Clinical events after transjugular intrahepatic portosystemic shunt:

correlation with hemodynamic findings. *Gastroenterology* 1998;114:1296–303.

68. Bureau C, Pagan JC, Layrargues GP, et al. Patency of stents covered with polytetrafluoroethylene in patients treated by transjugular intrahepatic portosystemic shunts: long-term results of a randomized multicentre study. *Liver Int* 2007;27:742–7.

69. Conn HO. Hemolysis after transjugular intrahepatic portosystemic shunting: the naked stent syndrome. *Hepatology* 1996;23:177–81.

70. Sanyal AJ, Freedman AM, Shiffman ML, Purdum PP, 3rd, Luketic VA, Cheatham AK. Portosystemic encephalopathy after transjugular intrahepatic portosystemic shunt: results of a prospective controlled study. *Hepatology* 1994;20: 46–55.

71. Riggio O, Merlli M, Pedretti G, et al. Hepatic encephalopathy after transjugular intrahepatic portosystemic shunt. Incidence and risk factors. *Dig Dis Sci* 1996;41:578–84.

72. Sanyal AJ, Freedman AM, Luketic VA, et al. Transjugular intrahepatic portosystemic shunts compared with endoscopic sclerotherapy for the prevention of recurrent variceal hemorrhage. A randomized, controlled trial. *Ann Intern Med* 1997;126:849–57.

73. Riggio O, Ridola L, Angeloni S, et al. Clinical efficacy of transjugular intrahepatic portosystemic shunt created with covered stents with different diameters: results of a randomized controlled trial. *J Hepatol* 2010;53:267–72.

74. Zhao H, Liu F, Yue Z, Wang L, Fan Z. Evaluation of mid- and long-term efficacy of shunt limiting for hepatic myelopathy after transjugular intrahepatic portosystemic shunt. *Clin Res Hepatol Gastroenterol* 2016;40:440–6.

75. Cho SW, Bhayani N, Newell P, et al. Umbilical hernia repair in patients with signs of portal hypertension: surgical outcome and predictors of mortality. *Arch Surg* 2012;147:864–9.

76. Marsman HA, Heisterkamp J, Halm JA, Tilanus HW, Metselaar HJ, Kazemier G. Management in patients with liver cirrhosis and an umbilical hernia. *Surgery* 2007;142:372–5.

77. Eker HH, van Ramshorst GH, de Goede B, et al. A prospective study on elective umbilical hernia repair in patients with liver cirrhosis and ascites. *Surgery* 2011;150:542–6.

78. Agarwal AK, Sharma D, Singh S, Agarwal S, Girish SP. Portal biliopathy: a study of 39 surgically treated patients. *HPB (Oxford)* 2011;13:33–9.

79. Bosch J, Berzigotti A, Garcia-Pagan JC, Abraldes JG. The management of portal hypertension: rational basis, available treatments and future options. *J Hepatol* 2008;48:S68–92.

80. Nicoll A. Surgical risk in patients with cirrhosis. *J Gastroenterol Hepatol* 2012;27:1569–75.

30

Complications after Liver Transplantation

G. Kumar, N. Goyal and S. Gupta

ABSTRACT

Most of the complications are similar between deceased-donor liver transplantation (DDLT) and living-donor liver transplantation (LDLT); however, each one has its own set of complications. For DDLT, primary nonfunction and ischaemia reperfusion injury are more common. For LDLT, small-for-size syndrome is an exclusive problem. Moreover, LDLT is also associated with additional risks of complication in donor population (30%), with about 20% minor and 10% major complications. The goal of the therapy should include minimisation of complications and then appropriate treatment. The complications after liver transplantation are divided into three parts: those associated with the surgery; those associated with the management of immunosuppression and, last, recurrence of underlying diseases. The surgical complications can be further divided into vascular, biliary and miscellaneous. Vascular complications include complications related to hepatic artery, portal vein and hepatic veins. The overall incidence of vascular complications, though dependent upon the expertise and volume of surgery in a transplant centre, is about 7% and 13% in DDLT and LDLT, respectively. The most common biliary complications include bile leak and biliary stricture. In this chapter, we discuss in detail the management of technical and surgical complications associated with both DDLT and LDLT.

KEYWORDS

Living-donor liver transplantation, deceased-donor liver transplantation, primary nonfunction, hepatic artery thrombosis, portal vein thrombosis, donation after cardiac death, small-for-size syndrome, hepatic venous outflow obstruction, biliary stricture

INTRODUCTION

Liver transplantation is a complicated operation, and its outcome not only depends upon the surgical technique but also on various immunological and infective factors. In deceased-donor liver transplantation (DDLT), the quality of the cadaveric graft has a significant impact on the outcome, and due to the shortage of donor organs, more and more organs from marginal donors such as those after cardiac death (DCD) are being used. This has further resulted in increased complications after DDLT. In addition, living-donor liver transplantation (LDLT), which was initially developed to overcome the poor cadaveric donation rates in eastern countries, is technically more demanding and is associated with potentially more complications, both in recipients and in donors. One

of the most dreaded complications after living donor hepatectomy is donor death. In this chapter, we will only describe surgical complications and their management and will not discuss immunological or infective complications such as rejection and cytomegalovirus (CMV) infection. In this chapter, surgical complications after DDLT will be described first and then the complications that occur after LDLT will be discussed (Table 30.1).

DECEASED-DONOR LIVER TRANSPLANTATION

Primary Nonfunction

Early graft failure followed by death or retransplantation of the patient in the first week after liver transplantation is called primary nonfunction (PNF).[1] It is more common in

Table 30.1 Recipient complications and their incidences

	Complications	Incidence
Graft dysfunction	PNF	6%
	IGF	16%
	SFSS	Rare
Vascular complications	HAT	3–8%
	PVT	0.3–3%
	HVOO	<1%
Biliary complications	Bile leak	8–9%
	Biliary strictures	12–13%

Abbreviations: HAT, hepatic artery thrombosis; HVOO, hepatic venous outflow obstruction; IGF, impaired graft function; PNF, primary nonfunction; PVT, portal vein thrombosis; SFSS, small-for-size syndrome.

DDLT than in LDLT, with its incidence been greatest with DCDs. The incidence of PNF has been less than 5% in most series.[2] Factors such as advanced donor age, prolonged cold and warm ischaemic times, high inotropic support in the donor before liver retrieval, marked hypernatraemia and steatosis in the graft are the contributing factors. Grafts, which have over 60% macrovascular steatosis, are more prone to PNF and should be rejected.[3] Visual appearance at the time of retrieval is quite accurate in predicting the extent of steatosis if the surgeon is experienced. However, in case of doubt, frozen section can be used to determine the extent of steatosis. The management of PNF is similar to that after acute liver failure with appropriate mechanical ventilation, haemodynamic monitoring and measures to prevent cerebral oedema. Infusion of N-acetyl cysteine (NAC), a glutathione precursor that restores endogenous stores of glutathione, may decrease the incidence of PNF.[4] Continuous renal replacement therapy is often needed, as coagulopathy, bleeding and disseminated intravascular coagulation (DIC) may require appropriate blood products. Prophylaxis for bacterial and fungal infections must be instituted. Some reports have suggested improvement using prostaglandin E$_1$ infusion, but its use cannot be universally recommended, as a meta-analysis has not shown it to be superior to placebo in preventing PNF, death and retransplantation.[5] Similarly, liver support devices such as the molecular adsorbent recirculating system (MARS) have very limited success.[6] Currently, these patients are listed for urgent retransplant, and in most cadaveric programs, along with hepatic artery thrombosis (HAT) and acute liver failure, PNF is accorded priority in organ allocation.

Impaired Graft Function

This is more common than PNF, with the incidence of about 16%,[1] and careful postoperative management

may help some of the patients to recover. A number of definitions are in use, and Ploeg et al has given the most popular definition.[2] In this definition, impaired graft function (IGF) is defined when the aspartate transaminase (AST) is >2000 IU/L, international normalised ratio (INR) >1.6 and ammonia level is >50 µmol/L between postoperative days 2 and 7. The factors contributing to IGF are similar to those that contribute to PNF. Poor general condition of the recipient as well as prolonged pretransplant hospitalisation are often associated with IGF. Technical complications should be ruled out by duplex USG Doppler (DUS) examination, and immune-related complications are further evaluated by liver biopsy and donor-specific antibody measurements. Plasmapheresis may help in removing preformed antibodies if antibody-mediated rejection is suspected.[7]

Hepatic Artery Thrombosis

This is the commonest technical complication after liver transplant, and about half of the immediate retransplants in recipients can be ascribed to HAT.[8] The overall incidence of early HAT in a systematic review was found to be 4.4% (adults, 2.9%, and paediatric, 8.4%). The causes of HAT can be due to the following reasons:

- Poor inflow from dissection of the recipient artery due to rough handling or from preoperative transarterial chemoembolisation for hepatocellular carcinoma (HCC) or from entrapment of the coeliac axis by median cruciate ligament and recipient hypotension with high vasopressor support.
- Multiple- or small-calibre donor arteries and absence of Carrel patch in donor artery.
- ABO-incompatible liver transplant, rejection episodes and fungal infection.
- Small underweight recipients such as in paediatric liver transplant with weight less than 10 Kg.

The regular use of microscope or loupe for arterial anastomosis can possibly decrease the incidence of HAT. Antiplatelet agents such as aspirin and clopidogrel have been recommended to prevent the development of HAT.[9] However, in the first postoperative week, poor graft function, low platelet count and risk of bleeding will often preclude the use of these agents when the risk for thrombosis is the highest.[10] Vascular complications are best detected by DUS (Figure 30.1a). Hence, with routine Doppler surveillance in the postoperative period, HAT can be detected before the development of symptoms or even before changes in blood biochemistry. Further routine ultrasound surveillance may be able to

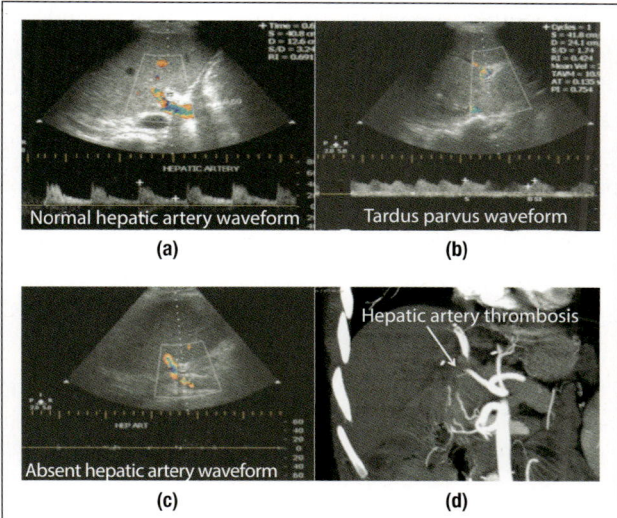

Figure 30.1 Duplex ultrasonography showing (a) normal hepatic artery flow with appropriate resistive index and peak velocity, (b) Tardus-Parvus pattern of hepatic artery flow suggestive of hepatic artery stenosis, (c) absent flow suggestive of hepatic artery thrombosis, (d) confirmatory computed tomography angiography shows no flow in hepatic artery, suggestive of hepatic artery thrombosis.

Courtesy: Goutham Kumar, Neerav Goyal and Subhash Gupta.

predict subsequent development of HAT by showing falling peak systolic velocity, falling resistive index and increasing systolic acceleration time (Figure 30.1b). If detected before complete occlusion (Figure 30.1c and d), angiographic intervention may help prevent complete HAT. The clinical presentation in the first week can vary from the patient being completely asymptomatic to being febrile or to that of graft failure. Blood biochemistry may show metabolic acidosis, with rising blood lactate levels. Transaminases may show a marked increase, and values may be in thousands. Once the diagnosis is suspected, it should be confirmed by a computed tomography (CT) angiogram. Endovascular therapies such as intra-arterial thrombolysis, percutaneous transluminal angioplasty (PTA) and surgical thrombectomy are used as urgent revascularisation strategies, with about 50% success, particularly if detected early with routine surveillance.[10] In rest of the patients, retransplant is needed for graft failure or after failed thrombectomy attempts.

On the other hand, late HAT occurs at the median of 6 months and may have an immunological component. Biliary tract complications are commoner in late HAT and present with stricture or liver abscesses. Risk factors for late hepatic artery stenosis include CMV donor recipient mismatch, usage of arterial conduit, variant arterial anatomy and retransplantation. Late HAT usually does not warrant retransplantation but is required in patients with recurrent cholangitis from ischaemic-type biliary strictures.

At our centre, the treatment in the first week is by operative thrombectomy and reanastomosis of the hepatic artery if the recipient is stable for a laparotomy. If the general condition of the recipient is poor, or thrombosis has been detected beyond the first week, angiographic intervention is carried out. The clots are usually soft, and thrombolysis can be done with either urokinase or streptokinase. Subsequent to the procedure, intra-arterial microcatheter is placed for continuous infusion of anticoagulation agents for 24 to 48 hours.

Portal Vein Thrombosis

Portal vein thrombosis (PVT) is an uncommon complication in adult transplantation, with a reported overall incidence of 0.3 to 2.6%. Although liver has dual blood supply, portal blood flow is necessary for liver regeneration and proper functioning.

In paediatric transplant, the incidence of PVT is much higher and is between 8 and 27% in high-risk patients, such as babies who are less than 10 Kg of weight, are diagnosed with biliary atresia with hypoplastic portal vein or have a history of multiple upper abdominal surgeries.[11] In this group, multiple techniques have been described such as branch patch anastomosis (creating a patch from the right and left portal vein branches) and placing an interposition graft between the donor portal vein and the junction of the splenic vein and superior mesenteric vein.[12] A graft with graft-to-recipient weight ratio (GRWR) >4% is more prone to PVT. Either grafts should be reduced in size or a monosegment graft should be used if the anteroposterior diameter of the recipient in the hepatic fossa is less than the anteroposterior diameter of the liver graft. Portal vein anastomosis can be done either with continuous suture with a growth factor or with interrupted sutures on the anterior wall and continuous suture in the posterior wall. Use of magnification will prevent PVT.

In our technique of portal vein anastomosis in infants, the porta is divided high up in the recipient. The branches are slit longitudinally to create a large opening for anastomosis. The connective tissue and lymph nodes around the portal vein are not disturbed. This provides support to the portal vein and prevents redundancy. After adopting this technique, our rates of PVT in infants have decreased dramatically.

If PVT is encountered on the table, it should be revised carefully after completing the arterial anastomosis.

Ueda et al have suggested that all collaterals in the abdomen should be disconnected in order to prevent PVT in small babies.[13] Quite often, this works, but in small babies with low-flow states, either it may be necessary to stent the portal vein through the segment IV portal vein branch that was tied while retrieving the left lateral segment graft (LLSG) in the donor or a hemiportocaval transposition can be done. The cava is divided below the hepatic vein anastomosis, and then, the cava above the renal veins is joined to the portal vein. The portal vein can be anastomosed to the cava to prevent development of subsequent portal hypertension. If detected postoperatively, apart from re-exploration, stenting can also be attempted via the hepatic or the splenic route.

In adult liver transplant also, PVT does happen, and the risk factors are hypercoagulability, operative thrombectomy for chronic PVT, previous splenectomy, large portosystemic shunts, redundancy or kinking in the anastomosis and the use of a venous conduit for reconstruction.[14,15]

In adults, if PVT is detected in the early postoperative period, the patient should be taken for re-exploration, operative thrombectomy should be carried out and the patient should be placed on anticoagulation thereafter.

Late thrombosis is usually difficult to treat but may respond to anticoagulation. Often, collaterisation will develop through the Roux limb or by the bile duct collaterals, and the patient may remain completely asymptomatic.

A Rex shunt between superior mesenteric vein and left portal vein may occasionally be possible if there is filling of intrahepatic portal vein through collaterals. If feasible, radiological intervention can be carried out either through hepatic vein canulation or percutaneously through liver parenchyma. Once the vein has been opened up, a stent may need to be placed in the portal vein (Figure 30.2a, b and c).

Hepatic Venous Outflow Obstruction

Hepatic venous outflow obstruction (HVOO) has catastrophic outcome in graft function and patient recovery. Piardi et al showed that the overall incidence of HVOO is 0.5 to 3.2%.[8] Early HVOO is usually a technical problem caused by kinking, stenosis or thrombosis, and late HVOO is due to intimal fibrosis or hyperplasia. The classical venous reconstruction with venovenous bypass had been associated with problems such as air embolism and clotting of the lines. With the introduction of piggyback venous reconstruction, total clamping of the IVC is prevented, but the risk of HVOO is increased.[16] Hepatic venous outlet obstruction should be excluded in grafts with poor function by ultrasound duplex examination (Figure 30.3a and b). If suspected, transjugular hepatic venous angiogram (Figure 30.3c and d) will establish the diagnosis and can also be used for treatment by gently dilating the anastomosis. Untreated hepatic venous outlet obstruction will result

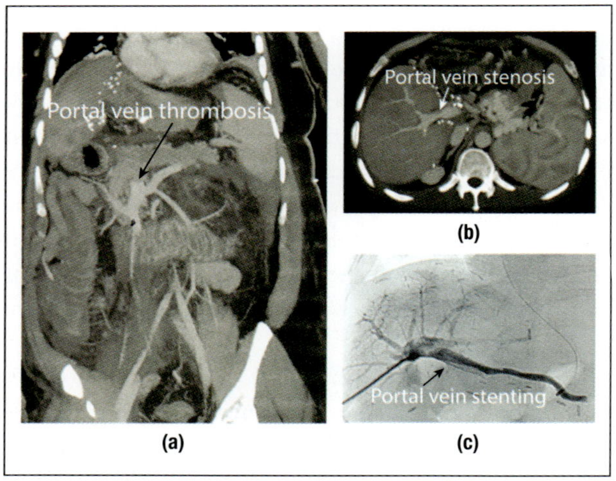

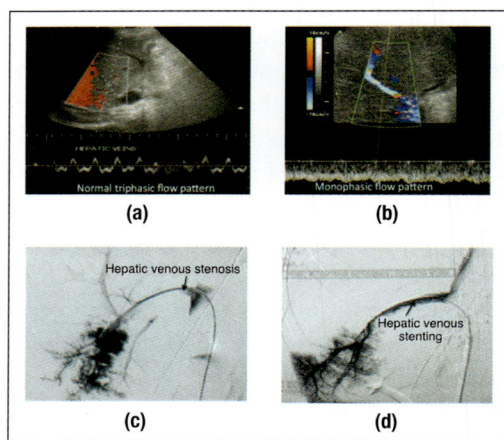

Figure 30.2 Computed tomography liver angiography shows (a) posttransplant development of portal vein thrombosis, (b) portal vein stenosis (small arrow) managed with (c) portal vein stenting accessed through the spleen.

Courtesy: Goutham Kumar, Neerav Goyal and Subhash Gupta.

Figure 30.3 (a) Duplex ultrasonography depicting normal flow. (b) Monophasic flow suggestive of hepatic vein stenosis. (c) Hepatic venogram shows significant narrowing of the right hepatic vein, with significant gradient managed with (d) right hepatic vein stenting.

Courtesy: Goutham Kumar, Neerav Goyal and Subhash Gupta.

in patient's death, and operative intervention should be attempted before listing for urgent retransplant. At surgery, endovascular stapler can be used to refashion the cavocavostomy.[17]

Persistent Ascites

Persistent ascites after liver transplantation is usually investigated if the ascites do not resolve after 4 weeks of successful transplantation. The usual causes are bacterial and fungal peritonitis, renal dysfunction, portal venous obstruction and HVOO.[18] Most cases will resolve with prolonged percutaneous drainage (PCD) and treatment with antimicrobial therapy. Minor bile leak and chylous ascites should be ruled out by biochemical examination of the ascitic fluid. Chylous ascites will usually resolve by drainage and medium-chain-triglyceride diet. Doppler examination and CT angiogram will help identify the aetiology in difficult cases that do not resolve on their own. Measurement of transjugular hepatic vein pressure gradient (HVPG) will provide further clarity in this situation and can be combined with liver biopsy. In case of HVOO, there will be a gradient across the anastomosis and a value >3 cm H_2O is regarded as significant.[19] The hepatic venous anastomosis can be either dilated or stented. In case of portal hyperperfusion, HVPG will be high, and in this situation, recurrent viral hepatitis should be considered. If the HVPG is low, portal vein stenosis should be considered. Portal vein stenosis can be corrected by percutaneous transhepatic portal vein dilatation, with or without endovascular stenting.

Bile Leak

In DDLT, bile leak usually occurs from the anastomosis, T-tube insertion site, the cystic duct or the gallbladder bed. The mean incidence of bile leak after transplantation is 8.2%, and with LDLT, the incidence is slightly higher than that with DDLT (9.5% vs. 7.8%). Hepatic artery thrombosis can result in necrosis of the bile duct and the hilar plate, resulting in a leak. The other risk factors include poor general condition of the recipient, advanced age, prolonged cold and warm ischaemic times and donor macrosteatosis.[20] In order to avoid bile leaks, strategies include better selection of a graft, prevention of bile duct denudation and dissection of hepatic artery only till the origin of gastroduodenal artery. Intraoperative cholangiogram reduces the incidence of bile leaks. The bile leaks associated with T-tube insertion can be treated successfully by endoscopy. On the other hand, leak from bile duct anastomosis has 50% success rate when treated

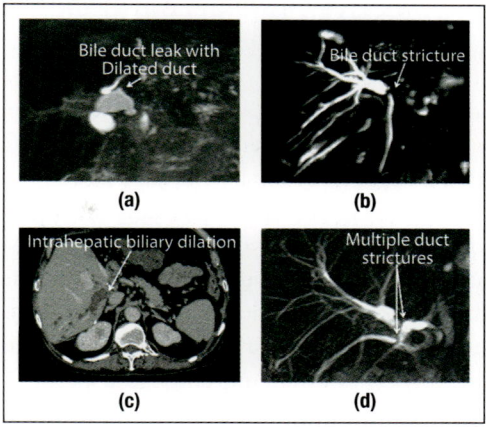

Figure 30.4 Postoperative magnetic resonance cholangiopancreatography shows (a) biloma with dilated duct and anastomotic site bile leak, (b) biliary stricture of single anastomotic site, (c) plain computed tomography scan shows intra hepatic biliary radicals dilatation indicative of biliary stricture and (d) magnetic resonance cholangiopancreatography showing multiple duct anastomotic stricture.

Courtesy: Goutham Kumar, Neerav Goyal and Subhash Gupta.

by endoscopic management.[21] Surgical management with refashioning of bile duct reconstruction is required in very few instances, only if all the above measures fail (Figure 30.4a).

Biliary Stricture

Biliary stricture is one of the commonest complications after liver transplantation. The overall incidence of biliary stricture is 12.8%, with LDLT having a higher incidence (19% vs. 12%).[20] There are two types of biliary strictures, namely anastomotic and nonanastomotic ischaemic strictures. Although the anastomotic strictures are associated with early anastomotic bile leak, nonanastomotic stricture is associated with an ischaemic aetiology such as ABO-incompatible liver transplant, prolonged cold ischaemia and grafts from DCDs, as well as with HAT. Anastomotic strictures are easy to treat with endoscopic retrograde cholangiopancreatography (ERCP) and stenting. If this fails, Roux-en-Y hepaticojejunostomy can also be carried out. If the primary biliary reconstruction was done with a Roux limb such as in primary sclerosing cholangitis, then biliary stricture is treated with revision surgery. Difficult ischaemic strictures will require endoscopic, radiological or even a combined approach. Recurrent cholangitis and biliary cirrhosis, despite adequate endoscopic therapy, are an indication for liver retransplantation.[21] (Figure 30.4b, c and d).

LIVING-DONOR LIVER TRANSPLANTATION

Complications in the Donor

Living-donor liver transplantation was introduced initially for children before subsequently being performed in adults. This procedure has had its fair share of criticism, mainly due to its high complication rates. However, it has survived the test of time to become a routine procedure in countries with poor cadaveric donation rates. The most dreaded complications are donor death and the need for liver transplantation for posthepatectomy liver failure. A systematic review showed mortality rate between 0.23 and 0.5% for right hemihepatectomy grafts (RHG) and 0.1% for an LLSG or left hemihepatectomy grafts (LHG).[22] The complication rates may now be lower due to innovations in surgical techniques (Figure 30.5); however, complications still remains a major concern.[23] Their overall rate is at a median of 16%.[22] Most of the complications after donor hepatectomy are similar to those of hepatectomy for other indications, and these have been dealt with in detail elsewhere in the book. In this section, we will describe those complications (Table 30.2) that are unique to donor hepatectomy.

Inadequate Remnant and Liver Failure

In RHG, the remnant liver volume should not be less than 30%[24] and is usually calculated using 3D-CT volumetric software. The required remnant volume may be higher in people with steatotic livers or in elderly donors. It is important to calibrate the accuracy of volumetry as an error in calculation may have untoward consequences. Donors with low remnant liver volumes (<30%) can alternatively undergo LHG or a right posterior section graft (RPSG) donation, provided the GRWR for the recipient is adequate. An inadequate remnant may lead

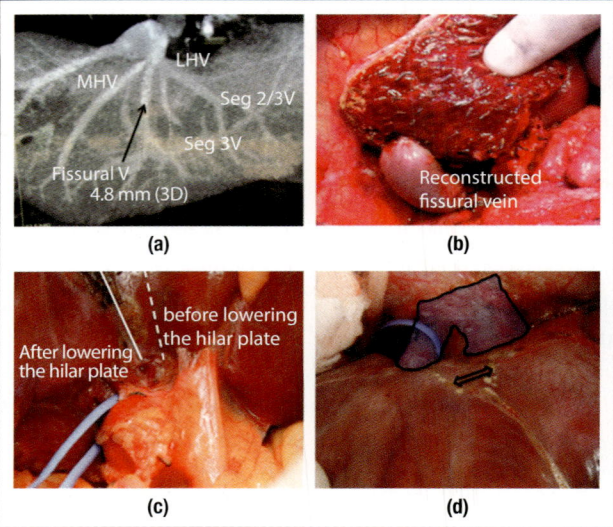

Figure 30.5 (a) Computed tomography scan reconstruction showing fissural vein that might be encountered when left lateral segment graft is procured. (b) Reconstruction of fissural vein by using a recipient's portal vein graft. (c) Lowered hilar plate and transection line can be shifted based the requisite graft size. (d) Transection line either along with middle hepatic vein (MHV) or 2 cm away from the junction of MHV and left hepatic vein (LHV).

Courtesy: Goutham Kumar, Neerav Goyal and Subhash Gupta.

to posthepatectomy liver failure, and at least four donors worldwide have needed urgent liver transplantation.[25]

Errors in the Plane of Transection

In donor hepatectomy, it is important to remember that portal inflow territory may not match outflow territory. Therefore, as one proceeds with transection, it may need to be altered to include branches that drain the graft that is

Table 30.2 Donor complications in our centre (n = 2000)

	Complications	Incidence
Intraoperative complications	Hepatic artery intimal dissection	4
	Damage to bile duct of the remnant	7
	Cystic duct patch	1
	Hepaticojejunostomy	
Postoperative complications	Surgical site infection	3.1%
	Bile leak	1.9%
	Neurological deficit	1%
	Pleural effusion	3%
	Biliary stricture	0.15%
	Deep vein thrombosis	0.3%
	Hernia	1%

being obtained. A precise line of transection is important, as it prevents excessive bleeding and postoperative bile leaks by avoiding pedicles, improves predictability of graft size and remnant volume and, most important, assists retrieval of the venous branches of the middle hepatic vein (MHV) for back table preparation.

In LLSG, excessive volume in the graft can be detrimental for recipient outcome as 'large-for-size' syndrome[26] may develop. If the GRWR is >4, the graft volume must be reduced in order to prevent large-for-size syndrome, which usually manifests by PVT. In left lobe grafts (LLG), the graft volume can be further augmented by inclusion of the caudate lobe, together with its draining short hepatic vein. In extended right lobe grafts (eRLG), the MHV is included in the graft. This graft should be taken only if the remnant liver volume exceeds 35% and has <5% steatosis, with a clearly identifiable large segment IVa vein. In modified right lobe graft (mRHG), an attempt should be made, whenever possible, to obtain a single VIII and a single V branch, so that reconstruction is easy and the drainage of the anterior sector is maintained. Segment V can often be obtained as a single trunk by transecting till the point where the different tributaries can be seen converging at a point. Oblique clamps may be placed, so that the entire drainage of segment V comes in a single cuff (Figure 30.6b). The segment VIII vein can often be obtained as a single branch if small IVa branches are ligated. Ligation of these small branches will not affect IVa drainage, as the entire MHV would have left with the graft. In RPSG, the transection line near the porta should run to the right of the right anterior portal vein and artery, in order to obtain a single posterior bile duct, or if there is early branching, then both segment 6 and segment 7 ducts can come in a single sheath. The right hepatic vein can get exposed during transection if care is not taken to maintain sufficient liver tissue to its left. This complication can be avoided if the plane of transection in the depth is directed to the left and parallel to the direction of the right hepatic vein (Figure 30.6c).

Excessive Bleeding During Transection

As parenchymal transection is done without inflow occlusion, catastrophic bleeding may need to be controlled quickly by temporary inflow occlusion. In case there is bleeding from a branch of MHV/MHV, it should be repaired by clamping the porta and the root of the middle and left hepatic veins, creating a situation of total remnant liver vascular occlusion, to leave a dry field, making the repair easy and controlled (Figure 30.6a). Transection may be faster after hanging the liver, as described by Belghiti

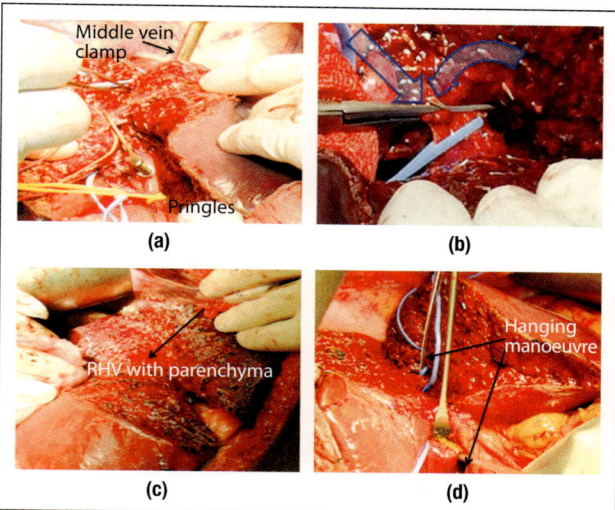

Figure 30.6 (a) Pringle's manoeuvre and middle hepatic vein clamping to repair the tear in segment IVa vein. (b) Oblique clamp placement on segment V vein for a single cuff. (c) Plane of transection for right posterior section graft. (d) Hanging the liver after looping segment V and segment VIII veins.

Abbreviation: RHV, right hepatic vein.

Courtesy: Goutham Kumar, Neerav Goyal and Subhash Gupta.

et al,[27] but there is a risk of avulsion of the segments V and VIII veins. Our policy is to continue transection till the segments V and VIII veins have been looped and divided and then use the hanging manoeuvre (Figure 30.6d).

Intimal Dissection of the Hepatic Artery

This is the most dreaded complication of donor hepatectomy and will usually lead to nonusability of the graft. Undue traction on the right hepatic artery or application of a traumatic bulldog clamp on the vessel may cause intimal separation. It can also be caused by avulsion of a branch of the hepatic artery and subsequent attempt to stitch it by superficial bites, resulting in continued bleeding within the arterial layers. On suspicion of intimal dissection, the artery may be clamped distally for a few minutes to limit the damage, and then, the artery may be carefully stitched under magnification. However, if an artery has a long intimal dissection, then it might be possible to dissect till the anterior and posterior branches of the right hepatic artery and then anastomosing them separately, as the intimal dissection usually stops at the branching point. Arterialisation of the portal vein has also been reported, but it is not clear whether it is actually beneficial.[28] Late portal hypertension may develop if the patient is salvaged.

Damage to the Bile Duct of the Remnant Liver

This is also a very dreaded complication and should be carefully avoided. If bile duct is damaged, an attempt should not be made to repair it transversely. A cystic duct patch can be applied on the bile duct in order to avoid narrowing (Figure 30.7a). Alternatively, a side-to-side hepaticojejunostomy can also be performed, so that the bile duct continuity is maintained and the defect in the bile duct can be repaired without narrowing it. Lowering the hilar plate and clearly marking the confluence with a radio-opaque marker can avoid this injury. The hilar plate can be lowered easily if the vein that runs from the confluence of the ducts to the liver parenchyma is identified and ligated.

Orphan Graft

Very rarely, the recipient may die soon after the graft has been removed from the donor. In such a situation, it is not clear what should be done with the graft. Consent from the donor and the Hospital Ethical Committee may allow it to be used in another recipient.[29] In over 2000 transplants, we have not yet faced this situation, as even if the recipient has a very low blood pressure, a

quick implantation may dramatically alter the situation. In two such cases in our series, when we were thinking of abandoning the recipient surgery, rapid anastomosis of right hepatic vein by using side clamps on the IVC and subsequent portal vein anastomosis salvaged the situation.

If the bile duct has been divided in the donor and then the recipient has died, it is not clear what should be the best course of action in the donor. The bile duct can be rejoined by a hepaticojejunostomy, or the lobe can be removed. Removal may theoretically increase the risk of posthepatectomy liver failure, but anastomosis to a Roux limb may lead to late stricture and recurrent cholangitis.

Bile Leaks

Along with superficial wound infection, bile leak is one of the most common complications after donor hepatectomy. The only intraoperative predictor for bile leak in one study was the amount of blood loss,[30] and this highlights the importance of maintaining the exact plane of transection. Bile leaks in donors will increase the recovery period and are usually managed by prolonged drainage. If the posthepatectomy cholangiogram has been satisfactory, most bile leaks would stop on their own. Occasionally, a small bile leak from an isolated caudate lobe duct may be missed, and a hepatobiliary iminodiacetic acid (HIDA) scan before drain removal can be useful in detecting these leaks. Late bilomas can be managed by prolonged PCD, if they are accessible. If the leak persists, then it may require either ERCP or laparotomy for further management.

Late Bile Duct Strictures

If the postoperative recovery has been smooth, then late bile duct strictures should not happen. However, we have had two late bile duct strictures after the donor had recovered fully and then presented with bile duct obstruction at 6 weeks. It is possible that as the left lobe hypertrophies, it can cause an acute angulation at the bile duct transection site and obstruction. Both the donors were treated by endoscopic stent placement for 3 months (Figure 30.7b and c).

Persistent Thrombocytopenia

This was reported from the Adult-to-Adult Living Donor Liver Transplantation Cohort Study (A2ALL) that donors could have persistent thrombocytopenia in the long term and splenomegaly.[31] However, in our own cohort, this has not been seen.

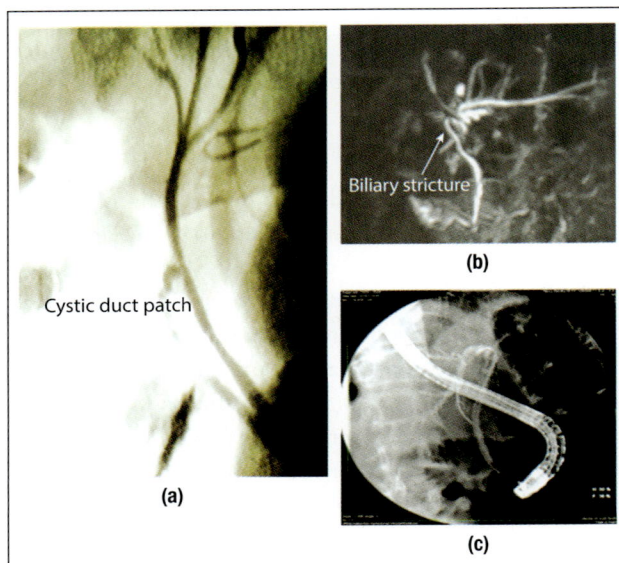

Figure 30.7 (a) Intraoperative cholangiogram delineating cystic duct patch repair for narrowing of the bile duct after primary stump closure. (b) Magnetic resonance cholangiopancreatography showing biliary stricture at the confluence 3 months post donor hepatectomy. (c) Endoscopic retrograde cholangiopancreatography showing dilatation of the stricture and stent placement.

Courtesy: Goutham Kumar, Neerav Goyal and Subhash Gupta.

Donor Death

The most unfortunate complication of a living donor hepatectomy is a donor's death. A systematic review showed the mortality rate to be approximately 0.23 to 0.5% for right lobe hepatectomy and 0.1% for left or left lateral lobe hepatectomy. An analysis of donor deaths showed that the common causes were postoperative sepsis, liver failure due to an inadequate remnant, massive haemorrhage and pulmonary embolism.[32] Table 30.3 summarises the steps taken to reduce near-miss events and mortality associated with liver donation.

RECIPIENT COMPLICATIONS UNIQUE TO LIVING-DONOR LIVER TRANSPLANTATION

Early Graft Dysfunction (EGD)

Early graft dysfunction (EGD) is the biggest challenge after LDLT, where smaller but better-quality grafts are used. About 5% of recipients will develop prolonged cholestasis (bilirubin >20 mg/dL). If this value is maintained for seven consecutive days after transplant and is also associated with an INR >2, mortality is very high.[33] Delayed functional cholestasis is not always related to size, and therefore, this syndrome is quite different from small-for-size syndrome (SFSS), discussed below. Some of the other factors that causes EGD are renal dysfunction, posttransplant infection, difficult operation with major blood loss, prolonged cold and warm ischaemia times, poor general condition of the recipient and suboptimal donor liver. Graft dysfunction may also result from less-than-perfect vascular or biliary anastomosis, immunological factors and recurrent viral hepatitis, and these conditions should be ruled out.

Small-for-Size Syndrome

Small-for-size syndrome (SFSS) is seen in partial liver grafts, where the transplanted lobe is unable to meet the recipient's metabolic demands.[34] As a result, there is prolonged cholestasis, raised INR, formation of ascites and encephalopathy. It is thought to occur either because of portal hyperperfusion or from HVOO. A GRWR of >0.8 may prevent this syndrome. Further, it is also known that higher portal pressure is necessary for adequate graft regeneration. It is not clear that at what point this increase in portal pressure becomes harmful for the graft. Younger grafts may tolerate high portal flows, without any ill effect. Small grafts may need inflow modulation

Table 30.3 Strategies to reduce morbidity and near-miss events in living liver donor

Inadequate remnant	Safer standards for CT volumetry Remnant >30% Intraoperative visual inspection, Portal pressure measurements and MHV clamp test Macrosteatosis <30%

Massive bleeding	• MHV bleeding:
	  – Inflow and outflow control, hanging of the liver only after adequate dissection of segment V and VIII veins
	• RHV bleeding
	  – RHV is looped after adequate mobilisation of the liver
	  – Phrenics veins are doubly ligated for adequate clamp space

Sepsis	Adequate antibiotic coverage Prevent bile leak
DVT and pulmonary embolism	Hypercoagulability work-up SCD for DVT ICU monitoring for 3 days
Gastrointestinal ulcers	Prophylactic PPI for a period of 1 month Minimal NSAIDs
Liver torsion	Proper fixation of the liver Uncongested and soft liver at the end of fixation
Liver quality	Judicious usage of biopsy

Abbreviations: CT, computed tomography; DVT, deep vein thrombosis; ICU, intensive care unit; MHV, middle hepatic vein; NSAIDs, nonsteroidal anti-inflammatory drugs; PPI, proton-pump inhibitor; RHV, right hepatic vein; SCD, sequential compression device.

such as splenic artery embolisation, hemiportocaval shunt or splenectomy. After completion of all anastomosis, ultrasound duplex examination is carried out and portal volume flow is measured. If the flow exceeds 400 mL/100 g of liver volume, inflow modulation may be is necessary.[35] This syndrome is more likely to develop if after reperfusion, the corrected portal pressure is >15 cmH$_2$O. As technical complications are common after LDLT, this must be ruled out before making a diagnosis of SFSS.

Biliary Complications

Biliary complications are common after LDLT and mark the major difference between DDLT and LDLT. In LDLT, bile ducts are quite often more than one and of smaller calibre. Apart from anastomotic leaks, leak can also happen from caudate ducts that have been left untied. Further, late leaks can also happen from graft regeneration and rotation. Bile leaks can be reduced substantially by careful technique and check cholangiogram after completing the anastomosis. The recipient bile duct should be cut as short as possible, and the right hepatic artery should remain adherent to it. In our centre, we routinely anastomose the donor artery to the left hepatic artery, so that the integrity of the recipient bile duct is maintained. Very early bile leak in the first few days posttransplant may be treated by re-exploration and revision of anastomosis, particularly if it is felt that this would be easy to do. However, most bile leaks are managed conservatively by refeeding of bile and by nonoperative management such as initial percutaneous drainage.

If conservative measures fail, ERCP and stenting should be attempted, preferably after 6 weeks. If done before this time, there is a risk of intra-abdominal infection and bleeding from the hepatic artery anastomosis site. Surgical management in the initial period should consist mainly of lavage and drain placement, as repair/revision of anastomosis is unlikely to be successful. In LDLT, it may be difficult to perform percutaneous transheptic biliary drainage (PTBD), as often, the bile duct is not dilated, and access may be limited, as there is a large cut-surface injury and a potential to injure vascular structures at the porta. At our centre, if there is minimal bile duct dilation, after failed endoscopic approach, open hepaticojejunostomy is preferred. In this procedure, a side-to-side anastomosis is preferred, as it is much easier to perform.

Bile strictures are managed, as in DDLT, with stent placement, dilatation and stent exchanges. In the great majority, this is successful, with only a small fraction requiring revisional surgery.

CONCLUSIONS

Complications after liver transplant are common, as liver transplant is a difficult surgery with massive blood loss and requirement for difficult vascular and biliary anastomoses. Frequently, the access is limited for shrunken liver and obese patients. Bowel may be dilated, and hepaticojejunostomy to edematous bowel may need to be done. Living-donor liver transplantation requires an even higher degree of technical refinement and is associated with a greater incidence of complications.

Apart from myriad surgical complications, liver transplant is often associated with rejection episodes, infection with opportunistic organisms, disease recurrence such as HCC and viral hepatitis, malignancy and renal dysfunction. Liver transplant recipients are looked after both by surgeons and by hepatologists, and therefore, these complications should be best dealt with in textbooks of hepatology.

REFERENCES

1. Johnson SR, Alexopoulos S, Curry M, Hanto DW. Primary nonfunction (PNF) in the MELD era: an SRTR database analysis. *Am J Transplant* 2007;7:1003–9.
2. Ploeg RJ, D'alessandro AM, Knechtle SJ, et al. Risk factors for primary dysfunction after liver transplantation-a multivariate analysis. *Transplantation* 1993;55:807–13.
3. Noujaim HM, de Goyet JD, Montero EF, et al. Expanding postmortem donor pool using steatotic liver grafts: a new look. *Transplantation* 2009;87:919–25.
4. Thies JC, Teklote J, Clauer U, et al. The efficacy of N-acetylcysteine as a hepatoprotective agent in liver transplantation. *Transplant International* 1998; 11:S390–2.
5. Cavalcanti AB, De Vasconcelos CP, Perroni de Oliveira M, Rother ET, Ferraz LJ. Prostaglandins for adult liver transplanted patients. *Cochrane Database Syst Rev* 2011;11: CD006006.
6. Faenza S, Baraldi O, Bernardi M, et al. Mars and Prometheus: our clinical experience in acute chronic liver failure. *Transplant Proc* 2008;40:1169–71.
7. Mandal AK, King KE, Humphreys SL, Maley WR, Burdick JF, Klein AS. Plasmapheresis: an effective therapy for primary allograft non-function after liver transplantation. *Transplantation* 2000;70:216–20.
8. Piardi T, Lhuaire M, Bruno O, et al. Vascular complications following liver transplantation: A literature review of advances in 2015. *World J Hepatol* 2016;8:36–57.
9. Shay R, Taber D, Pilch N, et al. Early aspirin therapy may reduce hepatic artery thrombosis in liver transplantation. *Transplant Proc* 2013;45:330–4.
10. Bekker, J, Ploem S, De Jong KP. Early hepatic artery thrombosis after liver transplantation: a systematic review of the incidence, outcome and risk factors. *Am J Transplant* 2009;9:746–57.

11. Gu LH, Fang H, Li FH, Zhang SJ, Han LZ, Li QG. Preoperative hepatic hemodynamics in the prediction of early portal vein thrombosis after liver transplantation in pediatric patients with biliary atresia. *Hepatobiliary Pancreat Dis Int* 2015;14:380–5.

12. Mizuno S, Murata Y, Kuriyama N, et al. Living donor liver transplantation for the patients with portal vein thrombosis: use of an interpositional venous graft passed posteriorly to the pancreatic parenchyma without using jump graft. *Transplant Proc* 2012;44:356–9.

13. Ueda M, Oike F, Kasahara M, et al. Portal vein complications in pediatric living donor liver transplantation using left-side grafts. *Am J Transplant* 2008;8:2097–105.

14. Kyoden Y, Tamura S, Sugawara Y, et al. Portal vein complications after adult-to-adult living donor liver transplantation. *Transpl Int* 2008;21:1136–44.

15. Langnas AN, Marujo W, Stratta RJ, Wood RP, Shaw BW. Vascular complications after orthotopic liver transplantation. *Am J Surg* 1991;161:76–82; discussion 82–3.

16. Belghiti J, Panis Y, Sauvanet A, Gayet B, Fekete F. A new technique of side to side caval anastomosis during orthotopic hepatic transplantation without inferior vena caval occlusion. *Surg Gynecol Obstet* 1992;175:270–2.

17. Quintini C, Miller CM, Hashimoto K, et al. Side-to-side cavocavostomy with an endovascular stapler: Rescue technique for severe hepatic vein and/or inferior vena cava outflow obstruction after liver transplantation using the piggyback technique. *Liver Transplant* 2009;15:49–53.

18. Cirera I, Navasa M, Rimola A, et al. Ascites after liver transplantation. *Liver Transplant* 2000;6:157–62.

19. Ikeda O, Tamura Y, Nakasone Y, et al. Percutaneous transluminal venoplasty after venous pressure measurement in patients with hepatic venous outflow obstruction after living donor liver transplantation. *Jap J Radiol* 2010;28:5202–6.

20. Akamatsu N, Sugawara Y, Hashimoto D. Biliary reconstruction, its complications and management of biliary complications after adult liver transplantation: a systematic review of the incidence, risk factors and outcome. *Transplant International* 2011;24:379–92.

21. Pfau PR, Kochman ML, Lewis JD, et al. Endoscopic management of postoperative biliary complications in orthotopic liver transplantation. *Gastrointest Endosc* 2000;52:55–63.

22. Middleton PF, Duffield M, Lynch SV, et al. Living donor liver transplantation—adult donor outcomes: a systematic review. *Liver Transplant* 2006;12:24–30.

23. Hwang S, Lee SG, Lee YJ, et al. Lessons learned from 1,000 living donor liver transplantations in a single center: how to make living donations safe. *Liver Transplant* 2006;12: 920–7.

24. Fong YK, Chan SC, Cheung TT, et al. Remnant left liver size and recovery of living right liver donors. *Hepatol Int* 2013;7:734–40.

25. Cheah YL, Simpson MA, Pomposelli JJ, Pomfret EA. Incidence of death and potentially life-threatening near-miss events in living donor hepatic lobectomy: A worldwide survey. *Liver Transplant* 2013;19:499–506.

26. Yamada N, Sanada Y, Hirata Y, et al. Selection of living donor liver grafts for patients weighing 6 kg or less. *Liver Transplant* 2015;21:233–8.

27. Belghiti J, Guevara OA, Noun R, Saldinger PF, Kianmanesh R. Liver hanging maneuver: a safe approach to right hepatectomy without liver mobilization. *J Am Coll Surg* 2001;193:109–11.

28. Bhangui P, Salloum C, Lim C, et al. Portal vein arterialization: a salvage procedure for a totally de-arterialized liver. The Paul Brousse Hospital experience. *HPB* 2014;16: 723–38.

29. Siegler J, Siegler M, Cronin DC. Recipient death during a live donor liver transplantation: who gets the "Orphan" Graft? *Transplantation* 2004;78:1241–4.

30. Ghobrial RM, Freise CE, Trotter JF, et al. Donor morbidity after living donation for liver transplantation. *Gastroenterology* 2008;135:468–76.

31. Trotter JF, Gillespie BW, Terrault NA, et al. Laboratory test results after living liver donation in the adult-to-adult living donor liver transplantation cohort study. *Liver Transplant* 2011;17:409–17.

32. Lo CM. Complications and long-term outcome of living liver donors: a survey of 1,508 cases in five Asian centers. *Transplantation* 2003;75:S12–5.

33. Ikegami T, Shirabe K, Yoshizumi T, et al. Primary graft dysfunction after living donor liver transplantation is characterized by delayed functional hyperbilirubinemia. *Am J Transplant* 2012;12:1886–97.

34. Kiuchi T, Kasahara M, Uryuhara K, et al. Impact of graft size mismatching on graft prognosis in liver transplantation from living donors 1, 2. *Transplantation* 1999;67:321–7.

35. Troisi R, Ricciardi S, Smeets P, et al. Effects of hemi-portocaval shunts for inflow modulation on the outcome of small-for-size grafts in living donor liver transplantation. *Am J Transplant* 2005;5:1397–404.

Pancreas

31

Management of Complications after Operations for Acute Pancreatitis

S. Pandanaboyana and J.A. Windsor

ABSTRACT

There has been a progressive decline in the overall mortality of acute pancreatitis in published reports. This realisation and the development of less-invasive treatment strategies, including the 'step-up' approach, have diminished the role of open surgical treatment for complicated acute pancreatitis. The complications that are most often the targets of interventions are infected walled-of necrosis (WON) and, less commonly, infected pseudocyst. The indications for the endoscopic drainage of WON and pseudocysts include the presence of symptoms, infection and cholestasis. The technical success rate of endoscopic ultrasound–guided drainage, which means achieving the intended deployment of the drains, is close to 100%, and the success of the procedure, which means complete resolution, is more than 90% for pseudocysts and 70 to 80% for WON. Current evidence indicates that the success rate and adverse events from endoscopic drainage appear to be similar with metal and plastic stents. Although percutaneous drainage was initially considered a secondary treatment of residual collections after surgical treatment, it has become increasingly important as a primary treatment and, in some cases, the sole treatment. Open surgical treatment has an ongoing, though more limited, role as a salvage approach when these less-invasive interventions have failed.

KEYWORDS

Acute pancreatitis, walled-off necrosis, pseudocyst, endoscopy, surgery

INTRODUCTION

There have been sweeping changes in the treatment of acute pancreatitis (AP) over the last few decades, because of a better understanding of the pathophysiology and complications of AP, the development of alternative interventions and improvements in the overall and intensive care of these patients.[1] As a result, there has been a progressive decline in the overall mortality of AP in published reports.[2]

Although it is not always possible to distinguish between treatment-related complications and disease-related complications, it is well accepted that open surgical treatment can make patients sicker, essentially adding 'injury to insult'. Evidence for this comes from the first randomised controlled trial conducted to evaluate surgical treatments of AP, in which open surgery was associated with a significant increase in 'new onset organ failure'.[3] A discussion on the management of organ failure as a complication of surgery is beyond the scope of this chapter. This realisation and the development of less-invasive treatment strategies, including the 'step-up' approach, have diminished the role of open surgical treatment for complicated AP. The focus of this chapter will be on the management of complications arising from the surgical treatment of AP, broadly defined to include endoscopic, radiological and surgical interventions, all of which are associated with the risk of complications. The successful treatment of these complications and achieving a low 'failure to rescue' rate require early detection, the timely engagement of specialist expertise and the delivery of appropriate treatment. In settings where these are not available, prompt transfer to a regional centre may be required to treat the complications of treatment or even deterioration of pancreatitis itself.

EVOLUTION OF SURGICAL TREATMENT

The history of the surgery for severe AP has been eloquently recorded[4] and includes some notable trends in the evolution of surgical treatment. Early attempts at the surgical resection for infected pancreatic necrosis, especially in the 1960s and 1970s, were abandoned because of an unacceptable mortality rate.[5,6] Collections secondary to pancreatic necrosis (pseudocyst) were successfully treated by surgical internal drainage.[7] It has been learnt that removing necrotic pancreatic tissue becomes easier after an interval, because it demarcates and separates from viable pancreatic tissue, like a 'sequestrum' in osteomyelitis. Thus, delayed surgical necrosectomy and debridement have replaced early surgical resection for the treatment of infected pancreatic necrosis. Further, it was learnt that it is often better to complete necrosectomy over two or more operations than to attempt complete necrosectomy at the 'first sitting'. Over time, it also became apparent that the placement of multiple wide-bore drains allowed for less-aggressive necrosectomy as long as adequate drainage could be maintained. It also became apparent that just the drainage of pus under pressure, without any necrosectomy, could arrest the clinical decline of a patient, allowing a delay for subsequent 'definitive' necrosectomy when the patient had become more stable and the infected necrosis had been better demarcated. Recognising that the wide exposure of open surgery carries its own risk of complications, there has been a drive to implement less-invasive access approaches to further improve clinical outcomes. The acceptance of laparoscopic surgery, interventional radiology and

interventional endoscopy with endosonography gave significant impetus to the move away from open surgery to minimally invasive treatments of infected pancreatic necrosis.

CLASSIFYING TREATMENTS AND THEIR TARGETS

Minimally invasive treatments for infected pancreatic necrosis proliferated in the 1990s, with multiple different approaches.[8] These used a range of imaging methods (e.g., laparoscopic, nephroscopic and flexible endoscopic) and different routes to the target lesion (e.g., transperitoneal, retroperitoneal and transgastric). These have been classified based on the method of visualisation, the access route and the purpose of intervention.[9] There have been no well-designed studies to compare different minimally invasive surgical interventions, but emerging contenders are videoscopic-assisted retroperitoneal debridement (VARD), which uses a 5 to 7 cm flank incision; the minimal-access retroperitoneal pancreatic necrosectomy (MARPN), which uses a dilated percutaneous track to insert a nephroscope; and endoscopic ultrasound (EUS)-guided endoscopic transgastric drainage and debridement.[10]

Along with the evolution of treatment strategies, the local complications of AP,[1,11] which are the targets of treatment, have also been redefined. These new definitions have been widely adopted (Table 31.1). The complications that are most often the targets of surgical treatment are infected walled-of necrosis (WON) and, less commonly, infected pseudocysts. There are other factors important in selecting the most appropriate intervention for one of these target lesions. The availability of expertise and the presence of experience and equipment are important considerations. In addition, the location, shape, complexity and anatomic relations of the target lesion are important. The decision as to the most appropriate intervention has a direct bearing on the spectrum and risk of complications.

Table 31.1   The classification of local complications of acute pancreatitis, as defined by Revised Atlanta criteria

	Acute (<4 weeks, no defined wall)		Chronic (>4 weeks, defined wall)	
Content	No infection	Infection	No infection	Infection
Fluid	Acute pancreatic fluid collection	Infected APFC	Pseudocyst	Infected pseudocyst
Solid ± fluid	Acute necrotic collection	Infected ANC	Walled off necrosis	Infected WON

Abbreviations: ANC, acute necrotic collection; APFC, acute pancreatic fluid collection; WON, walled-of necrosis.

SPECTRUM OF COMPLICATIONS AFTER SURGICAL TREATMENT OF ACUTE PANCREATITIS

The recently published Liverpool experience of the surgical treatment of severe AP provides an opportunity to review the spectrum of complications in the context of an evolving practice in a unit dedicated to the treatment of AP.[12] The large volume of cases (n = 394, with 73% tertiary referrals) and considerable experience with open surgical treatment have allowed them to help pioneer one of the less-invasive treatment strategies (i.e., MARPN). Figure 31.1 shows the rising number of patients treated per year and the increasing proportion of minimally invasive interventions, the relatively constant and low conversion rate and, more recently, the possible rise in open surgical necrosectomy, at least in Liverpool. Not included in this series are the complications associated with percutaneous drainage (which was used in only a quarter of patients) and endoscopic treatment (attempted in only three patients acutely), which will be discussed later.

In this series, there was a useful comparison of postoperative outcomes between MARPN and open pancreatic necrosectomy (OPN). Although this strongly suggests fewer procedure-related complications for the former, there is an acknowledged selection bias in the absence of randomisation. The 'overall complication' rate was 63% versus 82% (p < 0.001) for MARPN and OPN, respectively, and this difference holds true for 'operation-specific complications' (35% vs. 52%; p < 0.001) and 'operation-nonspecific complications' (17% vs. 27%; p < 0.001). The mortality was not significantly different between the groups (15% vs. 23%; p = 0.064). The specific complications were reported as persistent pancreatic fistulas (11.7% vs. 5.1%; p = 0.032) and postoperative sepsis with multiorgan failure (MOF) (25% vs. 12%; p = 0.003), which were significantly more prevalent after OPN, whereas MARPNs were associated with significantly higher postoperative deep venous thrombosis (DVT) rates (6.6% vs. 1.7%; p = 0.046) (Table 31.2). When complications directly attributable to both MARPN and OPN are combined, the most frequent complications, in order of frequency, are bleeding (n = 68; 17%), persistent sepsis/MOF (n = 63; 16%), gastrointestinal (GI) fistulae (n = 42; 11%) and pancreatic fistulae (n = 28; 7%). Although not strictly a complication, the conversion from MARPN to OPN was required in 13% of patients for poor access to the cavity (n = 16), bleeding (n = 8), perforation into hollow viscus or peritoneal cavity (n = 6), inadequate debridement (n = 4) and ischaemic colitis requiring colectomy (n = 2).

COMPLICATIONS OF OPEN AND MINIMALLY INVASIVE SURGICAL TREATMENT

Bleeding

Bleeding associated with local complications of AP (e.g., WON and pseudocyst) is usually due to a ruptured pseudoaneurysm and is almost always successfully managed by angiographic embolisation. Bleeding also occurs as a result of surgical treatment itself. Exposure of vessels to activated pancreatic enzymes results in softening of the vessel wall, erosive vasculitis and the risk of bleeding.

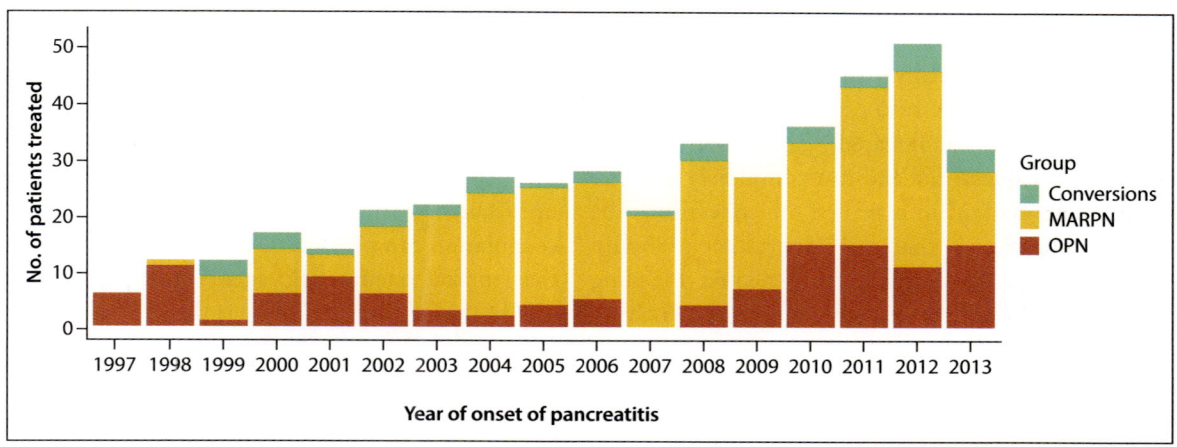

Figure 31.1 Minimal access retroperitoneal pancreatic necrosectomies (MARPNs), open pancreatic necrosectomies (OPNs), and conversion rate over a 17-year period in one institution.

Reprinted with permission from: Gomatos IP, Halloran CM, Ghaneh P, et al. Outcomes from minimal access retroperitoneal and open pancreatic necrosectomy in 394 patients with necrotizing pancreatitis. *Ann Surg* 2016;263:992–1001.

Table 31.2 Postoperative complications after minimal access retroperitoneal pancreatic necrosectomy (MARPN) and open pancreatic necrosectomy (OPN) for acute pancreatitis, excluding missing data[12]

Complications	Total (n = 394)	MARPN (n = 274)	OPN (n = 120)	p value
Bleeding*	68	50 (18.2%)	18 (15%)	0.470
Pseudoaneurysm	14	12 (4.4%)	2 (1.7%)	0.243
Persistent pancreatic fistula*	28	14 (5.1%)	14 (11.7%)	0.032
Upper gastrointestinal fistula*	18	9 (3.3%)	9 (7.5%)	0.113
Lower gastrointestinal fistula*	24	20 (7.3%)	4 (3.3%)	0.170
Biliary stricture	15	8 (2.9%)	7 (5.8%)	0.251
Ischaemic bowel	6	4 (1.5%)	2 (1.7%)	1.000
Clostridium difficile colitis	14	12 (4.4%)	2 (1.7%)	0.243
Ascites	31	25 (9.1%)	6 (5%)	0.222
Portal vein thrombosis	41	32 (11.7%)	9 (7.5%)	0.282
Superior mesenteric vein thrombosis	20	14 (5.1%)	6 (5%)	1.000
Myocardial infarction	8	4 (1.5%)	4 (3.3%)	0.257
Stroke	5	4 (1.5%)	1 (0.8%)	1.000
Other cardiac complications	9	5 (1.8%)	4 (3.3%)	0.465
Pulmonary embolus	8	3 (1.1%)	5 (4.2%)	0.061
Deep vein thrombosis	20	18 (6.6%)	2 (1.7%)	0.046
Nosocomial pneumonia	23	15 (5.5%)	8 (6.7%)	0.647
Persistent sepsis and multiorgan failure*	63	33 (12%)	30 (25%)	0.003
Total		**175 (63.9%)**	**98 (81.7%)**	**<0.001**

*Complications directly related to surgical treatment.

Reprinted with permission from: Gomatos IP, Halloran CM, Ghaneh P, et al. Outcomes from minimal access retroperitoneal and open pancreatic necrosectomy in 394 patients with necrotizing pancreatitis. *Ann Surg* 2016;263:992–1001.

The reported incidence of major haemorrhage after surgical debridement is 20%.[13] The splenic or mesocolic vessels and the portal vein are the most common sites of bleeding.

Bleeding is more likely when surgical debridement is attempted early in the disease course (<3 weeks). At this early stage, the hypoperfused tissue remains partially vascularised and the necrotic portions of the pancreas are often not well demarcated. Later, the necrotic tissue forms a 'sequestrum' and can completely separate from the pancreas within a walled-off collection. The practical implication is that early debridement should be avoided to prevent debridement-related bleeding and that later debridement is facilitated by demarcation and separation of the necrotic tissue. When OPN is performed, it is imperative that gentle debridement is performed, starting first with the 'educated finger', which is best able to distinguish the soft and removable dead tissue, and then, only using forceps to remove loosened necrosum. Sharp dissection is contraindicated. High volume irrigation of the cavity can be very helpful, but care must be taken to monitor for bacteraemia,

which is more likely to occur with high-pressure irrigation within a cavity. If bleeding does occur during OPN, then an attempt should be made to identify the source of bleeding, if possible. Access to the cavity can be restricted because of the inflamed and stiff tissues, and direct inspection may not be possible. Sometimes, a single bleeding vessel is apparent, and this can be ligated or clipped. Otherwise, the best strategy is to pack the cavity with a length of gauze (e.g., Macfarlane roll), systematically laying in portions to the periphery until haemostasis is achieved by pressure. Argon beam coagulation can be useful for oozing surfaces. It is likely that topical haemostatic agents and pads will have a role in this setting, but there is no published experience or guideline to date. Packing will require a return to the operating room for removal after an interval of less than 48 hours, and this can be facilitated by leaving the abdomen open, using a negative-pressure dressing. Packing increases the risk of GI fistulae (see below). If the bleeding is brisk and arterial, and even though temporary haemostasis has been achieved with packing, it is prudent to consider angiographic embolisation, if possible, before pack removal. Direct closure of the abdomen with postoperative drainage and lavage is associated with lower incidence of bleeding compared with laparostomies or repeat laparotomies.

Minimally invasive debridement is associated with lower rates of bleeding. When bleeding occurs during VARD through a small open flank incision, it is usually necessary to pack the cavity. There are two advantages when a nephroscope is used through an Amplatz sheath. Identification of the source of bleeding is facilitated by the high-flow irrigation within the closed collection and the bleeding is readily seen as a 'plume under water'. Tamponade of venous bleeding is also more likely to succeed with this more closed approach, compared with the VARD.

Persistent Sepsis

Strictly speaking, this is more of a failure of surgical treatment than a complication of it. It usually means the failure to control sepsis 'at source' or a failure to recognise a source of sepsis elsewhere. When focussing on the former, the reason for failure to control sepsis is usually the inability to adequately drain and debride infected pancreatic and peripancreatic tissue. The complexity, multiplicity and extent of infected pancreatic necrosis can limit the effectiveness of drainage (Figure 31.2). In addition, even when OPN is indicated because of this, there is often difficulty in completely debriding all extensions of the disease process, especially those that extend into the small bowel mesentery. Pursuing less-invasive approaches for too long can result in persisting sepsis. Recognising the limits of these approaches can be very difficult, but

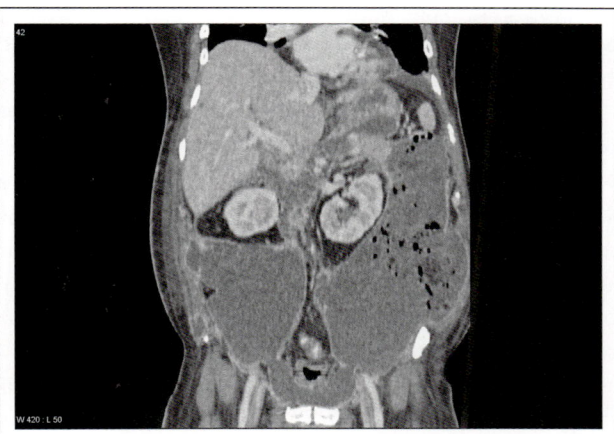

Figure 31.2 Computed tomography image of a patient with severe acute pancreatitis, with complex, infected retroperitoneal and intraperitoneal collections.

Courtesy: Sanjay Pandanaboyana and John A Windsor.

desisting and resorting to OPN can sometimes help prevent prolongation of sepsis and organ dysfunction. The practical implication is to ensure that all significant areas of infection are adequately drained. This means upsizing the drains, using multiple drains into complex collections, using irrigation to reduce the bacterial load and facilitating more efficient drainage. The current pigtail irrigation catheters that are commonly used for drainage fail frequently. The PANTER trial noted a 65% failure rate,[3] and this is usually due to blockage of the catheter side holes by particulate necrosum fragments. There is significant room for improvement of drainage techniques (see below).

Perforation and Gastrointestinal Fistulas

Perforation of the GI tract can occur with the placement of a drain. Inserting a drainage catheter along the pancreatic axis from the left and below the spleen puts the splenic flexure of the colon at risk. The insertion of a percutaneous transgastric drain is sometimes the safest route to a central collection in the lesser sac, when EUS-guided drainage is not available. This intentional perforation of the anterior and posterior walls of the stomach rarely causes a problem. This approach can be subsequently converted to an endoscopic transgastric drain through the posterior wall of the stomach or, even better, a direct endoscopic approach.

Perforation can also occur as a result of endoscopic retrograde cholangiopancreatography (ERCP) with sphincterotomy in severe AP. This may be more likely if ERCP is delayed, with significant inflammation and oedema of the ampulla and duodenal wall. The practical implication is that ERCP should be employed only if absolutely required. It is not indicated for transient cholestasis (because a stone is likely to have passed) or for predicted severe pancreatitis (because this has accuracy of only 70%, which exposes 30% to the risks of an unnecessary ERCP)[14] but only for severe cholangitis.

There is an increased risk of GI fistulae when packing is required to control bleeding. The key to reducing this risk is to not leave the packs too long (<48 hours) and to soak them thoroughly as the gauze is gently removed. Another way to reduce the risk is to separate the gauze from the tissue with a plastic sheet, reducing the risk of adherence to blood vessels in the cavity wall.

The colonic flexures are particularly at risk with retroperitoneal drainage catheters. With OPN, it is advised to surgically 'lower' the flexures before placing drains. This not only increases the exposure for debridement and allows the drains to be dependent but also reduces the risk of colonic fistulae from drain erosion. The duodenojejunal flexure is another part of the GI tract that is vulnerable to fistulation, sometimes forming part of the wall of the pancreatic collection. It is at risk from both debridement and drain erosion. The management of a GI fistula should be along standard lines, including the drainage of any associated collection not covered by the inserted drain and defining the anatomy of the fistula by contrast radiography.[15] Usually, the fistula is low-volume and is treated by the stepwise withdrawal of the drain once the tract has become established. Rarely, a self-expandable metal stent (SEMS) in the colon or duodenum will facilitate the management of a fistula at these sites.

COMPLICATIONS OF ENDOSCOPIC INTERVENTION

The indications for the endoscopic drainage of WON and pseudocysts include the presence of symptoms, infection and cholestasis. Endoscopic drainage is possible only when these local complications abut the stomach or proximal duodenum; otherwise, percutaneous drainage is usually preferable.[10] Success with drainage is more likely with a fluid-filled pseudocyst[1] than with WON, where solid necrosum can block catheters and stents. The technical success rate of EUS-guided drainage, which means achieving the intended deployment of the drains, is close to 100%, and the success of the procedure, which means complete resolution, is more than 90% for pseudocysts and 70 to 80% for WON.[10]

Significant innovation has occurred in relation to the technique of EUS-guided drainage, including the type, size and number of stents used. Traditionally, plastic pigtail stents have been used because of the low risk of migration, but the narrow internal diameter results in high occlusion rates and the narrow external diameter means that endoscopic access to the cavity requires subsequent dilation. Using multiple plastic pigtail stents has been shown to increase the efficacy of drainage.[16] More recently, SEMS (uncovered and covered) have been used, but the purpose-designed wall-opposing metal stents with a wider lumen appear to be most effective.[17] These include the NAGI™ stent (Taewoong Medical Co., Ltd., Seoul, Korea), BCF stent (M.I. Tech Co., Ltd., Seoul, Korea) and AXIOS™ stent (Xlumena Inc., Mountain View, CA, US).

Current evidence indicates that the success rate and adverse events from endoscopic drainage appear to be similar with metal and plastic stents. A recent systematic review (17 studies, n = 881 patients) comparing plastic and metal stents reported similar pooled success rates (80.7% vs. 81.9%, respectively).[18] There was also no difference in the pooled complication rates (including bleeding, secondary infection and stent migration) with

metal stents compared with plastic stents (23.3% vs. 16.1%). There were similar success rates for the treatment of pseudocysts (85.1% vs. 83.3%) and WON (69.5% vs. 77.9%) for plastic and metal stents, respectively.[18]

Complications of endoscopic drainage include perforation, bleeding, stent occlusion, stent migration and superinfection. The risk of perforation can be reduced by delaying intervention to allow an inflammatory wall to develop around the collection and for it to become adherent to the stomach or duodenum. Selecting the point for initial puncture, where the stomach and collection are best apposed, is aided by EUS, which is also useful to reduce the risk of bleeding by helping to select a window, without significant blood vessels. The risk of a perforation is probably reduced by the new designs of SEMS by applying an apposition force to the wall of the stomach and collection. When compared with other locations, perforation was more common with collections involving the uncinate region.[19] A perforation is not always immediately apparent, and intraperitoneal air adjacent to the site of drainage on subsequent imaging may be the only sign. Such patients require antibiotics, but more significant perforations may require percutaneous drainage or a laparotomy.

The treatment of bleeding may be successful with endoscopic balloon tamponade, adrenaline injection or endoscopic clipping.[20] The insertion of a SEMS may be sufficient to arrest bleeding from the puncture site. Bleeding from within the cavity itself, during debridement, is more challenging. It is either due to an overly vigorous debridement or due to a pseudoaneurysm. With endoscopic access to the cavity and using vigorous irrigation, it might be possible to identify the point of bleeding and treat it by adrenaline inject or clipping. More significant bleeding will require angiographic embolisation or a laparotomy.

Stent migration (into the stomach or into adjacent organs) is a problem with both plastic and metal stents but is more common with the former. Metals stents are less likely to migrate because of the anchoring effect of self-expansion and because of the addition of proximal and distal flanges. These more recent 'anchoring' fully covered metal stents have lower rates of migration (<10%) compared with plastic stents (up to 18%).[21]

Secondary infection of the collection can be due to the presence of a stent, but it is difficult to quantify this risk. Clinical evidence suggesting secondary infection may be due to stent occlusion rather than due to introduced infection. The use of a single plastic stent with narrow diameter (8.5 Fr or less) may have a lower secondary infection rate of 3.5%, whereas a larger stent diameter

(10 Fr or more) appears to have a higher secondary infection rate (17.2%).[22] The wide reported infection rates for plastic stents (2.7–12%), for covered metal stents (0–28%) and for purpose-designed metal stents (0–15.2%)[22] make it difficult to draw any conclusions. The management principle is to optimise drainage, whether the infection is native or introduced, and this might be by increasing the number of plastic stents or replacing the metal stent for a larger one. The insertion of a nasocystic irrigation catheter might also be helpful.

COMPLICATIONS OF PERCUTANEOUS DRAINAGE

The excitement generated by various minimally invasive approaches to the surgical treatment of AP tended to overshadow the expanding role of percutaneous drainage, initially pioneered by Freeny.[23] Although percutaneous drainage was initially considered a secondary treatment for residual collections after surgical treatment, it has become increasingly important as a primary treatment and, in some cases, as the sole treatment.[3] Not only does percutaneous treatment permit a delay in surgical treatment to allow maturation of the lesion and improvement in the clinical status of the patient, but also the evidence now shows that it can replace surgery in moderate proportion of patients.[23–25] The challenge now is to optimise drainage techniques in order to avoid surgical treatment and prevent its complications.[26] This may involve designed-for-purpose drains and the use of augmented irrigation to accelerate liquefaction of particulate necrosum, reduce drain blockage, establish more effective drainage and reduce the rate of persisting sepsis.[27] A recent systematic review highlighted significant room for improvement in the way that percutaneous drains are used.[27] For improved safety, efficacy and outcomes, it is important to use a guidewire for insertion (the Seldinger method), regular replacement (for blockage) and upsizing, and for continuous alternating irrigation, it is useful to have more than one drain in a complex collection.

Percutaneous drainage is beset with the same range of complications described for endoscopic drainage (above): perforation, bleeding, migration and infection. Perforation is sometime unavoidable, as puncture of organs may be required to access collections for drainage. The stomach can be transgressed with relatively low risk, whereas colon and small bowel puncture should be avoided. These are all treated in a similar way.

Bleeding can occur with the insertion of the drain, and delayed bleeding can occur because of erosion of drains into vessels or adjacent tissue. It is important to be aware of the 'sentinel bleed', which is usually a haemodynamically insignificant bleed evidenced by blood within the drain. This can sometimes herald a catastrophic subsequent bleed and needs prompt investigation before this occurs. A contrast CT followed by selective angiography is the diagnostic 'gold standard' for localising active bleeding. Although treatment of vascular complications by surgery was the mainstay in the past, the angiographic approach by catheter-directed embolisation is shown to detect the bleeding site in approximately 80% of cases[28] and arterial embolisation can achieve definite haemostasis in 35 to 50% (Figure 31.3a and b).

Pancreatic Fistula

External pancreatic fistulae are a common sequel after intervention in severe pancreatitis. These usually occur when a pancreatic or peripancreatic collection is drained externally and/or the collection is connected with the (main) pancreatic duct, especially if there is a stricture distally. Internal fistulae are less of a concern. Most external pancreatic fistulae are of low output and close spontaneously with conservative management. In a series of 210 patients with severe pancreatitis, 43 (20%) patients developed external pancreatic fistulae after intervention for infected pancreatic necrosis (n = 23) and pancreatic abscess (n = 20). Spontaneous closure of the fistulae occurred in 38 (88%) patients; however, 24% of patients with spontaneous closure developed pseudocyst during follow-up, requiring further intervention.[29] Data from the PENGUIN trial, which compared endoscopic transgastric and open necrosectomy, showed significantly lower incidence of postoperative pancreatic fistulae after an endoscopic approach (10% vs. 70%).[30] Similarly, nonrandomised larger series comparing minimally invasive approach with open approach have shown lower incidence

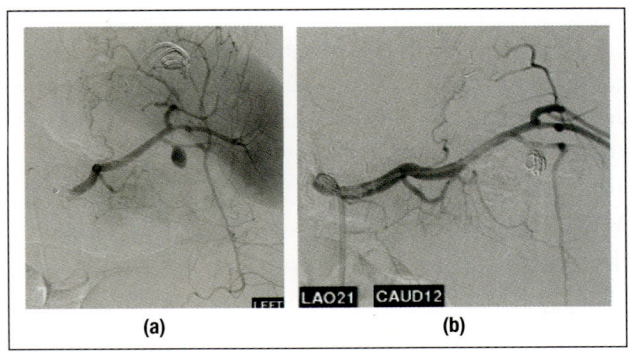

Figure 31.3 Catheter angiography images of (a) splenic artery pseudoaneurysm secondary to necrotising pancreatitis and (b) subsequent coiling of the pseudoaneurysm.

Courtesy: Sanjay Pandanaboyana and John A Windsor.

of pancreatic fistula with a minimally invasive approach.[12] For fistulas after open necrosectomy, the percutaneous catheter inserted at the time of surgery should not be removed as long as there is any significant drainage. Endoscopic retrograde cholangiopancreatography or magnetic resonance imaging (MRI) with magnetic resonance cholangiopancreatography is helpful for identifying the site of the leak and the presence of a stricture. Transpapillary stenting at the time of ERCP has been shown to accelerate the resolution of pancreatic fistulae if the anatomy is favourable (e.g., a tail leak or a disruption within the head that can be traversed by the stent). Convincing data on the role of octreotide in reducing and closing fistulous drainage are lacking. Two meta-analysis on the role of octreotide in reducing fistulae after pancreatoduodenectomy did not show a benefit in preventing postoperative fistula and complications.[31,32]

Persistent pancreatic fistula from pancreatic duct disruption leads to disconnected pancreatic duct syndrome (DPDS). It is a recognised complication of acute necrotising pancreatitis, and 30% of the patients who develop necrotising pancreatitis have disruption of the main pancreatic duct, predisposing them to DPDS. It is defined by complete discontinuity of the pancreatic duct, most often in the pancreatic neck and body region, leaving a viable left side of the pancreas that cannot drain into the duodenum.[33,34] The disconnected pancreatic duct permits the remnant of the body and/or tail to secrete pancreatic juice into the retroperitoneum, causing peripancreatic necrosis, and the development of either WON or a pseudocyst. The diagnosis of concurrent DPDS is predominantly made on contrast-enhanced computed tomography (CT), which shows necrosis of the neck and body of the pancreas but perfusion to the tail of the gland. Alternatively, a high-quality MRI with magnetic resonance cholangiopancreatography may demonstrate a duct cut-off in the proximal pancreas. Management of necrotising pancreatitis through a transgastric approach has the advantage of the distal pancreatic remnant draining internally into the stomach, which averts the need for a distal pancreatectomy.

Abdominal Compartment Syndrome and Incisional Herniae

Compartment syndrome occurs early in AP as a consequence of a profound systemic inflammatory response, with capillary leak and expansion of the interstitial fluid volume. Tissue oedema occurs throughout the body, increasing diffusion distance for oxygen and glucose at the cellular level, and may contribute to organ failure.[35] In the abdomen, oedema contributes to intra-abdominal hypertension and compartment syndrome. The problem is almost certainly compounded by overvigorous fluid resuscitation, and it is preferable to institute pressor support rather than overresuscitate to reduce this complication. The practical implication this complication is the optimisation of fluid resuscitation (not too much and too little) and early vasopressors and intensive care support. The consequence of compartment syndrome in some patients is the need to decrease intra-abdominal hypertension by laparostomy. Despite modern approaches with negative-pressure dressings, there is an increased risk of GI fistulae in the short term and incisional herniae in the long term, especially when full abdominal wall closure cannot be effected, and healing is by secondary intention.

CONCLUSIONS

There have been significant advances in the surgical treatment of the local complications of AP, especially with the increasing role of endoscopic and radiological techniques and the step-up approach. These have resulted in a reduction in the complications associated with treatment. Open surgical treatment has an ongoing, though more limited, role as a salvage approach when these less-invasive interventions have failed. The common complications of bleeding, perforation, fistula and infection are treated along standard lines. Complications related to less-invasive treatments are similar but may require additional techniques, as discussed.

REFERENCES

1. Banks PA, Bollen TL, Dervenis C, et al. Classification of acute pancreatitis – 2012: revision of the Atlanta classification and definitions by international consensus. *Gut* 2013; 62:102–11.

2. Russell PS, Mittal A, Brown L, et al. Admission, management and outcomes of acute pancreatitis in intensive care. *ANZ J Surg* 2016. doi: 10.1111/ans.13498.

3. van Santvoort HC, Besselink MG, Bakker OJ, et al; Dutch Pancreatitis Study Group. A step-up approach or open necrosectomy for necrotizing pancreatitis. *N Engl J Med* 2010;362:1491–502.

4. Bradley EL 3rd, Dexter ND. Management of severe acute pancreatitis: a surgical odyssey. *Ann Surg* 2010;251:6–17.

5. Hollender LF. Resection of the pancreas for acute hemorrhagic and necrotizing pancreatitis. *World J Surg* 1979;3:631–7.

6. Hollender LF, Kohler JJ, Klein A. Zur chirurgischen Behandlung der akuten nekrotischen pankreatitis. *Der Chirurg* 1972;43:256–61.

7. Warshaw AL, Rattner DW. Timing of surgical drainage for pancreatic pseudocyst. Clinical and chemical criteria. *Ann Surg* 1985;202:720–4.

8. Windsor JA. Minimally invasive pancreatic necrosectomy. Leading Article. *Br J Surg* 2007;2:132–3.

9. Loveday BP, Petrov MS, Connor S, et al. A comprehensive classification of invasive procedures for treating the local complications of acute pancreatitis based on visualization, route, and purpose. *Pancreatology* 2011;11:406–13.

10. Freeman M, Werner J, van Santvoort HC, et al. Interventions for necrotizing pancreatitis: summary of a multidisciplinary consensus conference. *Pancreas* 2012;41:1176–94.

11. Windsor JA, Petrov MS. Acute pancreatitis re-classified. Editorial. *Gut* 2013;62:4–5.

12. Gomatos IP, Halloran CM, Ghaneh P, et al. Outcomes from minimal access retroperitoneal and open pancreatic necrosectomy in 394 patients with necrotizing pancreatitis. *Ann Surg* 2016;263:992–1001.

13. Connor S, Alexakis N, Raraty MG, et al. Early and late complications after pancreatic necrosectomy. *Surgery* 2005;137:499–505.

14. Petrov MS, Uchugina AF, Kukosh MV. Does endoscopic retrograde cholangiopancreatography reduce the risk of local pancreatic complications in acute pancreatitis? A systematic review and meta-analysis. *Surg Endosc* 2008;22:2338–43.

15. Kaushal M, Carlson GL. Management of enterocutaneous fistulas. *Clin Colon Rectal Surg* 2004;17:79–88.

16. Jintao G, Linlin F, Siyu S, et al. Risk factors for infection after endoscopic ultrasonography-guided drainage of specific types of pancreatic and peripancreatic fluid collections (with video). *Surg Endosc* 2016;30:3114–20.

17. Téllez-Ávila FI, Villalobos-Garita Á, Ramírez-Luna MÁ. Use of a novel covered self-expandable metal stent with an anti-migration system for endoscopic ultrasound-guided drainage of a pseudocyst. *World J Gastrointest Endosc* 2013;5:297–9.

18. Bang JY, Hawes R, Bartolucci A, Varadarajulu S. Efficacy of metal and plastic stents for transmural drainage of pancreatic fluid collections: a systematic review. *Dig Endosc* 2015;27:486–98.

19. Varadarajulu S, Christein JD, Wilcox CM. Frequency of complications during EUS-guided drainage of pancreatic fluid collections in 148 consecutive patients. *J Gastroenterol Hepatol* 2011;26:1504–8.

20. Săftoiu A, Ciobanu L, Seicean A, Tantău M. Arterial bleeding during EUS-guided pseudocyst drainage stopped by placement of a covered self-expandable metal stent. *BMC Gastroenterol* 2013;24:93.

21. Kawakami H, Itoi T, Sakamoto N. Endoscopic ultrasound-guided transluminal drainage for peripancreatic fluid collections: where are we now? *Gut Liver* 2014;8:341–55.

22. Lin H, Zhan XB, Sun SY, et al. Stent selection for endoscopic ultrasound-guided drainage of pancreatic fluid collections: a multicenter study in china. *Gastroenterol Res Pract* 2014;2014:193562.

23. Freeny PC, Hauptmann E, Althaus SJ, Traverso LW, Sinanan M. Percutaneous CT-guided drainage of infected acute necrotising pancreatitis: techniques and results. *AJR* 1998;170:869–975.

24. Fotoohi M, D'Agostino HB, Wollman B, Chon K, Shahrokni S, van Sonnenberg E. Persistent pancreatocutaneous fistula after percutaneous drainage of pancreatic fluid collections: role of cause and severity of pancreatitis. *Radiology* 1999;213:573–8.

25. Baril NB, Ralls PW, Wren SM, Selby RR, Radin R, Parekh D. Does an infected peripancreatic fluid collection or abscess mandate operation? *Ann Surg* 2000;231:361–7.

26. Windsor JA. Infected pancreatic necrosis: drain first, but do it better. Leading article. *HPB* 2011;13:367–8.

27. van Baal MC, van Santvoort HC, Bollen TL, Bakker OJ, Besselink MG, Gooszen HG; Dutch Pancreatitis Study Group. Systematic review of percutaneous catheter drainage as primary treatment for necrotizing pancreatitis. *Br J Surg* 2011;98:18–27.

28. Beattie G, Hardman J, Redhead D, et al. Evidence for central role of selective mesenteric angiography in the management of the major vascular complications of pancreatitis. *Am J Surg* 2003;185:96–102.

29. Sikora SS1, Khare R, Srikanth G, Kumar A, Saxena R, Kapoor VK. External pancreatic fistula as a sequel to management of acute severe necrotizing pancreatitis. *Dig Surg* 2005;22:446–51.

30. Bakker OJ, van Santvoort HC, van Brunschot S, et al. Endoscopic transgastric vs surgical necrosectomy for infected necrotizing pancreatitis: a randomized trial. *JAMA* 2012;307:1053–61.

31. Alghamdi AA, Jawas AM, Hart RS. Use of octreotide for the prevention of pancreatic fistula after elective pancreatic surgery: a systematic review and meta-analysis. *Can J Surg* 2007;50:459–66.

32. Li-Ling J, Irving M. Somatostatin and octreotide in the prevention of postoperative pancreatic complications and the treatment of enterocutaneous pancreatic fistulas: a systematic review of randomized controlled trials. *Br J Surg* 2001;88:190–9.

33. Kozarek RA, Ball TJ, Patterson DJ, et al. Endoscopic transpapillary therapy for disrupted pancreatic duct and peripancreatic fluid collections. *Gastroenterology* 1991;100:1362–7.

34. Nealon WH, Bhutani M, Riall TS, et al. A unifying concept: pancreatic ductal anatomy both predicts and determines the major complications resulting from pancreatitis. *J Am Coll Surg* 2009;208:790–9.

35. Malbrain ML, Marik PE, Witters I, et al. Fluid overload, de-resuscitation, and outcomes in critically ill or injured patients: a systematic review with suggestions for clinical practice. *Anaesthesiol Intensive Ther* 2014;46:361–80.

32

Prevention and Management of Complications after Surgery for Chronic Pancreatitis

S. Burmeister, E. Jonas, S.R. Thomson and P.C. Bornman

ABSTRACT

Chronic pancreatitis (CP) is a multifactorial chronic disease, with alcohol as the predominant aetiological factor. Longstanding disease leads to exocrine and endocrine dysfunction and malnutrition, which add to the complexity of management. This requires a multidisciplinary team approach throughout the course of the patient's disease. Intractable pain is the predominant symptom that leads to the consideration of surgical therapy. When surgery is indicated, optimising patients' general condition before surgery is essential to minimise the risk for complications. Inconsistency in the reporting of complications for surgery of CP hampers the formulation of disease-specific recommendations as to how they should be managed. As a result, the data from pancreatic resection series for non-CP indications are used as surrogates. Postoperative pancreatic fistulae are less of a problem than in pancreatic resection for other indications and can be managed expectantly or by minimal access techniques. The infective and haemorrhagic complications are similarly best managed by percutaneous or angiographic interventions. Major complex surgery with its attendant high morbidity should be reserved for those in which the nonoperative approach has failed or is inappropriate.

KEYWORDS

Chronic pancreatitis, surgical treatment, complications, endoscopic retrograde cholangiopancreatography, endoscopic ultrasound, pancreatoduodenectomy

INTRODUCTION

Chronic pancreatitis (CP) is a pathological fibroinflammatory syndrome of the pancreas in patients with genetic, environmental and/or other risk factors, who develop persistent pathological responses to parenchymal injury or stress.[1,2] Although alcohol is the predominant aetiological factor, it is increasingly recognised that CP is a multifactorial disease in which the interplay between genetic and environmental factors plays an important role. In the alcohol-induced group, psychosocial and economic factors are often coupled with substance abuse, including tobacco, which adds to the complexity of its management.

The pathological features of CP are pancreatic atrophy, fibrosis, duct distortion, strictures, calcifications, fluid collections, ascites and obstruction of the adjacent structures. Some or all of these features may be present in individual cases but are more likely to be present in those with long-standing or advanced disease, when pancreatic exocrine and endocrine dysfunction is inevitable and there is an increased likelihood of malignancy.

Pain is the predominant symptom. Pain patterns vary from minimal to intermittent during flares to persistent and intractable, requiring opioids for control, resulting in impaired lifestyle and quality of life.[3] The exact pathogenesis of pain remains poorly understood.[4] Ductal obstruction and hypertension, parenchymal tissue fluid hypertension, inflammatory cytokines producing visceral and central nerve stimulation and sensitisation, and tissue hypoxia causing oxygen-derived free radicals damage are the major aetiopathogenic postulates. A recent review coalesces the role that these various factors play.[5]

Complications of CP occur not only in the gland but also in adjacent structures owing to extension of the inflammatory process, particularly to the common bile duct and the duodenum. Bile duct strictures are commonly seen in the presence of an inflammatory mass in the head of the pancreas and may cause various degrees of biliary obstruction. Pancreatic fluid collections (PFCs) may be the result of duct obstruction and/or disruption secondary to focal necrosis. Pancreatic fluid collections may be either intrapancreatic or extrapancreatic. In addition, rupture of the collection usually presents as ascites or rarely as an isolated pleural or pericardial effusion secondary to a retroperitoneal leak. Pancreatic fluid collections may cause duodenal or biliary obstruction or may become secondarily infected. Another serious complication may occur when these pancreatic enzyme-rich fluid collections result in erosion of neighbouring arterial vessels, with the creation of a false aneurysm. This may rupture with bleeding into the collection or via the pancreatic duct, presenting as an upper gastrointestinal (GI) bleed, commonly referred to as haemosuccus pancreaticus.

MANAGEMENT OF CHRONIC PANCREATITIS

Nonsurgical Management

The mainstay of medical management includes lifestyle modification, emphasising abstinence from alcohol, cessation of smoking and dietary modification by utilising a low-fat, balanced protein–carbohydrate diet, together with pancreatic enzyme replacement, if indicated. A step-up approach for pain relief is used with standard nonopioid analgesics and anti-inflammatory drugs, progressing to opioid-containing medications.[6] Minimal access options are now integrated into management algorithms. These include utilising endoscopic retrograde cholangiopancreatography (ERCP) and endoscopic ultrasound (EUS) for endotherapy of PFCs, ductal strictures and pancreatic calculi removal (with or without extracorporeal shock wave lithotripsy [ESWL]). Neurolysis

by thoracoscopy or by image-guided techniques is also employed in selected cases for pain control.[6,7]

Surgical Management

Surgery is an integral part of the multidisciplinary management of CP.[8] The surgical management of pain in CP is reserved for patients who do not respond to conservative measures. Surgical intervention of CP is performed to address pain and/or complications. Surgical procedures for pain can be classified as drainage procedures, resective procedures or a combination of both. In the absence of an inflammatory pancreatic head mass lateral pancreatojejunostomy (LPJ), the Partington-Rochelle operation remains a commonly performed procedure in the presence of a dilated main pancreatic duct. The simplest of the resections is a distal pancreatectomy when the disease is confined to the body and tail of the pancreas. Approximately 30% of patients presenting with CP will have an inflammatory mass in the head of the pancreas that can be addressed by resective procedures such as pancreatoduodenectomy (PD) or pylorus-preserving PD (PPPD). Duodenal-preserving pancreatic head resections (DPPHR) with or without drainage of the pancreatic duct are now increasingly performed. These were originally described by Frey and Smith[9] and Beger et al.[10] However, more recently, a number of modifications, often referred to as hybrid procedures, have been devised.[11–13] These DPPHR variations are schematically shown in Figure 32.1. Pylorus-preserving PD can lead to complete pain relief in about 75 to 82% of patients in the short and long terms, with a mortality rate of less than 3% and excellent long-term survival.[14–16] Ongoing exocrine and endocrine deteriorations appear to be unrelated to the type of resection or whether resection is combined with a drainage procedure.[17,18] Although no apparent difference in mortality rates has been found among standard PD, PPPD and DPPHR, the duodenal-preserving procedures are associated with significantly lower morbidity rates than PD (9–22% vs. 20–70%).[8] Therefore, the current trend is to favour drainage or combination procedures.[4–6,19] Total pancreatectomy with concomitant autologous transplant of islet cells is an option to consider when there is concern over malignant transformation or small duct disease, or it can be used as a salvage procedure.[20,21]

CLASSIFICATION OF COMPLICATIONS

Complications of surgery for CP can be divided into general and those specific to CP surgery, which are either early or late. The spectrum of complications of surgery for CP has changed with the trend over the last two decades towards

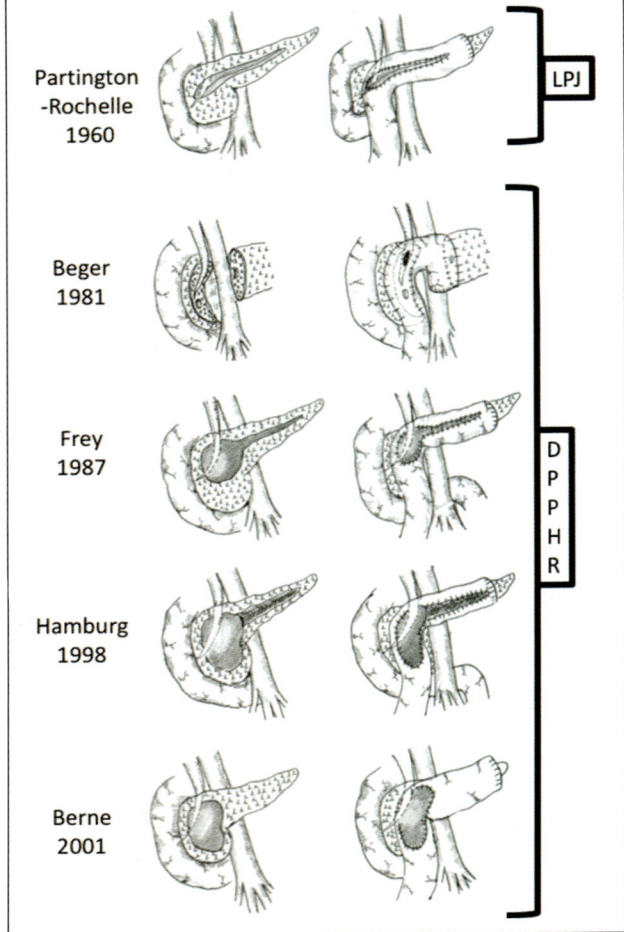

Figure 32.1 Schematic representation of the major drainage and hybrid procedures for chronic pancreatitis.

Abbreviations: LPJ, lateral pancreatojejunostomy; DPPHR, duodenal-preserving pancreatic head resection.

Adapted from: Aimoto T, Uchida E, Nakamura Y, et al. Current surgical treatment for chronic pancreatitis. *J Nippon Med Sch* 2011;78:352–9.

organ preserving/hybrid operations and the increasing popularity of minimal access options for their treatment.

INCIDENCE OF COMPLICATIONS

Papers reporting on the surgical treatment of CP have focussed mainly on the results of pain control; hence, the incidence of complications is not consistently specified for individual procedures.[22] There is also a lack of reporting on less serious complications.[23,24] Duration of follow-up, mainly due to poor compliance, varies significantly, affecting the validity of data on long-term complications. Furthermore, selective reporting of short- or long-term complications is frequent, and few publications use

standardised definitions and grading systems for reporting of complications such as delayed gastric emptying (DGE), postoperative bleeding and pancreatic fistulae. Definitions have now been standardised for these three complications to facilitate consistent recording in future studies.[25–27] The standardised definition of postoperative pancreatic fistula, as formulated by the International Study Group on Pancreatic Fistula (ISGPF), shown in Table 32.1, is most relevant. Exocrine and endocrine dysfunction is a of CP but can also be precipitated or exacerbated by surgical procedures. It can be difficult to assess whether worsening function is purely the result of the intervention or a manifestation of the natural course of the disease, uninfluenced by the procedure.[17,28] Combining procedures, for example, adding a biliary bypass to a DPPHR, further compound accurate assessment of the risk for complications for the specific procedures.[24] Another confounding factor is the use of sequential procedures in a step-up approach, which makes it difficult to attribute long-term complications to the most recent procedure.[14]

Table 32.2 summarises the complications as reported between 1990 and 2016 in randomised controlled trials (RCTs) or comparative cohort studies, where complications could clearly be assigned to specifically described operations. The data illustrate the deficits and variability in the reporting of complications.

PREVENTION OF COMPLICATIONS OF SURGERY

Centralisation of Care

Lower operative and/or 30-day mortalities have been reported in patients undergoing advanced pancreatic surgery in high-volume centres compared with those in low-volume centres.[37] Most of these series report the results of surgery for cancer patients. Nevertheless, the same benefits were observed in studies where CP patients were included in the cohorts.[37,38] A key factor in ensuring appropriate management and the reduction of complications from all interventions, including surgery, is early referral of patients with CP to dedicated high-volume institutions, where multidisciplinary teams can coordinate their care.

Optimising Comorbidities

The complications and comorbidities related to CP take a toll on the individual's physiological and nutritional reserve. The first step in reducing the risk and severity of surgical complications is the optimisation of these comorbidities, which is usually achievable as most of the procedures are elective. Malnutrition, resulting from the interplay of

Table 32.1 Standardised definition and grading of postoperative pancreatic fistula

A postoperative pancreatic fistula		Drain output of any measurable volume of fluid on or after postoperative day 3, with an amylase content >3 times the serum amylase activity	
Grade	**A**	**B**	**C**
Clinical conditions	Well	Often well	Ill-appearing /bad
Specific treatment*	No	Yes/no	Yes
US/CT (if obtained)	Negative	Negative/positive	Positive
Persistent drainage (after 3 weeks)	No	Usually yes	Yes
Reoperation	No	No	Yes
Death related to POPF	No	No	Possibly yes
Signs of infection	No	Yes	Yes
Sepsis	No	No	Yes
Readmission	No	Yes/no	Yes/no

*Parenteral nutrition, antibiotics, enteral nutrition, somatostatin analogue and/or minimal invasive drainage.
Abbreviations: CT, computed tomographic scan; POPF, postoperative pancreatic fistula; US, ultrasonography.
Adapted from: Bassi C, Dervenis C, Butturini G, et al. Postoperative pancreatic fistula: an international study group (ISGPF) definition. *Surgery* 2005;138:8–13.

Table 32.2 Complications as reported between 1990 and 2016 in randomised controlled trials or comparative cohort studies

	Operation type	n	Complications expressed as %						
			Intra-abdominal abscess	DGE	Pancreatic leak/ fistula	Biliary leak/ fistula	Bleeding	New-onset endocrine dysfunction	New-onset exocrine dysfunction
RCT									
Cahen DL, et al[29]*	LPJ	20	NR	NR	NR	NR	NR	20	13
Keck T, et al[30]	PPPD	45	NR	NR	5	NR	NR	19	21
	Beger	47	NR	NR	10	NR	NR	24	26
Izbicki J, et al[31]	Frey	22	NR	NR	0	NR	4.5	NR	NR
	Beger	20	NR	NR	5	NR	5	NR	NR
Büchler M, et al[32]	PPPD	20	NR	NR	5	NR	0	NR	NR
	Beger	20	NR	NR	0	NR	10	NR	NR
Farkas G, et al[33]	PPPD	20	NR	30	NR	NR	NR	NR	NR
	Berne**	20	NR	0	NR	NR	NR	NR	NR
Comparative cohorts									
Hildebrand P, et al[34]	PD	12	NR	NR	0	NR	16.7	25	30
	Frey	39	NR	NR	2.7	NR	2.7	13	2.7
Keck T, et al[35]	Frey	50	2	NR	4	NR	NR	34	34
	Beger	42	10	NR	5	NR	NR	17	33
Aimoto T, et al[36]	PPD	10	10	10	NR	NR	NR	20	NR
	Frey	6	NR	NR	17	NR	NR	NR	NR

*Randomised trial that compared endoscopic and surgical drainage of the pancreatic duct in patients with advanced chronic pancreatitis.
**Modification of Berne operation.
Abbreviations: DGE, delayed gastric emptying; LPJ, lateral pancreatojejunostomy; PD, pancreatoduodenectomy; PPPD, pylorus-preserving pancreatoduodenectomy; NR, not reported.

multiple factors, is common but is often underdiagnosed in patients with CP.[39,40] An adequate dietary intake must be ensured and tailored to the management of exocrine and endocrine capacity of a patient; this requires detection and active management throughout an individual patient's illness.[41] Major surgery requires nutritional optimisation in the perioperative period. This is best achieved by the enteral route, with intravenous nutritional support being reserved for the few whose critical illness precludes, or is a contraindication to, the adequate provision of nutrients via the GI tract.

Exocrine Insufficiency

Although the production of all pancreatic digestive enzymes is reduced in long-standing disease, it is the lack of lipase that is the most clinically significant. The degree of exocrine insufficiency may vary, ranging from frank steatorrhoea and weight loss to subclinical, as determined by a variety of pancreatic function tests. The gold standard for the diagnosis of exocrine insufficiency is direct testing by secretin stimulation of enzyme output. Owing to the technical complexity of this method, its use is limited to referral centres. Despite their lack of sensitivity in mild to moderate disease, indirect methods of testing using serum pancreolauryl values, stool fat quantification and faecal elastase levels are more frequently used in the clinical setting.[6,42,43]

Dietary management by an experienced dietician is essential. Lifestyle and nutritional modifications are important and should include limitation of alcohol intake, cessation of smoking and avoidance of fatty foods. The therapeutic mainstay of patients with exocrine insufficiency is pancreatic enzyme replacement therapy (PERT), which aims to normalise gut absorption and correct nutritional deficiencies.[42] Pancreatic enzyme replacement therapy is clearly indicated when fat malabsorption is clinically evident.[7] There is increasing evidence that it should also be used in those with subclinical evidence of malabsorption.[41] Enzyme replacement for exocrine insufficiency is best done by using enteric-coated preparations that protect the synthetic lipase from digestion by gastric acid.[6,44] The current trend is to use larger doses than originally recommended, which has been shown to be nutritionally effective in treating fat and nitrogen maldigestion in the short and intermediate terms, with few side effects.[45,46] Recommended doses utilise 25,000 to 75,000 units of lipase with meals and 10,000 to 25,000 units with snacks. It has been recommended that doses should not exceed 10,000 units/Kg of body weight per meal. Enzyme replacement should

be taken before or during meals and dosage should be adjusted according to weight gain and solidification of stools.[6,47] Where there is failure of therapy, GI factors such as gastroduodenal passage disturbance, bacterial overgrowth and hyperacidity of the stomach should be addressed before a stepwise increase in dosage is considered. The introduction of medium-chain triglycerides and acid reduction with a proton-pump inhibitor can be used in those refractory to PERT.[6,43] Vitamin supplementation, particularly the fat-soluble vitamins A, D, E and K, should be instituted early to prevent clinical vitamin deficiencies.

Endocrine Insufficiency

The diagnosis of diabetes as a consequence of endocrine insufficiency is based on criteria proposed by the American Diabetes Association: an $HBA_{1C} \geq 6.5\%$; fasting plasma glucose of 7.0 mmol/L (126 mg/L); 2 hour plasma glucose ≥ 11.1 mmol/L (200 mg/L) during an oral glucose tolerance test or a random plasma glucose of ≥ 11.1 mmol/L (200 mg/L), associated with symptoms of hyperglycaemia.[48] Diabetics with CP whose glycaemic control is refractory to dietary manipulation will eventually require insulin. Oral hypoglycaemic agents have little role to play in advanced disease.[49] Pancreatic diabetics are at higher risk of severe hypoglycaemia as a consequence of impaired glucagon secretion, malnutrition and low glycogen stores from hepatic dysfunction, owing to alcohol abuse. Hence, patients with one or more episodes of severe hypoglycaemia may benefit from relaxation of glycaemic targets. Optimising glucose control periprocedurally is best managed by insulin infusion. The involvement of an experienced diabetic team in managing these patients is desirable.

Jaundice and Cholangitis

Although significant biliary obstruction with clinically evident jaundice is not a common complication, it increases the risk of major surgery. This is particularly pertinent when it contributes to suboptimal nutrition or presents with cholangitis, which may be subtle in presentation due to the incomplete biliary obstruction. In these patients, effective endoscopic internal biliary drainage, appropriate antimicrobial therapy and nutritional support are logical stepping stones to safer surgery.

Surgical Prevention of Endocrine and Exocrine Deterioration

Cessation of alcohol consumption and smoking is key in preventing deterioration of physiological function of the gland in all phases of treatment. This is particularly true for those who have long-standing disease with already-advanced parenchymal loss but is also relevant in young patients in whom the remainder of the pancreas has to last a lifetime. Exocrine and endocrine insufficiencies deteriorate gradually during the course of the disease but rarely manifest clinically in under 10 years.[50] Surgery can accelerate this deterioration by removal of the pancreatic tissue that is not contributing to the patient's symptomatology.[51] As a result, drainage procedures or DPPHR, which sacrifice less pancreatic tissue, have gained favour over resective procedures.[19]

Total pancreatectomy and autologous islet cell transplantation are increasingly being performed in highly selected patient groups.[20,21] Adequate islet cell function, indicated by exogenous insulin independence, can be attained in approximately 50% of patients in 3 years. The likelihood of not requiring insulin is directly related to the yield of islets from the initial harvest, which is better in those whose CP is not due to alcohol and in whom the operations are performed at a young age.[20,52] This is a function of the number of islets not destroyed by the disease and the technical aspects of the collagenase extraction. Dunderdale et al[53] showed that the islet yield in alcoholic chronic pancreatitics was so poor and the likelihood of sustained functioning islets was so low that the procedure should be abandoned for CP. Until efficacy in preventing long-term diabetes in CP is established, selection for this therapy needs to be confined to those patients who are predicted to have a high islet yield and to institutions that have perfected islet cell harvesting.

Prevention of Intraoperative Complications

The prevention of operative complications starts with a detailed preoperative assessment of the morphology of the diseased pancreas. When a resection of the head of the pancreas is planned, imaging is important to identify arterial anomalies such as aberrant or accessory hepatic arteries coming from the superior mesenteric artery. The presence of segmental portal hypertension would also favour the performance of operations such as the Frey procedure, where the dissection is confined to the pancreas. Severe peripancreatic inflammation increases the risks of both arterial and major venous injuries (portal and superior mesenteric veins) when resections are performed. Thus, when performing a pancreatic head resection, it is often wise not to isolate the pancreas neck from the underlying superior mesenteric vein. As this is not a cancer operation, one can leave a sliver of pancreas on the superior mesenteric vein and avoid dissection close to the superior mesenteric artery. When performing

a coring-out procedure of the pancreas head, special precautions should be undertaken to ensure haemostasis of the pancreatic remnant, while avoiding injury or devascularisation of the duodenum.[54]

Open or Laparoscopic Surgery

Distal pancreatectomy for all pancreatic pathologies is increasingly being performed laparoscopically. Recent meta-analyses of the comparative trials of distal pancreatectomy showed better outcomes in terms of lower blood loss, reduced hospital stay and reduced risks of complications for laparoscopic operations.[55,56] In a meta-analysis by Mehrabi et al,[56] only 7% of the laparoscopic resections were performed for CP. This calls into question the notion that a laparoscopic approach has a reduced complication rate in CP. Drainage of PFCs is also being performed laparoscopically, but there is only one study comparing the outcome of EUS-guided versus laparoscopic versus open drainage.[57] In this series, only 16 out of 83 patients were drained laparoscopically. The surgical drainage methods had a better primary resolution than the endoscopic methods, but the complication rates were not significantly different. The Partington-Rochelle operation and the DPPHR procedures are being performed laparoscopically, but there are no RCTs available regarding either of these types of operations to reliably compare their complication rates with conventional open surgery.[58,59] The information on robotic surgery on the pancreas remains too scanty to draw any inference regarding its benefits over open or conventional laparoscopic surgery.[60]

Prophylaxis for Pancreatic Fistula

Risk factors for breakdown of the pancreatic anastomosis are a soft parenchymal texture, small duct size, large size of the remnant pancreas and normal pancreatic exocrine function.[61–64] By virtue of the fibrotic remnant, the risk of a pancreatic leak after resection or drainage operation for CP is appreciably less than that observed after resections for pancreatic cancer. In a review of 2664 pancreatic resections, the pancreatic fistula rate in CP was 5%, compared with 12%, 15% and 33% for pancreatic cancer, ampullary cancer and bile duct cancer, respectively.[65] Somatostatin and its analogues have been used extensively to prevent pancreatic fistula in various types of pancreatic surgery. The cohorts used to study these analogues are either exclusively or predominantly composed of patients who had a surgery for pancreatic neoplasia. Hence, assessing the evidence for the efficacy of these antisecretagogues in surgery for CP remains problematic. There is only one study from 1995 that specifically addresses the use of somatostatin analogues in CP.[66] Using octreotide Friess et al[66] concluded that the drug reduced the risk of complications, including pancreatic fistula, and the length of hospital stay and recommended its routine use. However, the limitation in this and other studies before 2005 was the lack of standardisation of the definition of postoperative pancreatic fistulae.[62] A recent Cochrane review on the use of prophylactic somastatin analogues included 2348 patients from 21 trials, 19 of which had a high risk of bias. When analysing only clinically significant fistulae (grade C, Table 32.1), there was no difference in the incidence between the somatostatin analogue and the placebo groups.[25,67] In a recent RCT of surgery for pancreatic neoplasia, another long-acting somatostatin analogue, pasireotide, which has a greater binding capacity, has been shown to halve the pancreatic fistula rate.[68] The low incidence of pancreatic fistula in patients with CP undergoing surgery questions the need for somatostatin or its analogues outside of clinical trials.

MANAGEMENT OF COMPLICATIONS OF SURGERY FOR CHRONIC PANCREATITIS

Data on the management of complications of surgery for CP are lacking. It is most often combined with the reporting of management of complications of pancreatic surgery for neoplasia, which is performed far more frequently. Hence, management strategies for complications are mostly extrapolated from the evidence available for neoplastic resections. These complications are most frequent and problematic for PDs or PPPDs, which are now being performed less frequently for CP.

Anastomotic Leaks and Sequelae

Anastomotic leakage, when it occurs after CP surgery, remains problematic, with the potential for significant morbidity and mortality. It may result in the development of an intra-abdominal fluid collection, which in turn can become secondarily infected, leading to intra-abdominal sepsis and abscess formation. Enzyme-rich pancreatic fluid may erode the surrounding tissues, including vascular structures, and thereby result in major haemorrhage. Alternatively, persistent anastomotic leaks that have been successfully drained externally either by operatively placed drains or by radiologically guided percutaneous catheters may result in the formation of pancreatic or biliary fistulae. Pancreatic leaks should be suspected when there is clinical and biochemical evidence of inflammation or sepsis, especially in the presence of perianastomotic fluid collections on imaging. The diagnosis is confirmed by aspiration of enzyme-rich pancreatic fluid collections,

with biochemical analysis of the fistula effluent and/or the demonstration of a pancreatic anastomotic breakdown by fistulogram. Fluid collections should be drained promptly under ultrasound or computed tomography (CT) guidance. This approach is supported by a recent study showing shorter hospital stay (33 days vs. 47 days) and a reduction in mortality (0% vs. 37%) associated with interventional drainage when compared with reoperation as the initial treatment of the fluid collection.[69]

The treatment principles for fistulae after surgery for CP are similar to those occurring after surgery for pancreatic neoplasia. The rare high-volume pancreatic fistula may lead to fluid and electrolyte disturbances and nutritional deficiencies. Initial management is aimed at correcting fluid and electrolyte abnormalities, treating sepsis and ensuring adequate nutrition support. The choice of nutritional support should be determined by an experienced nutritional support team. Intravenous nutrition may be required as a bridge to enteral nutrition in the critically ill. The latter is safer, relatively cheaper and has improved maintenance of the gut mucosal barrier. In patients with an established fistula, normal intake may be limited by patient factors such as anorexia and nausea, and in such cases, fine-bore enteral feeding should be commenced to achieve defined nutritional goals.[70]

Fortunately, the majority of pancreatic leaks after surgery run a benign course, requiring only supportive management and maintenance of drains placed percutaneously or at the initial surgery.[71,72] Accordingly, in the absence of peritonitis, sepsis, haemorrhage or organ failure, this conservative approach should apply.[61,72–74] There is no evidence as yet that somatostatin analogues such as octreotide will accelerate closure of pancreatic fistula.[72,75] Some success has been shown with the use of fibrin glues, but this has not yet found widespread use.[76,77]

Should the fistula persist, a surgical treatment strategy should be devised, based on the general condition of the patient and the anatomical position of the fistula. Options include drainage of the fistula via a Roux-en-Y loop or as a last resort, resection. Repeat surgery can be hazardous, as there is likely to be extensive postsurgical inflammatory change in the region of the fistula, together with altered surgical anatomy. Owing to the infrequency with which redo surgery is required, there is little data to guide the choice of operation in such circumstances.

Delayed Gastric Emptying

Delayed gastric emptying is more often seen after duodenal resection than after duodenum-preserving operations. It most commonly occurs in the presence of other associated complications such as pancreatic leaks and infected intra-abdominal collections and, as such, these should be addressed as the initial management.[78,79] A recent meta-analysis showed that DGE was reduced by the placement of the gastro- or duodenojejunostomy away from the pancreatojejunostomy by means of an antecolic reconstruction.[80]

Subsequent management is largely supportive, including nasogastric drainage, maintenance of fluid and electrolyte balance and nutritional support. The role of promotility agents, such as intravenous erythromycin and metoclopramide, often used for other causes of gastroparesis, is unclear in this setting.[81] Adhesive bowel obstruction or compromised passage at the site of anastomoses should be excluded by contrast meal or cross-sectional imaging using water-soluble contrast. In most instances, DGE resolves spontaneously, albeit in some patients, only after prolonged conservative management.

Vascular Complications

Postoperative vascular complications can be arterial or venous. Arterial complications generally relate to either misadventure at the time of surgery or technical error, or occur as the result of arterial erosion, with bleeding or false aneurysm formation. Early postoperative haemorrhage (within 24–72 hours) into the peritoneal cavity is best managed by urgent reoperation. In the presence of a pancreatojejunostomy, in isolation or as part of DPPHR, the bleeding may originate from the suture line or the intraluminal exposed pancreatic surface. The bleeding then occurs into the Roux-en-Y loop and presents with melaena rather than haematemesis, which can delay the diagnosis. It is prudent to exclude other sources of upper GI bleeding by endoscopy. The source of the bleeding then needs to be established by CT angiography or direct catheter angiography, which offers therapeutic options. However, in most cases, early bleeds cannot be controlled nonoperatively and surgery should not be delayed, particularly in haemodynamically unstable patients.

Delayed haemorrhage is most often the consequence of anastomotic leakage, with or without associated sepsis, and may occur up to weeks after the initial surgery. If the patient is haemodynamically stable, contrast-enhanced triple-phase CT scan should be performed to identify the site of haemorrhage and to guide angiographic therapy.[82] Results from retrospective comparative studies suggest that angiographic methods are safer and more effective than difficult repeat surgery.[83,84] Historically, bleeding vessels were embolised using coils, but in current practice,

placement of a covered stent is preferred in order to avoid ischaemic complications.[82]

Portomesenteric thrombosis is the most often early postoperatively encountered venous complication. The clinical presentation varies from patients being asymptomatic to those with symptoms of acute venous mesenteric ischaemia. This also reflects in the clinical findings, which can vary from being minimal to the presence of an acute abdomen. Doppler ultrasound and contrast-enhanced ultrasound have reasonable sensitivity and specificity but may be limited by patient factors and are operator-dependant, making triple-phase contrast-enhanced CT the special investigation of choice.[85]

Treatment is aimed at preventing propagation and promoting recanalisation of the thrombus and treating complications.[86] This is determined by severity of the disease process, based on the clinical picture and the findings of special investigations. After resuscitation and the administration of broad-spectrum antibiotics and anticoagulation therapy, close patient monitoring, preferably in a high-care environment, is mandatory. A high suspicion of compromised bowel should prompt surgical exploration. At operation, thrombectomy may be an option, but usually, resection is the only salvage option.[85,86]

CONCLUSIONS

The overall management of CP requires a multidisciplinary team, as the decision-making and technical aspects around therapy for CP can be challenging. When surgery is indicated, it is important to be aware that patients usually have a number of comorbidities, which increase their risk for postoperative complications. The role of optimising patients before surgery in order to prevent complications cannot be overemphasised. The treatment of exocrine and endocrine failure requires special attention throughout the course of the disease. Complications of surgery for CP are inconsistently reported, and management is largely based on data from series of pancreatic resections for pancreatic neoplasms. Many of the complications of surgery can be managed with effective support and a variety of minimally invasive adjuncts, without having to resort to major complex surgery with it's attendant risks. All surgical therapy remains an interlude in the disease, which requires life-long follow-up.

REFERENCES

1. Lerch MM, Gorelick FS. Models of acute and chronic pancreatitis. *Gastroenterology* 2013;144:1180–93.
2. Whitcomb DC, Frulloni L, Garg P, et al. Chronic pancreatitis: an international draft consensus proposal

for a new mechanistic definition. *Pancreatology* 2016;16: 218–24.

3. Pezzilli R, Bini L, Fantini L, Baroni E, et al. Quality of life in chronic pancreatitis. *World J Gastroenterol* 2006;12: 6249–51.

4. Bornman PC, Marks IN, Girdwood AW, Berberat PO, Gulbinas A, Buchler MW. Pathogenesis of pain in chronic pancreatitis: ongoing enigma. *World J Surg* 2003;27:1175–82.

5. Braganza JM, Lee SH, McCloy RF, McMahon MJ. Chronic pancreatitis. *Lancet* 2011;377:1184–97.

6. Bornman PC, Botha JF, Ramos JM, et al. Guideline for the diagnosis and treatment of chronic pancreatitis. *S Afr Med J* 2010;100:845–60.

7. Forsmark CE. Management of chronic pancreatitis. *Gastroenterology* 2013;144:1282–91.e3.

8. Schafer M, Mullhaupt B, Clavien PA. Evidence-based pancreatic head resection for pancreatic cancer and chronic pancreatitis. *Ann Surg* 2002;236:137–48.

9. Frey CF, Smith GJ. Description and rationale of a new operation for chronic pancreatitis. *Pancreas* 1987;2:701–7.

10. Beger HG, Krautzberger W, Bittner R, Buchler M, Limmer J. Duodenum-preserving resection of the head of the pancreas in patients with severe chronic pancreatitis. *Surgery* 1985;97:467–73.

11. Izbicki JR, Bloechle C, Broering DC, Kuechler T, Broelsch CE. Longitudinal V-shaped excision of the ventral pancreas for small duct disease in severe chronic pancreatitis: prospective evaluation of a new surgical procedure. *Ann Surg* 1998;227:213–9.

12. Hatori T, Imaizumi T, Harada N, et al. Appraisal of the Imaizumi modification of the Beger procedure: the TWMU experience. J *Hepatobiliary Pancreat Sci* 2010;17:752–7.

13. Gloor B, Friess H, Uhl W, Buchler MW. A modified technique of the Beger and Frey procedure in patients with chronic pancreatitis. *Dig Surg* 2001;18:21–5.

14. Frey CF. The surgical management of chronic pancreatitis: the Frey procedure. *Adv Surg* 1999;32:41–85.

15. Beger HG, Schlosser W, Siech M, Poch B. The surgical management of chronic pancreatitis: duodenum-preserving pancreatectomy. *Adv Surg* 1999;32:87–104.

16. Sohn TA, Campbell KA, Pitt HA, et al. Quality of life and long-term survival after surgery for chronic pancreatitis. *J Gastrointest Surg* 2000;4:355–64; discussion 64–5.

17. Bachmann K, Tomkoetter L, Erbes J, et al. Beger and Frey procedures for treatment of chronic pancreatitis: comparison of outcomes at 16-year follow-up. *J Am Coll Surg* 2014;219:208–16.

18. Bachmann K, Tomkoetter L, Kutup A, et al. Is the Whipple procedure harmful for long-term outcome in treatment of chronic pancreatitis? 15-years follow-up comparing the outcome after pylorus-preserving pancreatoduodenectomy and Frey procedure in chronic pancreatitis. *Ann Surg* 2013;258:815–20; discussion 20–1.

19. Burmeister S BP, Krige JEJ, Thomson SR. The Surgical Management of Chronic Pancreatitis, 2012. Available from: http://www.intechopen.com/books/new-advances-in-the-basic-and-clinical-gastroenterology/the-surgical-management-of-chronic-pancreatitis

20. Chinnakotla S, Beilman GJ, Dunn TB, et al. Factors Predicting Outcomes after a total pancreatectomy and islet autotransplantation lessons learned from over 500 cases. *Ann Surg* 2015;262:610–22.

21. Tanhehco YC, Weisberg S, Schwartz J. Pancreatic islet autotransplantation for nonmalignant and malignant indications. *Transfusion* 2016;56:761–70.

22. Jawad ZA, Kyriakides C, Pai M, et al. Surgery remains the best option for the management of pain in patients with chronic pancreatitis: a systematic review and meta-analysis. *Asian J Surg* 2016;pii:S1015-9584(15)00153-0.

23. Sudo T, Murakami Y, Uemura K, et al. Short- and long-term results of lateral pancreaticojejunostomy for chronic pancreatitis: a retrospective Japanese single-center study. *J Hepatobiliary Pancreat Sci* 2014;21:426–32.

24. Rebibo L, Yzet T, Cosse C, Delcenserie R, Bartoli E, Regimbeau JM. Frey procedure for the treatment of chronic pancreatitis associated with common bile duct stricture. *Hepatobiliary Pancreat Dis Int* 2013;12:637–44.

25. Bassi C, Dervenis C, Butturini G, et al. Postoperative pancreatic fistula: an international study group (ISGPF) definition. *Surgery* 2005;138:8–13.

26. Wente MN, Bassi C, Dervenis C, et al. Delayed gastric emptying (DGE) after pancreatic surgery: a suggested definition by the International Study Group of Pancreatic Surgery (ISGPS). *Surgery* 2007;142:761–8.

27. Wente MN, Veit JA, Bassi C, et al. Postpancreatectomy hemorrhage (PPH): an International Study Group of Pancreatic Surgery (ISGPS) definition. *Surgery* 2007;142:20–5.

28. Cauchy F, Regimbeau JM, Fuks D, Balladur P, Tiret E, Paye F. Influence of bile duct obstruction on the results of Frey's procedure for chronic pancreatitis. *Pancreatology* 2014;14:21–6.

29. Cahen DL, Gouma DJ, Laramee P, et al. Long-term outcomes of endoscopic vs surgical drainage of the pancreatic duct in patients with chronic pancreatitis. *Gastroenterology* 2011;141:1690–5.

30. Keck T, Adam U, Makowiec F, et al. Short- and long-term results of duodenum preservation versus resection for the management of chronic pancreatitis: a prospective, randomized study. *Surgery* 2012;152:S95–102.

31. Izbicki JR, Bloechle C, Knoefel WT, Kuechler T, Binmoeller KF, Broelsch CE. Duodenum-preserving resection of the head of the pancreas in chronic pancreatitis. A prospective, randomized trial. *Ann Surg* 1995;221:350–8.

32. Buchler MW, Friess H, Muller MW, Wheatley AM, Beger HG. Randomized trial of duodenum-preserving pancreatic head resection versus pylorus-preserving Whipple in chronic pancreatitis. *Am J Surg* 1995;169:65–9; discussion 9–70.

33. Farkas G, Leindler L, Daroczi M, Farkas G, Jr. Prospective randomised comparison of organ-preserving

pancreatic head resection with pylorus-preserving pancreaticoduodenectomy. *Langenbecks Arch Surg* 2006;391:338–42.

34. Hildebrand P, Dudertadt S, Czymek R, et al. Different surgical strategies for chronic pancreatitis significantly improve long-term outcome: a comparative single center study. *Eur J Med Res* 2010;15:351–6.

35. Keck T, Wellner UF, Riediger H, et al. Long-term outcome after 92 duodenum-preserving pancreatic head resections for chronic pancreatitis: comparison of Beger and Frey procedures. *J Gastrointest Surg* 2010;14:549–56.

36. Aimoto T, Uchida E, Matsushita A, Kawano Y, Mizutani S, Kobayashi T. Long-term outcomes after Frey's procedure for chronic pancreatitis with an inflammatory mass of the pancreatic head, with special reference to locoregional complications. *J Nippon Med Sch* 2013;80:148–54.

37. van Heek NT, Kuhlmann KF, Scholten RJ, et al. Hospital volume and mortality after pancreatic resection: a systematic review and an evaluation of intervention in the Netherlands. *Ann Surg* 2005;242:781–8, discussion 8–90.

38. Balzano G, Zerbi A, Capretti G, Rocchetti S, Capitanio V, Di Carlo V. Effect of hospital volume on outcome of pancreaticoduodenectomy in Italy. *Br J Surg* 2008;95:357–62.

39. Bachmann J, Buchler MW, Friess H, Martignoni ME. Cachexia in patients with chronic pancreatitis and pancreatic cancer: impact on survival and outcome. *Nutr Cancer* 2013;65:827–33.

40. Sikkens EC, Cahen DL, van Eijck C, Kuipers EJ, Bruno MJ. Patients with exocrine insufficiency due to chronic pancreatitis are undertreated: a Dutch national survey. *Pancreatology* 2012;12:71–3.

41. Rasmussen HH, Irtun O, Olesen SS, Drewes AM, Holst M. Nutrition in chronic pancreatitis. *World J Gastroenterol* 2013;19:7267–75.

42. Dominguez-Munoz JE. Pancreatic enzyme replacement therapy for pancreatic exocrine insufficiency: when is it indicated, what is the goal and how to do it? *Adv Med Sci* 2011;56:1–5.

43. Lohr JM, Oliver MR, Frulloni L. Synopsis of recent guidelines on pancreatic exocrine insufficiency. *United European Gastroenterol J* 2013;1:79–83.

44. Krishnamurty DM, Rabiee A, Jagannath SB, Andersen DK. Delayed release pancrelipase for treatment of pancreatic exocrine insufficiency associated with chronic pancreatitis. *Ther Clin Risk Manag* 2009;5:507–20.

45. Gubergrits N, Malecka-Panas E, Lehman GA, et al. A 6-month, open-label clinical trial of pancrelipase delayed-release capsules (Creon) in patients with exocrine pancreatic insufficiency due to chronic pancreatitis or pancreatic surgery. *Aliment Pharmacol Ther* 2011;33:1152–61.

46. Whitcomb DC, Lehman GA, Vasileva G, et al. Pancrelipase delayed-release capsules (CREON) for exocrine pancreatic insufficiency due to chronic pancreatitis or pancreatic surgery: a double-blind randomized trial. *Am J Gastroenterol* 2010;105:2276–86.

47. Fieker A, Philpott J, Armand M. Enzyme replacement therapy for pancreatic insufficiency: present and future. *Clin Exp Gastroenterol* 2011;4:55–73.

48. Standards of medical care in diabetes—2015: summary of revisions. *Diabetes Care* 2015;38:S4.

49. Rickels MR, Bellin M, Toledo FG, et al. Detection, evaluation and treatment of diabetes mellitus in chronic pancreatitis: recommendations from PancreasFest 2012. *Pancreatology* 2013;13:336–42.

50. Ahmed SA, Wray C, Rilo HL, et al. Chronic pancreatitis: recent advances and ongoing challenges. *Curr Probl Surg* 2006;43:127–238.

51. Kahl S, Malfertheiner P. Exocrine and endocrine pancreatic insufficiency after pancreatic surgery. *Best Pract Res Clin Gastroenterol* 2004;18:947–55.

52. Bellin MD, Freeman ML, Gelrud A, et al. Total pancreatectomy and islet autotransplantation in chronic pancreatitis: recommendations from PancreasFest. *Pancreatology* 2014;14:27–35.

53. Dunderdale J, McAuliffe JC, McNeal SF, et al. Should pancreatectomy with islet cell autotransplantation in patients with chronic alcoholic pancreatitis be abandoned? *J Am Coll Surg* 2013;216:591–6; discussion 6–8.

54. Bornman PC, Krige JEJ. Chronic pancreatitis surgery commentary. In: Mantke R LH, Buchler MW, Sarr MG, editors. *International Practices in Pancreatic Surgery*. Heidelberg, Germany: Springer; 2013. p. 89.

55. Jin T, Altaf K, Xiong JJ, et al. A systematic review and meta-analysis of studies comparing laparoscopic and open distal pancreatectomy. *HPB (Oxford)* 2012;14:711–24.

56. Mehrabi A, Hafezi M, Arvin J, et al. A systematic review and meta-analysis of laparoscopic versus open distal pancreatectomy for benign and malignant lesions of the pancreas: it's time to randomize. *Surgery* 2015;157:45–55.

57. Melman L, Azar R, Beddow K, et al. Primary and overall success rates for clinical outcomes after laparoscopic, endoscopic, and open pancreatic cystgastrostomy for pancreatic pseudocysts. *Surg Endosc* 2009;23:267–71.

58. Khaled YS, Ammori MB, Ammori BJ. Laparoscopic lateral pancreaticojejunostomy for chronic pancreatitis: a case report and review of the literature. *Surg Laparosc Endosc Percutan Tech* 2011;21:e36–40.

59. Tantia O, Jindal MK, Khanna S, Sen B. Laparoscopic lateral pancreaticojejunostomy: our experience of 17 cases. *Surg Endosc* 2004;18:1054–7.

60. Zureikat AH, Moser AJ, Boone BA, Bartlett DL, Zenati M, Zeh HJ, 3rd. 250 robotic pancreatic resections: safety and feasibility. *Ann Surg* 2013;258:554–9; discussion 9–62.

61. Berberat PO, Friess H, Kleeff J, Uhl W, Buchler MW. Prevention and treatment of complications in pancreatic cancer surgery. *Dig Surg* 1999;16:327–36.

62. Buchler M, Friess H, Klempa I, et al. Role of octreotide in the prevention of postoperative complications following pancreatic resection. *Am J Surg* 1992;163:125–30; discussion 30–1.

63. Yeo CJ, Cameron JL, Lillemoe KD, et al. Does prophylactic octreotide decrease the rates of pancreatic fistula and other complications after pancreaticoduodenectomy? Results of a prospective randomized placebo-controlled trial. *Ann Surg* 2000;232:419–29.

64. Suc B, Msika S, Piccinini M, et al. Octreotide in the prevention of intra-abdominal complications following elective pancreatic resection: a prospective, multicenter randomized controlled trial. *Arch Surg* 2004;139:288–94; discussion 95.

65. Bartoli FG, Arnone GB, Ravera G, Bachi V. Pancreatic fistula and relative mortality in malignant disease after pancreaticoduodenectomy. Review and statistical meta-analysis regarding 15 years of literature. *Anticancer Res* 1991;11:1831–48.

66. Friess H, Beger HG, Sulkowski U, et al. Randomized controlled multicentre study of the prevention of complications by octreotide in patients undergoing surgery for chronic pancreatitis. *Br J Surg* 1995;82:1270–3.

67. Gurusamy KS, Koti R, Fusai G, Davidson BR. Somatostatin analogues for pancreatic surgery. *Cochrane Database Syst Rev* 2013;4:CD008370.

68. Allen PJ, Gonen M, Brennan MF, et al. Pasireotide for postoperative pancreatic fistula. *N Engl J Med* 2014;370:2014–22.

69. Hackert T, Hinz U, Pausch T, et al. Postoperative pancreatic fistula: We need to redefine grades B and C. *Surgery* 2016;159:872–7.

70. Blatnik JA, Hardacre JM. Management of pancreatic fistulas. *Surg Clin North Am* 2013;93:611–7.

71. Cullen JJ, Sarr MG, Ilstrup DM. Pancreatic anastomotic leak after pancreaticoduodenectomy: incidence, significance, and management. *Am J Surg* 1994;168:295–8.

72. Ho CK, Kleeff J, Friess H, Buchler MW. Complications of pancreatic surgery. *HPB (Oxford)* 2005;7:99–108.

73. Halloran CM, Ghaneh P, Bosonnet L, Hartley MN, Sutton R, Neoptolemos JP. Complications of pancreatic cancer resection. *Dig Surg* 2002;19:138–46.

74. Buchler MW, Wagner M, Schmied BM, Uhl W, Friess H, Z'Graggen K. Changes in morbidity after pancreatic resection: toward the end of completion pancreatectomy. *Arch Surg* 2003;138:1310–4; discussion 5.

75. Gans SL, van Westreenen HL, Kiewiet JJ, Rauws EA, Gouma DJ, Boermeester MA. Systematic review and meta-analysis of somatostatin analogues for the treatment of pancreatic fistula. *Br J Surg* 2012;99:754–60.

76. Fischer A, Benz S, Baier P, Hopt UT. Endoscopic management of pancreatic fistulas secondary to intraabdominal operation. *Surg Endosc* 2004;18:706–8.

77. Cothren CC, McIntyre RC, Jr., Johnson S, Stiegmann GV. Management of low-output pancreatic fistulas with fibrin glue. *Am J Surg* 2004;188:89–91.

78. Horstmann O, Markus PM, Ghadimi MB, Becker H. Pylorus preservation has no impact on delayed gastric emptying after pancreatic head resection. *Pancreas* 2004;28:69–74.

79. van Berge Henegouwen MI, van Gulik TM, DeWit LT, et al. Delayed gastric emptying after standard pancreaticoduodenectomy versus pylorus-preserving pancreaticoduodenectomy: an analysis of 200 consecutive patients. *J Am Coll Surg* 1997;185:373–9.

80. Su AP, Cao SS, Zhang Y, Zhang ZD, Hu WM, Tian BL. Does antecolic reconstruction for duodenojejunostomy improve delayed gastric emptying after pylorus-preserving pancreaticoduodenectomy? A systematic review and meta-analysis. *World J Gastroenterol* 2012;18:6315–23.

81. Kim YH. Management and prevention of delayed gastric emptying after pancreaticoduodenectomy. *Korean J Hepatobiliary Pancreat Surg* 2012;16:1–6.

82. Cazejust J, Raynal M, Bessoud B, Tubiana JM, Menu Y. Diagnosis and radiological treatment of digestive haemorrhage following supramesocolic surgery. *Diagn Interv Imaging* 2012;93:e148–58.

83. Schafer M, Heinrich S, Pfammatter T, Clavien PA. Management of delayed major visceral arterial bleeding after pancreatic surgery. *HPB (Oxford)* 2011;13:132–8.

84. Kalva SP, Yeddula K, Wicky S, Fernandez del Castillo C, Warshaw AL. Angiographic intervention in patients with a suspected visceral artery pseudoaneurysm complicating pancreatitis and pancreatic surgery. *Arch Surg* 2011;146:647–52.

85. Lang SA, Loss M, Wohlgemuth WA, Schlitt HJ. Clinical management of acute portal/mesenteric vein thrombosis. *Viszeralmedizin* 2014;30:394–400.

86. Wijaya R, Ng JH, See AH, Kum SW. Open thrombectomy for primary acute mesentericoportal venous thrombosis–should it be done? *Ann Vasc Surg* 2015;29:1454 e21–5.

33

How to Prevent, Diagnose and Treat Major Complications after Pancreatic Head Surgery

G. Gemenetzis, C.L. Wolfgang and A.A. Javed

ABSTRACT

Pancreatoduodenectomy is the standard treatment of benign and malignant diseases located in the head of the pancreas. The complexity of the regional surgical anatomy and the demanding surgical technique (at least three anastomoses need to be performed) have historically led to increased postoperative complications. Improvements in patient selection, surgical approach and perioperative management have resulted in a significant decrease in mortality after pancreatoduodenectomy. However, surgeons continue to deal with major postoperative complications that contribute to a morbidity rate of as high as 50%. The most common complications after pancreatoduodenectomy are delayed gastric emptying and pancreatic fistula; surgical site infections, haemorrhage and cardiopulmonary complications also affect significantly the postoperative course of patients who undergo pancreatic head surgery. Prevention, early diagnosis and treatment of these complications significantly improve patient outcomes.

KEYWORDS

Pancreatoduodenectomy, Whipple, postoperative complications, morbidity, DGE, pancreatic fistula, bleeding, SSI

INTRODUCTION

Surgical resection is the standard treatment of benign and malignant diseases located in the pancreas. Lesions in the head of the pancreas are excised with a pancreatoduodenectomy (PD), as described by Whipple et al.[1] The complexity of the surgical anatomy around the pancreatic head and the demanding postoperative treatment resulted initially in high postoperative morbidity and mortality rates. Over the years, improvements in patient selection, surgical technique and perioperative management have resulted in a significant decrease in PD-associated mortality from 25 to less than 2%.[2] However, this decrease was not paralleled in postoperative morbidity, where the complication rates remain high, ranging between 25 and 55%, even at high-volume reference centres.[3] The most common complications

after pancreatic head surgery are postoperative pancreatic fistula (POPF) and delayed gastric emptying (DGE); when combined, they affect more than 50% of the patients who undergo this procedure. Formation of intra-abdominal abscesses and subsequent sepsis, surgical site infections (SSIs), acute and delayed bleeding, acute pancreatitis and cardiopulmonary events also account for postoperative complications observed after PD (Table 33.1). Their impact on patient outcomes is significant and is associated with prolonged patient recovery, increased length of stay and hospitalisation costs, delays in initiation of adjuvant therapy in cases of malignant disease and, occasionally, patient death. Prevention of possible postoperative complications has been under investigation from many surgical scientific groups that focus on both variations in surgical technique and enhanced postoperative care

Table 33.1 Postoperative complications in pancreatoduodenectomy

Delayed gastric emptying
Postoperative pancreatic fistula
Surgical site infection
Postpancreatectomy haemorrhage
Biliary leak
Acute cholangitis
Chyle leak/chylous ascites
Cardiac events
Pneumonia

protocols. Early diagnosis and treatment also contribute significantly to the reduction of postoperative morbidity.

DELAYED GASTRIC EMPTYING

Delayed gastric emptying is one of the most common postoperative complications affecting patients who undergo a PD, with a reported incidence in large series of as high as 60%.[4] Delayed gastric emptying, also known as 'functional gastroparesis' was first reported by Warshaw and Torchiana.[5] Over the years, various definitions of DGE have been developed; most of them referred to DGE as the nasogastric tube (NGT) producing 200 to 500 mL/day after postoperative day (POD) 10. In 2007, the International Study Group of Pancreatic Surgery (ISGPS) classified DGE into three grades: grade A is defined as the need for use of NGT beyond POD 3, reinsertion of NGT after POD 3 or the inability of the patient to tolerate solid diet after POD 7; grade B refers to nasogastric intubation lasting up to POD 14, intolerance of solid diet for the same time period or reinsertion of the NGT after POD 7; and grade C constitutes of continued NGT use after POD 14, reinsertion after POD 14 or intolerance of solid food intake by POD 21[6] (Table 33.2). The majority of patients experiencing DGE fall into grade A classification

and their condition resolves quickly after a few days with nutritional support.

The pathophysiology of DGE remains unclear. Several physiological and anatomical mechanisms have been proposed as being causative (Table 33.3); duodenal resection and intraoperative injury of the vagus nerve may lead to reduced gastric motility due to lower concentrations of motilin and pancreatic polypeptide or limited parasympathetic innervation, respectively.[7] Patient comorbidities, reflected in higher American Society of Anesthesiologists (ASA) scores, and postoperative complications have also been suggested to be causative factors for DGE; diabetes mellitus and development of POPF or sepsis have been found to be the most clinically significant.[8,9] Moreover, it appears that the surgical approach for pancreatic head resection is a key factor in DGE development. A wide range of surgical resection techniques has been investigated in an attempt to prevent DGE.

Surgical Technique Variations for Reduction of Delayed Gastric Emptying Incidence

The development of pylorus-preserving PD (PPPD) as a more physiological modification of the standard operation has led to a change in the rates of DGE compared with the classic PD (Table 33.4). Numerous retrospective studies have been published on the subject and provide contradictory conclusions: DGE rates are reported to be higher, lower or similar between classic PD and PPPD. Van Berge Henegouwen et al compared 200 consecutive patients who underwent PD and PPPD and found no statistically significant difference in DGE incidence between the two groups (34% vs. 37%, $p > 0.05$).[10] On the other hand, in a recent study, Hackert et al reported a higher rate of DGE in the PPPD group (42.5% vs. 15%; $p = 0.006$).[11]

After a PPPD, the jejunum can be mobilised on the top and in front of the transverse colon (antecolic

Table 33.2 International Study Group for Pancreatic Surgery's classification of delayed gastric emptying

DGE grade	NGT required	Unable to tolerate solid oral intake by POD	Vomiting/gastric distention
A	4–7 days or reinsertion >POD 3	7	+/–
B	8–14 days or reinsertion >POD 7	14	+
C	>14 days or reinsertion >POD 14	21	+

Abbreviations: DGE, delayed gastric emptying; NGT, nasogastric tube; POD, postoperative day.
Adapted from: Wente MN, Bassi C, Dervenis C, et al. Delayed gastric emptying (DGE) after pancreatic surgery: a suggested definition by the International Study Group of Pancreatic Surgery (ISGPS). *Surgery* 2007;142:761–8.

Table 33.3 Risk factors associated with development of delayed gastric emptying after pancreatoduodenectomy

Preoperative diabetes mellitus
Increased body mass index
Pancreatitis
Increased intraoperative blood loss
Increased length of operation
Postoperative complications • Pancreatic fistula • Intra-abdominal collection • Biliary leakage

Table 33.4 Surgical technique variations studied for effect on delayed gastric emptying

Pylorus-preserving pancreatoduodenectomy • Antecolic reconstruction of duodenojejunostomy • Retrocolic reconstruction of duodenojejunostomy
Subtotal stomach-preserving pancreatoduodenectomy • Billroth II reconstruction of gastrojejunostomy • Modified Roux-en-Y reconstruction of gastrojejunostomy
Braun enteroenterostomy

approach) or through the right side of the transverse mesocolon (retrocolic approach) for reconstruction of the duodenojejunostomy. The two anastomotic techniques have been compared extensively in the literature with regards to DGE rates; large prospective randomised trials have found no significant differences between them.[12,13] However, Hanna et al recently performed a meta-analysis of all studies comparing the two duodenojejunostomy anastomotic techniques and concluded that the antecolic reconstruction is associated with lower rates of DGE.[14]

Several surgical variations in anastomotic reconstruction, extent of stomach resection and regional lymph node dissection have also been studied. In subtotal stomach-preserving PD (SSPPD), only the pyloric ring is removed and more than 90% of the stomach is preserved; comparison of DGE rates between PPPD and SSPPD in a meta-analysis suggests that the latter is associated with less DGE.[15] Preservation of the left gastric vein, Billroth II reconstruction for gastrojejunostomy and duodenojejunostomy with Braun enteroenterostomy have also been independently associated with lower DGE rates.[16–18]

It appears that DGE can present after all types of PD, with some techniques having more favourable results. The surgeon's experience and familiarisation with a specific surgical approach is more important in perfecting the technique and achieving consistent surgical outcomes.[19]

Diagnosis and Management of Delayed Gastric Emptying

The diagnosis of DGE is straightforward: the NGT produces a significant amount of usually biliary content (>300 mL daily), and the patient cannot tolerate solid food intake by POD 3. The clinical diagnosis of DGE must be followed up by imaging studies to investigate a possible mechanical obstruction, for example, kinking or oedema of the gastrojejunostomy or duodenojejunostomy site. Routinely, an abdominal computed tomography (CT) is a fast and reliable way to investigate the possible cause of DGE. When the CT does not provide sufficient information, gastric-emptying scintigraphy is considered the gold standard for assessing gastric motility and objectively grading the severity of DGE.[20] Diagnostic modalities, such as manometry and breath test, can also be used but are infrequently performed.

The subsequent decrease in motilin circulating levels and in motilin receptor numbers after PD is strongly associated with gastric atony and DGE. Motilin agonists include erythromycin and metoclopramide and can be utilised for the treatment of DGE. Erythromycin further stimulates phase III of gastric emptying movement in the fasting state and can improve DGE symptoms. Treatment dosage must be kept low (<3 mg/Kg/h), since erythromycin is occasionally linked to symptoms of abdominal cramping, diarrhoea, nausea and, most importantly, prolongation of the QT interval. Utilisation of erythromycin has been supported by randomised controlled trials (RCTs)[21]; however, its impact in the clinical setting is limited. Metoclopramide is a Food and Drug Administration (FDA)-approved dopamine D_2 receptor antagonist that accelerates antral contractility and increases the lower oesophageal sphincter tone. Metoclopramide passes through the blood–brain barrier and may cause extrapyramidal neurological disorders, such as parkinsonism. Somatostatin and its analogues, such as octreotide, reduce exocrine pancreatic secretions and have been used post PD for containment of complications associated with pancreatic leakage. Administration of somatostatin has been associated with a significantly increased incidence of DGE due to the suppression of plasma motilin levels and prolongation of the gastric emptying phases.[22]

POSTOPERATIVE PANCREATIC FISTULA

Postoperative pancreatic fistula is the second most common major postoperative complication observed in patients undergoing pancreatic head surgery, and its reported rate is 10 to 28%.[23] It can lead to considerable morbidity and has been reported to be associated with an increase in the length of stay and higher rates of readmissions, reoperations and deaths. Despite considerable effort to study this complication, including multiple prospective randomised trials, its rate has not changed significantly over time; however, its severity has been reduced. Postoperative pancreatic fistula results from the leakage of pancreatic exocrine secretions at the site of anastomosis, in a PD. Its diagnosis is predominantly based on the amylase levels of the drain fluid; however, it can present with nonspecific symptoms, including nausea, abdominal pain and distention, and in certain cases of DGE. Although not required for the diagnosis of POPF, radiological imaging can be performed to identify fluid collection around the pancreatojejunal anastomosis site.

In the past, multiple definitions of POPF have been proposed. Currently, the most widely accepted and clinically relevant definition is the one proposed in 2005 by the International Study Group on Pancreatic Fistula (ISGPF).[24] This classification system defines POPF as a drain amylase of over three times that of the serum amylase at or beyond POD 3. Once the diagnosis of POPF has been established, it can be classified into three grades, based on the clinical impact and the subsequent management required (Table 33.5). The least severe form of POPF is known as a Grade A POPF, which is a short-lived fistula presenting with no clinical symptoms in the presence of a high drain amylase levels. In these cases, POPF does not require any significant alterations in the management of the patient. A Grade B fistula is associated with clinical symptoms and radiographical imaging that may demonstrate peripancreatic fluid collections. For Grade B POPF, the clinical management can include antibiotic administration, placement of a postoperative percutaneous drain, supplemental nutrition or readmission to the hospital.[25] Patients with most severe form of this complication, that is, with a Grade C fistula, are clinically unstable and present with sepsis or multiorgan dysfunction—often warranting a reoperation and exploration—and can even lead to death. Recently, the classification has been adapted by the ISGPS.

Approaches to Reduction of Rate and Severity of Postoperative Pancreatic Fistula

In the past, both surgical and nonsurgical interventions have been studied in the setting of large prospective studies and randomised control trials to determine their effect on the rate and severity of POPF. These interventions include the type of anastomosis performed, technique of stump closure, placement of stents, application of both biological and nonbiological agents to the site of anastomosis, drain placement, duration of drain usage, postoperative feeding and the use of pharmacological agents. One of the most commonly evaluated surgical factors is the technique of performing the pancreatojejunal anastomosis. The two

Table 33.5 Parameters for grading of postoperative pancreatic fistula, proposed by the International Study Group of Pancreatic Fistula

	Grade A	Grade B	Grade C
Clinical conditions	Well	Often well	Ill appearing/bad
Specific treatment*	No	Yes/no	Yes
US/CT (if obtained)	Negative	Negative/positive	Positive
Persistent drainage (after 3 weeks)**	No	Usually yes	Yes
Reoperation	No	No	Yes
Death related to POPF	No	No	Possibly yes
Signs of infection	No	Yes	Yes
Sepsis	No	No	Yes
Readmission	No	Yes/no	Yes/no

*Partial (peripheral) or total parenteral nutrition, antibiotics, enteral nutrition, somatostatin analogues and/or minimally invasive drainage.
**With or without a drain in situ.
Abbreviations: CT, computed tomographic scan; POPF, postoperative pancreatic fistula, US, ultrasonography.
Adapted from: Bassi C, Dervenis C, Butturini G, et al. Postoperative pancreatic fistula: an international study group (ISGPF) definition. *Surgery* 2005; 138:8–13.

categories of techniques are used: duct-to-mucosa or invagination. Randomised controlled trials have generally found no significant difference in rates of POPF between the two techniques.[26] However, Berger et al reported that invagination results in significantly lower rates of POPF.[27] Another aspect of the pancreatojejunostomy (PJ) anastomosis is the stenting of the main pancreatic duct, which has been evaluated in multiple studies. Winter et al in an RCT failed to demonstrate any difference in rates and severity of POPF between patients who did and did not undergo pancreatic duct stenting.[28] Contrastingly, Motoi et al reported a reduction in the rate of clinically significant POPF in patient who had stent placement. However, on detailed analysis, this finding remained true only for patients who had nondilated ducts.[29]

The PJ anastomosis drains the pancreatic secretions from the pancreatic remnant into the gastrointestinal tract and can be performed in either an end-to-end or an end-to-side manner. There is a potential risk of breakdown of the anastomosis due to the activation of pancreatic enzymes by both gastric and biliary secretions.[30] To prevent this, a Roux-en-Y reconstruction with isolated pancreatic drainage has been evaluated, given that such a reconstruction minimises the exposure of pancreatic secretion to the gastric and biliary output, thus limiting the activation of the pancreatic enzymes. In an RCT performed by Ke et al, no significant difference was observed in the rates of POPF between the two techniques; interestingly, there was a decrease in the severity of POPF and length of stay in patients undergoing Roux-en-Y reconstruction.[30] Another study compared isolated loop pancreatojejunostomy (IRPJ) with pancreatogastrostomy (PG) after PD, with the rationale that this would limit the exposure of pancreatic secretions to the biliary secretions. While demonstrating no effect on rates of POPF, the authors did report a significantly lower rate of steatorrhoea and early return to oral feeding in patients undergoing IRPJ.

Pancreatogastrostomy is a less common method of pancreatic anastomosis.[31] Multiple RCTs have compared PJ with PG and presented contradicting results. Duffas et al found no difference in rates of POPF between the two groups, also concluding that PJ was safer than PG.[32] On the other hand, Bassi et al reported reduced rates of surgical complications, biliary fistula, DGE and postoperative collections in the PG group.[33] The application of topical sealing agents such as fibrin glue at the pancreatic anastomotic site has also been investigated. In an RCT performed by Lillemoe et al, a trend towards decreased rates of POPF was observed; however, this difference was not significant.[34] The inability of the

sealing agents to prevent POPF can be attributed to their poor adherence and degradation, due to the pancreatic enzyme activity. Van Buren et al recently evaluated intraperitoneal drainage, and although there was no significant difference in rates of POPF, higher rates and severity of other postoperative complications occurred, and subsequently the study had to be stopped prematurely, given the significant increase in mortality in patients who did not receive drain placement.[35]

Postoperatively, early drain removal (<POD 3) was also evaluated. Molinari et al compared early (POD 3) and late (>POD 5) drain removal in patients at low risk of having POPF; early drain removal demonstrated a significant decrease in the incidence of POPF, abdominal complications, median hospital stay and hospital costs.[36] Studies on the use of somatostatin and its analogues for pancreatic secretion inhibition have demonstrated conflicting results. In most of them, somatostatin analogues such as vapreotide and octreotide did not decrease the POPF rate significantly.[37,38] The most significant reduction in rates of POPF was reported in a study on pasireotide, a somatostatin analogue with a longer half-life and broader binding profile.[25]

Management of Postoperative Pancreatic Fistula

The management of a majority of patients experiencing POPF is usually conservative and consists of nutritional support, use of somatostatin analogues and antibiotic therapy (Table 33.6). Postoperative pancreatic fistula results in increased catabolic activity and basal energy expenditure, along with fluid, electrolyte and nutritional depletion; nutritional supplementation is therefore essential. Total parenteral nutrition (TPN) can be utilised, as it eliminates gastrointestinal hormone production. However, prolonged use can lead to gastrointestinal and

Table 33.6 Interventions to reduce postoperative pancreatic fistula rates after pancreatic head surgery

Surgical interventions
Invagination versus duct-to-mucosa pancreatoenteric anastomosis
Stenting of the main pancreatic duct
Roux-en-Y reconstruction with isolated pancreatic drainage
Pancreatojejunostomy versus pancreatogastrostomy
Application of topical sealing agents
Intraperitoneal drainage
Nonsurgical interventions
Early drain removal
Use of somatostatin and its analogues

pancreatic functional and morphological changes and can also increase the risk for wound infections and subsequent sepsis. An alternative approach is to use no- or low-fat enteral nutrition, which reduces pancreatic secretions and has been shown to result in a quicker recovery and higher rates of fistula closure. In case of fluid collections near the pancreatojejunal anastomosis presenting with clinical symptoms, including fever, pain and sepsis, image-guided percutaneous or endoscopic drainage may be warranted. The fluid can be aspirated and analysed for amylase levels and cultured to direct the antimicrobial therapy. Reoperation is required in a few select patients and is the treatment of choice for those with refractory POPF. Furthermore, surgery is indicated when the intra-abdominal fluid collections cannot be aspirated by interventional radiology or in case of visceral perforation, bleeding from a pseudoaneurysm or sepsis.[39] Based on the intraoperative findings, the type and extent of surgical management may vary from debridement and drainage of the peripancreatic region to a completion pancreatectomy.

SURGICAL SITE INFECTIONS

Surgical site infections are a commonly reported complication of PD. Their rates vary from 7 to 32%, and they often contribute to a prolonged recovery, delay of adjuvant therapy and higher hospitalisation costs.[40] Surgical site infections have been classified by the Centers for Disease Control and Prevention (CDC) into three categories: superficial incisional, deep incisional and organ space SSIs (Table 33.7).[41] The majority of SSIs are contaminated by the patient's own endogenous flora originating in the hollow viscera, the mucous membrane or the skin. Contaminating pathogens from the intrinsic bowel flora include gram-negative bacilli or anaerobic bacteria (e.g., *Escherichia coli*) and from the skin include gram-positive cocci (e.g., *Staphylococcus aureus*).

A wide range of risk factors has been associated with SSIs, in patients who undergo pancreatic head surgery (Table 33.8). Malnutrition and hypoalbuminaemia—common findings in patients with pancreatic cancer—are characterised by decreased collagen synthesis and granuloma formation, which lead to delayed tissue healing and increase in the dead space within the wound, making it susceptible to infection.[42,43] Preoperative biliary drainage is a common practice in patients who present with painless jaundice, caused by solid pancreatic head lesions. In these patients, a correlation between stenting of the common bile duct preoperatively and an increase in SSI incidence has been previously reported[44,45] through matching bacteria present in both the SSI and intraoperative bile cultures[46]; however, there are studies that suggest that preoperative stenting does not affect the postoperative SSI rate.[47] In addition, increased length of operation, poor surgical technique, intraoperative contamination and a number of postoperative surgical complications of PD, such as POPF and postoperative bleeding, have also been associated with SSIs.[48] Pancreatic leakage from the PJ, in particular, may work as a fertile ground for bacteria propagation and intra-abdominal abscess formation. Postoperatively, ineffective regulation of blood glucose, body temperature and tissue oxygenation may also be associated with SSIs.[49–51]

Diagnosis of SSIs is based on clinical findings characteristic for each classification'—purulent drainage through the incision, local signs of inflammation (erythema, pain or tenderness and warmth) and, in deeper-layer SSIs, fever, abdominal discomfort, inability to tolerate food and, occasionally, signs of systemic sepsis. Diagnosis can be confirmed by abdominal imaging

Table 33.7 Centers for Disease Control and Prevention's classification of surgical site infections

	Infection involves
Superficial incisional SSIs	Skin and subcutaneous tissue
Deep incisional SSIs	Deep tissues, such as fascial and muscle layers; also includes organ/space SSI draining through the incision
Organ/space SSIs	Any part of the organ and space anatomy opened or manipulated during operation, other than the incision

Abbreviation: SSIs, surgical site infections.

Table 33.8 Risk factors associated with development of surgical site infections post pancreatoduodenectomy

Malnutrition/hypoalbuminaemia
Diabetes mellitus
Preoperative steroid use
Increased length of operation
Hypothermia
Poor surgical technique
Intraoperative contamination
Postoperative complications • Pancreatic fistula • Haemorrhage/haematoma
Poor blood glucose regulation postoperatively
Inadequate tissue oxygenation postoperatively

(ultrasound and CT) for verification of intra-abdominal fluid collections. For superficial SSIs, a culture from a swab for both aerobic and anaerobic bacteria can identify specific microorganisms and direct antibiotic treatment. A Gram stain is also a quick and effective way to assess the infective microorganisms.

Treatment of SSIs is composed of drainage of abscesses or fluid collections and antibiotics for cellulitis. For the majority of patients, the management is limited to changes of dressing of the opened wound, to optimise healing. Suture removal and drainage through the incision, evacuating the pus and cleansing the wound, may be indicated.[52] Inspection of deeper tissues for integrity and identification of possible infection is also important.

Percutaneous drainage and culturing of the collection content are the treatments of choice for deep or organ space infections and help direct the antimicrobial therapy, accordingly. In less than one-third of the patients, organ space SSIs are not amenable to percutaneous drainage; in very few cases, when the patient's status does not improve with the antibiotic regimen, a laparotomy may be necessary.

The choice of antibiotics for the treatment of SSIs is based on two key factors—the patient and the identified or probable infecting microorganism. Hepatic and renal functions, possible allergies documented in the patient's personal history and interactions with other administered medications may limit the arsenal of antibiotics that can be utilised. The main driver for the regimen of choice is the identified bacteria; first- or second-generation cephalosporin and/or metronidazole are routinely administered intravenously (i.v.) for gram-positive cocci and anaerobic bacteria, respectively, until wound or blood cultures become negative for colonisation. Prophylactic antibiotic use in pancreatic head surgery falls within the standardised protocol for gastrointestinal surgery: a bolus (with or without extracorporeal shock wave lithotripsy [ESWL]). administration of a first-generation cephalosporin immediately before incision, followed by 48 hours of i.v. administration of the same regimen.[53]

Surgical site infections have a strong impact on patient's postoperative morbidity; they result in an increase in length of stay and hospitalisation costs and, in cases of pancreatic cancer, a significant delay in receiving adjuvant therapy. Prevention of SSIs is feasible with the preservation of optimal patient management perioperatively and containment of any postoperative complications.

POSTOPERATIVE BLEEDING

Postoperative haemorrhage is a rare, yet severe complication after pancreatic head surgery, with an overall mortality of up to 45%.[54] The ISGPS proposed a universal definition and classification of postpancreatectomy haemorrhage (PPH).[55] All postoperative bleeding episodes are stratified into three different grades (A, B and C) based on onset, location and the severity of haemorrhage (Table 33.9). Early PPH occurs within 24 hours from the operation and is most likely caused by an underlying coagulopathy, surgical technique or inadequate haemostasis; late PPH is defined as occurring beyond POD 2 and is usually the result of a concurrent postoperative complication such as pancreatic fistula formation.[56] This may cause erosion of the wall of a peripancreatic blood vessel due to enzymatic digestion by trypsin and other pancreatic exocrine enzymes. Pseudoaneurysm of an artery due to

Table 33.9 International Study Group for Pancreatic Surgery's classification for postpancreatectomy haemorrhage

Grade	Time of onset, location and severity of bleeding	Clinical presentation	Diagnostic flowchart	Therapeutic intervention
A	Early, intra- or extraluminal, mild	Unremarkable	Observation, haemoglobin measurement, US/CT	None
B	Early, intra- or extraluminal, severe Late, intra- or extraluminal, mild	Tachycardia, hypotension	Observation, haemoglobin measurement, US/CT, angiography, upper GI endoscopy	Fluid resuscitation, blood transfusion, optional follow-up in ICU, therapeutic endoscopy, vessel embolisation, reoperation
C	Late, intra- or extraluminal, severe	Oliguria, hypovolaemic shock	CT, angiography, upper GI endoscopy	Fluid resuscitation, blood transfusion, ICU hospitalisation, bleeding localisation, therapeutic endoscopy, vessel embolisation, reoperation

Abbreviations: CT, computed tomographic scan; GI, gastrointestinal; ICU, intensive care unit; US, ultrasonography.

Adapted from: Wente MN, Veit JA, Bassi C, et al. Postpancreatectomy hemorrhage (PPH): an International Study Group of Pancreatic Surgery (ISGPS) definition. *Surgery* 2007;142:20–5.

Table 33.10 Most common sites of postpancreatectomy haemorrhage

Gastroduodenal artery stump
Branches of the superior mesenteric artery • Jejunal mesenteric arterial branches • Inferior pancreatoduodenal artery
Branches of the hepatic artery
Portal vein tributaries
Superior mesenteric vein tributaries
Pancreatic cut surface/pancreatojejunostomy suture line
Duodenojejunostomy suture line after PPPD
Gastrojejunostomy suture line after classic PD
Gallbladder fossa after cholecystectomy
Retroperitoneal area of pancreatic resection

Abbreviations: PD, pancreatoduodenectomy; PPPD, pylorus-preserving pancreatoduodenectomy.

intraoperative injury (gastroduodenal, splenic or branches of the superior mesenteric artery) and ulceration at the gastrojejunostomy anastomotic site are also risk factors for late PPH[55] (Table 33.10). Most importantly, PPH is categorised into mild and severe; the latter accounts for significant blood loss that results into the need for transfusion and, occasionally, invasive treatment.

The diagnosis of PPH depends on a high level of suspicion in the postoperative period. The presence of small amounts of blood in the abdominal drains or the NGT, haematochezia or haematemesis are the first signs of intra- or extraluminal haemorrhage. This is also known as 'sentinel bleeding' and may be the precursor of an upcoming massive blood loss.[57] Clinical signs such as unexplained tachycardia and hypotension can be indicative of PPH and may lead to oliguria and hypovolaemic shock in severe cases. A haemoglobin drop of greater than 3 mg/dL in the arterial blood gas or a blood test can help with the diagnosis. Imaging modalities such as upper GI endoscopy, CT and angiography can also be utilised for establishing the diagnosis.

The treatment of PPH is regulated according to its onset and severity. Early mild PPH usually requires no therapeutic intervention; close patient monitoring is sufficient for the majority of cases. Patients with grade B PPH (early severe/late mild) will often present with clinical signs of hypovolaemia, and intensive care unit (ICU) transfer may be indicated for monitoring. Volume resuscitation with fluids and blood transfusion of up to 3 units of packed reb blood cells (pRBCs) within 24 hours are adequate for patient stabilisation. In the presence of

intraluminal haemorrhage, a therapeutic endoscopy can be helpful. Severe cases of early PPH may need reoperation for definitive management of the cause.

Delayed severe PPH is the most dangerous for the patient, since it is almost always the result of a pseudoaneurysm and can occur weeks after surgery, after the patient is discharged. Massive haemorrhage in this setting causes acute hypovolaemia, a life-threatening situation. The patient needs to be supported immediately with blood transfusion and fluid resuscitation, and the site of bleeding must be identified as soon as the patient is stabilised haemodynamically. The ICU-level care is indicated. An emergency percutaneous angiogram can provide information about the bleeding site, and embolisation can be performed in cases of a pseudoaneurysm or a confirmed contrast agent leak.[58] This is the preferred initial management over reoperation. Reoperation in grade C patients is rare and is utilised when all other therapeutic modalities have been exhausted.

OTHER POSTOPERATIVE COMPLICATIONS AFTER PANCREATIC HEAD SURGERY

There is an abundance of complications that may occur after pancreatic head surgery, and they have been studied extensively in the literature (Table 33.1). Biliary complications are uncommon and include biliary leak from the hepaticojejunostomy, acute cholangitis and transient postoperative jaundice. Biliary leak is diagnosed by the presence of biliary content in the abdominal drainage within a week from surgery and is usually a result of technique's technical failure. Acute cholangitis presents with fever and chills, right upper quadrant pain and jaundice. Bacteraemia is found with positive blood cultures in more than 50% of the patients. When cholangitis occurs early in the postoperative period, it is related to surgical field contamination; delayed cholangitis may be due to stricture of the hepaticojejunostomy. In both occasions, the treatment is antibiotics for the microorganisms identified through the bile or blood culture. Hepatic abscess development may further complicate the patient's postoperative course.[59,60]

Chyle leak and subsequent chyloperitoneum have also been reported as very uncommon postoperative surgical complications after PD. Chyle leak is defined as the leakage of lymphatic fluid, which is rich in triglycerides, into the peritoneal cavity. In surgery of the pancreatic head, chyle leak is usually associated with disruption of the cisterna chyli or its major lymphatic tributaries— located at the same level behind the pancreas—during extended retroperitoneal lymph node dissection.[61] The development of chylous ascites from a chyle leakage can prove detrimental to the patient's well-being; it is rich in nutrients, and the constant flow in the abdomen can lead to severe malnutrition, electrolyte imbalance and dehydration. Immunological disturbances are also possible, due to the increased concentration of lymphocytes and immunoglobulins in the lymphatic fluid. Treatment of chyle leak includes dietary modifications, such as a very-low-fat diet or TPN. Leaks refractory to the dietary support can be addressed with somatostatin administration. In extreme cases of chylous ascites, utilisation of external beam radiotherapy has been reported with mixed outcomes.[62]

Adverse cardiopulmonary events, such as pneumonia, atrial fibrillation and hypertension, are also observed in the postoperative course, and their incidence can be as high as 5%.[19] The incidence of these complications is not higher in PD than in other major operations; however, they contribute significantly to increased length of stay and may rarely result in patient's death. Close monitoring of the patients according to their personal history of cardiopulmonary disease, early return to outpatient medications and pulmonary physiotherapy can significantly reduce the occurrence of these complications.[63]

CONCLUSIONS

Over the past three decades, pancreatic head surgery has become safer to perform because of a multitude of factors, including improved operative techniques, surgeon experience and hospital care. Although postoperative mortality has decreased significantly, PD still ranks very high in terms of morbidity. More than 50% of these cases may present with some kind of postoperative complication of varying severity. Prevention, early diagnosis and treatment of these complications after PD are challenging; however, standardised perioperative protocols developed at high-volume centres can significantly decrease their incidence and contribute to reduced length of stay, low hospital costs and improved patient outcomes.

REFERENCES

1. Whipple AO, Parsons WB, Mullins CR. Treatment of carcinoma of the ampulla of vater. *Ann Surg* 1935;102: 763–79.

2. Wolfgang CL, Pawlik TM. Pancreatoduodenectomy: time to change our approach? *Lancet Oncol* 2013;14:573–5.

3. Wu W, He J, Cameron JL, et al. The impact of postoperative complications on the administration of adjuvant therapy following pancreaticoduodenectomy for adenocarcinoma. *Ann Surg Oncol* 2014;21:2873–81.

4. Gangavatiker R, Pal S, Javed A, Dash NR, Sahni P, Chattopadhyay TK. Effect of antecolic or retrocolic reconstruction of the gastro/duodenojejunostomy on delayed gastric emptying after pancreaticoduodenectomy: a randomized controlled trial. *J Gastrointest Surg* 2011;15:843–52.

5. Warshaw AL, Torchiana DL. Delayed gastric emptying after pylorus-preserving pancreaticoduodenectomy. *Surg Gynecol Obstet* 1985;160:1–4.

6. Wente MN, Bassi C, Dervenis C, et al. Delayed gastric emptying (DGE) after pancreatic surgery: a suggested definition by the International Study Group of Pancreatic Surgery (ISGPS). *Surgery* 2007;142:761–8.

7. Kim DK, Hindenburg AA, Sharma SK, et al. Is pylorospasm a cause of delayed gastric emptying after pylorus-preserving pancreaticoduodenectomy? *Ann Surg Oncol* 2005;12: 222–7.

8. Qu H, Sun GR, Zhou SQ, He QS. Clinical risk factors of delayed gastric emptying in patients after pancreaticoduodenectomy: a systematic review and meta-analysis. *Eur J Surg Oncol* 2013;39:213–23.

9. Haltmeier T, Kaderli RM, Kurmann A, et al. Delayed Gastric Emptying after pancreaticoduodenectomy: analysis of associated risk factors. *Am Surg* 2015;81:392–4.

10. van Berge Henegouwen MI, van Gulik TM, et al. Delayed gastric emptying after standard pancreaticoduodenectomy versus pylorus-preserving pancreaticoduodenectomy: an analysis of 200 consecutive patients. *J Am Coll Surg* 1997;185:373–9.

11. Hackert T, Hinz U, Hartwig W, et al. Pylorus resection in partial pancreaticoduodenectomy: impact on delayed gastric emptying. *Am J Surg* 2013;206:296–9.

12. Eshuis WJ, van Eijck CHJ, Gerhards MF, et al. Antecolic versus retrocolic route of the gastroenteric anastomosis after pancreatoduodenectomy: a randomized controlled trial. *Ann Surg* 2014;259:45–51.

13. Qian D, Lu Z, Jackson R, et al. Effect of antecolic or retrocolic route of gastroenteric anastomosis on delayed gastric emptying after pancreaticoduodenectomy: a meta-analysis of randomized controlled trials. *Pancreatology* 2016;16:142–50.

14. Hanna MM, Tamariz L, Gadde R, et al. Delayed gastric emptying after pylorus preserving pancreaticoduodenectomy-does gastrointestinal reconstruction technique matter? *Am J Surg* 2016;211:810–9.

15. Hanna MM, Hanna M, Gadde R, et al. Delayed gastric emptying after pancreaticoduodenectomy: is subtotal stomach preserving better or pylorus preserving? *J Gastrointest Surg* 2015;19:1542–52.

16. Kurosaki I, Hatakeyama K. Preservation of the left gastric vein in delayed gastric emptying after pylorus-preserving pancreaticoduodenectomy. *J Gastrointest Surg* 2005;9: 846–52.

17. Shimoda M, Kubota K, Katoh M, Kita J. Effect of billroth II or Roux-en-Y reconstruction for the gastrojejunostomy on

delayed gastric emptying after pancreaticoduodenectomy: a randomized controlled study. *Ann Surg* 2013;257:938–42.

18. Nikfarjam M, Houli N, Tufail F, Weinberg L, Muralidharan V, Christophi C. Reduction in delayed gastric emptying following non-pylorus preserving pancreaticoduodenectomy by addition of a Braun enteroenterostomy. *JOP* 2012;13:488–96.

19. Cameron JL, He J. Two thousand consecutive pancreaticoduodenectomies. *J Am Coll Surg* 2015;220:530–6.

20. Samaddar A, Kaman L, Dahiya D, Bhattachyarya A, Sinha SK. Objective assessment of delayed gastric emptying using gastric scintigraphy in post pancreaticoduodenectomy patients. *ANZ J Surg* 2015. [Epub ahead of print]. doi: 10.1111/ans.13360

21. Ohwada S, Satoh Y, Kawate S, et al. Low-dose erythromycin reduces delayed gastric emptying and improves gastric motility after Billroth I pylorus-preserving pancreaticoduodenectomy. *Ann Surg* 2001;234: 668–74.

22. Shan Y-S, Sy ED, Tsai M-L, Tang L-Y, Li PS, Lin P-W. Effects of somatostatin prophylaxis after pylorus-preserving pancreaticoduodenectomy: increased delayed gastric emptying and reduced plasma motilin. *World J Surg* 2005;29:1319–24.

23. Vin Y, Sima CS, Getrajdman GI, et al. Management and outcomes of postpancreatectomy fistula, leak, and abscess: results of 908 patients resected at a single institution between 2000 and 2005. *J Am Coll Surg* 2008;207: 490–8.

24. Bassi C, Dervenis C, Butturini G, et al. Postoperative pancreatic fistula: an international study group (ISGPF) definition. *Surgery* 2005;138:8–13.

25. Allen PJ, Gönen M, Brennan MF, et al. Pasireotide for postoperative pancreatic fistula. *N Engl J Med* 2014;370:2014–22.

26. El Nakeeb A, El Hemaly M, Askr W, et al. Comparative study between duct to mucosa and invagination pancreatojejunostomy after pancreaticoduodenectomy: a prospective randomized study. *Int J Surg* 2015;16:1–6.

27. Berger AC, Howard TJ, Kennedy EP, et al. Does type of pancreatojejunostomy after pancreaticoduodenectomy decrease rate of pancreatic fistula? A randomized, prospective, dual-institution trial. *J Am Coll Surg* 2009;208:738–47; discussion 747–9.

28. Winter JM, Cameron JL, Campbell KA, et al. Does pancreatic duct stenting decrease the rate of pancreatic fistula following pancreaticoduodenectomy? Results of a prospective randomized trial. *J Gastrointest Surg* 2006;10:1280–90; discussion 1290.

29. Motoi F, Egawa S, Rikiyama T, Katayose Y, Unno M. Randomized clinical trial of external stent drainage of the pancreatic duct to reduce postoperative pancreatic fistula after pancreatojejunostomy. *Br J Surg* 2012;99:524–31.

30. Ke S, Ding X-M, Gao J, et al. A prospective, randomized trial of Roux-en-Y reconstruction with isolated pancreatic drainage versus conventional loop reconstruction after pancreaticoduodenectomy. *Surgery* 2013;153:743–52.

31. Klaiber U, Probst P, Knebel P, et al. Meta-analysis of complication rates for single-loop versus dual-loop (Roux-en-Y) with isolated pancreatojejunostomy reconstruction after pancreaticoduodenectomy. *Br J Surg* 2015;102:331–40.

32. Duffas J-P, Suc B, Msika S, et al. A controlled randomized multicenter trial of pancreatogastrostomy or pancreatojejunostomy after pancreatoduodenectomy. *Am J Surg* 2005;189: 720–9.

33. Bassi C, Falconi M, Molinari E, et al. Reconstruction by pancreatojejunostomy versus pancreatogastrostomy following pancreatectomy: results of a comparative study. *Ann Surg* 2005;242:767–71; discussion 771–3.

34. Lillemoe KD, Cameron JL, Kim MP, et al. Does fibrin glue sealant decrease the rate of pancreatic fistula after pancreaticoduodenectomy? Results of a prospective randomized trial. *J Gastrointest Surg* 2004;8:766–72; discussion 772–4.

35. Van Buren G 2nd, Bloomston M, Hughes SJ, et al. A randomized prospective multicenter trial of pancreaticoduodenectomy with and without routine intraperitoneal drainage. *Ann Surg* 2014;259:605–12.

36. Bassi C, Molinari E, Malleo G, et al. Early versus late drain removal after standard pancreatic resections: results of a prospective randomized trial. *Ann Surg* 2010;252: 207–14.

37. Sarr MG; Pancreatic Surgery Group. The potent somatostatin analogue vapreotide does not decrease pancreas-specific complications after elective pancreatectomy: a prospective, multicenter, double-blinded, randomized, placebo-controlled trial. *J Am Coll Surg* 2003;196:556–64; discussion 564–5; author reply 565.

38. Fernández-Cruz L, Jiménez Chavarría E, Taurà P, Closa D, Boado M-AL, Ferrer J. Prospective randomized trial of the effect of octreotide on pancreatic juice output after pancreaticoduodenectomy in relation to histological diagnosis, duct size and leakage. *HPB* 2013;15:392–9.

39. Malleo G, Pulvirenti A, Marchegiani G, Butturini G, Salvia R, Bassi C. Diagnosis and management of postoperative pancreatic fistula. *Langenbecks Arch Surg* 2014;399: 801–10.

40. Nanashima A, Abo T, Arai J, et al. Clinicopathological parameters associated with surgical site infections in patients who underwent pancreatic resection. *Hepatogastroenterology* 2014;61:1739–43.

41. National Nosocomial Infections Surveillance (NNIS) report, data summary from October 1986-April 1996, issued May 1996. A report from the National Nosocomial Infections Surveillance (NNIS) System. *Am J Infect Control* 1996;24:380–8.

42. La Torre M, Ziparo V, Nigri G, Cavallini M, Balducci G, Ramacciato G. Malnutrition and pancreatic surgery: prevalence and outcomes. *J Surg Oncol* 2013;107:702–8.

43. Shinkawa H, Takemura S, Uenishi T, et al. Nutritional risk index as an independent predictive factor for the development of surgical site infection after pancreaticoduodenectomy. *Surg Today* 2013;43:276–83.

44. Sohn TA, Yeo CJ, Cameron JL, Pitt HA, Lillemoe KD. Do preoperative biliary stents increase postpancreaticoduodenectomy complications? *J Gastrointest Surg* 2000;4:258–67; discussion 267–8.

45. Gavazzi F, Ridolfi C, Capretti G, et al. Role of preoperative biliary stents, bile contamination and antibiotic prophylaxis in surgical site infections after pancreaticoduodenectomy. *BMC Gastroenterol* 2016;16:43.

46. Herzog T, Belyaev O, Akkuzu R, Hölling J, Uhl W, Chromik AM. The impact of bile duct cultures on surgical site infections in pancreatic surgery. *Surg Infect* 2015;16:443–9.

47. Sewnath ME, Birjmohun RS, Rauws EA, Huibregtse K, Obertop H, Gouma DJ. The effect of preoperative biliary drainage on postoperative complications after pancreaticoduodenectomy. *J Am Coll Surg* 2001;192:726–34.

48. Sugiura T, Uesaka K, Ohmagari N, Kanemoto H, Mizuno T. Risk factor of surgical site infection after pancreaticoduodenectomy. *World J Surg* 2012;36:2888–94.

49. Kurz A, Sessler DI, Lenhardt R. Perioperative normothermia to reduce the incidence of surgical-wound infection and shorten hospitalization. Study of Wound Infection and Temperature Group. *N Engl J Med* 1996;334:1209–15.

50. Barreto SG, Singh MK, Sharma S, Chaudhary A. Determinants of surgical site infections following pancreatoduodenectomy. *World J Surg* 2015;39:2557–63.

51. Wetterslev J, Meyhoff CS, Jørgensen LN, Gluud C, Lindschou J, Rasmussen LS. The effects of high perioperative inspiratory oxygen fraction for adult surgical patients. *Cochrane Database Syst Rev* 2015;6:CD008884.

52. Bressan AK, Roberts DJ, Edwards JP, et al. Efficacy of a dual-ring wound protector for prevention of incisional surgical site infection after Whipple's procedure (pancreaticoduodenectomy) with preoperatively-placed intrabiliary stents: protocol for a randomised controlled trial. *BMJ Open* 2014;4:e005577.

53. Kondo K, Chijiiwa K, Ohuchida J, et al. Selection of prophylactic antibiotics according to the microorganisms isolated from surgical site infections (SSIs) in a previous series of surgeries reduces SSI incidence after pancreaticoduodenectomy. *J Hepatobiliary Pancreat Sci* 2013;20:286–93.

54. Yekebas EF, Wolfram L, Cataldegirmen G, et al. Postpancreatectomy hemorrhage: diagnosis and treatment: an analysis in 1669 consecutive pancreatic resections. *Ann Surg* 2007;246:269–80.

55. Wente MN, Veit JA, Bassi C, et al. Postpancreatectomy hemorrhage (PPH): an International Study Group of Pancreatic Surgery (ISGPS) definition. *Surgery* 2007;142:20–5.

56. Ricci C, Casadei R, Buscemi S, Minni F. Late postpancreatectomy hemorrhage after pancreaticoduodenectomy: is it possible to recognize risk factors? *JOP* 2012;13:193–8.

57. Tien Y-W, Lee P-H, Yang C-Y, Ho M-C, Chiu Y-F. Risk factors of massive bleeding related to pancreatic leak after pancreaticoduodenectomy. *J Am Coll Surg* 2005;201:554–9.

58. Chen J-F, Xu S-F, Zhao W, et al. Diagnostic and therapeutic strategies to manage post-pancreaticoduodenectomy hemorrhage. *World J Surg* 2015;39:509–15.

59. Malgras B, Duron S, Gaujoux S, et al. Early biliary complications following pancreaticoduodenectomy: prevalence and risk factors. *HPB* 2016;18:367–74.

60. Parra-Membrives P, Martínez-Baena D, Sánchez-Sánchez F. Late biliary complications after pancreaticoduodenectomy. *Am Surg* 2016;82:456–61.

61. Assumpcao L, Cameron JL, Wolfgang CL, et al. Incidence and management of chyle leaks following pancreatic resection: a high volume single-center institutional experience. *J Gastrointest Surg* 2008;12:1915–23.

62. Corradini S, Liebig S, Niemoeller OM, Zwicker F, Lamadé W. Successful radiation treatment of chylous ascites following pancreaticoduodenectomy. *Strahlenther Onkol* 2015;191:448–52.

63. Junejo MA, Mason JM, Sheen AJ, et al. Cardiopulmonary exercise testing for preoperative risk assessment before pancreaticoduodenectomy for cancer. *Ann Surg Oncol* 2014;21:1929–36.

34

Complications after Laparoscopic Distal Pancreatectomy

S. Sánchez Cabús and L. Fernández-Cruz

ABSTRACT

The excellent results obtained with the laparoscopic approach in the surgical treatment of localised lesions in the body and tail of the pancreas have led to the acceptance of laparoscopic distal pancreatectomy (LDP) as the preferred approach today. The accumulated scientific evidence after 20 years of use of LDP have shown that it is able to significantly reduce intraoperative blood loss and postoperative hospital stay as well as improve postoperative quality of life, without adversely affecting postoperative complications—both overall and pancreatic-specific complications. However, the laparoscopic approach has unique connotations, which imply the need for a learning curve, the need for conversion to conventional open surgery in a number of cases and the presence of specific complications that must be taken into account. The treatment of these complications depends on the type thereof and the team's experience. If these complications require surgical treatment, such as a significant postoperative bleeding, presence of peripancreatic collections, splenic ischaemia and others, it is possible in a large proportion of cases to solve them laparoscopically or at least start the intervention by the laparoscopic approach. However, in these cases, patient safety and the resolution of the complication should be the priority. Finally, the long-term oncological results seem to be equivalent to those obtained after conventional surgery, so the use of the LDP is fully valid in patients with pancreatic malignancy.

KEYWORDS

Distal pancreatectomy, laparoscopy, postoperative complications, pancreatic fistula, delayed gastric emptying, postpancreatectomy haemorrhage, ISGPS, learning curve, oncological principles

INTRODUCTION

Surgical procedures for resection of lesions located in the body and tail of the pancreas are less challenging than those needed for resection of the pancreatic head. The reasons behind this are the very different anatomical relationships between those two pancreatic regions and the surrounding organs and major vessels, and the absence of the need for complex reconstructions. These factors favoured the introduction and subsequent development of the laparoscopic approach for distal pancreatectomy, and many years later, it has progressively become the preferred approach in most of the high-volume centres, given its advantages in terms of postoperative pain, intraoperative blood loss and cosmetic results over its open counterpart.

However, pancreatic surgery, no matter which approach is selected, is associated with a high complication rate. The main difference between laparoscopic surgery and open pancreatic surgery is the trauma to the abdominal wall, and these two approaches do not necessarily mean different surgical managements. Therefore, the expected differences between these two approaches should not affect the pancreatic-specific complications, unless the way of performing a particular surgical step is different from open surgery.

In this chapter, we will describe the most common complications after laparoscopic distal pancreatectomy (LDP) and compare its results against open distal pancreatectomy (ODP), discussing the pancreatic-specific, laparoscopy-specific and other complications and their management.

THE POSTOPERATIVE COMPLICATION RATE AFTER LAPAROSCOPIC DISTAL PANCREATECTOMY IS IT DIFFERENT FROM OPEN SURGERY?

Since the extended implementation of LDP, there have been many reports describing the outcomes associated with the technique. However, to date, there has been no benchmark study for complications after LDP. In 2014, the group from Verona tried to validate the complication risk score (CRS) in a series of 100 consecutive LDPs. Their results showed that the overall postoperative complication rate was 49%, with a major complication rate of 12% and a clinically relevant pancreatic postoperative pancreatic fistula (POPF) rate of 13%. Interestingly, their study showed that the CRS failed to adequately assess the postoperative complications, since they did not significantly change when the CRS increased. Their conclusion, after a multivariate analysis of their cohort of patients, showed that the male sex and a blood loss higher that 150 mL were independent factors associated with postoperative complications and pancreatic fistula (PF).[1]

However, more than just a mere description of the outcomes after LDP, it has been interesting to compare the results of ODP against LDP. Until now, the introduction of LDP has been done in a very progressive way, and results have been published showing its superiority compared with ODP. There have not been any randomised controlled trials comparing both techniques; however, there are many retrospective studies comparing both approaches. In 2014, a multicentre study led by a group in Philadelphia included 655 patients and aimed to define the postoperative complications after distal pancreatectomy by using a scoring system named the Postoperative Morbidity Index (PMI) for assessing complications. They had a mortality rate of 0.6% and a morbidity rate of 27%, which included operative bleeding and need for transfusion (15.4%) and organ-specific complications (7.2%). Postoperative pancreatic fistula was present in 22.7% of the patients, and the rate of clinically relevant POPF was 9.2%. The laparoscopic approach was used in 21.7% of the patients, and most importantly, there were no differences in PMI between ODP and LDP, showing, in this study, a comparable outcome between the classical open approach and the LDP.[2]

A comparative study published in 2015 of 100 patients undergoing LDP with a 100 propensity score–matched patients that received ODP concluded that there were no differences in terms of postoperative complications between the two approaches. However, there was an extra cost of €775 per patient in the LDP, even if patients with LDP who had an uneventful postoperative course had an earlier rehabilitation than their ODP counterparts.[3] Baker et al compared the ODP's and LDP's postoperative complications classified by the Clavien-Dindo score and, additionally, by using *poor-quality outcomes*, based on complications equal or above Clavien-Dindo IIIb, as well as any II or IIIa complications requiring a significantly prolonged overall length of stay (including readmissions within 90 days or more than one invasive intervention). They found an equivalent complication profile according to the Clavien-Dindo system grading, but since LDP was related with a reduced hospital stay and transfusion rate, it revealed a reduced incidence of severe adverse poor-quality postoperative outcomes.[4] In a multiinstitutional study published by Cho et al, the outcomes after 439 ODPs and 254 LDPs were analysed. They found that patients with a body mass index ≤27, without pancreatic ductal adenocarcinoma (PDAC) and with pancreatic specimen length ≤8.5 cm had significantly higher rates of significant POPF after ODP than after LDP; in contrast, no preoperative variables were associated with a higher likelihood of significant POPF after LDP versus ODP. They concluded that risk factors for complications and pancreatic POPF after left pancreatectomy differed when open versus laparoscopic techniques were employed, so LDP might be the procedure of choice.[5]

Given the high number of comparative studies, a few meta-analyses have been performed. Nakamura et al performed a meta-analysis on 24 comparative studies between ODP and LDP and found the latter to be associated with a lower blood loss, lower transfusion rates, lower wound infection rates, lower morbidity rates and a shorter hospital stay. On the other hand, LDP showed significantly longer operative times compared with ODP. There was no significant difference in oncological outcomes between the LDP and the open technique.[6] Jin et al performed a systematic review and meta-analysis in 2012, comparing ODP and LDP for a total of 1456 patients, showing again no differences in terms of postoperative complications or POPF, with a benefit in LDP of less intraoperative blood loss, fewer blood transfusions, a shorter hospital stay, a higher rate of splenic preservation, earlier oral intake and fewer surgical site infections.[7] The systematic review and meta-analysis of case-matched studies comparing ODP and LDP published by Pericleous et al is one of those at a higher level of evidence in the literature; it showed that LDP was associated with a longer operative time and lower hospital stay, without any differences in postoperative morbidity, POPF rate and mortality as compared with ODP, concluding that LDP is a safe alternative to ODP; however, there is a need for randomised controlled trials in order to provide level 1 evidence as to the safety and efficacy of LDPs.[8] However, systematic review and meta-analysis by Venkat et al in the same year, which included 1814 patients, showed a benefit in LDP of reduced blood loss, a shorter length of stay and less postoperative complications (33.9% vs. 44.2%; odds ratio [OR]: 0.73; 95% confidence interval [CI]: 0.57–0.95), without differences for POPF rate and margin positivity, which suggests that this technique is a reasonable approach in selected cancer patients.[9] A recent meta-analysis by Mehrabi et al, including 29 observational studies and 5 systematic reviews, demonstrated the superiority of LDP over ODP in terms of estimated blood loss (EBL) (308 mL less), time to first oral intake (1.3 days less) and length of hospital stay (3.8 days less). However, no difference between the techniques was found in terms of PF (21.8% vs. 21.6%) and postoperative morbidity (34% vs. 38%) and mortality (0.4% vs 1.1%). Again, their conclusion is that LDP seems to be a safe and effective alternative to ODP, and a large, randomised trial is warranted and should focus on oncological effectiveness, defined endpoints and cost-effectiveness.[10]

LAPAROSCOPY-RELATED COMPLICATIONS

Laparoscopy has shown a reduction in the abdominal wall trauma, which leads to a faster mobilisation of the patient, less postoperative pain and an improved cosmetic result. However, LDP may be associated with some complications that are very rare in open surgery.

Inadvertent Intra-Abdominal Lesions

Inherent to the laparoscopic access is that in some parts of the surgical procedure, the attention of the surgical team is often focussed on a very specific part of the abdomen, thus leaving the rest of the abdominal cavity without surveillance while surgical instruments are constantly entering and leaving the abdominal cavity. One of the complications that may happen, though exceedingly rare in open surgery, is inadvertent bowel or hepatic injury, which can be repaired if noticed during the surgical procedure; if not noticed, a major postoperative complication may occur, which may warrant early surgical exploration due to intra-abdominal bleeding or peritonitis.

Inadvertent bowel lesions are a rare complication and are not frequently described in the published series. Recently, the combined experience of LDP from two high-volume pancreatic surgery centres reported inadvertent bowel injury in two cases.[11] However, if present, these lesions constitute a major complication needing a surgical reintervention.

Intraoperative Bleeding

One of the concerns when performing pancreatic surgery is the anatomical relationship of the pancreas with the surrounding vascular structures. Preoperative planning is indispensable, since knowing the exact location of the pancreatic lesion and its surroundings may avoid an unnecessary vascular injury. On the other hand, laparoscopy enables the surgeon to have a more precise vision of the operative field and helps identify small vessels, which can be safely controlled.

The general consensus is that overall intraoperative bleeding is reduced in LDP compared with ODP. This may be the result of the better identification of the vessels and also an effect of the elevated intraperitoneal pressure due to the pneumoperitoneum. One aspect that could influence the presence of bleeding is the way in which small vessels are treated. In open surgery, haemostasis consists of vessel ligation or direct suturing, whereas in laparoscopic surgery, it is achieved, in most situations, with energy devices (bipolar diathermy or harmonic scalpel), endostaplers or the use of metallic or plastic clips. Results from the majority of comparative studies, systematic reviews and meta-analysis in the literature show an advantage of LDP over ODP in terms of operative blood loss and transfusion rate.[3,6–10,12–17] In addition, in spleen-preserving LDP, there exists some evidence that the so-called Warshaw technique (WT) may be associated with a less significant blood loss.

PANCREAS-RELATED COMPLICATIONS

Postoperative Pancreatic Fistula

Of all the possible complications after pancreatic surgery, one that is most feared for its potentially important clinical implications is the appearance of a POPF. Since 2005, diagnosis of POPF has been well described by the International Study Group of Pancreatic Fistula as the 'output via an operatively placed drain (or a subsequently placed, percutaneous drain) of any measurable volume of drain fluid on or after postoperative day 3, with an amylase content greater than three times the upper normal serum value',[18] and its consequences have been graded, according to the severity, into three groups, ranging from grade A, which does not entail any clinical complications, to grades B and C, also named clinically relevant POPFs, which correspond to patients that have to undergo a change in the clinical management, especially the latter, in which the patient is severely ill and an intervention is warranted in order to treat the POPF.

According to the available evidence from meta-analysis of comparative studies, the surgical approach is not considered an independent factor for the presence of overall POPF, since it is not significantly different between ODP and LDP,[6–8,10,19,20] despite the fact that there is a considerable variation among published data, with most series describing it to be in the range of 15 to 35% and the clinically relevant POPF rate to be about 8 to 10%.

One factor that potentially could influence the appearance of POPF is the pancreatic transection method and the closure of the pancreatic stump. Given the peculiarities of the laparoscopic approach, the preferred transection method is the use of endostaplers. Endostapler method has proved to be an easy and reproducible way of an all-in-one transection and closure method in comparison with the most used alternative, that is, scalpel or diathermy pancreatic section and closure of the pancreatic stump by means of suturing—a technically demanding procedure to perform laparoscopically. A few studies have addressed this issue, and it is generally concluded that the endostapler method is superior to the conventional technique in terms of operative time and POPF. However, the technique needs to be very accurate in order to avoid crushing the pancreatic parenchyma; in fact, endostapler manufacturers advocate for a progressive closure of the stapler for a number of seconds and then to maintain the stapler closed before firing it for about 20 to 30 seconds, in order to keep the transection line free of pancreatic fluid, making the stapling and section procedure easier. Another strategy to prevent PF is to transect the pancreas and reinforce the stapler with a patch of plastic material, hoping for the pancreatic stump to remain tightly closed. Results from the use of this technical refinement are somewhat controversial in the literature. In 2014, Kurahara et al published a trial of 50 consecutive patients undergoing distal pancreatectomy and showed a decreased leakage of postoperative pancreatic juice into the abdominal cavity in patients that were treated by the reinforced stapler, which may lead to a reduced inflammatory reaction, low incidence of PF and early hospital discharge. However, the use of one or other type of stapler depended on the surgeon's choice, so a selection bias might have been present.[21] Other authors have shown less positive results with the use of the reinforced stapler.

It has been pointed out that the site of pancreatic transection has a direct influence on the development of a PF, and since the neck of the pancreas corresponds to the point where the pancreas is narrowest, a reduction in the PF rate is expected in these situations. In 2015, Sell et al demonstrated the influence of the transection site on the occurrence of POPF, comparing the outcomes of 244 patients who were transected at the pancreatic neck with the outcomes of 50 patient who were transected at the pancreatic tail. The PF rates were significantly lower when the transection was done at the pancreatic neck (28% vs. 15.6%; p = 0.04). However, the large majority of PF in tail transections were grade A PF, since there were no differences between groups in the clinically relevant PF rates.[22] There is another factor that may be related to POPF: the thickness of the pancreas. Independently of the transection point, a POPF is more prone to happen if there is a bulky and somewhat rigid pancreas. In those cases, stapler pressure may lead to pancreatic crushing, which will result in a POPF (Figure 34.1).

The management of the pancreatic stump may play a role in the POPF rate. A review article from 2012 from the Heidelberg group evaluated the influence of different methods of pancreatic stump closure that have been tried and reported, such as scalpel and suture, stapler with or without reinforcement, fibrin glue, artificial or extrapancreatic organ patches, anastomoses, ultrasound dissection and Ligasure™ transection.[23] In the laparoscopic approach, the preferred transection method is the stapler method, and most of the large series published show a POPF rate around 30%, which is consistent with the results of the DISPACT trial, in which a stapler was used.[24] Zhang et al performed a systematic review and meta-analysis of more than 5000 patients regarding the outcomes of the three main methods: stapler closure, anastomotic closure and manual suture of the

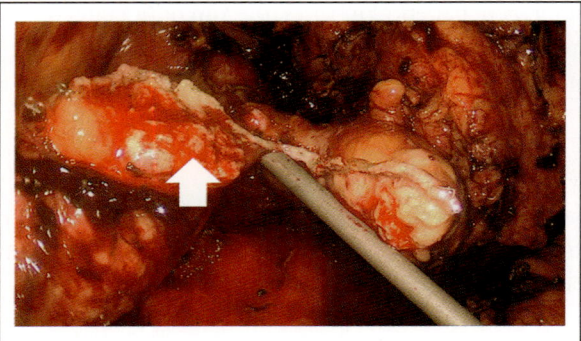

Figure 34.1 Image of crushed pancreatic parenchyma (white arrow) after transection with endostapler.

Courtesy: Santiago Sánchez Cabús and Laureano Fernández-Cruz.

pancreatic remnant. Their conclusion was that POPF rate was significantly lower when stapler closure or pancreatic stump anastomosis was performed compared with suture closure.[25]

Finally, there are some possible future perspectives that may help in the future to lower the POPF rate. In 2012, Blansfield et al published their experience in a comparative study that aimed to achieve a lower POPF rate in patients undergoing stump closure by using a saline-coupled radiofrequency dissector (RF dissector) (Salient Surgical Technologies) compared with what they called *traditional stump closure*, which, in reality, was a heterogeneous group of methods such as stapling, suturing and fibrin glue, amongst others. Both groups had a significant proportion of patients operated on laparoscopically. They demonstrated a reduction of POPF in the experimental group (10% vs. 36%; p < 0.02), as well as less operative time and blood loss.[26] In addition, in an effort to minimise POPF, there have also been a few studies that have addressed the influence of the local application of a fibrin sealant in order to prevent leakage of the pancreatic fluid. However, the level of evidence from these studies is low, with some authors reporting clinical benefit from the use of fibrin sealant, whereas others showing no differences in the appearance of PF.

The treatment of a clinically significant PF may need, in some cases, a surgical exploration of the patient in order to evacuate peripancreatic fluid collections, performing a peritoneal lavage and, in some cases, treatment of the pancreatic stump, either by replacing intra-abdominal drains or by performing a proximal pancreatic transection. The choice of the surgical approach must be determined by its nature, the clinical status of the patient and the experience of the surgical team, but in most cases, these reinterventions can be successfully accomplished by laparoscopy, which will ultimately have a positive effect on a severely ill patient. However, the aim of the intervention must be, above all, the patient's safety and solving the complication.

Delayed Gastric Emptying

Another pancreatic-specific complication, delayed gastric emptying (DGE) has been again well documented and described since the publication in 2007 by Wente et al,[27] and it is actually a frequent postoperative complication, presenting in 19 to 57% of the patients undergoing pancreatic surgery. Delayed gastric emptying is the inability to return to a standard diet by the end of the first postoperative week and includes prolonged nasogastric

intubation of the patient. It is classified at three levels as PF, depending on the duration of the symptoms and the need for other alternatives of oral nutrition. Before defining a patient as having DGE, it is of utmost importance to discard the presence of postoperative ileus, which may share some clinical aspects with DGE, the latter being an absence of small bowel/colon normal peristalsis after surgery, which may be induced by visceral mobilisation or peritoneal irritation.

Although some postoperative factors might be implicated in the appearance of DGE, such as the presence of a PF and postoperative dyselectrolytemia, its actual physiopathology is largely unknown. However, one of the most important factors that has been related with DGE is duodenal resection. As is noted in many reports, this may be an important reason why DGE is frequently seen after a pancreatoduodenectomy (PD) but is rarely present after distal pancreatectomy.

As a result of the low frequency of DGE occurring after LDP, it is a complication that is rarely mentioned in series of patients' data published. In fact, data from the available meta-analyses show a consistent advantage of LDP over ODP in terms of oral intake, which is one of the factors that may influence a reduced length of hospital stay.[6–8,10,17,19]

Postpancreatectomy Haemorrhage

The pancreatic gland, as all endocrine organs, has very rich vascularisation. When performing a pancreatic surgical resection, this phenomenon adds complexity to the procedure and can be the origin of the third pancreatic-specific complication, postpancreatectomy haemorrhage (PPH).[28] Although a rather infrequent complication, which is thought to happen in about 1 to 8% of pancreatic resections, its implications are very important, since mortality rates derived from PPH are 11 to 38%.

Most part of the published data of PPH after LDP come from single-institution, retrospective studies, and the reported PPH rate is between 0 and 12.5%.[11,13,29–32] One of the supposed benefits of the laparoscopic approach for distal pancreatectomy is an improved field of view due to the magnification from the optics. Theoretically, this might lead to a more accurate dissection, identification and control of the little vessels, thus lowering the PPH rate in comparison with ODP.

Just like POPF, surgical treatment of a clinically significant PPH can be safely accomplished by means of laparoscopy as long as the patient's clinical and haemodynamic status and the surgical team's expertise allows.

OTHER COMPLICATIONS

Influence of the Learning Curve

The influence of a learning curve was evident in a Swedish retrospective study that showed a significant reduction in operative time (195 minutes vs. 143 minutes; p = 0.04) as well as major postoperative complications (37% vs. 6%; p = 0.02) when a comparison between the first and the last patient of the series was done; however, the authors did not find any differences in terms of oncological outcomes and overall complications between patients undergoing LDP and ODP, even though malignancy was present in only 6 out of 37 patients undergoing LDP and 12 out of 45 patients undergoing ODP.[33] The completion of the learning curve seems to be mainly associated with a decrease in the operative time. However, conversion rate, overall morbidity and length of stay do not seem to be affected by the learning curve, as stated by the report from the University of Bologna in a retrospective analysis of 32 patients.[13] Similar findings had been published earlier by the Milan group regarding blood loss, postoperative morbidity rate and hospital stay; however, conversion rate was reported to be higher in the first 10 patients.[34]

Splenic Complications

In recent years, there has been a trend towards preservation of the spleen when performing a distal pancreatectomy, since splenectomy has proven to be associated with an increase in infectious complications.[35] The spleen has important haematological and immunological roles, and nowadays, its removal in the setting of a distal pancreatectomy is encouraged only for oncological reasons, in cases of proven malignant neoplasms located in the left pancreas.[36]

There are two surgical techniques for performing a spleen-preserving distal pancreatectomy:

1. Spleen-preserving distal pancreatectomy, with preservation of the splenic vessels (Kimura Technique [KT]): This surgical technique consists of a full dissection and preservation of the splenic artery and vein, ligating and sectioning all the pancreatic small vessels. Since spleen vascularisation is ensured by the splenic vessels, the spleen can be safely preserved, without having a significant number of ischaemic events, and in addition, the short gastric vessels can be safely sacrificed, if necessary. This is considered a challenging procedure, and therefore, there are a percentage of cases that cannot be finally completed using this technique.

2. Spleen-preserving distal pancreatectomy, without preservation of the splenic vessels (WT): A posterior modification of the KT aims to preserve the spleen through the short gastric vessels. In this procedure, after the pancreas is transected at the neck, both artery and splenic vein are dissected and cut at the same level and then in the splenic hilum. After performing this technique, splenic vascularisation is impaired, given that it mostly depends on the splenic artery and vein, and in some cases, splenic infarction can occur, which ultimately will lead to splenectomy. In addition, some patients will postoperatively develop segmental portal hypertension, with the appearance of perigastric and perioesophageal varicose veins, despite the reported instances of upper gastrointestinal bleeding being rare. The WT has proven to be technically less demanding than the preservation of the splenic vessels. Because of this, in many centres, it has become the technique of choice for performing a spleen-preserving LDP.

There exists an abundance of comparative studies in the literature between KT and WT, aiming to clarify which procedure is superior in terms of operative bleeding, operative time and postoperative complications. One study that aimed specifically to compare the short-term outcomes of both techniques in LDP in 140 patients from Bordeaux and Barcelona was published in 2013 by Adam et al.[37] This retrospective comparative study confirmed the feasibility of both procedures, and the operative time, blood loss and rate of conversion were equal. However, patients undergoing WT had worse results than KT, with splenic preservation rate: 84.7% vs. 96.4% (p = 0.03) and splenic complications: 10.5% vs. 0% (p = 0.03); delayed splenectomy was seen in 4.7% of the patients, and it even showed a longer hospital stay than KT (10.5 days vs. 8.2 days; p = 0.01). The authors' conclusion was that, whenever possible, the splenic vessel preservation technique should be the procedure of choice. On the other hand, performing KT does not mean long-term splenic vessel patency in all cases. Yoon et al compared splenic vessel patency after open versus laparoscopic KT and found that the patients with the latter had worse long-term splenic vein patency than those operated on by open surgery (64.3% vs. 87.0%; p = 0.022). In addition, in this study, the splenic vein patency rate was significantly better in the late period (n = 34) than in the early period (n = 35) (79.4% vs. 48.6%; p = 0.008).[38]

There are four recent meta-analysis and systematic reviews that compare both techniques and their outcomes. All of them coincide in showing no differences in pancreatic-specific complications, in particular, POPF.

The WT seems to be associated with a reduction in blood loss, especially laparoscopically, and a trend towards a reduction in operative time. In addition, all studies confirm an increased rate of splenic infarction associated with WT, which, sometimes, can lead to a delayed splenectomy. In most studies, the appearance of gastric varices is a radiological finding rather than a clinically relevant event, since variceal bleeding in this setting is thought to be exceedingly rare.[39–42]

Conversion to Open Surgery

Nowadays, the laparoscopic approach in left pancreatectomy is considered to be advantageous for patients in terms of postoperative recovery, hospital stay, postoperative pain and improved cosmetics, amongst others. However, given that LDP is a challenging surgical procedure to accomplish, sometimes, it cannot be be performed completely laparoscopically, forcing a switch to the open approach.

Conversion should be performed in any situation where surgical progression is not feasible for whatever reason (adhesions, bleeding andtumoural infiltration to the surrounding organs), and although the advantages of laparoscopy may be lost, it is rather desirable to finish the intervention safely.

Unlike other issues that really are complications, most published articles on LDP pay attention to the conversion rates, which can range between series from 0 to 35%.[3,6,11–13,20,30,32,34,43] There are many factors that can influence conversion to open surgery rate, the most important being the learning curve (which is believed to be accomplished after 10 to 17 performed procedures[13]) and the presence of malignancy, in which microscopic tumoural clearance is essential.[33,34]

DOES THE COMPLICATION RATE AFTER LAPAROSCOPIC DISTAL PANCREATECTOMY DIFFER, DEPENDING ON MALIGNANCY?

After the introduction of LDP for benign or borderline malignant lesions and the good results obtained, it has been progressively been adopted for patients with malignant lesions of the pancreas, mainly PDAC.[44,45] In this setting, oncological principles must be followed, and a formal left splenopancreatectomy with a complete regional lymphadenectomy must be performed.[46] Since this is a more extended intervention than what is usually performed in benign lesions, the fact whether LDP for PDAC is related to a higher complication rate is a reasonable question. However, up to now, there is a lack of a randomised controlled trial on LDP for PDAC,

so the evidence level is still low and comes mainly from retrospective comparative studies with ODP for PDAC.

Kooby et al published the results of a multicentre comparative study for ODP (189 patients) versus LDP (23 patients) for patients having PDAC. In a matched analysis of these patients, there were no significant differences in positive margin rates, number of nodes examined, number of patients with at least one positive node or overall survival, and the surgical approach was not independently associated with a worse survival. However, this study did not analyse postoperative complications.[47] A systematic review by Anderson et al[48] in 2014 studied the existing evidence of the outcomes of patients undergoing laparoscopic surgery for PDAC. In their analysis of LDP, they concluded that outcomes were fairly equivalent to ODP in almost every aspect. For instance, short-term oncological outcomes appear comparable and the overall appearance of postoperative complications are no different, even when comparing PF rates independently of the pancreatic stump closure method. There was even reported advantage in terms of postoperative stay in case of LDP, which may ultimately affect total costs ($10,842 vs. $13,656 for LDP and ODP, respectively), a phenomenon previously noted regarding LDP versus ODP for all indications.[49] In conclusion, despite the fact that long-term oncological outcomes are still unavailable, the laparoscopic approach does not seem to be associated with an increase in postoperative complications in patients with left-sided PDAC. In the same way, a review was done regarding the overall outcomes between the open approach and the laparoscopic approach with patients with PDAC; it had the same findings as the previous review but with the added benefit of less intraoperative blood loss.[50] However, currently, there are no randomised prospective controlled trials between ODP and LDP for PDAC. Therefore, the ongoing evidence of oncological equivalence without an increase of postoperative complications should be taken with caution, for there may exist a selection bias in the patients operated on laparoscopically.

Recently, authors from Florida have published a comparative study between ODP (28 patients) and LDP (44 patients) in patients with left-sided PDAC. They showed no differences between the two approaches in terms of operative time, but at the same time, LDP was advantageous since intraoperative blood loss, transfusion rate and hospital stay were significantly shortened. One important benefit associated with LDP in patients with PDAC was a reduced period of time from the surgical procedure to the start of the adjuvant chemotherapy treatment, a factor that may have positively influenced the unusually high survival rate (41% at 5 years); however, there does not seem to be a significant difference with the open approach.[32] A recent paper combining experiences from Tokyo and Paris showed outcomes after LDP 'en bloc' in 23 patients with PDAC. They found 47% of overall complications, with 17% complications above Clavien-Dindo IIIa and with a clinical PF rate of 17%. Survival rates for these patients at 1, 3 and 5 years were 67%, 49% and 33%, respectively, even though they did not perform splenectomy in many cases, which is a very controversial issue nowadays.[51]

A recent paper summarised a multicentre experience of 196 patients undergoing LDP for PDAC and showed a postoperative complication rate of 31.9%, while having a clinical PF rate of 15.7%. They also showed a lack of benefit in patients undergoing extended resections; however, this might well be because of more advanced tumours in these patients. It is of note that even in patients with PDAC, some institutions reported a retrieval of zero lymph nodes, which clearly reflects insufficient oncological surgery.[52]

Shin et al recently published a study regarding the outcomes of LDP in patients with PDAC and compared them with a cohort of patients operated by the open approach, as well as performed a matched comparison of 102 patients. They showed equivalent outcomes in terms of operative time, length of stay, postoperative complications and even a comparable survival between groups.[14]

CONCLUSIONS

Laparoscopic distal pancreatectomy has proven, from its introduction to its adoption, to be a feasible, reproducible and safe procedure by a large number of centres performing pancreatic surgery. High levels of evidence from randomised controlled trials is lacking, but its overall complication profile is equivalent to ODP, including the POPF rate, with some added benefits that are mainly lower blood loss and transfusion rate, shorter length of hospital stay and an improved quality of life. Even if these complications occur, their treatment can be achieved laparoscopically in most cases.

Results from LDP performance in patients with PDAC are equally attractive, with a low complication profile and equivalence in terms of patient survival compared with ODP.

REFERENCES

1. Malleo G, Salvia R, Mascetta G, et al. Assessment of a complication risk score and study of complication profile in laparoscopic distal pancreatectomy. *J Gastrointest Surg* 2014;18:2009–15. doi: 10.1007/s11605-014-2651-9.

2. Lee MK, Lewis RS, Strasberg SM, et al. Defining the post-operative morbidity index for distal pancreatectomy. *HPB (Oxford)* 2014;16:915–23. doi: 10.1111/hpb.12293.

3. Braga M, Pecorelli N, Ferrari D, Balzano G, Zuliani W, Castoldi R. Results of 100 consecutive laparoscopic distal pancreatectomies: postoperative outcome, cost-benefit analysis, and quality of life assessment. *Surg Endosc* 2015;29:1871–8. doi: 10.1007/s00464-014-3879-x.

4. Baker MS, Sherman KL, Stocker S, et al. Defining quality for distal pancreatectomy: does the laparoscopic approach protect patients from poor quality outcomes? *J Gastrointest Surg* 2013;17:273–80. doi: 10.1007/s11605-012-2104-2.

5. Cho CS, Kooby DA, Schmidt CM, et al. Laparoscopic versus open left pancreatectomy: can preoperative factors indicate the safer technique? *Ann Surg* 2011;253:975–80. doi: 10.1097/SLA.0b013e3182128869.

6. Nakamura M, Nakashima H. Laparoscopic distal pancreatectomy and pancreatoduodenectomy: is it worthwhile? A meta-analysis of laparoscopic pancreatectomy. *J Hepatobiliary Pancreat Sci* 2013;20:421–8. doi: 10.1007/s00534-012-0578-7.

7. Jin T, Altaf K, Xiong JJ, et al. A systematic review and meta-analysis of studies comparing laparoscopic and open distal pancreatectomy. *HPB (Oxford)* 2012;14:711–24. doi: 10.1111/j.1477-2574.2012.00531.x.

8. Pericleous S, Middleton N, McKay SC, Bowers KA, Hutchins RR. Systematic review and meta-analysis of case-matched studies comparing open and laparoscopic distal pancreatectomy: is it a safe procedure? *Pancreas* 2012;41:993–1000. doi: 10.1097/MPA.0b013e31824f3669.

9. Venkat R, Edil BH, Schulick RD, Lidor AO, Makary MA, Wolfgang CL. Laparoscopic Distal pancreatectomy is associated with significantly less overall morbidity compared to the open technique. *Ann Surg* 2012;255:1048–59. doi: 10.1097/SLA.0b013e318251ee09.

10. Mehrabi A, Hafezi M, Arvin J, et al. A systematic review and meta-analysis of laparoscopic versus open distal pancreatectomy for benign and malignant lesions of the pancreas: it's time to randomize. *Surgery* 2015;157:45–55. doi: 10.1016/j.surg.2014.06.081.

11. Sánchez-Cabús S, Adam J-P, Pittau G, Gelli M, Cunha AS. Laparoscopic left pancreatectomy: early results after 115 consecutive patients. *Surg Endosc* 2016;30:4480–88. doi: 10.1007/s00464-016-4780-6.

12. De Rooij T, Jilesen AP, Boerma D, et al. A nationwide comparison of laparoscopic and open distal pancreatectomy for benign and malignant disease. *J Am Coll Surg* 2015;220:263–70.e1. doi: 10.1016/j.jamcollsurg.2014.11.010.

13. Ricci C, Casadei R, Buscemi S, et al. Laparoscopic distal pancreatectomy: what factors are related to the learning curve? *Surg Today* 2015;45:50–6. doi: 10.1007/s00595-014-0872-x.

14. Shin SH, Kim SC, Song KB, et al. A comparative study of laparoscopic vs. open distal pancreatectomy for left-sided ductal adenocarcinoma: a propensity score-matched analysis. *J Am Coll Surg* 2015;220:177–85. doi: 10.1016/j. jamcollsurg.2014.10.014.

15. Mardin WA, Schleicher C, Senninger N, Mees ST. Laparoscopic versus open left pancreatectomy: can preoperative factors indicate the safer technique? *Ann Surg* 2014;259:e60. doi: 10.1097/SLA.0000000000000400.

16. Iacobone M, Citton M, Nitti D. Laparoscopic distal pancreatectomy: up-to-date and literature review. *World J Gastroenterol* 2012;18:5329–37. doi: 10.3748/wjg.v18.i38.5329.

17. Nigri GR, Rosman AS, Petrucciani N, et al. Metaanalysis of trials comparing minimally invasive and open distal pancreatectomies. *Surg Endosc* 2011;25:1642–51. doi: 10.1007/s00464-010-1456-5.

18. Bassi C, Dervenis C, Butturini G, et al. Postoperative pancreatic fistula: An international study group (ISGPF) definition. *Surgery* 2005;138:8–13. doi: 10.1016/j.surg.2005.05.001.

19. Sui C-J, Li B, Yang J-M, Wang S-J, Zhou Y-M. Laparoscopic versus open distal pancreatectomy: a meta-analysis. *Asian J Surg* 2012;35:1–8. doi: 10.1016/j.asjsur.2012.04.001.

20. Ricci C, Casadei R, Lazzarini E, et al. Laparoscopic distal pancreatectomy in Italy: a systematic review and meta-analysis. *Hepatobiliary Pancreat Dis Int* 2014;13:458–63. doi: 10.1016/S1499-3872(14)60297-6.

21. Kurahara H, Maemura K, Mataki Y, et al. Closure of the pancreas in distal pancreatectomy: comparison between bare stapler and reinforced stapler. *Hepatogastroenterology* 2014;61:2367–70. Accessed 2016 March 8. Available from: http://www.ncbi.nlm.nih.gov/pubmed/25699384.

22. Sell NM, Pucci MJ, Gabale S, et al. The influence of transection site on the development of pancreatic fistula in patients undergoing distal pancreatectomy: A review of 294 consecutive cases. *Surgery* 2015;157:1080–7. doi: 10.1016/j.surg.2015.01.014.

23. Hackert T, Büchler MW. Remnant closure after distal pancreatectomy: current state and future perspectives. *Surgeon* 2012;10:95–101. doi: 10.1016/j.surge.2011.10.003.

24. Diener MK, Seiler CM, Rossion I, et al. Efficacy of stapler versus hand-sewn closure after distal pancreatectomy (DISPACT): a randomised, controlled multicentre trial. *Lancet* 2011;377:1514–22. doi: 10.1016/S0140-6736(11)60237-7.

25. Zhang H, Zhu F, Shen M, et al. Systematic review and meta-analysis comparing three techniques for pancreatic remnant closure following distal pancreatectomy. *Br J Surg* 2015;102:4–15.

26. Blansfield J a, Rapp MM, Chokshi RJ, et al. Novel method of stump closure for distal pancreatectomy with a 75% reduction in pancreatic fistula rate. *J Gastrointest Surg* 2012;16:524–8. doi: 10.1007/s11605-011-1794-1.

27. Wente MN, Bassi C, Dervenis C, et al. Delayed gastric emptying (DGE) after pancreatic surgery: a suggested definition by the International Study Group of Pancreatic Surgery (ISGPS). *Surgery* 2007;142:761–8. doi: 10.1016/j.surg.2007.05.005.

28. Wente MN, Veit J a, Bassi C, et al. Postpancreatectomy hemorrhage (PPH): an International Study Group of Pancreatic Surgery (ISGPS) definition. *Surgery* 2007;142:20–5. doi: 10.1016/j.surg.2007.02.001.

29. Soh YF, Kow AWC, Wong KY, et al. Perioperative outcomes of laparoscopic and open distal pancreatectomy: our institution's 5-year experience. *Asian J Surg* 2012;35:29–36. doi: 10.1016/j.asjsur.2012.04.005.

30. Malleo G, Damoli I, Marchegiani G, et al. Laparoscopic distal pancreatectomy: analysis of trends in surgical techniques, patient selection, and outcomes. *Surg Endosc* 2015;29:1952–62. doi: 10.1007/s00464-014-3890-2.

31. de Rooij T, Tol JA, van Eijck CH, et al. Outcomes of distal pancreatectomy for pancreatic ductal adenocarcinoma in the Netherlands: a nationwide retrospective analysis. *Ann Surg Oncol* 2016;23:585–91. doi: 10.1245/s10434-015-4930-4.

32. Stauffer JA, Coppola A, Mody K, Asbun HJ. Laparoscopic versus open distal pancreatectomy for pancreatic adenocarcinoma. *World J Surg* 2016;40:1477–84. doi: 10.1007/s00268-016-3412-6.

33. Hasselgren K, Halldestam I, Fraser MP, et al. Does the introduction of laparoscopic distal pancreatectomy jeopardize patient safety and well-being? *Scand J Surg* 2016;pii:1457496915626838. [Epub ahead of print]. doi: 10.1177/1457496915626838.

34. Braga M, Ridolfi C, Balzano G, Castoldi R, Pecorelli N, Di Carlo V. Learning curve for laparoscopic distal pancreatectomy in a high-volume hospital. *Updates Surg* 2012;64:179–83. doi: 10.1007/s13304-012-0163-2.

35. Shi N, Liu SL, Li YT, You L, Dai MH, Zhao YP. Splenic preservation versus splenectomy during distal pancreatectomy: a systematic review and meta-analysis. *Ann Surg Oncol* 2016;23:365–74. doi: 10.1245/s10434-015-4870-z.

36. Fernández-Cruz L, Martínez I, Gilabert R, Cesar-Borges G, Astudillo E, Navarro S. Laparoscopic distal pancreatectomy combined with preservation of the spleen for cystic neoplasms of the pancreas. *J Gastrointest Surg* 2004;8:493–501. doi: 10.1016/j.gassur.2003.11.014.

37. Jean-Philippe Adam, Alexandre Jacquin, Christophe Laurent, et al. Laparoscopic spleen-preserving distal pancreatectomy: splenic vessel preservation compared with the Warshaw technique. *JAMA Surg* 2013;148:246–52. doi: 10.1001/jamasurg.2013.768.

38. Yoon YS, Lee KH, Han HS, et al. Effects of laparoscopic versus open surgery on splenic vessel patency after spleen and splenic vessel-preserving distal pancreatectomy: a retrospective multicenter study. *Surg Endosc* 2015;29:583–8. doi: 10.1007/s00464-014-3701-9.

39. Partelli S, Cirocchi R, Randolph J, Parisi A, Coratti A, Falconi M. A systematic review and meta-analysis of spleen-preserving distal pancreatectomy with preservation or ligation of the splenic artery and vein. *Surgeon* 2016;14:109–18. doi: 10.1016/j.surge.2015.11.002.

40. Elabbasy F, Gadde R, Hanna MM, Sleeman D, Livingstone A, Yakoub D. Minimally invasive spleen-preserving distal pancreatectomy: Does splenic vessel preservation have better postoperative outcomes? A systematic review and meta-analysis. *Hepatobiliary Pancreat Dis Int* 2015;14: 346–53. Accessed 2016 March 22. Available from: http://www.ncbi.nlm.nih.gov/pubmed/26256077.

41. Yu X, Li H, Jin C, et al. Splenic vessel preservation versus Warshaw's technique during spleen-preserving distal pancreatectomy: a meta-analysis and systematic review. *Langenbeck's Arch Surg/Dtsch Gesellschaft für Chir* 2015;400:183–91. doi: 10.1007/s00423-015-1273-3.

42. Jain G, Chakravartty S, Patel AG. Spleen-preserving distal pancreatectomy with and without splenic vessel ligation: a systematic review. *HPB (Oxford)* 2013;15:403–10. doi: 10.1111/hpb.12003.

43. Kim H, Song KB, Hwang DW, et al. A single-center experience with the laparoscopic Warshaw technique in 122 consecutive patients. *Surg Endosc* 2016;30:4057–64. doi: 10.1007/s00464-015-4720-x.

44. Hilal MA, Takhar AS. Laparoscopic left pancreatectomy: current concepts. *Pancreatology* 2013;13:443–8. doi: 10.1016/j.pan.2013.04.196.

45. Kneuertz PJ, Patel SH, Chu CK, et al. Laparoscopic distal pancreatectomy: trends and lessons learned through an 11-year experience. *J Am Coll Surg* 2012;215:167–76. doi: 10.1016/j.jamcollsurg.2012.03.023.

46. Fernández-Cruz L, Cosa R, Blanco L, Levi S, López-Boado M-A, Navarro S. Curative laparoscopic resection for pancreatic neoplasms: a critical analysis from a single institution. *J Gastrointest Surg* 2007;11:1607–21; discussion 1621–2. doi: 10.1007/s11605-007-0266-0.

47. Kooby D a, Hawkins WG, Schmidt CM, et al. A multicenter analysis of distal pancreatectomy for adenocarcinoma: is laparoscopic resection appropriate? *J Am Coll Surg* 2010;210:779–85, 786–7. doi: 10.1016/j.jamcollsurg.2009.12.033.

48. Anderson B, Karmali S. Laparoscopic resection of pancreatic adenocarcinoma: dream or reality? *World J Gastroenterol* 2014;20:14255–62. doi: 10.3748/wjg.v20.i39.14255.

49. Rutz DR, Squires MH, Maithel SK, et al. Cost comparison analysis of open versus laparoscopic distal pancreatectomy. *HPB (Oxford)* 2014;16:907–14. doi: 10.1111/hpb.12288.

50. Björnsson B, Sandström P. Laparoscopic distal pancreatectomy for adenocarcinoma of the pancreas. *World J Gastroenterol* 2014;20:13402–11. doi: 10.3748/wjg.v20.i37.13402.

51. Kawaguchi Y, Fuks D, Nomi T, Levard H, Gayet B. Laparoscopic distal pancreatectomy employing radical en bloc procedure for adenocarcinoma: Technical details and outcomes. *Surgery* 2015;157:1106–12. doi: 10.1016/j.surg.2014.12.015.

52. Sahakyan MA, Kazaryan AM, Rawashdeh M, et al. Laparoscopic distal pancreatectomy for pancreatic ductal adenocarcinoma: results of a multicenter cohort study on 196 patients. *Surg Endosc* 2016;30:3409–18. doi: 10.1007/s00464-015-4623-x.

Prevention and Management of Complications after Ablative Therapies on the Pancreas

S. Paiella, R. Salvia, G. Marchegiani, M. D'Onofrio and C. Bassi

ABSTRACT

Since the advent of modern radiology, the use of ablative therapies for pancreatic cancer has become more common. The underlying rationale is the need to offer an alternative treatment option to the locally advanced stage of this lethal disease, the one most common diagnosed. Several types of ablation have been introduced, using different kinds of energy and conveying devices. The continuous development and introduction of new ablative techniques can be explained by the peculiar structure of the pancreatic parenchyma and peripancreatic structures. In fact, each attempt to ablate the tumour carry with itself a certain risk of damaging the surrounding vital pancreas or peripancreatic vessels or organs. The complications arising after the application of ablative therapies are potentially serious and even life-threatening. For these reasons, these should be used after multidisciplinary decisions by expert pancreatologists. This chapter provides an insight on the prevention and management of complications arising after radiofrequency ablation and irreversible electroporation on locally advanced pancreatic cancer, the two most used ablative therapies on pancreas.

KEYWORDS

Pancreatic cancer, radiofrequency ablation, irreversible electroporation, tumour ablation, pancreatic surgery complications

INTRODUCTION

The continuing progress of oncology research in the study of the genome of cancers and improvements in surgical techniques are a constant encouragement to those involved in surgical oncology. While waiting to discover new methods for early diagnosis of cancer, the surgeon has the task of providing the best care possible to patients, even if only in terms of palliation of symptoms.

The use of ablative therapies over the years has gained the interest of the scientific community, insofar, that with proper precautions and in selected cases, ablative therapies may represent a valuable new treatment option in the arsenal of the surgeon. Advances in science have brought many innovations that have enabled the development of different types of ablation, such as radiofrequency ablation (RFA), irreversible electroporation (IRE), microwave ablation (MWA), cryoablation and high-intensity focussed ultrasound (HIFU). The possibility of using different types of energy directed towards the tumour responds to different needs to be addressed, depending on the organ that must be treated—liver or pancreas.

The scientific literature shows encouraging data for each of these ablative therapies. However, it must be kept in mind that the ablation is, in fact, in most cases, a nonselective activity, potentially accountable for damage to healthy tissue around the tumour. Complications after ablative therapies are potentially very dangerous, and therefore, they must be applied by experienced and well-trained specialists. The selection of patients to be submitted to ablative procedures must be done after decisions in multidisciplinary settings. This chapter will provide an overview of the potential risks associated with the application of ablative therapies on the pancreas, the organ that, in the last years, has received considerable interest in this field. Directions on how to prevent and manage the potential complications will also be provided.

ABLATIVE THERAPIES AND PANCREAS

Pancreatic adenocarcinoma (PDAC) is the fourth leading cause of death from cancer in Western countries.[1] By the time that PDAC is diagnosed, the majority of patients have disease that has spread to distant locations. Only about 20 to 30% of patients are candidates for surgical resection. In 40% of cases, the PDAC is a locally advanced pancreatic cancer (LAPC), for a more or less extended involvement of the mesentericoportal arteriovenous axis. Vascular involvement can make surgery difficult and with a high risk of not being radical, without providing real advantages in terms of survival.[2,3] Ablative therapies are an increasingly popular therapeutic choice in the multimodal treatment of LAPC. The rationale of the use of ablative procedures is the possibility of inducing a local tumour cytoreduction (already demonstrated by RFA)[4] through the use of various forms of energy, which, in the end, permit complete tumour ablation. Considering also the potential systemic effects arising from the application of these local therapies, their application looks even more attractive.[5] Their application should be restricted to selected cases and should be made by pancreatologists (surgeons, interventional radiologists and endoscopists) working in high-volume pancreatic treatment centres. In fact, the ablative procedures are not free from complications; they are sometimes serious, life threatening and difficult to manage if not carried out by teams who have already gained enough confidence in pancreatic surgery.

Over the years, different types of ablative procedures have been applied to LAPC, such as RFA, IRE, HIFU, MWA and cryotherapy. Since the vast majority of publications in the literature on ablative therapies and LAPC deals with RFA and IRE, this discussion will focus primarily on these two techniques.

HINTS OF TECHNIQUE

Radiofrequency Ablation

Radiofrequency ablation is a thermal technique. A special generator creates a medium-frequency alternating current, delivered into the core of the tumour by proper needle electrodes, that induces ionic agitation. The ionic agitation produces friction and therefore heat that leads to coagulative necrosis and denaturation of proteins within the tumour. Inside the needle electrodes, there are tiny thermocouples that allow a constant adjustment of the local temperature, according to the preprocedure settings.

Different types of needle electrodes have been produced, single- or multitip, fixed or expandable and monopolar or bipolar, with different types of inner cooling. The temperatures applied range from 30°C to 105°C, whereas the duration of the application of heat ranges from 5 minutes to 15 minutes, according to various reports.[6] There are several different ways in which an RFA may be performed, that is, by laparoscopy, percutaneously, endoscopically and open, but it is always performed under ultrasound or computed tomography (CT) guidance. When applied under ultrasound guidance, an instantaneous effect of the procedure can be appreciated (gas bubbles formation within the tumour; Figure 35.1).

Figure 35.2 shows a decentralised needle electrode placement on purpose. Owing to the morphology of the tumour, the treatment was divided into two halves (left and right). It is necessary to centre the lesion as much as possible, to optimise the delivery of energy and to avoid the spreading of head to the surrounding tissues, except when the shape of the tumour is complex.

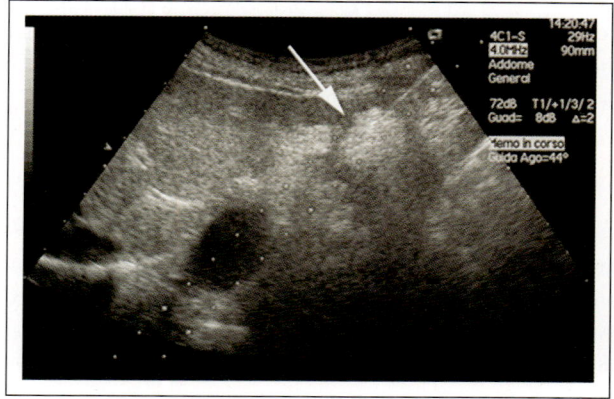

Figure 35.1 Gas bubbles formation during radiofrequency ablation of the pancreas.

Courtesy: Salvatore Paiella, Roberto Salvia, Giovanni Marchegiani, Mirko D'Onofrio and Claudio Bassi.

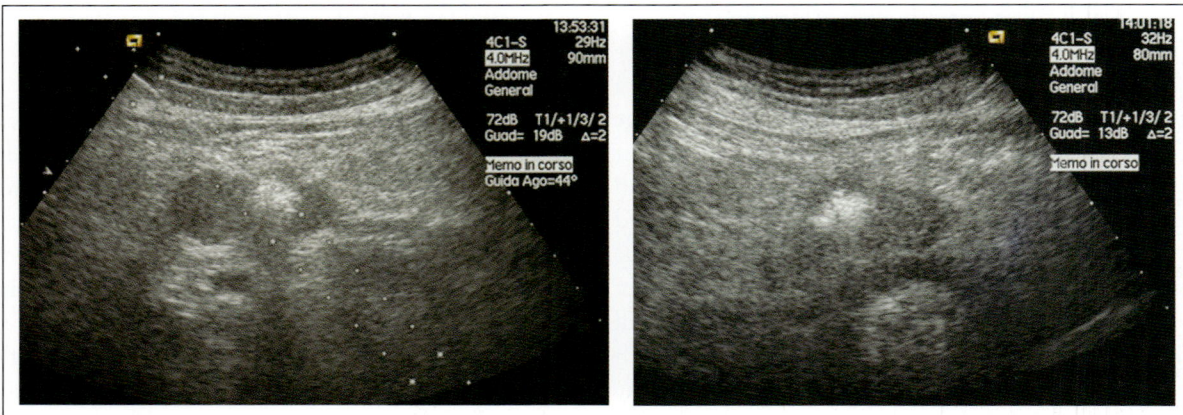

Figure 35.2 Decentralised needle electrode placement on purpose.

Irreversible Electroporation

Irreversible electroporation is considered a nonthermal ablative therapy. Short high-voltage electric current fields developed between couples of monopolar electrodes (or single bipolar electrodes) are able to induce irreversible cell damage and death.[7,8] It has a different mode of action from the RFA in that it does not damage the extrapancreatic surrounding structures such as blood vessels, nerves and bile ducts.[9–11] Even the extracellular matrix is spared, so after ablation, it can act as a scaffold for tissue regeneration.

Although under high-energy intensity, the IRE develops high local temperatures, using the common settings used in the clinical scenarios (e.g., 70–100 pulses, 90 microseconds for pulse, 1.5 KV/cm and spacing of up to 2 cm between probe pairs), local temperatures are around 50°C, a temperature developed already sufficient to induce cell death via apoptosis.[12,13] Like RFA, it can be applied through the open surgical, laparoscopic or percutaneous approaches. For this reason, IRE is considered a 'nonthermal' ablative therapy. The technique of application of IRE has been described in detail by Martin.[14]

PITFALLS AND POTENTIAL RISKS

Every medal has its reverse, and when planning to use ablative therapies, careful attention must be paid to the ablation program to avoid incurring severe complications related to uncontrolled heat diffusion. The choice of the proper ablative therapy to use must be based on the type of cancer, the patient characteristics and the expertise of the operators.

Radiofrequency Ablation

The strength of RFA is the heat generated, but at the same time, this is its weakness (Figure 35.3). The thermal

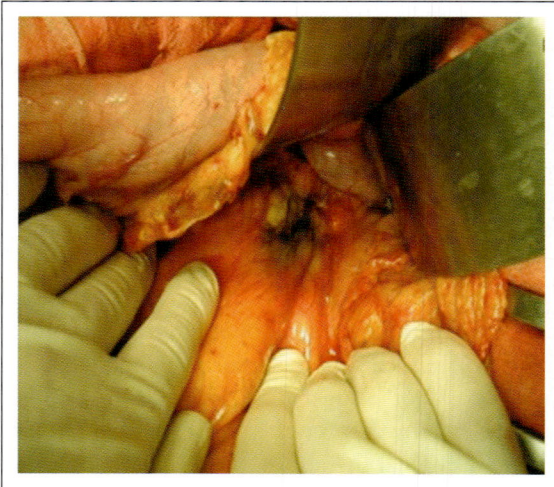

Figure 35.3 Result of the application of radiofrequency ablation on pancreas. A burn of the pancreatic surface can be appreciated at the end of the procedures.

Courtesy: Salvatore Paiella, Roberto Salvia, Giovanni Marchegiani, Mirko D'Onofrio and Claudio Bassi.

damage done by RFA is not selective, and although one can 'predict' the volume of the ablated area, considering the setting chosen before RFA, it is not possible to predict precisely the diffusion of the heat to the surrounding structures. In addition, the pancreatic parenchyma is particularly sensitive to a thermal insult and responds with an inflammatory process that may progress towards severe pancreatitis and is surrounded by the stomach, duodenum and large peripancreatic vessels; complications arising from an injury of these structures are potentially life threatening. The thermocouples located at the tips of the needle electrodes ensure the maintenance of the set temperature but not the control of its spread to the surrounding tissues. An experimental animal model has clearly demonstrated the histopathological effects of heat on the duodenum, the pancreatic parenchyma and peripancreatic vessels with the phenomena of pancreatic and duodenal necrosis and thrombosis of small venous peripancreatic wall.[15]

Although in the application of RFA on the liver, it is essential to include a safety margin—from oncological point of view, of 0.5 cm of peritumoural tissue, on the pancreas—in our opinion, based on our clinical experience, this is very difficult as well as risky. In fact, by definition, the LAPC extensively involves the peripancreatic arteriovenous vascular axis, and it is almost impossible to get complete tumour ablation, at least for tumours of the head of the pancreas, without visceral or vascular damages. Furthermore, the pancreatic tumour is not round and the margins are not always clear and, often, are lost in the peripancreatic surrounding structures.

In theory, the presence of metallic stents, at least those uncovered, within the bile duct may make the spread of the heat to the surrounding tissues, induced by the same stent overheated, even more unpredictable. However, this aspect has never been proved experimentally or clinically.

The heat produced by RFA is also able to activate the vascular endothelium and to cause different grades of thrombotic phenomena on the mesentericoportal axis.

Unlike other solid organs,[16] as far as we know, the phenomenon of needle track seeding after the application of RFA on the pancreas has never been reported. An increase in temperature within 24 to 48 hours after RFA, without any clinical symptom, is common and probably a reabsorption fever.

Irreversible Electroporation

The underlying physical principles make the IRE more secure than RFA. Lower local temperatures produced and the peculiar mechanism of action reduce the possibility of causing postablation adverse events. Despite the fact that IRE does not damage the extracellular matrix and the vascular, biliary and nervous structures,[9–11] temperatures are high enough to cause both pancreatitis from thermal damage and progression of a mesentericoportal thrombosis.[17] Although some studies warned that the IRE can overheat metal stents,[18] recently, a study has clarified that there is no direct metal stent overheating as a result of the IRE, but rather, this may occur as an indirect heat diffusion to the stent by the overheated surrounding tissues.[13] In parallel, the presence of a metal stent may change the desired therapeutic effects by distorting the electric fields and making tumour ablation ineffective.[13,19]

Irreversible electroporation is performed by introducing multiple needle electrodes to create the desired ablation.[14]

This increases the risk of producing traumatic injuries to the duodenum (for the lateromedial transduodenal placement), the pancreatic and the bile duct.

In addition, for RFA, the phenomenon of tumour seeding has never been reported after the application of IRE on the pancreas.

TRICKS FOR PREVENTING COMPLICATIONS

In general, the preparation of a patient for an ablative procedure is comparable to that of any major surgery. An accurate radiological study of the tumour is of utmost importance to plan the ablation, the goals to achieve and the needle-electrode positioning strategy. The placement of the needle electrodes, guided by ultrasound or CT, should be accurate and should take into account the size and the shape of the tumour, as well as its relations with the vascular structures and the surrounding organs.

Radiofrequency Ablation

Radiofrequency ablation can be applied to tumours localised throughout the pancreas. Its safety and efficacy mostly depend on the experience of the operator who inserts the needle electrodes. The ideal settings are up to 25 Watts of power and a temperature of 85°C to 90°C for 5 minutes.[6] An ablation zone ranging from 1 to 4 cm can be obtained according to the pre-RFA setting and the type of needle electrodes used (to increase the size of the area, it is possible to move the needle electrodes and repeat the treatment). Although all available needle electrodes are fitted with a system of irrigation water, used to minimise possible damage caused by heat diffusion, in case of pancreatic head tumours, it is important to perform a concurrent cooling of the duodenal lumen through endovisceral instillation of saline cooled down to 5°C through a feeding tube. A direct endoluminal cooling of blood through a mesentericoportal catheter is also possible.[15] Moreover, to reduce the risk of damaging the surrounding structures, it is fundamental to maintain a safety distance of 10 mm from the duodenum and of 15 mm from the mesentericoportal axis.[6]

To prevent tumour seeding, the track should be ablated. In our institution we place a soft laminar drain near the ablation area.

Irreversible Electroporation

The number of needle electrodes that can be positioned to perform the IRE ranges from two to six, depending on the location, the form and the size of the tumour. A tumour diameter greater than 5 cm represents an absolute contraindication to IRE and 1 cm of healthy tissue within the area of tumour ablation should be included.[14]

However, the ideal settings of IRE sometimes collide with the clinical scenario. Locally advanced pancreatic cancers are often ellipsoid rather than spherical and may surround the peripancreatic vessels. The placement of multiple needle electrodes may be difficult, especially if it is necessary to realise more pullbacks in order to obtain the maximum possible ablation. Besides, we must also point out that, in an animal model, a certain risk of tumour progression in case of incomplete ablation has been reported.[20] For these considerations, the planning of the procedure is of paramount importance to perform a complete ablation and to avoid thermal damage.

If necessary, a fully covered metallic stent should be selectively chosen to drain cholestasis, so that it can be easily removed before ablation.

Owing to induction of an electric current, IRE is contraindicated in the presence of pacemakers or defibrillators, recent myocardial infarction and a history of epilepsy.

MANAGEMENT OF COMPLICATIONS

Ablative procedures should be regarded as surgical or radiological interventional high-risk treatments. The mortality and morbidity rates after the use of RFA on the pancreas range from 0 to 11% and from 4 to 22%, respectively. For IRE, more encouraging numbers have been reported, with mortality and morbidity rates of 2% and 13%, respectively.[21] Table 35.1 shows all types of ablative therapies–related complications reported in the literature after the use of RFA and IRE. Complications most likely related to surgical procedures associated with ablative therapies were not included.

Table 35.1 All-encompassing list of all types of complication reported in literature after the application of radiofrequency ablation and irreversible electroporation on pancreas

Complication	Radiofrequency ablation			Irreversible electroporation		
	Yes/No	References	%	Yes/No	References	%
Bleeding/haematoma	Yes	25–27, 43	0.7–18.7	Yes	28–30, 39, 40, 42	1.3–8
Duodenal ulcer/perforation	Yes	26, 43	4–4.4	Yes	18, 31, 32, 39	0.5–8.1
Pancreatic fistula	Yes	25, 26, 43	2.7–18.8	Yes	28, 31, 32, 42	4.7–5.4
Gastric ulcer/perforation	No			Yes	39	2
Pancreatitis	Yes	26, 33, 34	3.3–100	Yes	29, 31, 40, 41	7.1–20
PM thrombosis	Yes	26, 43	2.6	Yes	29–31, 32, 40, 42	0.6–12.5
Duodenal fistula	No			Yes	32, 35	8.1–10
Pseudoaneurysm	No			Yes	31	NA
Abdominal abscess (drained)	Yes	26, 34, 43	1.1–3	Yes	28	9.5
Reoperation	Yes	26, 43	0.5–1.6	Yes	28	9.5
Arterial thrombosis	No			Yes	31, 42	2
Pancreatic abscess	No			Yes	35	10
Cholangitis	No			Yes	28	4.7
Liver abscess	No			Yes	28	4.7
Biliary peritonitis	No			Yes	28	4.7
Ascites	Yes	36, 37	28.5–66.6	Yes	31, 42	4.1
Biliary fistula	Yes	36, 43	2.2–6	Yes	41, 42	6.2–20
Fistula/abscess abdominal wall	No			Yes	28	4.7
Lymphatic fistula	Yes	26	0.5	No		
Pseudocyst	Yes	27	33.3	No		
Bile duct stricture	No			Yes	31, 39	2
90-day mortality	Yes	26, 27, 43	1.5–25	Yes	18, 30, 38, 39	1.5–11

Abbreviations: PM, portomesenteric; NA: not available.

As can be seen from Table 35.1, adverse events that may occur after application of RFA and IRE can be serious and sometimes life threatening. Hence, again, ablative therapies must be applied only by well-trained specialists in high-volume centres of pancreatic surgery.

The early identification of postprocedural complications relies principally on case studies. Postoperative abdominal pain that does not respond to analgesia may ring an alarm bell, especially when surgical procedures were not performed together with the ablation. A rapidly evolving intrapancreatic haematoma (often resulting from a lesion of the gastroduodenal artery or one of its branches) may not be highlighted by the drain; in such cases (and especially for percutaneous treatments), a contrast-enhanced CT scan of the abdomen may be useful in identifying bleeding complications. Once haemodynamic stability is achieved and the cause of the haemorrhage identified, a medical endoscopic approach can help in arresting the bleeding from duodenum or stomach, whereas endovascular embolisation may be required to stop bleeding from the splanchnic vessels. The last choice, in case the previous approaches failure, is urgent surgery, even if it means performing a pancreatic resection.

Duodenal and gastric ulcers and perforations can occur as a consequence of the application of ablative therapies (Figure 35.4). In such cases, when the extent of the damage is minimal, endoscopy and interventional radiology (to drain fluid collections) can be attempted

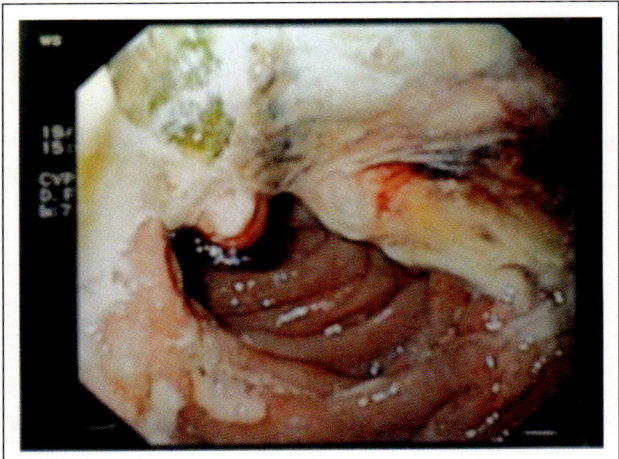

Figure 35.4 Endoscopic vision of a duodenal burn after radiofrequency ablation of a pancreatic head cancer. An urgent pancreatoduodenectomy was then performed due to further massive bleeding from pancreas and duodenum, which was uncontrollable with endovascular approaches.

Courtesy: Salvatore Paiella, Roberto Salvia, Giovanni Marchegiani, Mirko D'Onofrio and Claudio Bassi.

initially. Surgical treatment should be saved only for those that cannot be managed conservatively.

Young patients may have a normal peritumoural pancreas, more sensitive to thermal injury, and this can increase the risk of iatrogenic acute pancreatitis. The pancreatitis from thermal damage potentially developed must be diagnosed and treated according to the Atlanta guidelines.[22] An asymptomatic temporary rise in postoperative amylase and lipase, rapidly responsive to fasting and moisturising, sometimes occurs.

External iatrogenic pancreatic fistulae must be treated promptly, so it is important to diagnose them early. A patient who has undergone ablative therapy and presents with a clear pancreatic discharge or one that is typically brown as a result of pancreatitis and one that has a high amylase level most likely has an iatrogenic pancreatic fistula. However, although possible, it is rare to find clear pancreatic output from the drain, as a consequence of a selective rupture of the main pancreatic duct. In the vast majority of cases, the output is brown as result of the underlying pancreatic inflammation. A three-phase CT of the abdomen performed early in the first days after the procedure can be helpful in determining the degree of pancreatitis and the possible presence of undrained peripancreatic fluid collections. If a selective rupture of the main pancreatic duct is suspected, several types of diagnostic radiological examinations can help reach the diagnosis [selective fistulography through the drain, endoscopic retrograde cholangiopancreatography (ERCP) and magnetic resonance cholangiopancreatography (MRCP) with or without secretin enhancement]. Most patients with iatrogenic external pancreatic fistulae respond well to conservative treatment with gut rest, fluid and electrolyte balance, nasojejunal feeding and broad-spectrum antibiotic therapy to prevent or treat infectious complications. Drain placement using interventional radiology can be indicated to remove fluid collections.

There are no specific studies on the management of postablation mesentericoportal thrombosis; hence, there is need to borrow the experience from the application of RFA on the liver. A nonoccluding mesentericoportal thrombus can be considered a minor complication. In most cases, it is not associated with symptoms or an increase in liver enzymes and does not require an increased dosage of anticoagulants. Radiological monitoring with a contrast-enhanced CT scan of the abdomen at 1 month and every 3 months may be useful to track its evolution.[23] Complete occlusion of the portal and superior mesenteric veins by a thrombus can be very dangerous and responsible for an acute impairment of liver function and intestinal infarction. In such cases, early appropriate anticoagulant therapy is mandatory to stop the otherwise-irreversible necrosis.[24] In our experience (unpublished data), we no longer have encountered phenomena of mesentericoportal thrombosis after reducing the temperature to 85°C and maintaining 10 to 15 mm of distance from the mesentericoportal axis.

An early postoperative CT scan (24–48 hours after the ablation) may be performed to investigate early complications such as mesentericoportal thrombosis, intra- or extrapancreatic haematomas and gross fluid collections. At our institution, we usually run a radiological control by CT 1 week after the procedure or at discharge if earlier. Radiological scanning should be performed subsequently to investigate the possible progression of the disease (local or systemic) or the potential development of long-term postablation adverse events (progression of pre-existent mesentericoportal thrombosis).

CONCLUSIONS

Ablative therapies such as RFA and IRE are intriguing and promising treatment options for the multimodal approach to LAPC. However, their use is not devoid of risks, and possible ablative-related complications may occur and even be life threatening. They should be used by well-trained specialists after careful and multidisciplinary planning, involving surgeons, oncologists, gastroenterologists and interventional radiologists. The identification of complications is entrusted to the clinical evaluation assisted by radiology; however, their management is equal to the typical postoperative care applied to pancreatic surgery.

REFERENCES

1. American Cancer Society Cancer Facts & Figures 2013. [Online] 2013. Available from: http://www.cancer.org/research/cancerfactsfigures/cancerfactsfigures/cancer-facts-figures-2013.
2. Giovinazzo F, Turri G, Katz MH, Heaton N, Ahmed I. Meta-analysis of benefits of portal-superior mesenteric vein resection in pancreatic resection for ductal adenocarcinoma. *Br J Surg* 2016;103:179–91.
3. Mollberg N, Rahbari NN, Koch M, et al. Arterial resection during pancreatectomy for pancreatic cancer: a systematic review and meta-analysis. *Ann Surg* 2011;254:882–93.
4. D'Onofrio M, Barbi E, Girelli R, et al. Variation of tumoral marker after radiofrequency ablation of pancreatic adenocarcinoma. *J Gastrointest Oncol* 2016;7:213–20.
5. Chu KF, Dupuy DE. Thermal ablation of tumours: biological mechanisms and advances in therapy. *Nat Rev Cancer* 2014;14:199–208.
6. Fegrachi S, Molenaar IQ, Klaessens JH, Besselink MG, Offerhaus JA, van Hillegersberg R. Radiofrequency ablation of the pancreas with and without intraluminal duodenal cooling in a porcine model. *J Surg Res* 2013;184:867–72.
7. Rubinsky B, Onik G, Mikus P. Irreversible electroporation: a new ablation modality–clinical implications. *Technol Cancer Res Treat* 2007;6:37–48.
8. Al-Sakere B, Andre F, Bernat C, et al. Tumor ablation with irreversible electroporation. *PloS One* 2007;2:e1135.
9. Maor E, Ivorra A, Leor J, Rubinsky B. Irreversible electroporation attenuates neointimal formation after angioplasty. *IEEE Trans Biomed Eng* 2008;55:2268–74.
10. Schoellnast H, Monette S, Ezell PC, et al. Acute and subacute effects of irreversible electroporation on nerves: experimental study in a pig model. *Radiology* 2011;260:421–7.
11. Silk MT, Wimmer T, Lee KS, et al. Percutaneous ablation of peribiliary tumors with irreversible electroporation. *J Vasc Interv Radiol* 2014;25:112–8.
12. Faroja M, Ahmed M, Appelbaum L, et al. Irreversible electroporation ablation: is all the damage nonthermal? *Radiology* 2013;266:462–70.
13. Scheffer HJ, Vogel JA, van den Bos W, et al. Comment to: Mansson C, Nilsson A, Karlson B-M. Severe complications with irreversible electroporation of the pancreas in the presence of a metallic stent: a warning of a procedure that never should be performed. *Acta Radiologica Short Reports* 2014;3:1–3. *Acta Radiol Open* 2015;4:2058460115584111.
14. Martin RC. Irreversible electroporation of locally advanced pancreatic head adenocarcinoma. *J Gastrointest Surg* 2013;17:1850–6.
15. Geranios A, Pikoulis E, Papalois A, et al. Radiofrequency ablation of the pancreas: protective effect of local cooling techniques. *Am Surg* 2015;81:483–91.
16. Howenstein MJ, Sato KT. Complications of radiofrequency ablation of hepatic, pulmonary, and renal neoplasms. *Semin Intervent Radiol* 2010;27:285–95.
17. Scheffer HJ, Nielsen K, de Jong MC, et al. Irreversible electroporation for nonthermal tumor ablation in the clinical setting: a systematic review of safety and efficacy. *J Vasc Intervent Radiol* 2014;25:997–1011; quiz.
18. Mansson C, Nilsson A, Karlson BM. Severe complications with irreversible electroporation of the pancreas in the presence of a metallic stent: a warning of a procedure that never should be performed. *Acta Radiol Short Rep* 2014;3:2047981614556409.
19. Dunki-Jacobs EM, Philips P, Martin RC, 2nd. Evaluation of thermal injury to liver, pancreas and kidney during irreversible electroporation in an in vivo experimental model. *Br J Surg* 2014;101:1113–21.
20. Philips P, Li Y, Li S, St Hill CR, Martin RC. Efficacy of irreversible electroporation in human pancreatic adenocarcinoma: advanced murine model. *Mol Ther Methods Clin Dev* 2015;2:15001.
21. Rombouts SJ, Vogel JA, van Santvoort HC, et al. Systematic review of innovative ablative therapies for the

treatment of locally advanced pancreatic cancer. *Br J Surg* 2015;102:182–93.

22. Banks PA, Bollen TL, Dervenis C, et al. Classification of acute pancreatitis–2012: revision of the Atlanta classification and definitions by international consensus. *Gut* 2013;62:102–11.

23. Kim AY, Rhim H, Park M, et al. Venous thrombosis after radiofrequency ablation for hepatocellular carcinoma. *AJR Am J Roentgenol* 2011;197:1474–80.

24. de Baere T, Risse O, Kuoch V, et al. Adverse events during radiofrequency treatment of 582 hepatic tumors. *AJR Am J Roentgenol* 2003;181:695–700.

25. Wu Y, Tang Z, Fang H, Gao S, et al. High operative risk of cool-tip radiofrequency ablation for unresectable pancreatic head cancer. *J Surg Oncol* 2006;94:392–5.

26. Frigerio I, Giardino A, Girelli R, Regi P, Scopelliti F. RFA and pancreatic cancer: 5 years experience from a single center. *Eur J Surg Oncol* 2013;39:S46.

27. Matsui Y, Nakagawa A, Kamiyama Y, Yamamoto K, Kubo N, Nakase Y. Selective thermocoagulation of unresectable pancreatic cancers by using radiofrequency capacitive heating. *Pancreas* 2000;20:14–20.

28. Lambert L, Horejs J, Krska Z, et al. Treatment of locally advanced pancreatic cancer by percutaneous and intraoperative irreversible electroporation: general hospital cancer center experience. *Neoplasma* 2016;63:269–73.

29. Narayanan G, Hosein PJ, Arora G, et al. Percutaneous Irreversible electroporation for downstaging and control of unresectable pancreatic adenocarcinoma. *J Vasc Interv Radiol* 2012;23:1613–1621.

30. Philips P, Hays D, Martin RC. Irreversible electroporation ablation (IRE) of unresectable soft tissue tumors: learning curve evaluation in the first 150 patients treated. *PloS One* 2013;8:e76260.

31. Martin RC, 2nd, Kwon D, Chalikonda S, et al. Treatment of 200 locally advanced (stage III) pancreatic adenocarcinoma patients with irreversible electroporation: safety and efficacy. *Ann Surg* 2015;262:486–94; discussion 92–4.

32. Martin RC, Philips P, Ellis S, Hayes D, Bagla S. Irreversible electroporation of unresectable soft tissue tumors with vascular invasion: effective palliation. *BMC Cancer* 2014;14:540.

33. Elias D, Baton O, Sideris L, Lasser P, Pocard M. Necrotizing pancreatitis after radiofrequency destruction of pancreatic tumours. *Eur J Surg Oncol* 2004;30:85–7.

34. Singh, V, Varshney S, Sewkani A, et al. Radiofrequency ablation of unresectable pancreatic carcinoma: 10-year experience from single centre. *Pancreatology* 2011; 11:52.

35. Paiella S, Butturini G, Frigerio I, et al. Safety and feasibility of Irreversible Electroporation (IRE) in patients with locally advanced pancreatic cancer: results of a prospective study. *Dig Surg* 2015;32:90–7.

36. Casadei R, Ricci C, Pezzilli R, et al. A prospective study on radiofrequency ablation locally advanced pancreatic cancer. *Hepatobiliary Pancreat Dis Int* 2010;9:306–11.

37. Varshney S, Sewkani A, Sharma S, et al. Radiofrequency ablation of unresectable pancreatic carcinoma: feasibility, efficacy and safety. *J Pancreas* 2006;7:74–8.

38. Martin RC, 2nd, McFarland K, Ellis S, Velanovich V. Irreversible electroporation therapy in the management of locally advanced pancreatic adenocarcinoma. *J Am Coll Surg* 2012;215:361–9.

39. Kluger MD, Epelboym I, Schrope BA, et al. Single-institution experience with irreversible electroporation for T4 pancreatic cancer: first 50 patients. *Ann Surg Oncol* 2016;23:1736–43. doi: 10.1245/s10434-015-5034-x.

40. Mansson C, Brahmstaedt R, Nilsson A, Nygren P, Karlson BM. Percutaneous irreversible electroporation for treatment of locally advanced pancreatic cancer following chemotherapy or radiochemotherapy. *Eur J Surg Oncol* 2016;42:1401–6.

41. Nielsen K, Scheffer HJ, Vieveen JM, et al. Anaesthetic management during open and percutaneous irreversible electroporation. *Br J Anaesthesia* 2014;113:985–92.

42. Kwon D, McFarland K, Velanovich V, Martin R, 2nd. Borderline and locally advanced pancreatic adenocarcinoma margin accentuation with irreversible electroporation. *Surgery* 2014;156:910–22.

43. Paiella S, Salvia R, Girelli R, et al. (Role of local ablative techniques (Radiofrequency ablation and Irreversible Electroporation) in the treatment of pancreatic cancer. *Updates Surg* 2016;68:307–11.

Postoperative Complications after Resection of Pancreatic Neuroendocrine Tumours

E.J.M. Nieveen van Dijkum and C.H.J. van Eijck

ABSTRACT

Patients with neuroendocrine pancreatic tumours are treated with standard pancreatic resections and/or enucleations. Postoperative complications in this specific patient group are described according to the Clavien-Dindo classification. Complications related to hormonal overproduction of pancreatic neuroendocrine tumours occur sporadically. Complications described are pancreatic fistula, bleeding, delayed gastric emptying and long-term complications such as endocrine and exocrine pancreatic dysfunctions and nonalcoholic fatty liver disease.

KEYWORDS

Neuroendocrine tumours, postoperative complications, long-term complications, Clavien-Dindo, pancreatic fistula, bleeding, delayed gastric emptying, endocrine and exocrine dysfunctions, NAFLD, nonalcoholic fatty liver disease

INTRODUCTION

Patients with resected pancreatic neuroendocrine tumours (pNETs) have a better 5-year survival rate compared with patients with a resected pancreatic adenocarcinoma (90% vs. 20%). However, pancreatic resection is associated with complications, which do occur frequently and have major impact on patients' quality of life. As survival is promising, limited resections and even enucleations, only 'peeling-out' the pNET from the surface of the pancreas, have been advocated as a way of preventing major complications. We will therefore focus on complications after pancreatic resections as well as on enucleations for pNETs.

Searching literature for pNET-specific postoperative complications is cumbersome, since most studies describe postoperative complications of all pancreatic resections, including pNET resections. However, a recent systematic review searched for specific pNET studies and described complications rates specific for patients who underwent pancreatic resections or enucleations for pNETs.[1] A second important point is that clear distinctions should be made between pancreatic head resections (or pancreatoduodenectomy [PD]), pancreatic tail resections (or distal pancreatectomy) and central pancreatectomy, since these types of procedures have specific associated postoperative complications. Finally, all complications should be scored by international definitions to improve data presentation, comparability and the possibility to perform meta-analyses. Knowledge of survival data as well as data on the incidence and outcomes of postoperative complications will facilitate shared decision making with a patient. Especially patients with small pNET should outweigh the survival benefit of a pancreatic resection against the risk of postoperative complications and subsequent impact on quality of life.

COMPLICATIONS DUE TO HORMONAL OVERPRODUCTION

The most frequent hormone-producing neuroendocrine pancreatic tumours are insulinoma and gastrinoma. Both tumour types cause specific hormonal syndromes and have distinct preoperative diagnostic strategies. Perioperative measures are only necessary for patients with an insulinoma, owing to the autonomous insulin releases, which can be dangerous in a patient without glucose availability before and during surgery. Therefore, continuous glucose infusion is essential before and during surgery in case of an insulinoma.

Hormone-related postoperative complications after resection of an insulinoma are very rare. Rebound hyperglycaemia is described as a marker for successful insulinoma removal but cannot be defined as a postoperative complication. Resection of other functioning pNETs can resolve or diminish the preoperative-associated syndromes, and rebound hormonal effects do not cause postoperative problems. Treatment with somatostatin analogues can often be discontinued during or directly after surgery for pNET. This is contrary to operations performed on patients with small bowel neuroendocrine tumours and liver-related disease, who often need high dosage of somatostatin analogues to prevent serotonin-related complications during and after surgery. These carcinoid crises are not expected in patients with pNETs.

CLASSIFICATION OF COMPLICATIONS

The International Study Group of Pancreatic Surgery (ISGPS's) experts studied the complications of pancreatic surgery and presented international definitions for the most common complications. Included are the definitions of pancreatic fistula, delayed gastric emptying (DGE) and haemorrhage.[2–4]

Another method of reporting postoperative complications is the Clavien-Dindo system.[5] The original Clavien-Dindo system is shown in Table 36.1. The Clavien-Dindo system is a grading system based on the severity and therapy used to overcome postoperative complications.

Finally, surgical mortality or 30-day mortality is included as a measure of postoperative complications, as it is the worst outcome encountered after surgery.

Pancreatic Fistula

Pancreatic fistula is defined as a failure of healing/sealing of a pancreatic-enteric anastomosis or a parenchymal leak not directly related to an anastomosis. An all-inclusive definition is a drain output of any measurable volume of fluid on or after postoperative day 3, with an amylase content greater than three times the serum amylase activity. Three different grades of postoperative pancreatic fistula (POPF) (grades A, B and C) are defined according to the clinical impact on the patient's hospital course (Table 36.2).

The most important known risk factors for pancreatic fistula are soft consistency of the pancreatic parenchyma, small pancreatic duct size (<3 mm) and a fatty pancreas. The pNET are known to cause less pancreatic duct obstruction and parenchyma reaction such as fibrosis and inflammation, thereby increasing the risk of pancreatic fistula postoperatively. A patients' body mass index (BMI) is also known to be an independent risk factor for pancreatic fistula development, as BMI is related to the fat contents of the pancreas.

When resections for adenocarcinoma and other indications were compared with resections for pNET in a series of 744 patients versus 88 patients, the incidence of

Table 36.1 Classification of surgical complications according to Clavien-Dindo system

Grade	Definition
Grade 1	Any deviation from the normal postoperative course, without the need of pharmacological treatment or surgical, endoscopic and radiological interventions. Allowed therapeutic regimens are drugs as antiemetics, analgesics, diuretics, electrolytes and physiotherapy. This grade also includes wound infections opened at the bedside.
Grade 2	Requiring pharmacological treatment with drugs other than those allowed for grade 1 complications. Blood transfusions and total parenteral nutrition are also included.
Grade 3 • Grade 3a • Grade 3b	Requiring surgical, endoscopic or radiological treatment. • Intervention not under general anaesthesia • Intervention under general anaesthesia
Grade 4 • Grade 4a • Grade 4b	Life-threatening complications (including CNS complications) requiring IC/ICU management • Single-organ dysfunction (including dialysis) • Multiorgan dysfunction
Grade 5	Death of a patient
Suffix 'd'	If the patients suffers from a complication at discharge (suffix 'd' for disability)

Abbreviations: CNS, central nervous system; IC/ICU = intermediate care/intensive care unit.
Adapted from: Stolzenburg JU, Rabenalt R, Do M, et al. Categorisation of complications of endoscopic extraperitoneal and laparoscopic transperitoneal radicalprostatectomy. *World J Urol* 2006;24:88–93.

Table 36.2 Pancreatic fistula grade criteria suggested by International Study Group of Pancreatic Fistula

Criteria	No. fistulas	Grade A	Grade B	Grade C
Drain amylase	<3 × normal serum amylase	>3 × normal serum amylase	>3 × normal serum amylase	>3 × normal serum amylase
Drain >21 days	No	No	Yes	Yes
Clinical condition	Well	Well	Well	Sick
US/CT (if obtained)	Negative	Negative	Negative/positive	Positive
Percutaneous drain	No	No	Yes/no	Yes/no
Nonoperative specific treatments	No	No	Yes/no	Yes
Signs of infection	No	No	Yes/no	Yes
Sepsis	No	No	No	Yes
Reoperation	No	No	Yes/no	Yes
Readmission	No	No	Yes/no	Yes
Death related to fistula	No	No	No	Yes

Abbreviations: CT, computed tomography; US, ultrasonography.
Adapted from: Bassi C, Dervenis C, Butturini G, et al. Postoperative pancreatic fistula: an international study group (ISGPF) definition. *Surgery* 2005;138:8–13.

pancreatic fistula was 17.2% versus 22.7%, respectively, for pNET.[6] This confirms the principle of more pNET patients with normal pancreas parenchyma. Often, the pancreas parenchyma consistency and the diameter of the main pancreatic duct are related to the risk of pancreatic fistula occurrence. Pancreatic tumours with invasive growth patterns, such as adenocarcinomas, tend to change the pancreatic parenchyma, mainly due to duct obstruction, which leads to a more fibrotic parenchyma. A fibrotic pancreatic parenchyma seems to be less susceptible to pancreatic fistula. Small neuroendocrine tumours of the pancreas are mostly noninvasive tumours, causing no duct obstruction and subsequently no change in the structure of the pancreatic parenchyma and therefore increasing the rate of pancreatic fistula. Larger neuroendocrine tumours, in general, lead to pancreas parenchymal atrophy, which is also less vulnerable to pancreatic fistula postoperatively.

The systematic review of postoperative complications in pNET describes a pancreatic fistula rate of 45% after enucleation, 14% after distal pancreatectomy, 14% after PD and 58% after central pancreatectomy.[1] Especially the high incidence of pancreatic fistula after enucleations and central pancreatic resections is surprising. Patients are often informed that an enucleation is a less-invasive procedure compared with pancreatic resections.

Possible explanations for the high incidence of pancreatic fistula are the same for enucleations as for resections, with BMI, fatty pancreas and normal pancreatic parenchyma being also the risk factors, and all these factors are often present in patients with small pNET undergoing enucleations. As for the rate of pancreatic fistula after

central pancreatic resections, high fistula rates can be explained by the fact that after a central pancreatectomy, two pancreatic transection areas need to heal.

Long-term outcome of patients after enucleation should be considered, as the burden of treatment of the initial postoperative complications is weighed against the long-term prevention of exocrine and endocrine dysfunctions.[7]

As shown in a Cochrane systematic review, prophylactic use of somatostatin analogues decreased the overall number of pancreatic fistulae (RR 0,63) and showed a lower incidence of postoperative complications (RR 0,69).[8] However, somatostatin analogues did not reduce the incidence of clinically significant pancreatic fistulae. No data are currently available as to whether these analogues reduce the rate of pancreatic fistula in patients operated for pNETs. Newer somatostatin analogues, such as pasireotide, possibly reduce the incidence of pancreatic fistulae even more, but larger studies are needed, and specific studies on patients with surgical resections for pNETs will be difficult to perform, since these tumours are relatively rare.[9]

A recent study performed on costs of pancreatic fistula after pancreatectomy showed a median total hospital costs of $90,673.50 ($59,979–$743,667) for patients who developed a POPF versus $86,563 ($39,190–$463,601) for those who did not (p = 0.004).[10] Costs were also calculated for patients who received somatostatin analogues. Although these patients had less pancreatic fistulae, the costs were comparable for those with and without somatostatin analogues.

Sealants for closure of the pancreatic stump after distal pancreatectomy have not yet decreased the incidence of pancreatic fistulae or other postoperative complications such as bleeding.[11,12] One possible explanation for the lack of effect of the sealant is the time to dissolve. Sealants are known to be effective for 2 to 4 days. After the first days after pancreatectomy, pancreas production is low due to lack of food intake and low parasympathetic function. Pancreas fluid production returns to normal from day 3 or sometimes later, at the moment the sealant already starts to lose its sealing capacity.

Other preventive measures such as specific surgical techniques for anastomoses, for example, pancreatogastric anastomoses or specific stapling techniques for distal pancreatectomy, and other innovative techniques have not yet improved the occurrence of POPFs.[13]

Delayed Gastric Emptying

Postoperative paralytic ileus is common, caused by the gastric or pyloric anastomosis in PD or just by surgery and anaesthesia. Haemostasis of the normal gastroduodenal motility is disturbed, and a prolonged nasogastric tube is necessary to prevent vomiting and aspiration.

If gastroparesis remains for more than 1 week postoperatively, by definition of the ISGPS, this should be scored as DGE. Delayed gastric emptying represents the inability to return to a standard diet by the end of the first postoperative week and includes prolonged nasogastric intubation of the patient. Three different grades (A, B and C) were defined, based on the impact on the clinical course and on postoperative management (Table 36.3).

Delayed gastric emptying is most common, secondary to other complications such as pancreatic fistula and intra-abdominal abscess. Treatment of gastroparesis should focus on the underlying causes. Primary DGE, with no other associated complications, is more difficult to treat. Disturbed feedback mechanisms between the duodenum and stomach are thought to cause this complication.

The main driver for gastric emptying is a peristaltic wave, the gastroduodenal migrating motor complex (MMC).[14] This wave originates at the proximal stomach and propagates to the pylorus. The peristaltic waves originate from electrical waves initiated by the interstitial cells of Cajal (ICC). These ICC are a network in the wall of the stomach, duodenum and small intestines. When the peristaltic wave moves over the middle of the antrum, the pylorus opens and duodenal contractions are inhibited; thus, food from the stomach can be delivered to the duodenum. Motilities of the stomach and duodenum are related, and this collaboration is damaged by duodenum resection, as is performed during PD.

Some trials showed that removal of the pylorus could result in a lower incidence of DGE. Matsumoto et al

Table 36.3 Definition of delayed gastric emptying and its grades according to the International Study Group for Pancreatic Surgery

DGE grade	NGT required	Unable to tolerate solid oral intake by POD	Vomiting/ gastric distension	Use of prokinetics
A	4–7 days or reinsertion >POD 3	7	±	±
B	8–14 days or reinsertion >POD 7	14	+	+
C	>14 days or reinsertion >POD 14	21	+	+

Abbreviations: DGE, delayed gastric emptying; NGT, nasogastric tube; POD, postoperative day.
Adapted from: Wente MN, Bassi C, Dervenis C, et al. Delayed gastric emptying (DGE) after pancreatic surgery: a suggested definition by the International Study Group of Pancreatic *Surgery* (ISGPS). *Surgery* 2007;142:761–8.

performed a prospective randomised comparison between pylorus-preserving PD (PPPD) and modified classical PD and assessed the effects of stomach-preserving PD on postoperative DGE occurrence and long-term nutritional status. They observed that the incidence of DGE was similar (20% vs. 12%; p = 0.414), with comparable long-term nutritional status, indicated by serum albumin levels, serum total cholesterol levels and BMI during the 3-year follow-up.[15] Another study comparing PD with and without preservation of the pylorus showed that pylorus preservation was associated with a low incidence of DGE; however, during a 6-month follow-up period, comparable outcomes for quality of life, weight loss and nutritional status between the two groups were observed.[16]

Enterogastric reflexes and release of intestinal hormones perform the feedback regulation of gastric emptying. Among them, motilin is a 22-amino-acids peptide that is primarily localised in enterochromaffin cells of the duodenum and proximal jejunum; this peptide is known to be responsible for phase III activity of the gastroduodenal MMC. Once food has entered the duodenum, intestinal hormones signal the stomach to slow down on peristalsis until the duodenum can receive more food. These signals are lost after duodenectomy, and the stomach lacks feedback on peristalsis, causing a complete but temporarily paresis in some patients.

Delayed gastric emptying occurs most frequently after PD and secondary to other complications after pancreatic surgery. The incidence of DGE after various pancreatic resections for pNET was 5% after enucleation, 5% after distal pancreatectomy, 16% after central pancreatectomy and 18% after PD.[1]

Treatment of primary DGE is patience, since over time, all patients will be able to tolerate oral intake. Erythromycin may be started but should be discontinued if not effective in 5 days. Prolonged nasogastric tube treatment and feeding with a nasointestinal feeding tube or by parenteral feeding might be necessary in some cases. Secondary DGE should be treated the same way, but obviously, it includes treating the intra-abdominal fistula or abscess as well.

Postoperative Haemorrhage

Bleeding complications are divided into early and late haemorrhage. Late haemorrhage is related to pancreatic fistula and abdominal sepsis, whereas early bleeding complications are related to surgical technique or coagulation disorders. Overall, postoperative mortality after pancreatic surgery is often related to late haemorrhage. Postoperative bleeding is not only divided into early or late bleeding but also into intraluminal versus extraluminal bleeding and into mild versus severe bleeding.

Early bleeding occurs within 24 hours after the operation. Bleeding can be intraluminal, for example, when an anastomosis has a venous or arterial bleeding and a patient is losing blood into the intestines. Another cause may be an intraluminal ulcer, causing intraluminal postoperative blood loss. In most cases, early bleeding is extraluminal, causing visible blood loss, as seen in the postoperative intra-abdominal drain, or is caused by an increased abdominal volume, with a visible tensed abdomen. Depending on the amount of blood loss, a quick return to the operative theatre can save lives. Radiological interventions can be time consuming and harbours also potential risks such as liver ischaemia and small bowel necrosis in case of overstenting vital arteries. Therefore, patients with fulminant postoperative early bleeding are preferably treated operatively. In less-fulminant blood loss postoperatively, correction of haemostasis and coagulation and supportive care may stop the bleeding.

Late postoperative bleeding, bleeding after more than 24 hours postoperatively, usually occurs sometime after pancreatic fistula, together with intra-abdominal sepsis, has been diagnosed. Bile leakage can also be the cause of late postoperative haemorrhage. Possible pathophysiological explanations for late haemorrhage include enzymatic digestion of the blood vessel wall by

trypsin, elastase and other pancreatic exocrine enzymes secondary to a pancreatic leak; intra-abdominal infection, with involvement of peripancreatic vessels; and vascular injury during resection that leads to a pseudoaneurysm.

Grade A results only in a temporary and marginal variation of the standard postoperative course of the patient after pancreatectomy. In general, postpancreatectomy haemorrhage (PPH) grade A has no major clinical impact, and its occurrence should not be associated with a major delay of the patient's hospital discharge.

Postpancreatectomy haemorrhage grade B requires adjustment of a given clinical pathway, including further diagnostics and intervention; this grade of haemorrhage will lead to therapeutic consequences such as the need for transfusion, the (re)admission to an intermediate or intensive care unit and potential invasive therapeutic interventions, such as relaparotomy and embolisation. Most likely, the occurrence of haemorrhage grade B will prolong the patient's hospital stay.

Postpancreatectomy haemorrhage grade C leads to severe impairment of the patient and should always be considered potentially life-threatening. Immediate diagnostic and therapeutic consequences are mandatory and often needed. The hospital stay of this group of patients is always prolonged and sometimes necessitates that the patient stay longer in the intensive care unit.

The patient suddenly starts losing some fresh blood in one of the drains or through the nasogastric tube. This is also known as a sentinel bleed, a first sign of a serious bleeding coming soon. After some time, ranging from minutes to hours, clinical deterioration occurs, with tachycardia or hypotension preceding a full-blown bleeding, causing hypovolaemic shock. In most patients, this blood loss is caused by a pseudoaneurysm breaking through. This pseudoaneurysm is the consequence of persistent intra-abdominal leakage of pancreatic and/or bile fluids. Preferred locations for a pseudoaneurysm and bleeding are the hepatic artery and the gastroduodenal artery stump after a PD and bleeding from the splenic artery after a distal pancreatectomy. Especially arterial blood loss causes hypovolaemic shock, but one should never underestimate the amount of blood loss caused by venous bleeding.

In the systematic review of postoperative complications after pNET resections, postoperative haemorrhage could not be divided into early/late, extra-/intraluminal and mild/severe bleeding. The overall incidence rates were 6% after enucleations, 1% after distal pancreatectomy, 4% after central pancreatectomy and 7% after PD.

A recent study showed an incidence of late haemorrhage after PD of 4.5%, with a more severe bleeding if they suffered pancreatic fistula (odds ratio: 10.2) or extra luminal bleed (odd ratio: 5.6) and if preceded by a sentinel bleed (odd ratio: 6.6).[17] The mortality in these patients was high (13%) and occurred before an intervention was performed. Some 80% of interventions were radiological, and the remaining interventions were surgical.

Sentinel bleeding is an urgent predictor of late severe haemorrhage and should be taught to staff and nurses taking care of the patients in the wards, since early intervention can save lives. Treatment options for haemorrhage include embolisation or stenting techniques and, less frequently, surgical interventions. However, in some patients with persistent bleeding, a rest pancreatectomy is sometimes the only remaining option to avoid further infection and persistent bleeding.

IN-HOSPITAL MORTALITY

Mortality after pNET resection was 3% after enucleation, 4% after distal pancreatectomy, 4% after central pancreatectomy and 6% after PD.[1] As is known from many studies, high-volume centres have better outcomes for postoperative complications and mortality.[18] Neuroendocrine tumours are rare tumours, and patients are often referred and treated in expert centres for neuroendocrine tumours. However, these centres are not necessarily pancreatic expert centers. In case of surgical treatment, pancreatic surgery is preferably performed in expert pancreas centres, as is shown by the lower morbidity and mortality figures in these centres.

LONG-TERM COMPLICATIONS AFTER PANCREATECTOMY OR ENUCLEATION

Since survival is excellent for patients with resected pNET, some emphasis must also be given on the long-term outcomes after surgery.

Pancreatic remnant function is related to pancreatic atrophy and main pancreatic duct dilation in the remnant pancreas after PD.[19] Pancreatic atrophy tended to develop over time, and patients with atrophy had reduced levels of faecal-1 elastase associated with exocrine dysfunction. Therefore, morphological changes can show that exocrine function in the remnant pancreas remain after PD. Exocrine dysfunction is associated with a decreased quality of life, caused by abdominal pain; food intolerance; frequent bowel movements and medication dependence.[20]

Nonalcoholic fatty liver disease (NAFLD) is thought to be associated with excessive nutrition and is one of the most common forms of chronic liver disease. A few clinical investigations correlating fatty liver and PD reported that PD can influence hepatic fat content, which was associated with frequent hepatic steatosis.[21] In severe cases, even steatohepatitis, leading to hepatic decompression, can develop because of malnutrition after PD. Therefore, surgeons need to be concerned about this condition, especially in patients expecting long-term survival after PD.

One study described postoperative long-term follow-up after enucleation versus pancreatic resection for pNET.[22] Functional follow-up was available for all included patients, with a median follow-up time of 29 months (interquartile range [IQR]: 10–64). Significantly, more patients developed endocrine insufficiency (19%) and exocrine insufficiency (55%) after PD compared with tumour enucleation (7 and 5%) or distal pancreatectomy (13 and 8%) (p < 0.001). There were no significant differences between tumour enucleation and distal pancreatectomy regarding the rate of pancreatic insufficiency.

CONCLUSIONS

Complications after resection of pancreatic neuroendocrine tumors occurs frequently (up to 58%) and is mainly caused by pancreatic fistula, delayed gastric emptying and hemorrhage. Postoperative complications are rarely caused by hormonal overproduction.

REFERENCES

1. Jilesen AP, van Eijck CH, In't Hof KH, van Dieren S, Gouma DJ, Nieveen van Dijkum EJ. Postoperative complications, in-hospital mortality and 5-year survival after surgical resection for patients with a pancreatic neuroendocrine tumor: a systematic review. *World J Surg* 2016;40:729–48. doi: 10.1007/s00268-015-3328-6.

2. Bassi C, Dervenis C, Butturini G, et al; International Study Group on Pancreatic Fistula Definition. Postoperative pancreatic fistula: an international study group (ISGPF) definition. *Surgery* 2005;138:8–13.

3. Wente MN, Bassi C, Dervenis C, et al. Delayed gastric emptying (DGE) after pancreatic surgery: a suggested definition by the International Study Group of Pancreatic Surgery (ISGPS). *Surgery* 2007;142:761–8.

4. Wente MN, Veit JA, Bassi C, et al. Postpancreatectomy hemorrhage (PPH): an International Study Group of Pancreatic Surgery (ISGPS) definition. *Surgery* 2007; 142:20–5.

5. Dindo D, Demartines N, Clavien PA. Classification of surgical complications: a new proposal with evaluation in a cohort of 6336 patients and results of a survey. *Ann Surg* 2004;240:205–13.

6. Atema JJ, Jilesen AP, Busch OR, van Gulik TM, Gouma DJ, Nieveen van Dijkum EJ. Pancreatic fistulae after

pancreatic resections for neuroendocrine tumours compared with resections for other lesions. *HPB (Oxford)* 2015;17:38–45. doi: 10.1111/hpb.12319.

7. Cherif R, Gaujoux S, Couvelard A, et al. Parenchyma-sparing resections for pancreatic neuroendocrine tumors. *J Gastrointest Surg* 2012;16:2045–55. doi: 10.1007/s11605-012-2002-7.

8. Gurusamy KS, Koti R, Fusai G, Davidson BR. Somatostatin analogues for pancreatic surgery. *Cochrane Database Syst Rev* 2012;6:CD008370. doi: 10.1002/14651858.CD008370.pub2.

9. Allen PJ, Gönen M, Brennan MF, et al. Pasireotide for postoperative pancreatic fistula. *N Engl J Med* 2014;370:2014–22. doi: 10.1056/NEJMoa1313688.

10. Anderson R, Dunki-Jacobs E, Burnett N, Scoggins C, McMasters K, Martin RC. A cost analysis of somatostatin use in the prevention of pancreatic fistula after pancreatectomy. *World J Surg* 2014;38:2138–44. doi: 10.1007/s00268-014-2512-4.

11. Hüttner FJ, Mihaljevic AL, Hackert T, Ulrich A, Büchler MW, Diener MK. Effectiveness of Tachosil® in the prevention of postoperative pancreatic fistula after distal pancreatectomy: a systematic review and meta-analysis. *Langenbecks Arch Surg* 2016;401:151–9.

12. Cheng Y, Ye M, Xiong X, et al. Fibrin sealants for the prevention of postoperative pancreatic fistula following pancreatic surgery. *Cochrane Database Syst Rev* 2016;2:CD009621. doi: 10.1002 /14651858.CD009621.pub2.

13. Schoellhammer HF, Fong Y, Gagandeep S. Techniques for prevention of pancreatic leak after pancreatectomy. *Hepatobiliary Surg Nutr* 2014;3:276–87. doi: 10.3978/j.issn.2304-3881.2014.08.08.

14. Kang CM, Lee JH. Pathophysiology after pancreaticoduodenectomy. *World J Gastroenterol* 2015;21:5794–804. doi: 0.3748/wjg.v21.i19.5794.

15. Matsumoto I, Shinzeki M, Asari S, et al. A prospective randomized comparison between pylorus- and subtotal stomach-preserving pancreatoduodenectomy on postoperative delayed gastric emptying occurrence and long-term nutritional status. *J Surg Oncol* 2014;109:690–6.

16. Kawai M, Tani M, Hirono S, Okada K, Miyazawa M, Yamaue H. Pylorus-resecting pancreaticoduodenectomy offers long-term outcomes similar to those of pylorus-preserving pancreaticoduodenectomy: results of a prospective study. *World J Surg* 2014;38:1476–83.

17. Jilesen AP, Tol JA, Busch OR, et al. Emergency management in patients with late hemorrhage after pancreatoduodenectomy for a periampullary tumor. *World J Surg* 2014;38:2438–47. doi: 10.1007/s00268-014-2593-0.

18. Tol JA, van Gulik TM, Busch OR, Gouma DJ. Centralization of highly complex low-volume procedures in upper gastrointestinal surgery. A summary of systematic reviews and meta-analyses. *Dig Surg* 2012;29:374–83. doi: 10.1159/000343929.

19. Lemaire E, O'Toole D, Sauvanet A, Hammel P, Belghiti J, Ruszniewski P. Functional and morphological changes in the pancreatic remnant following pancreaticoduodenectomy with pancreaticogastric anastomosis. *Br J Surg* 2000;87:434–8.

20. Bruno MJ, Haverkort EB, Tytgat GN, van Leeuwen DJ. Maldigestion associated with exocrine pancreatic insufficiency: implications of gastrointestinal physiology and properties of enzyme preparations for a cause-related and patient-tailored treatment. *Am J Gastroenterol* 1995;90:1383–93.

21. Nirei K, Ogihara N, Kawamura W, Kang W, Moriyama M. Rapid recovery from acute liver failure secondary to pancreatoduodenectomy-related non-alcoholic steatohepatitis. *Case Rep Gastroenterol* 2013;7:49–55.

22. Jilesen AP, van Eijck CH, Busch OR, van Gulik TM, Gouma DJ, Nieveen van Dijkum EJ. Postoperative Outcomes of Enucleation and Standard Resections in Patients with a Pancreatic Neuroendocrine Tumor. *World J Surg* 2016;40:715–28. doi: 10.1007/s00268-015-3341-9.

Index

Page numbers followed by *f* indicate figures; and those followed by *t* indicate tables.